PRACTICAL HANDBOOK OF SCHOOL PSYCHOLOGY

Practical Handbook of School Psychology

Effective Practices for the 21st Century

edited by
Gretchen Gimpel Peacock
Ruth A. Ervin
Edward J. Daly III
Kenneth W. Merrell

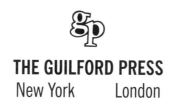

THE GUILFORD PRESS
New York   London

© 2010 The Guilford Press
A Division of Guilford Publications, Inc.
72 Spring Street, New York, NY 10012
www.guilford.com

Printed in the United States of America

This book is printed on acid-free paper.

Last digit is print number: 9 8 7 6 5 4 3 2 1

The authors have checked with sources believed to be reliable in their efforts to provide
information that is complete and generally in accord with the standards of practice that
are accepted at the time of publication. However, in view of the possibility of human error
or changes in medical sciences, neither the authors, nor the editor and publisher, nor any
other party who has been involved in the preparation or publication of this work warrants
that the information contained herein is in every respect accurate or complete, and they
are not responsible for any errors or omissions or the results obtained from the use of such
information. Readers are encouraged to confirm the information contained in this book
with other sources.

Library of Congress Cataloging-in-Publication Data
Practical handbook of school psychology: effective practices for the 21st century / editors,
Gretchen Gimpel Peacock . . . [et al.].
     p. cm.
   Includes bibliographical references and index.
   ISBN 978-1-59385-697-7 (hardcover: alk. paper)
   1. School psychology—United States.   I. Gimpel Peacock, Gretchen.
   LB1027.55.P72 2010
   370.15—dc22
                                                    2009025323

About the Editors

Gretchen Gimpel Peacock, PhD, is Professor of Psychology at Utah State University, where she has coordinated the specialist-level program in school psychology approved by the National Association of School Psychologists and is on the program faculty of the Combined Psychology (School/Clinical/Counseling) American Psychological Association-accredited PhD program. Dr. Gimpel Peacock is both a licensed psychologist and educator licensed school psychologist. She has been the faculty internship supervisor for the school psychology students and also supervises students' practicum experiences in the department's community clinic. Dr. Gimpel Peacock's publications and professional presentations focus on child behavior problems and family issues as related to child behaviors, as well as professional issues in school psychology. She currently serves on the editorial advisory boards of several school psychology and related journals.

Ruth A. Ervin, PhD, is Associate Professor at the University of British Columbia. Dr. Ervin has established a line of research that addresses the research-to-practice needs of local school districts and promotes a preventative and problem-solving approach to addressing the academic and emotional–behavioral needs of children and adolescents. Her professional teaching and research interests lie within the following major domains: promoting systems-level change to address research-to-practice gaps in school settings; collaborative consultation with school personnel, parents, and other service providers for the prevention and treatment of emotional–behavioral disorders (attention-deficit/hyperactivity disorder, oppositional defiant disorder); and linking assessment to intervention to promote academic performance and socially significant outcomes for school-age children. Dr. Ervin has served as associate editor of the *School Psychology Review* and the *Journal of Evidence-Based Practices for Schools* and on the editorial boards of the *School Psychology Review*, the *Journal of Applied Behavior Analysis*, the *Journal of Behavioral Education*, and the *Journal of Positive Behavioral Interventions*.

Edward J. Daly III, PhD, is Professor of Educational (School) Psychology at the University of Nebraska–Lincoln. Dr. Daly's research is in the areas of developing functional assessment methods for reading problems and the measurement and evaluation of academic and behavioral interventions. He has coauthored two texts and numerous chapters and journal articles on these topics. Dr. Daly is currently editor of the *Journal of School Psychology*. He also has served as associate editor for both the *School Psychology Review* and the *School Psychology*

Quarterly. In addition, he serves on a number of editorial boards and is a Fellow of Division 16 of the American Psychological Association. He worked for 5 years as a school psychologist before taking a faculty position in 1995 and trained school psychologists at the University of Cincinnati and Western Michigan University.

Kenneth W. Merrell, PhD, is Professor of School Psychology at the University of Oregon, where he has served as head of the Department of Special Education and Clinical Sciences and as director and codirector of the School Psychology Program. Dr. Merrell's research and scholarly work in social–emotional assessment and intervention in schools has been published widely in the field of school psychology, and he has been interviewed extensively in the popular media as well. Currently, Dr. Merrell serves as editor of The Guilford Press's *Practical Intervention in the Schools* book series. In addition, he is President of the Board of Directors at the Oregon Social Learning Center in Eugene.

Acknowledgments

We appreciate and acknowledge all of the support and assistance we have received from numerous individuals as we compiled this edited volume. We are grateful to the editors at The Guilford Press, in particular, Craig Thomas and Natalie Graham, who encouraged and supported us throughout the process. In addition, we are indebted to the many excellent professionals in school psychology and related fields who contributed to the volume. We appreciate everyone's patience and responsiveness throughout the editing process. We are also thankful for the support of our colleagues and graduate students at our respective universities. And last, but certainly not least, we would like to express our appreciation to our families for allowing us the time needed to devote to the book. School psychology is an exciting field to be part of, and we appreciate the opportunities to work with accomplished colleagues and to help educate future practitioners and trainers.

Contributors

Amanda Albertson, MA, University of Nebraska–Lincoln, Department of Educational Psychology, Lincoln, Nebraska

Keith D. Allen, PhD, University of Nebraska Medical Center, Munroe–Meyer Institute for Genetics and Rehabilitation, Omaha, Nebraska

Brent Alsop, PhD, University of Otago, Department of Psychology, Dunedin, New Zealand

Melissa Andersen, MEd, University of Nebraska–Lincoln, Department of Educational Psychology, Lincoln, Nebraska

Theresa Andreou, MEd, University of British Columbia, Department of Educational and Counseling Psychology and Special Education, Vancouver, British Columbia, Canada

Scott P. Ardoin, PhD, University of Georgia, Department of Educational Psychology and Instructional Technology, Athens, Georgia

Scott K. Baker, PhD, Pacific Institutes for Research, Eugene, Oregon

Elizabeth Barkley, MEd, University of Cincinnati, Division of Human Services, Cincinnati, Ohio

David W. Barnett, PhD, University of Cincinnati, Division of Human Services, Cincinnati, Ohio

Jaime L. Benson, MEd, Lehigh University, Department of Education and Human Services, Bethlehem, Pennsylvania

Carrie A. Blevins, MA, University of Nebraska–Lincoln, Department of Educational Psychology, Lincoln, Nebraska

Genery D. Booster, MEd, Lehigh University, Department of Education and Human Services, Bethlehem, Pennsylvania

Matthew K. Burns, PhD, University of Minnesota, Department of Educational Psychology, Minneapolis, Minnesota

Bryan Bushman, PhD, McKay–Dee Behavioral Health Institute, Ogden, Utah

David J. Chard, PhD, Southern Methodist University, Simmons School of Education and Human Development, Dallas, Texas

Nathan H. Clemens, MEd, Lehigh University, Department of Education and Human Services, Bethlehem, Pennsylvania

Edward J. Daly III, PhD, University of Nebraska–Lincoln, Department of Educational Psychology, Lincoln, Nebraska

Anna Dawson, MA, University of Otago, Department of Psychology, Dunedin, New Zealand

Jennifer L. DeSmet, MS, University of Wisconsin–Milwaukee, Department of Educational Psychology, Milwaukee, Wisconsin

Ronnie Detrich, PhD, Wing Institute, Oakland, California

George J. DuPaul, PhD, Lehigh University, Department of Education and Human Services, Bethlehem, Pennsylvania

Ruth A. Ervin, PhD, University of British Columbia, Department of Educational and Counseling Psychology and Special Education, Vancouver, British Columbia, Canada

Randy G. Floyd, PhD, University of Memphis, Department of Psychology, Memphis, Tennessee

Lynae J. Frerichs, MA, University of Nebraska–Lincoln, Department of Educational Psychology, Lincoln, Nebraska

Patrick C. Friman, PhD, Father Flanagan's Boys Home, Clinical Services and Research, Boys Town, Nebraska

Kristin A. Gansle, PhD, Louisiana State University, Department of Educational Theory, Policy, and Practice, Baton Rouge, Louisiana

Donna Gilbertson, PhD, Utah State University, Department of Psychology, Logan, Utah

Gretchen Gimpel Peacock, PhD, Utah State University, Department of Psychology, Logan, Utah

Jami E. Givens, MA, University of Nebraska–Lincoln, Department of Educational Psychology, Lincoln, Nebraska

Barbara A. Gueldner, PhD, The Children's Hospital, Department of Psychiatry and Behavioral Sciences, Aurora, Colorado

Kimberly A. Haugen, PhD, Father Flanagan's Boys Home, Clinical Services and Research, Boys Town, Nebraska

Renee O. Hawkins, PhD, University of Cincinnati, Division of Human Services, Cincinnati, Ohio

Keith C. Herman, PhD, University of Missouri, Department of Educational, School, and Counseling Psychology, Columbia, Missouri

Thomas S. Higbee, PhD, Utah State University, Department of Special Education and Rehabilitation, Logan, Utah

John M. Hintze, PhD, University of Massachusetts at Amherst, Department of Student Development and Pupil Personnel Services, Amherst, Massachusetts

Kathryn E. Hoff, PhD, Illinois State University, Department of Psychology, Normal, Illinois

Kristi L. Hofstadter, EdS, University of Nebraska–Lincoln, Department of Educational Psychology, Lincoln, Nebraska

Kenneth W. Howell, PhD, Western Washington University, Department of Special Education, Bellingham, Washington

Kevin M. Jones, PhD, Louisiana State University in Shreveport, Department of Psychology, Shreveport, Louisiana

Kathleen Jungjohann, MA, University of Oregon, Department of Special Education and Clinical Services, Eugene, Oregon

Lee Kern, PhD, Lehigh University, Department of Education and Human Services, Bethlehem, Pennsylvania

Leanne R. Ketterlin-Geller, PhD, Southern Methodist University, Department of Educational Policy, Dallas, Texas

David A. Klingbeil, PhD, University of Minnesota, School Psychology Program, Minneapolis, Minnesota

Sara Kupzyk, MA, University of Nebraska–Lincoln, Department of Educational Psychology, Lincoln, Nebraska

Verity H. Levitt, PhD, Glenview School District, Glenview, Illinois

Sylvia Linan-Thompson, PhD, University of Texas at Austin, Department of Special Education, Austin, Texas

Leslie MacKay, MA, University of British Columbia, Department of Educational and Counseling Psychology and Special Education, Vancouver, British Columbia, Canada

Katie L. Magee, MA, University of Nebraska–Lincoln, Department of Educational Psychology, Lincoln, Nebraska

Amanda M. Marcotte, PhD, University of Massachusetts at Amherst, Department of Student Development and Pupil Personnel Services, Amherst, Massachusetts

Brian K. Martens, PhD, Syracuse University, Department of Psychology, Syracuse, New York

Rebecca S. Martinez, PhD, Indiana University, Department of Counseling and Educational Psychology, Bloomington, Indiana

Merilee McCurdy, PhD, University of Nebraska–Lincoln, Department of Educational Psychology, Lincoln, Nebraska

Kent McIntosh, PhD, University of British Columbia, Department of Educational and Counseling Psychology and Special Education, Vancouver, British Columbia, Canada

Kenneth W. Merrell, PhD, University of Oregon, Department of Special Education and Clinical Sciences, Eugene, Oregon

David N. Miller, PhD, University at Albany, State University of New York, Division of School Psychology, Albany, New York

Julie Q. Morrison, PhD, University of Cincinnati, Division of Human Services, Cincinnati, Ohio

Shobana Musti-Rao, PhD, National Institute of Education, Early Childhood and Special Needs Education, Singapore, Singapore

Bradley C. Niebling, PhD, Heartland Area Education Agency, Johnston, Iowa

George H. Noell, PhD, Louisiana State University, Department of Psychology, Baton Rouge, Louisiana

Alecia Rahn-Blakeslee, PhD, Heartland Area Education Agency, Johnston, Iowa

Wendy M. Reinke, PhD, University of Missouri, Department of Educational, School, and Counseling Psychology, Columbia, Missouri

Robert L. Rhodes, PhD, New Mexico State University, Department of Special Education and Communicative Disorders, Las Cruces, New Mexico

Kristin D. Sawka-Miller, PhD, Siena College, Department of Psychology, Loudonville, New York

Elizabeth Schaughency, PhD, University of Otago, Department of Psychology, Dunedin, New Zealand

Stephanie Schmitz, EdS, University of Nebraska–Lincoln, Department of Educational Psychology, Lincoln, Nebraska

Joan Schumann, MEd, University of Utah, Department of Special Education, Salt Lake City, Utah

Susan M. Sheridan, PhD, University of Nebraska–Lincoln, Department of Educational Psychology, Lincoln, Nebraska

Mark D. Shriver, PhD, University of Nebraska Medical Center, Munroe–Meyer Institute for Genetics and Rehabilitation, Omaha, Nebraska

Rebecca Sonnek, EdS, Utah State University, Department of Psychology, Logan, Utah

Karen Callan Stoiber, PhD, University of Wisconsin–Milwaukee, Department of Educational Psychology, Milwaukee, Wisconsin

Michelle S. Swanger-Gagné, MA, University of Nebraska–Lincoln, Department of Educational Psychology, Lincoln, Nebraska

Susan M. Swearer, PhD, University of Nebraska–Lincoln, Department of Educational Psychology, Lincoln, Nebraska

W. David Tilly III, PhD, Heartland Area Education Agency, Johnston, Iowa

Amanda M. VanDerHeyden, PhD, Education Research and Consulting Inc., Fairhope, Alabama

Sharon Vaughn, PhD, University of Texas at Austin, Department of Special Education, Austin, Texas

Jennifer L. Volz, PhD, Father Flanagan's Boys Home, Clinical Services and Research, Boys Town, Nebraska

Lisa L. Weyandt, PhD, University of Rhode Island, Department of Psychology, Kingston, Rhode Island

Katherine F. Wickstrom, PhD, Louisiana State University in Shreveport, Department of Psychology, Shreveport, Louisiana

Contents

PART I

THE SCHOOL PSYCHOLOGIST AS A PROBLEM SOLVER

Establishing a Foundation and a Vision

Chapter 1

The School Psychologist as a Problem Solver in the 21st Century

Rationale and Role Definition

Ruth A. Ervin
Gretchen Gimpel Peacock
Kenneth W. Merrell

> To exist is to change, to change is to mature, to mature is to go on creating oneself endlessly.
> —HENRI BERGSON

> The future is not some place we are going to, but one we are creating, the paths are not to be found but made.
> —JOHN SCAAR

If the future is created from our present-day actions, as these quotes suggest, then who we are and what we do as school psychologists *now* will determine our *future roles*. In other words, the actions we take in the present and the thinking that guides our decision making set the stage regarding who we, as a profession, become. In our introductory text, *School Psychology for the 21st Century: Foundations and Practices* (Merrell, Ervin, & Gimpel, 2006), we argued that the practice of school psychology should follow a data-guided problem-solving approach consistent with the role posited for school psychologists over 40 years ago (Gray, 1963) and currently advocated as "best practice" by leading scholars in the field (e.g., Tilly, 2008; Reschly, 2008; Ysseldyke et al., 2006). In this edited handbook, intended to be used as a stand-alone text or as a companion volume to *School Psychology for the 21st Century*, we have brought together the work of experts in school psychology and special education to demonstrate in a practical manner what the problem-solving model

looks like at the individual-child, small-group, and larger (e.g., whole-school) levels. This introductory chapter frames school psychology practice within the problem-solving model and presents a broad vision for what the role of a problem-solving school psychologist looks like. Later chapters address specific aspects of applying this model in practice. Whereas *School Psychology for the 21st Century* presented a general overview of school psychology practice, this edited volume provides broader and more specific coverage through 34 chapters that demonstrate to readers in a very practical manner what the problem-solving model looks like and how this model can be implemented in practice across a variety of issues and problems school psychologists may encounter. Our aim is to show what is possible for school psychology practice and to ask readers to consider "trying on" this role in their own practice.

To establish a vision of the problem-solving role, we have asked ourselves the following questions:

- What would a day in the life of a problem-solving school psychologist look like?
- How would such a school psychologist approach professional tasks?
- What theoretical stance would this psychologist adopt or hold?
- What tools would he or she use for assessment and intervention purposes?
- How would the school psychologist interact with and be perceived by others in his or her work environment?
- What challenges would he or she face?

To answer these questions, this chapter begins with a broad vision of what we believe a problem-solving school psychologist looks like. We then discuss the evolution of the problem-solving model, including the philosophical and theoretical underpinnings of this approach, with an emphasis on how this approach shapes the psychologist's actions, as well as how this model fits within a response-to-intervention (RTI) approach to multi-tiered service delivery (see also Hawkins, Barnett, Morrison, & Musti-Rao, Chapter 2). Following this discussion, we briefly review the problem-solving steps and discuss the layout of the remaining chapters in this book. To further illustrate the application of the problem-solving model in practice, we end with several vignettes from practicing school psychologists. This chapter provides a framework for the remaining chapters in this volume, which expand on areas of competency important to a problem-solving approach to school psychology.

The Vision: Problem-Solving School Psychologists in the 21st Century

According to the Blueprint III model of school psychology (Ysseldyke et al., 2006) school psychologists should possess the "ability to use problem-solving and scientific methodology to create, evaluate, and apply appropriately empirically validated interventions at both an individual and a systems level" (p. 14). Further, they should "be good problem solvers who collect information that is relevant for understanding problems, make decisions about appropriate interventions, assess educational outcomes, and help others become accountable for the decisions they make" (Ysseldyke et al., 2006, pp. 17–

18). Although talk of a shift away from the historical test-and-place model to a problem-solving, data-driven model has floated about for years, many school psychologists continue to perform the same, historical functions. It is our hope and our belief that through increased exposure to and experience with the problem-solving model, school psychologists are truly starting to "walk the walk" and not just "talk the talk."

In this section, we summarize what we believe is possible for the practice of school psychology. Specifically, we provide a vision of what a successful problem-solving school psychologist looks like. To do so, we describe what he or she believes and values and how he or she thinks and approaches problems. The descriptors we use are not intended to be mutually exclusive, and many aspects of the problem solver could be subsumed under multiple areas. We hope that this vision will help illustrate to current and future school psychologists the key characteristics of a problem solver to provide an overall framework for the specific problem-solving activities that are discussed throughout this book.

School psychologists who are successful problem solvers:

- *Are open, flexible, and responsive to new information or changing circumstances.* To effectively solve problems of a human nature (i.e., to understand a situation and to act in a manner to make things better), successful problem solvers remain attentive and responsive to new information and changing circumstances. They view each problem situation and problem context as unique and do not assume that they know the solutions to problems a priori. "To assume that you know when you don't and to act on that assumption is a path toward error. To assume that you don't know, even when you might, and to act on that assumption, will more likely occasion a more measured, tentative, and humble set of actions that place one on a path toward correct action in the long run" (Joseph Lucyshyn, personal communication, December 19, 2008).
- *Are willing to recognize when they fail.* Problem-solving school psychologists are open to feedback, and when developing interventions, they always ask the question, "Did it work?" If the answer is "no, it didn't

work," the school psychologist is willing to acknowledge this to and continue to work toward a problem resolution. Thus, in their search for answers, problem-solving school psychologists are less concerned with "being right" (i.e., confirmation of an a priori hypothesis) than they are with finding a workable solution. Lack of progress or an unconfirmed hypothesis is not viewed as a failure but as new and important information about the problem situation. The problem-solving school psychologist admits when an intervention is not working and continues to engage in the problem-solving process to find a solution that does work.

• *Are "optimistic."* Successful problem solvers expect that problems can be solved, and they believe that all children can learn and can demonstrate appropriate behavior given the right supports. They are persistent in their efforts to improve the lives of the children they serve, and they keep trying until a solution is achieved.

• *Are outcome-focused, goal-oriented, and solution-focused.* Problem-solving school psychologists develop goals and outcomes to guide their work—they know the problem they are working to solve and the desired solution—so they will know when they have "solved" the problem.

• *Are self-questioning and data-driven.* Problem-solving school psychologists make use of empirical data in an ongoing manner as they evaluate problems and develop and implement potential solutions. They engage in self-questioning throughout the problem-solving process to define and analyze the problem and the problem context, to develop interventions, and to evaluate the effectiveness of these interventions.

• *Are committed to evidence-based practice.* Problem-solving school psychologists are informed about the empirical literature on how learning occurs and how behaviors are developed and maintained. They also are knowledgeable about evidence-based strategies for improving learning and behavior problems and about how to gather, interpret, and use data to make decisions.

• *Recognize that learning and behavior do not occur in isolation.* The problem-solving school psychologist understands that learning and behavior take place in a context (or multiple contexts) and that data on the problem, as well as the context (e.g.,

with whom, where, when, during what activities), are important for effective problem resolution.

• *Focus on assessment and analysis of alterable variables (what we can change) to improve the problem.* Problem-solving school psychologists do not become sidetracked describing variables that might be correlated with problems but that cannot be altered (e.g., a child's family history). Instead, they focus on identifying the variables that can be altered to improve the problem situation (e.g., the instruction a child receives).

• *Strive to work well with others.* Problem-solving school psychologists, particularly those who are successful, know that problems can rarely be solved by one person working alone. They recognize the importance of working as a team in a collaborative manner and understand that working with others requires flexibility.

Problem-solving school psychologists are able to ingrate these various traits and skills to:

• *Address problems that present themselves along a continuum.* They utilize their skills and put forth efforts to solve problems that are already occurring (i.e., tertiary and secondary prevention), as well as to reduce risk and prevent problems from occurring.

• *Address problems for large groups, small targeted groups, and/or individuals.* They recognize that a problem-solving approach is applicable not only to individual child-centered cases. They know that data-based problem solving can and should also be applied to all spheres of activity (e.g., multi-tiered models, schools as the unit of analysis).

Evolution of the Problem-Solving Model in School Psychology Practice

It is worthwhile noting that although much has been written and said about the problem-solving approach in education during the past decade, this way of conducting school psychology practice did not suddenly spring forth from an intellectual void. Rather, it is a manifestation of a long line of predecessor ideas, models, and viewpoints. This section provides a brief overview of some of the "then and now" aspects of the problem-solving model: how this approach has evolved and how it is currently making an impact in the day-to-day work of school psychologists who are guided by it.

As noted earlier, Susan Gray, a prominent school psychology scholar and trainer, advocated that school psychologists should be "data-oriented problem solvers" in their day-to-day practices (e.g., Gray, 1963). Given that she promoted this notion more than 40 years ago, Gray's view of what problem-solving school psychology practice should look like obviously has some differences in comparison with our current conceptions. Such differences are to be expected. How could even the most astute prognosticator of that time have possibly anticipated future developments that have proved to have such a major impact on our field? The advent of the first iteration of the Individuals with Disabilities Education Act in 1975, the subsequent dramatic expansion and professionalization of the field of school psychology, the increased pressure for practitioners to function in a "gatekeeper" role, the unprecedented increase in the number of students identified as having educational disabilities, the refinement of consultation models, the development of improved intervention techniques, the expansion of function-based approaches to assessment, and the more recent articulation and inclusion of RTI methods of identifying and supporting students are examples of mostly unanticipated changes in our field that have shaped the demands of practice. But even given the passage of time and the considerable changes in our field, Gray's influential views that practice should be guided by meaningful assessment and outcome data are remarkably consistent with what we are now advocating as best practice.

In his widely cited chapter on problem solving as a "best practice," Deno (2002) traced the roots of the current problem-solving paradigm in our field to as early as the 1950s, noting that psychologists of that era were influenced by "dissonance reduction" theories of how people go about the challenge of dealing with the difference between what they want and what they get. This idea is quite consistent with current conceptualization of problem solving as being an effort to help resolve the distance between "what is wanted" and "what is happening" (Tilly, 2002, 2008). Deno also noted that in the late 1960s, the then president of the American Psychological Association, Donald Campbell, advised psychologists to consider that our approaches to change should be thought of as "hypotheses to be tested," given that the outcomes of new programs and interventions were typically unpredictable. Again, we see a clear connection between this early advocacy of best practice and current efforts to approach individual cases from an idiographic, data-driven approach to what was later termed "short-run empiricism" (Cronbach, 1975) that seems to form the basis of the modern problem-solving approach. From a theoretical standpoint, we view the problem-solving approach to school psychology as fitting within the philosophical assumptions of *functional contextualism*. This approach places value on the use of scientific analysis not only to *predict* but also to *influence* behavior to *achieve a goal* (Biglan, 2004).

Perhaps the closest historical precursor to our modern conception of problem-solving was Bransford and Stein's (1984) formulation of the essential components of a hypothesis-driven and data-based approach to solving problems, which was termed the IDEAL problem-solving model. The title of this model reflects an acronym for the five essential steps that Bransford and Stein articulated: Identify the problem, Define the problem, Explore alternative solutions to the problem, Apply a solution, and Look at the impact or outcome of the particular application that was selected. Our view is that virtually all of the current influential approaches to problem solving in school psychology are essentially refinements of this earlier model, clearly derived from its basic components.

The most recent development in the evolution of the problem-solving model in school psychology practice is the integral pairing of the three-tiered model of service delivery and the RTI methods of assessing and supporting students who have learning problems (e.g., Shinn & Walker, in press; Tilly, 2008). RTI is a service delivery model in which students' responsiveness to instruction and intervention dictates the intensity of services they receive. According to Gresham

(2007), "the most important concept in any RTI model is the idea of matching the *intensity* of the intervention to the *severity* of the problem and *resistance* of that problem to change" (p. 17). The three-tiered model of service delivery, which is discussed extensively by Hawkins et al., in Chapter 2 of this volume, fits with this approach to matching intervention intensity to problem severity. As discussed in Chapter 2 as well as in numerous other sources (e.g., Batsche et al., 2006), the multi-tiered model involves a first tier in which assessment and intervention occur at a universal level (e.g., schoolwide or classwide). All students are screened multiple times a year, and preventative intervention strategies (e.g., improving schoolwide discipline procedures, changing the math curriculum to ensure that prerequisite skills are taught early on) are implemented and delivered to all students. Intervention efforts at this level are expected to meet the needs of approximately 80–90% of students. At the second tier, students who do not respond to Tier 1 interventions are identified and provided with small-group interventions that target the students' particular area of need. For the small portion (approximately 1–5%) of students who do not respond to Tier 1 or Tier 2 interventions, Tier 3 interventions that provide more intensive and individualized support (and that may consist of special education services) are provided.

At each tier, school psychologists should be engaged in the problem-solving process to ensure that problems are accurately identified and that the interventions implemented are effective for the majority of students to whom they are provided (or are changed if this is not the case). Although the problem-solving process and RTI are not synonymous, the problem-solving process is typically seen as integral to an efficient and effective multi-tiered model of service delivery. The chapters included in this book address the use of the problem-solving model within a multi-tiered service delivery model. As will be seen by readers, in some areas (e.g., assessment and intervention for internalizing disorders) this framework is newer, with less research on its use. For other areas (e.g., academic assessment and intervention, especially in reading) a more abundant literature exists. Overall, we hope that readers come away with the perspective that the problem-solving model (and its use within an RTI framework) is simultaneously simple and elegant and that it is both fluid and adaptable. The fact that the problem-solving approach continues to evolve and that it can be integrated with developing methods of educational practice speaks volumes about its utility.

Steps in the Problem-Solving Process as a Framework for This Volume

As noted earlier, we believe the problem-solving model provides an excellent framework for the provision of school psychology services. Thus we have chosen to use this model as an organization framework for this book, with the chapters falling into sections that correspond with the problem-solving model. To provide a context for the chapter discussions, we give a brief overview of the problem-solving steps here. According to Tilly (2008), within a problem-solving approach, decision making is guided by answering a series of questions:

- What is the problem?
- Why is it occurring?
- What can be done about it?
- Did it work?

A problem-solving school psychologist is able to work though each of these steps with the vision described earlier in mind. Thus the problem-solving school psychologist focuses on behaviors that are amenable to change and clearly identifies these, ensures that measureable outcomes are in place, and uses data to continually guide the process (i.e., the use of formative feedback rather than just summative feedback). Next we elaborate on each of these problem-solving stages.

What Is the Problem?

To answer the first question in the problem-solving process, it is important to determine the discrepancy between actual, or current, performance and desired outcomes. Discrepancies should be quantified in a manner that is useful in determining the severity of the problem and in goal setting. Objective and clear descriptions are important to ensure that everyone in the process is talking about the same behaviors and working toward the same goal. Because problems occur in context, the contextual factors surrounding the problem also need to be assessed and described; this information will lead into the second stage, determining why the problem is occurring.

Within this book, the six chapters in the section titled "Assessment and Analysis: Focus on Academic Outcomes," as well as the four chapters in the section titled "Assessment and Analysis: Focus on Social–Emotional and Behavioral Problems," address this first stage in the problem-solving process. These chapters provide information on assessment at the schoolwide level (VanDerHeyden, Chapter 3, and McIntosh, Reinke, & Herman, Chapter 9), as well as assessment of specific skills at all levels of the prevention and intervention process.

Why Is It Occurring?

Once the problem is identified, the school psychologist needs to focus on why the problem is occurring from a functional point of view. The "why" at this stage does not involve variables that cannot be changed (e.g., the child has a low scores on a test of cognitive abilities or the child is "biologically predisposed" to be depressed) but instead focuses on contextual and environmental circumstances that can be altered to address the problem. For example, maybe a child scored low on a test of cognitive abilities, but he is not learning to read because he is not allotted enough time to practice reading in school and at home. Or an adolescent with a family history of depression may be experiencing a significant amount of depression because she is telling herself she is worthless and she is not engaging in any pleasurable activities. All these variables are ones that (with appropriate intervention) can be changed so that the student can learn and can feel better. The chapters in the two "Assessment and Analysis" sections also address this second phase of the problem-solving process. In particular, Chapter 8 (Daly, Hofstadter, Martinez, & Andersen) and Chapter 12 (Jones & Wickstrom) address specifically the process of using assessment data to determine the function of the problem, which, in turn, allows the problem-solving school psychologist to develop interventions that are functionally related to the behavior in need of change.

What Can Be Done about It?

When selecting an intervention strategy to address a specific problem, it is important that the intervention is likely to improve the problem (i.e., reduce the discrepancy between actual and desired performance). Thus interventions should be selected because of their functional relevance (i.e., their link to the reasons the problem is occurring), their likelihood of success (i.e., they are based on evidence within the research literature), and their contextual fit (i.e., their fit with the problem situation and setting). Let us assume that information collected about the problem and the reason it is occurring point to a hypothesis that a particular strategy is likely to help to improve the problem situation. At this point, it is important to carefully plan the strategy.

An intervention plan should delineate various aspects of the intervention. For example, a very thorough intervention plan might describe (1) the steps and procedures of the intervention (what the intervention will look like); (2) the resources and materials needed and their availability; (3) the roles and responsibilities of those involved in delivering the intervention (e.g., who will implement the intervention, prepare materials, collect outcome data); (4) the intervention schedule (at what times in the day, for what duration, how may times per week) and situation (where, during what activities, with whom); (5) how the intervention and its outcomes will be monitored (what measures, collected by whom, and on what schedule); (6) timelines for implementation and for achieving desired goals; and (7) how the information will be analyzed and modification made.

Each of the 16 chapters in the section titled "Implementing Prevention and Intervention Strategies" addresses this third phase of the problem-solving process. This section begins with a chapter that provides an overview of the evidence-based practice and prevention and intervention strategies, and the chapters that follow emphasize the use of evidence-based techniques as well as ongoing data collection to determine whether the prevention and intervention strategy is working for the specific target (e.g., school, class, small group, individual child).

Did the Intervention Work?

We can know whether an intervention was effective for a specific problem situation only after we actually implement the intervention and evaluate its outcomes. To determine students' responsiveness to an intervention strategy, it is important to collect ongoing information on the degree to which the intervention was implemented as planned (i.e., intervention integrity) and, relative to this, whether student outcomes improved (i.e., whether there was a reduction in the discrepancy between desired and actual performance). Continuous monitoring and evaluation are essential aspects of any problem-solving process. Data should be collected on: (1) targeted student outcomes, (2) proper implementation of the intervention, and (3) social validity (practicality and acceptability) of the intervention and student outcomes. The two chapters in the section titled "Evaluating Interventions" address this final stage of the problem-solving process.

Implementing Problem Solving at a Systems Level

Not only is it important for problem-solving school psychologists to be knowledgeable about each step in the problem-solving process, but it is also important that they be aware of (and contribute to) building districtwide and schoolwide practices that support the ongoing use of the problem-solving model. In the section titled "Building Systems to Support the Problem-Solving Model," four chapters are included that cover systems-level issues in ensuring that the problem-solving model is adequately implemented. The last chapter in this section (and in the volume) provides an overview of the problem-solving model in practice. Within each of the individual chapters in these different sections, the authors have framed their discussions to be consistent with the problem-solving model of school psychology.

Vignettes: Walking the Problem-Solving Walk

Perhaps the most engaging way to understand the reasons that we have emphasized problem solving within this volume and how this model is influencing the delivery of school psychology services is to profile actual practitioners whose day-to-day work is heavily guided by the problem-solving approach. This section includes brief profiles or vignettes of three early-career school psychologists (each of them has been out of graduate school and practicing for less than 5 years) who were trained in problem-solving methods of service delivery and whose practice is clearly influenced in this direction. Jennifer Geisreiter is a school psychologist with the Catholic Independent Schools of Vancouver Archdiocese in British Columbia, Canada. Jon Potter is a school psychologist with the Heartland Area Education Agency in Johnston, Iowa. Moira McKenna is a school psychologist and RTI specialist for the Southern Oregon Education Service District, in Medford, Oregon. Each of them graciously agreed to our request for an interview and to allow us a small window into their efforts to make a difference in the lives of the students, families, and educators they are committed to supporting.

Jennifer noted that "the majority of my work is based within a problem-solving model," adding that "sometimes I am trying to solve problems at a systems level rather than at the school level." As an example of how she uses problem-solving strategies in delivering services, she described her involvement in her school's recent efforts to modify educational planning for students. "The district that I work for has just recently changed the process of writing individual education plans for children to make them more effective documents. One way that I utilize problem-solving strategies is by attending IEP meetings of children … and trying to develop clear, measurable, and appropriate goals for these students." In terms of the advantages she sees in practicing within a problem-solving orientation, Jennifer identified both efficiency and the opportunity to intervene earlier as key benefits. "It seems to be a more efficient and effective way to deal with issues that arise, particular for certain academic issues … it allows problems to be addressed at a much earlier stage, long before they become serious enough to merit more intensive efforts." Related to this last issue, she emphasized that traditional school psychology practice orientation may not offer her the same opportunity, noting that "I get to be involved with children long before I would in a traditional model."

Moira's current work includes a majority of her time assigned as an RTI specialist, meaning that she is more heavily involved in consultation, training, and systems-level efforts than she was in her internship and first position as a school psychologist. One interesting aspect of her problem-solving orientation to her work illustrates that problem solving is a flexible approach, amenable to appropriate variations rather than a rigid or monolithic model. As a graduate student at the University of Oregon, Moira worked closely with Roland Good, who helped develop the outcomes-driven model (ODM; Good, Gruba, & Kaminski, 2002), a more expansive way of approaching problem solving than some variations of this approach. Moira noted, "The problem-solving model and the preventative, systems-oriented evolution of the outcomes driven model have been essential to informing the development and implementation [of my efforts] for both schoolwide systems and individual student intervention." She sees several key advantages to using the problem-solving approach and ODM in her work, including "the ability to assess student performance as compared to a local and larger normative peer group, and to use a preventative and systemic approach to intervention by providing students with needed supports early," and she also notes that this approach allows the use of "measure(s) that [are] sensitive enough to determine whether students are making growth from week to week, with the use of decision-making guidelines." Although Moira has been careful in her career choices to select work environments that provide opportunities for her to practice using the skills she was trained in, she formerly worked for several years as a special education teacher and has been exposed to various models of school psychology, including the traditional gatekeeper/psychometrician model. She clearly sees the advantages

that a problem-solving orientation to school psychology practice offers: "Assessment in traditional school psychology practice does not often address intervention."

Like Jennifer's and Moira's, Jon's day-to-day work is heavily influenced by a problem-solving orientation: "The problem-solving orientation drives most everything that I do. All of the educational decisions I make ... are guided by the problem-solving process." As an example of how this process actually plays out into action day to day, Jon noted how he uses the problem-solving orientation to guide his thinking and practices: "when addressing a student with behavioral concerns, the initial steps I take are to define specifically what the problem behaviors are through interviews with teachers and staff, and observations of the student. I then validate that the student is having a significant problem through comparisons to the behavior of typical peers and what the behavioral expectations are." He then focuses on understanding why the problem behaviors are occurring, which involves "identifying what events reliably predict the behavior, and what variables in the classroom are reinforcing the behavior. All of this information really helps me to understand why the problem behavior is occurring, and if I understand why the problem behavior is occurring, I can help develop an intervention that will be effective in reducing (problem) behavior. Once that intervention is developed, we will implement the intervention and evaluate the effectiveness of the intervention over time." Jon sees a great difference between how he and his colleagues work and how traditional school psychology has operated in many instances. "In my opinion, the main difference is that in working within the problem-solving model, all of the evaluation and assessment that I do is for the purpose of intervention development. Though part of my practice is to evaluate students for special education eligibility, the focus is much more on determining what instructional strategies work for the student, rather than simply do they qualify?"

Although Jennifer, Moira, and Jon all agree that there are many advantages to the problem-solving orientations they espouse to guide their practice as school psychologists, they also acknowledge that the road is not always easy. Jon commented that a common misconception he has seen regarding problem-solving practice in our field is that "it delays the provision of extra support for children who need it" and that "there still exists a general thinking that special education is the most appropriate support for all students who struggle." Likewise, Jennifer notes that many educators with whom she works "view the assessment as the intervention rather than part of the problem-identification process" and recognizes that "data-based decision making is still difficult to get people on board with." In addition, Moira notes that she has sometimes observed "teacher resistance to change," admitting that it "requires more thinking, work, and accountability" and that many educators' approaches to student learning "continue to depend upon within-child orientations to problem solving, versus considering changes to the environment and thinking about how to reallocate resources and adjust variables to create predictable and safe environments." Regardless of the challenges they face in their work, these three early-career practitioners are all convinced that their efforts to support students, families, and teachers—which are clearly based on the problem-solving approach—are rewarding and that they are making a positive difference. And given that they each employ processes that are based on data, when they perceive positive results, it is probably more than a feeling.

Final Thoughts

To accomplish great things we must first dream, then visualize, then plan ... believe ... act!
—ALFRED A. MONTAPERT

In this introductory chapter, our primary aims were to provide a broad vision of what the role of a problem-solving school psychologist looks like and a framework for the remaining chapters in this volume that expand on areas of competency important to a problem-solving approach to school psychology. We have gone to great lengths to create a book that provides a vision and practical descriptions of the knowledge and tools necessary to carry out the role of a

problem-solving school psychologist. We are united in our enthusiasm for what this type of approach can offer for the practice of psychology in the schools and for making a real difference in promoting better educational and mental health outcomes for students. It is our hope that readers of this volume—whether they be newly trained or currently practicing school psychologists— are inspired to try out and ultimately adopt and enact the vision we are promoting.

References

Batsche, G., Elliott, J., Graden, J. L., Grimes, J., Kovaleski, J. F., Prasse, D., et al. (2006). *Response to intervention: Policy considerations and implementation.* Alexandria, VA: National Association of State Directors of Special Education.

Biglan, A. (2004). Contextualism and the development of effective prevention practices. *Prevention Science, 5,* 15–21.

Bransford, J. D., & Stein, B. S. (1984). *The IDEAL problem solver.* New York: Freeman.

Cronbach, L. J. (1975). Beyond the two disciplines of scientific psychology. *American Psychologist, 30,* 116–127.

Deno, S. L. (2002). Problem-solving as "best practice." In A. Thomas & J. Grimes (Eds.), *Best practices in school psychology* (4th ed., Vol. 1, pp. 37–55). Bethesda, MD: National Association of School Psychologists.

Good, R. H., III, Gruba, J., & Kaminski, R. A. (2002). Best practices in using Dynamic Indicators of Basic Early Literacy Skills (DIBELS) in an outcomes-driven model. In A. Thomas & J. Grimes (Eds.), *Best practices in school psychology* (4th., Vol. 1, pp. 699–720). Bethesda, MD: National Association of School Psychologists.

Gray, S. W. (1963). *The psychologist in the schools.* New York: Holt, Rinehart, & Winston.

Gresham, F. M. (2007). Evolution of the response-to-intervention concept: Empirical foundations and recent developments. In S. R. Jimerson, M. K. Burns, & A. M. VanDerHeyden (Eds.), *Handbook of response to intervention: The science and practice of assessment and intervention* (pp. 10–24). New York: Springer.

Merrell, K. W., Ervin, R. A., & Gimpel Peacock, G. A. (2006). *School psychology for the 21st century: Foundations and practices.* New York: Guilford Press.

Reschly, D. J. (2008). School psychology paradigm shift and beyond. In A. Thomas & A. J. Grimes (Eds.), *Best practices in school psychology* (5th ed., Vol. 1, pp. 3–15). Bethesda, MD: National Association of School Psychologists.

Shinn, M. R., & Walker, H. M. (Eds.). (in press). *Interventions for achievement and behavior in a three-tier model including RTI* (3rd ed.). Bethesda, MD: National Association of School Psychologists.

Tilly, W. D. (2002). Best practices in school psychology as a problem-solving enterprise. In A. Thomas & J. Grimes (Eds.), *Best practices in school psychology* (4th ed., Vol. 1, pp. 21–36).

Bethesda, MD: National Association of School Psychologists.

Tilly, W. D. (2008). The evolution of school psychology to science-based practice: Problem-solving and the three-tiered model. In A. Thomas & A. J. Grimes (Eds.), *Best practices in school psychology* (5th ed., Vol. 1, pp. 17–36). Bethesda, MD: National Association of School Psychologists.

Ysseldyke, J., Burns, M., Dawson, P., Kelley, B., Morrison, D., Ortiz, S., et al. (2006). *School psychology: A blueprint for training and practice: 3*. Bethesda, MD: National Association of School Psychologists.

Chapter 2

Choosing Targets for Assessment and Intervention

Improving Important Student Outcomes

Renee O. Hawkins
David W. Barnett
Julie Q. Morrison
Shobana Musti-Rao

This chapter was written to help guide professionals through key decision points in identifying problems that should be targeted for intervention and in determining how to measure the targets. Each of these decision points has a direct impact on student interventions and outcomes and is guided by available research and data-based problem solving.

Target variable selection refers to problem-solving teams identifying targets for intervention and ways to measure those targets, whether the problem occurs at an individual student, class, or schoolwide level. *Target variables are derived from constructs of educational risk and yield specific measures or observations to identify students in need of intervention support and to track intervention outcomes. Both target variables and measures need to be carefully selected by teams because the measures are used to construct the database for monitoring and evaluating intervention programs.* Thus target variables and measures set the course of action by teams and act as the "heart monitor" for educational services, allowing for timely modifications as needed by showing initial risk for academic or behavioral difficulties, as well as ongoing intervention effectiveness.

In most cases, target *variable* selection is used instead of the more traditional target "behavior" because data-based problem solving is increasingly linked to school, classroom, or setting characteristics that may be outcomes of problem solving and schoolwide programmatic changes. These intervention setting characteristics may be progress-monitored when students are referred or screened for concerns about their behavior or academic performance in school. For example, students may be referred for academic failure problems, but schools may need to measure not only student progress but also the amount and quality of instruction provided to students, as instruction may need to be changed and monitored. In keeping with traditional discussions, specific instructional procedures are the *intervention* for a targeted student, and the student's performance is the *behavior*. However, the need for ongoing selection, monitoring, and modification of instruction programs at school, class, and individual levels blurs the traditional distinctions in what is typically targeted for change (i.e., student behavior or instruction). Measurement focusing on targeted variables includes *behavior in environment* and functions of behavior, and in educational programming key features of instructional environments may be significant targets for change.

The importance of decisions for students and stakeholders related to target variable selection may be quite high, and teams will wonder about the adequacy of different variables or alternative methods of measuring variables. Technical adequacy (e.g., reliability and validity, sampling) of target variable measurement is discussed as a way to increase team confidence that sound decisions have been made.

A related task for problem-solving teams is identifying *students* requiring intervention based on specific risk indicators. Relying on target variable data related to school success, teams use data to decide not only which students are in need of support but also how many students and at which levels to intervene in order to effectively measure and interpret outcomes (i.e., school, class, group, and individual levels). *Risk indicators* are factors or measures that suggest the likelihood of students' school success or failure. Teams make efforts to ensure the accurate identification of students in need of intervention to prevent students from falling further behind and to improve the use of school resources through effective programming, as, for example, raising school or class performance if many students are at risk.

First, an overview of target selection basics and guidelines for choosing target variables is provided. Second, methods of selecting students for interventions are described, as the methods and outcomes affect which variables are targeted and the appropriate level of intervention and monitoring. Third, advances in target variable selection are discussed in the context of response to intervention (RTI).

Target Variable Selection

Generally, problem-solving teams start with broad targets for change and use a "funneling" process (Hawkins, 1986) to narrow the focus in selecting target variables. The measurement of target variables is direct, contextualized by settings, and functional: What is happening in a specific situation that is concerning? and What can and should be changed? Changes in socially significant performance are what matters. Data regarding

environmental and instructional variables, as well as technical adequacy (e.g., reliability and validity evidence), may be needed to defend specific team decisions concerning variables targeted for change. Students and situations can be highly challenging, and target variable selection is approached step by step, repeating problem-solving steps as needed.

Overview: The Basics of Target Variable Selection through Problem Solving

Target variables are selected based on the use of intervention research and behavioral problem solving. School psychologists trained in consultation team with teachers and, as appropriate, specialized professionals, students, and parents to resolve problem situations. Problem solving may be used repeatedly to help meet long-term objectives, as for a student with comprehensive socially and educationally related disabilities (Kratochwill & Bergin, 1990).

In classic discussions, a student's unique characteristics and situations are guiding factors in target variable selection. Kanfer (1985) wrote: "Each client presents the clinician anew with the fundamental task of deciding on a focus for the most effective intervention" (p. 7). Target variable selection steps generally include problem identification and analysis and continue with plan development, plan implementation, and evaluation. There is a creative process in which alternatives are considered and a rigorous progression links all steps with the best available empirical evidence.

In the problem identification step, teams clarify the problem behavior and desired alternative. In problem analysis, decisions also may be made to monitor environmental variables related to problem situations as significant factors that contribute to differences between observed and desired behavior and performance become understood. In applied behavior analysis (ABA), from which fundamental intervention methods are derived, an emphasis is on the use of high-quality data for decision making and the evaluation of interventions using single-case methods (baseline followed by intervention; see Daly, Barnett, Kupzyk, Hofstadter, & Barkley, Chapter 29, this volume). In addition, functional relationships are considered when making predictions about behavior. Through functional behavioral assessment (FBA; see Jones & Wickstrom, Chapter 12, this volume) and analysis methods, functional hypotheses are generated to understand relationships between target behaviors and environmental variables. A *functional hypothesis* is a proposed explanation as to the reason that problem behaviors occur and persist, such as gaining attention or escaping difficult tasks (expanded later in the chapter). ABA also emphasizes achieving *social validity*, which means in part that persons in close contact with students have a voice in considering the goals, methods, and outcomes of prevention and intervention programs (Wolf, 1978).

The Scope of Target Variables Has Appropriate Focus

Following careful selection of significant variables, teams must make measurement decisions. *Comprehensiveness* as used here refers to the many possible and intervention-relevant considerations related to academic and social performance in schooling (e.g., medical problems; home setting events that interfere with sleep, nutrition, homework completion; generalization of social or academic skills; etc.; Gresham, 2007). With the idea of *level of analysis*, picture using "zoom in" or "zoom out" when examining situations or behaviors. *Splitting* or *lumping* occurs as complex skills are used as variables targeted for change and as teams focus on specific hypothesized variables of importance in problem solving. For example, social competence is made up of many social skills (e.g., social problem solving, eye contact) that must be contextually and developmentally appropriate for intervention plans. Reading can be broken down into requisite skills such as vocabulary, phonemic awareness, and so on, based on functional and empirical hypotheses of what is needed. Teams monitor progress at the construct level (e.g., "reading and social behavior are improving") by using measures validly related to the improvements and the intervention methods (e.g., greater reading fluency through more practice time, fewer arguments with peers based on applying problem-solving skills).

Some concerns may require measuring a *constellation of behaviors* (Kazdin, 1985). For example, student anxiety or depression may have various degrees and expressions of overt behavior and covert events that may be exacerbated by incidents in school or home.

Stimulus and response patterns or *covariations* (Kazdin, 1985) may need to be measured. For example, to measure student compliance as a targeted variable, teams may need to look at the following: clarity of classroom rules or expectations; a student's fluency with behavioral expectations; various qualities of a teacher's request, such as whether it is said nicely but firmly, with eye contact, and in proximity to the student, whether it can be done without supports, and whether wait time is appropriate; student's behavior or compliance with requests; peer norms for compliance (Bell & Barnett, 1999); teacher's reinforcement of compliance; and sustained compliance. Decisions about what to target and selection of interventions to improve compliance are linked to what the data say about a student's compliance in context.

Scheduling Targeted Variable Measurements for Progress Monitoring

After variables and measures are selected, teams decide *when* and *how much* to measure and *at what point to analyze the data*. Targeted variables are measured to establish a baseline of current performance and to closely monitor intervention effects or "what is happening" so that timely changes can be made to plans as needed. In practice, *decision rules* are set with team members about what constitutes adequate plan implementation, how long to try the plan, and measurable goals or criteria for performance. A decision rule is used to link data to instructional decision making through carefully planned instructional trials to see whether changes in methods or content are needed (e.g., Fuchs & Fuchs, 1986). Thus a decision rule is an agreement or plan to carefully try an intervention for a set time (or number of trials, etc.) to see what changes in plans may be needed based on the data. Decision rules can improve decision making by providing timely feedback to teams on "what works." New decision rules are reset after each point-of-intervention evaluation.

Schedules for collecting data on targeted variables may vary widely. The schedule for monitoring should be based on specific research with the intervention and target variable measures and on the realities of situations. Also, teams should evaluate the amount of risk associated with the ongoing occurrence of the problem behavior for the targeted student, as well as for others in the environment. For guidelines, high-risk behaviors may be monitored every day to once per week or every 2 weeks for academic performance to allow for measurable growth to triannually for academic screening programs. As examples, it may be acceptable to monitor writing fluency weekly, whereas highly disruptive behavior or physical aggression toward peers may be monitored daily to quickly identify an effective intervention plan and ensure the safety of all students. Schedules are modified as needed based on what the data indicate (e.g., changes in level or trend). To help with the scheduling challenges, different data sources are used, and, as situations improve, follow-up measures become less frequent. For example, for challenging behaviors, a teacher daily report is used, along with periodic direct observation by a consultant (the data sources should not be combined but should show separate results). Schedules and organization of data collection also are linked to single-case designs (see Daly et al., Chapter 29, this volume).

Guidelines for Selecting Target Variables

Guidelines help teams with sound decisions regarding target variable selection. Target variables should be linked to direct measures of the problem that are reliable, sensitive enough to measure change resulting from the intervention, and related to valid outcomes (Macmann et al., 1996). Table 2.1 summarizes practical guidelines for selecting targeted variables and measures building on classic discussions (e.g., Hawkins, 1986; Kratochwill, 1985). Basic reliability and validity information and other measurement qualities are ways to help with the choices in target variable measure selection.

Target Variables Are Clearly Defined

Target variables are defined in observable and measurable terms and in ways that all members of the problem-solving team can understand. Operational definitions clearly and objectively describe the observable fea-

tures of the behavior. They include examples and nonexamples of behavior and provide a complete picture of what the target behavior looks like (Hawkins & Dobes, 1975).

Target Variables Can Be Significantly Changed

Teams select target variables that can be meaningfully changed in that they are influenced by the environment. Target variable measures should be sensitive enough to reflect changes in behavior resulting from prevention and intervention programming. Many examples show why the idea of changeability is important. Personalities, temperament, intelligence, and self-concept are mentioned frequently as concerns or explanations in consultations with parents or teachers. However, these attributes are not easily modifiable as targets of interventions, and typically measures of these constructs are not useful for progress monitoring. Through effective problem solving, variables can be selected that satisfy concerns but that also yield measures that are practical and valuable for progress monitoring. Examples include targeting and improving academic and classroom functioning and social competence skills, as well as supports for teachers and students. Taking broadly stated concerns of parents and teachers, finding sound ways to select target variables related to valid concerns, and progress-monitoring interventions are basic functions of problem solving.

Target Variables Can Be Directly Measured

Target variables are directly linked to the problem situation by carefully selected measurement methods. Intervention research is used to help achieve confidence in measurement and intervention plans by using high-quality data to evaluate instructional and behavioral outcomes. For academic concerns, curriculum-based measurement (CBM) is a well-researched, reliable, and direct method for measuring student performance in core academic areas including reading, math, written expression, and spelling (Deno, Marston, & Tindal, 1985–1986; see also Marcotte & Hintze, Chapter 5; Burns & Klingbeil, Chapter 6; and Gansle & Noell, Chapter 7, this volume). Table 2.2 describes common CBM variables. CBM allows the

TABLE 2.1. Practice Guidelines for Target Variable Selection

Professional standard	What to look for
Target variable measures meet scientific and professional standards of "high-quality data"	• Validity: teams use variables linked to specific prevention and intervention research or establish the functional validity of the variables (i.e., demonstrate its validity for an individual; demonstrate causal relationship)
Problem solving is used to form empirically valid plans	• Targeted variables may include environmental, instructional, and student measures of change as needed. • Validity and level of inference: Outcomes are directly observable and meaningful. • Validity and sensitivity: Teams use measures that can track changes in behavior or performance in increments that are useful for ongoing and timely decisions. • Social validity: Consumers of services (i.e., teachers, parents, and students) also evaluate intervention goals, methods, and outcomes. • Reliability: Teams use measures with known and acceptable reliability or ensure reliability through ongoing checks (i.e., agreement checks between observers).
Cost–benefit and sustainability are considered in making selections	• Costs are estimated by also considering potential outcomes. High-quality data may be needed to obtain high-quality results that can produce ultimate "savings" for students and schools. Intervention failure is costly.
Decisions are monitored carefully	• Decision rules are used whereby teams set goals and try out interventions for an agreed-on number of sessions based on research with the intervention. • Graphs are used to show the ongoing decision process, including baseline (if possible) and results of each condition.
Does the intervention work?	• Interventions are examined through an internally valid research design. Alternatively, schools can use an "accountability design" by looking at changes in performance or behavior as measured by carefully selected target variables with the intervention in place (see Daly et al., Chapter 29, this volume).
How well does it work?	• Questions that can be addressed by teams include the size and significance of effects, as compared with benchmarks, peer norms, and judgments by consumers. These data lead to the next steps by teams. • Broader consequences are considered, including planned as well as unplanned outcomes that may be positive or negative or may occur over longer time periods.

frequent collection of data to evaluate interventions. For example, students selected for small-group math instruction based on low performance on math CBM continue to be monitored weekly using math CBM.

For behavioral concerns, a high-quality data source for evaluating interventions is direct observation. There are several likely methods of collecting observational data, all based on selecting significant and consistent settings, times, conditions, or activities for observations. First, *time-sampling* procedures often are used to improve the technical adequacy of observational data. Observation sessions are divided into intervals (e.g., 10–30 seconds), and the variable of interest is recorded by set procedures (Cooper, Heron, & Heward, 2007). Observers record whether or not the behavior occurred continuously during the interval (e.g., 10 seconds) for *whole-interval recording*, at any point during the interval for *partial-interval recording*, or at the end of the interval for *momentary time sampling*. Second, in *event-recording* procedures, observers record features of behavior such as frequency. For both time sampling and event recording, the session is summarized using the data collected (e.g., student was engaged as a percent of intervals during a 20-minute session; the

TABLE 2.2. Academic Target Variables and Curriculum-Based Measurement

Variable	CBM
Reading fluency	Words correct per minute: Number of words correctly read aloud during 1-minute timed-reading probe
Math fluency	Digits correct per minute: Number of correct digits on timed (2–5 minutes) computation probe
Writing fluency	Total words written: Number of words written following a story starter during timed (3–5 minutes) probe
Spelling fluency	Correct letter sequences: Number of correct letter sequences during timed, dictated spelling probe

student talked out five times during a 20-minute lesson) over baseline and intervention sessions. Figure 2.1 shows an example of an observation system for engagement and how data would be graphed. As discussed in the following subsection, the graph also shows the results of a reliability check by a second observer, as noted by squares representing additional data points in the figure. Multiple variables can be measured simultaneously with more complex codes. For example, positive engagement is illustrated in Figure 2.1, a replacement behavior for inattentive, disruptive, or other concerning behavior that also may be measured in a code, along with instructional variables or a teacher's effective use of positive managerial practices. The variable of engagement also may be refined by measuring qualities of practice activities (e.g., Daly, Martens, Barnett, Witt, & Olson, 2007).

Target Variables Are Reliably Measured

At one level, teams agree on variables targeted for change and how to measure them and examine and resolve differences; this is the reliability or *consistency* of targeted variable *selection* across team members (Macmann et al., 1996). Evidence suggests that agreement on what to target may be a critical step, as team members may have

different beliefs about causes of behavior and therefore about what to measure (e.g., Wilson & Evans, 1983). As selected, and throughout the problem-solving process, teams check the reliability of target variable measures. Reliability is estimated for some targeted variable measures (i.e., CBM) based on prior research. Ongoing reliability checks, also known as *agreement* checks, allow problem-solving teams increased confidence in measuring targeted variables (e.g., agreement on performance, frequency, duration, discrepancy from typical peer performance) and intervention effects. Reliability checks involve comparing the results of two observers independently coding or scoring the same sample of behavior for consistency. For example, two professionals may co-observe a classroom and compare data at the end of the observation session. Permanent products, such as a completed math CBM probe, may be independently scored and compared. Additional ongoing samples of CBM or observations can improve the reliability of individual decisions.

Technical adequacy checks for educational programming—as when targeted variables are curriculum, instructional skills, and behavioral management—are known variously as intervention adherence, fidelity of implementation, or intervention integrity. These checks are typically based on agreement indices showing the consistency of steps as carried out compared with implementation plans, scripts, and schedules (Barnett et al., 2007).

The operational definition of the target variable and the assessment system selected can significantly affect reliability. The reliability of data on the target variable and the validity of decisions made based on those data are improved when a precise behavioral definition is established. If the definition of the behavior is unclear, data are more likely to be unreliable, and teams will not be able to interpret the effects of interventions with confidence.

The method selected to assess the target variable also affects the reliability of data (Cooper et al., 2007). For example, for behaviors without a discrete beginning and end, such as student engagement, a time-sampling approach (as discussed earlier) would be most appropriate. Using a frequency count for such behaviors would likely re-

Code	Behavior	Definition	Recording Method
✓	Engagement	Student is attending to assigned task/activity by writing, reading, raising hand, asking or answering questions, talking to peers on topic, listening to the teacher or peers, looking at academic material	10-second, whole-interval recording

Minute	1	2	3	4	5	6
1						
2						
3						
4						
5						
6						
7						
8						
9						
10						

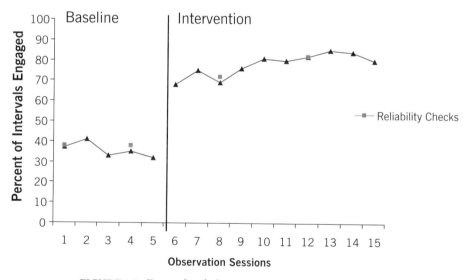

FIGURE 2.1. Example of observation code and graphed data.

sult in low reliability, as the observer would have difficulty determining when one occurrence of engagement ended and another began. Self-reports of teachers' adherence to intervention plans may not be equivalent to observational data by a consultant. Adequate training of those responsible for data collection and reliability checks can help improve reliability. Figure 2.1 provides an example of an operational definition for engagement and shows how reliability data can be coplotted to evaluate consistency of decisions that would be made by primary and other observers. Intervention adherence data also may be coplotted or summarized, along with student outcome data (Barnett et al., 2007).

Guidelines from research (e.g., Kennedy, 2005) suggest that reliability checks should occur for approximately 20–33% of the sample of observations across baseline and intervention, often using a criterion of at least 80% agreement. However, early in problem solving, more frequent reliability checks may help teams evaluate the adequacy of operational definitions of targeted variables and of the data collection system and provide feedback to observers. The frequency of reliability checks also may depend on the amount of risk or severity of the problem behavior. For problem behaviors that require intense interventions, reliability checks can increase confidence in decisions concerning the use of resources to produce positive student outcomes.

Target Variables Are Linked to Meaningful Present and Future Outcomes

Direct and reliable measurements are necessary, but validity evidence related to positive outcomes for students adds even stronger criteria to target variable selection. Intervention research guides teams toward target variables that are linked to both short- and long-term positive outcomes (Kazdin, 1985). To accomplish this task, the selection of target variables and measures should be associated with evidence-based intervention methods that lead to meaningful change (Barnett et al., 2007). Teams weigh evidence by being up to date on specific intervention research to accurately judge current risk and make predictions about future consequences and to help select measurement methods. For example, numerous studies link specific intervention procedures with improved performance on curriculum-based assessment and measurement variables (Shapiro, 2004; Shinn, Walker, & Stoner, 2002). Thus, although increasing "engagement" is frequently selected as a target variable, the quality of practice opportunities afforded by increased engagement is the likely active ingredient in intervention success and can be progress-monitored (Daly et al., 2007). Teams may select opportunities to respond to academic stimuli (e.g., Greenwood, 1991) as a target variable leading to interventions that focus on providing students additional guided, independent, and generalized practice of skills, progress-monitored on progressively more natural and difficult material, all of which are linked to positive outcomes (e.g., Daly et al., 2007). As examples, selecting oral reading fluency as a target variable would lead to empirically supported interventions, such as repeated readings, peer tutoring, previewing strategies, taped-word procedure, and so on,

and, through more practice on familiar and nonfamiliar material, to improved chances of school success (see Linan-Thompson & Vaughn, Chapter 16, this volume). Furthermore, although referral concerns may be extremely specific (e.g., hitting), targeted variables may be broader to ensure more significant positive behavior change (e.g., problem solving for increased social competence). Other criteria include possible benefits not only to the student but also to others in the environment, such as teachers and peers. The social validity of target variables is established when team members and data sources agree that targets, methods, and goals for change are acceptable (Wolf, 1978).

Functional Hypotheses Are Used to Critically Examine Possible Targeted Variables

Through FBA, information from a variety of methods, including interviews, questionnaires, rating scales, and direct observation, is used to hypothesize functional relationships between problem behaviors and features of the environment. Behavior or performance can "look" the same on the surface but can occur for very different reasons. FBA methods are a means of identifying these reasons to create effective interventions. Functional information about variables is used to develop intervention plans to decrease problem behavior and increase appropriate behavioral alternatives (see Jones & Wickstrom, Chapter 12, this volume; Gresham, Watson, & Skinner, 2001; Watson & Steege, 2003). The intensity of the FBA varies depending on the severity of the problem behavior. From relying solely on interviews to conducting multiple direct observations, teams can tailor the FBA process to meet students' needs. Furthermore, functional hypotheses can be directly evaluated to more clearly establish function. To establish *function* means that specific reasons for challenging behavior are tested. In a functional analysis, antecedent and consequence variables are experimentally manipulated to verify the function of behavior (Gresham et al., 2001; Horner, 1994). In some cases, teams also may conduct a brief experimental analysis in which different intervention conditions are presented and the effects compared to increase the validity of intervention selection decisions (see Daly, Hofstadter, Martinez, & Andersen, Chapter 8, this volume). In this way functionally significant target variables linked to interventions can be clarified.

Prioritizing and Combining Target Variables

Teams consider research indicating which target variables are associated with positive outcomes and linked to specific interventions. The idea of *keystone* variables prioritizes those having relatively *narrow targets for change with the possibility of widespread benefits* to clients (e.g., Barnett, Bauer, Ehrhardt, Lentz, & Stollar, 1997). Common examples include teachers' effective instruction and managerial skills and students' reading fluency, engagement with practice opportunities, social problem solving, compliance with adult requests, and independence with classroom routines through self-management. Selecting a keystone variable as the initial target may result in positive accompanying effects that reduce the need for additional interventions.

In many cases, students exhibit more than one problem behavior, presenting more than one possible target variable. Team members can prioritize targets based on a number of considerations or include more than one target variable. First, teams may consider the severity of problem behaviors. Dangerous and high-risk behavior would be targeted immediately. Behaviors most significantly discrepant from those of peers may be targeted early, providing more time for intervention efforts to have effects.

Sometimes teams may elect to target more than one variable right from the start. For example, a student may demonstrate academic skills deficits in math and reading. Both academic areas are keys to school success and may warrant immediate intervention. In such cases, teams must be careful to ensure that they have the resources necessary to target both variables meaningfully or develop plans in a sequence based on relative risk (e.g., reading, then math). As another example of possible multiple target variables, the relationship between poor academic performance and increased rates of problem social behavior has been well documented (Sugai, Horner, & Gresham, 2002). When a student is referred for academic and behavior problems, options for teams include deciding to intervene with academics and seeing whether social behavior changes without direct intervention, or vice versa, before implementing two distinct intervention plans. To help with this decision, teams would carry out a functional assessment to plan target variables based on hypotheses, confirmed with data, about whether or not a student has the needed skills to perform academic tasks or whether student performance variables need to be targeted (e.g., planning reinforcement).

Selecting Students for Intervention

Should schools select students based on concerning behaviors or performance, and then figure out target variables, measures, and interventions? Or should schools first select key variables and measures related to behavior and performance and educational risk, then screen all students and select students for interventions based on results? Both strategies have merit, and recent developments in screening and decision making now make both within reach. This section describes methods of student selection for intervention services, applying the foundation already discussed in target variable selection.

Schools often select students for intervention based on a concerning behavior or performance as typically determined by teachers or parents or by a student's self-referral. There are advantages to receiving referrals directly from those having the most knowledge about a situation and applying problem-solving steps to identify significant variables and to achieve needed outcomes. At the same time, the process of individual referral has led to great variability in who is selected to receive intervention services and what happens to them. The unfortunate tradition has involved waiting for students to fall behind peers or to fail and then applying cultural, local, or personal ideas about failure and what to do about it, including what to target for change. It is very common in schools for students referred for academic or behavior problems to be tested, classified, and placed in special programs. Inconsistent guidelines about selection, idiosyncratic and indefensible measurement decisions, weak systems-level interventions such as grade retention, group and individual interventions uneven in quality and of often-unknown effectiveness, and the lament "he or she just fell through the cracks" have been commonplace. In the end, the system of individual referrals, diagnostic testing for educational problems, and resulting classification and placement has been widely criticized with respect to systematic and effective special services to students (e.g., Heller, Holtzman, & Messick, 1982). Additionally, many argue that this flawed process has led to the overrepresentation of some minority groups in special education and that strengthening prevention, educational, and behavioral interventions without unnecessary and potentially stigmatizing labels is highly promising (e.g., Hosp & Reschly, 2004; Newell & Kratochwill, 2007; Skiba et al., 2008).

This section includes a discussion of various approaches to selecting students for intervention services, including strengths and weaknesses of teacher nominations, use of curriculum-based norms, and indicators of risk. Decision rules also are needed in cases in which intervention assistance is needed not for an individual student but for the class or even the school, and these decisions are informed by estimates of prevalence or base rates of the targeted variable.

Methods of Selection

Identifying Students in Need of Intervention Using Teacher Nominations

Teachers are significant participants in problem solving, and their observations about student performance are vital to the process because of their frequent and unique contacts with students under natural classroom demands. Teachers generally show a moderate to high level of accuracy in reporting student academics and behavior (e.g., Feinberg & Shapiro, 2003; Gresham, Reschly, & Carey, 1987). However, variations among teachers' goals, expectations, and tolerances for student behavior and academic performance can lead to different reasons for referral across teachers and referral rates. Factors such as the performance or behavior of peers in a class can affect how a teacher perceives an individual student and the likelihood that the student will be referred or not (e.g., VanDerHeyden & Witt, 2005).

Also, teachers unknowingly may be interacting with students in ways that exacerbate problem behavior or low performance. Regarding intervention decisions, VanDerHeyden, Witt, and Naquin (2003) showed that teachers' predictions of who will and will not have an adequate response to intervention are not very accurate, but many teachers also may have limited specific intervention experience. Nonetheless, when used in conjunction with direct measures of student performance (e.g., academic performance data, direct observation behavior data), information obtained from teacher observations can help effectively identify students in need of intervention support. To achieve the quality of data needed for accurate student selection, teacher information is supported with data on student performance relative to peers (locally and nationally), such as CBM and independent observations.

Curriculum-Based Approaches to Selection

Introduced earlier, CBM is commonly used to select students for academic intervention programs and to monitor student progress during intervention (Deno et al., 1985–1986). CBM is now used widely for academic screening (e.g., Ardoin et al., 2004; Glover & Albers, 2007). Advantages of CBM for screening include brevity (i.e., 1–5 minutes), repeatability, and sensitivity to student progress. For example, in CBM reading, students read aloud a grade-level passage for 1 minute as the administrator records the words read correctly and incorrectly. CBM is interpreted by using various norms and performance criteria from research, discussed next.

Identifying Students Using National Norms

Historically, comparing student performances with national norms from published norm-referenced tests has guided decisions about student need for intervention and/or special education. National norms provide information about the relative performance of students compared with same-age and same-grade peers. However, national norm groups do not necessarily reflect the educational and social environment of a particular school, classroom, and/or student, and they do not directly indicate the degree of possible risk for academic failure. Furthermore, the use of national norms may present problems with respect to interpreting the performance of some culturally and linguistically diverse students. National norms must enable meaningful comparisons with school and student demographics and must be useful in setting goals and evaluating progress. National norms are used with other norms, such as school, grade, classroom, or peer norms, and with valid criteria for identifying students at risk, depending on the prevention and intervention purpose.

Today, large-scale norms are available for most CBM measures (available from DIBELS [*dibels.uoregon.edu*] and AIMSweb [*aimsweb.com*]) based on data from schools subscribing to the Dynamic Indicators of Basic Early Literacy Skills (DIBELS) and AIMSweb data systems. Although these norms can provide a broader point of comparison for student performance, schools must take into account differences in student populations and resources, which contribute to significantly different performance. Schools included in the DIBELS and AIMSweb databases may not be representative of national student performance, even though they are geographically diverse. Schools subscribing to these systems are more likely to emphasize reading achievement, including adopting a research-based curriculum and using screening and progress monitoring (Good, Wallin, Simmons, Kame'enui, & Kaminski, 2002).

Identifying Students Using Local Norms

A local norm is a description of a school population's performance on a set of tasks developed to represent students from that particular school or school system (Habedank, 1995). The rationale for developing local norms is that behavior and academic performance are products of the ongoing interactions between students and their specific and unique environments. Local norms can be used to evaluate the performance of schools and classrooms over time when compared with national norms and risk indicators and to establish appropriate short-term goals for low-performing schools, classrooms, or students.

For example, schools may use CBM screening data to determine the average oral reading fluency of students at each grade, or schools may use archival data to determine the average number of office referrals per student (i.e., per month, semester, year). Local norms allow the comparison of an individual student's performance with the performances of peers within the same instructional context. As such, local norms provide a more direct and appropriate point of comparison than national norms for many intervention decisions, including student selection. However, local norms should be interpreted along with valid risk indicators that can reliably estimate the likelihood that a student will be successful or require intervention (e.g., Kame'enui, Good, & Harn, 2005) or that a class or group, and not necessarily an individual student, would be the focus of intervention efforts.

In summary, when selecting students for intervention assistance and when setting achievement goals for schools and individual students, it is important to consider national and local norms linked to valid indicators of educational risk. Local norms can be used to accurately identify struggling students within the context of the specific school setting. In addition, once students are selected for intervention, local norms can set initial performance goals that are attainable, and goals can be gradually increased to reduce risk based on national norms and empirically derived performance criteria associated with school success. Behavioral target variables, measurement methods, and goals likewise are set within a local context (e.g., numbers of students with disruptive behaviors in a classroom or other school context; Bell & Barnett, 1999).

Identifying Students Using Valid Indicators of Educational Risk

Researchers have identified numerous indicators of educational risk that may contribute to a student's school performance. Students also move in and out of risk situations. Thus schools cannot possibly assess all potential indicators of risk. However, by carefully selecting risk indicators with strong empirical support, problem-solving teams can increase the chances that they are correctly identifying many students who will need intervention assistance to achieve school success. Academic failure is preventable to a degree by early screening, with accurate risk appraisal and effective programming. Although local and national norms can provide valuable information about student performance relative to peers, the relative performance of the student may be less significant than risk estimates.

When selecting students for intervention, data should allow an empirical prediction or likelihood either that the student will be successful with additional supports or that the supports are not needed at that point. The selection of students should be both norm and criterion-referenced, taking into account comparisons between target student and peer performance, as well as comparisons with specific performance levels that are predictive of need for intervention or continued success. A *benchmark* is an empirical method of indicating that a student is on track if the current level of instruction is continued; similarly, levels of risk can be indicated for specific performances on measures (Kame'enui et al., 2005). Risk can also be estimated from repeating CBM measures and determining whether at-risk students are catching up to peers and grade-level benchmarks by noting changes in level and trend (or slope of progress) of performance.

As examples, DIBELS benchmarks are based on research correlating performance on various early-reading measures with later literacy outcomes. The benchmarks provide a criterion from which to evaluate student performance. Unlike screening based on comparisons only with national or local norms, criterion-based screening provides problem-solving teams with empirical estimates of risk levels that can be used for school planning (Kame'enui et al., 2005). Also, the AIMSweb system can help problem-solving teams conduct criterion-based screening by reporting percentile ranks for performance levels on various CBM measures across grade levels. Knowing that there is empirical evidence that performance on the CBM measures is linked to short- and long-term academic outcomes, teams can select students for interventions, set goals, and monitor progress using these data.

Why Base Rates Are Important

Base-rate estimates can help make the most of screening programs by appropriately focusing instruction or intervention efforts, including what variables to target, as well as methods of screening, selection, and program design (Macmann & Barnett, 1999; VanDerHeyden & Witt, 2005). Base rates are estimates of the prevalence of an objectively defined characteristic, such as risk for reading failure; social risk, such as dropping out of school; or a diagnostic category, such as learning disabilities. These specific base rates are estimated for a population or setting, such as a school (Meehl & Rosen, 1955). When deciding which students need intervention services, schools should consider base-rate estimates of the proportion of students expected to demonstrate academic or behavioral difficulties of interest. If base rates are very high or low, screening itself and program decisions need to be altered. For example, based on past graduation rates, two schools estimate the base-rate occurrence of dropping out of high school. School 1 has a base rate of 10%, whereas School 2 has a base rate of 60%. For School 1, with a relatively low base rate for dropout, intervention would focus on individual and small groups of students who are at risk for dropping out. In contrast, based on the high base-rate estimate for dropping out at School 2, planning would emphasize schoolwide prevention programming. In such a case, the focus is not only on individual students but also on the school as a system and on what can be done to effectively screen and better support the student population to increase graduation rates. By considering base rates, teams can evaluate an early screening process to ensure that students who need services are not being overlooked and that students who do not need intervention are not unnecessarily receiving additional support (Glover & Albers, 2007). When classrooms have high or low rates of academic problems, considering base rate helps ensure that appropriate screening methods are used and that interventions and support programs are targeting school needs effectively by addressing target variables and interventions, as appropriate, at class, group, or individual levels (e.g., Newell & Kratochwill, 2007; Skiba et al., 2008; VanDerHeyden & Witt, 2005).

In summary, student selection is based on improving *accuracy* and *usefulness* of targeted variables, measurement methods, and decisions about who needs help and what is helpful to students. In some cases, *schools* or *classrooms* may be selected for intervention if performance of many students is alarming, such as high rates of school failure or discipline referrals.

The RTI Context

RTI (response to intervention) changes the landscape of target variable selection due to its purposes and methods. At present, RTI is an option identified in Federal law (Individuals with Disabilities Education Improvement Act, 2004) for local educational agencies to help identify students with specific learning disabilities (SLD), but RTI's possible impact is much broader (e.g., Batsche et al., 2005). In contrast to starting with a student referral and figuring out target variables and next steps, the defining quality of RTI is an approach to decision making using universal early screening and outcomes of empirically defensible prevention programs and sequences of interventions as the database for service delivery determination. Selecting target variables and students for intervention is based on objective criteria derived from research. Concepts and measures of risk (e.g., poor reading fluency, challenging behaviors) are supported with data indicating that targets can be influenced by environmental changes *and* have evidence of positive outcomes for children. Research-based prevention programs and interventions are used to judge needed program qualities in schools. Thus target variable selection, as well as the selection of students for intervention services, starts with the premise of effective schools, research-based constructs of risk, and research on what works.

First, schools using RTI screen all students and offer appropriate services without delays. That is, schools assess the performance of all students on systemwide, high-priority target variables and assign students identified as "at risk" to valid instructional programs or interventions. This is in contrast to the approach taken by many schools in the past, in which target variables were identified idiosyncratically by the person making the referral and, more specifically, after a student had been referred for assistance. Second, a student's RTI intervention progress through established and research-based tiers of services may be used as evaluation data for more specialized service decisions or for decisions to fade intervention assistance when no longer necessary. These intervention data would be used instead of diagnostic test results collected at one point in time and questionably related to interventions. The dataset is different and would include detailed information on the research-based interventions implemented, reliable and valid data on the student's response to interventions, and evidence that interventions were carried out carefully. The result of a tiered intervention progression is a valid data-based description of targeted variables and needed interventions based on prior outcomes that can be used for planning next steps, as necessary, at all levels (school, class, group, and individual).

RTI is evolving, but generally, the first tier of RTI models is intended to be universal, school- and classwide, influencing the greatest number of children through prevention, sound curriculum, and evidence-based instructional and classroom managerial practices. Guidelines suggest that effective schoolwide supports should meet the needs of 80–90% of students in a given student population, with 10–20% of students requiring additional support (e.g., Kame'enui et al., 2005; Sugai et al., 2002). Students requiring additional support are served in a second tier consisting of short-term empirically based *selected* or *targeted* interventions (e.g., Batsche et al., 2005). More common examples of Tier 2 programs are based on standard protocols for valid instructional interventions that increase practice opportunities in small groups (i.e., reading skills) based on curriculum, data, and decision rules from Tier 1 (e.g., Vaughn, Wanzek, Woodruff, & Linan-Thompson, 2007; see also Linan-Thompson & Vaughn, Chapter 16, this volume). For the approximately 1–5% of students who are not sufficiently helped by the first two tiers, Tier 3 includes more intensive individualized services, or services delivered to smaller groups of students, and a focus on increased practice of specific skills related to the Tier 1 curriculum. Figure 2.2 shows a typical tiered model.

Data and team decisions would demonstrate need for intervention changes that increase or decrease in intervention intensity (e.g., time, specialized resources). Student performance ideally would be tracked

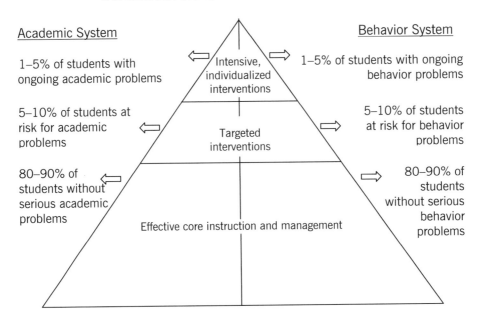

FIGURE 2.2. Typical tiered model.

or monitored in ways that are as close as schools can come to high-quality intervention research *within each tier* in order to expect results similar to the research from which it was derived. Multiple goals may be set that include immediate as well as long-term objectives, such as outcomes for success in typical environments and, ultimately, successfully maintained performance of targeted variables and generalization of responses to new situations. Teaming and problem solving are used to increase the chances of success for RTI by addressing planning and the logistics of intervention implementation (e.g., how often, where, who will implement, schedule for reliability and intervention adherence checks), as well as outcomes at the levels of both school and individual student. Problem solving also is used to help with needed instructional variations and unique student situations.

Similarly, the framework of positive behavior support (PBS) conceptualizes prevention and intervention efforts for social behaviors, calling for high-quality programming built on empirically validated interventions and tiered services (Sugai et al., 2002). First, an effective schoolwide system is developed and implemented. In Tier 1, classrooms are well designed and managed, behavioral expectations are directly taught, and all stu-

dents receive competent instruction on key social skills. In Tier 2, more practice is given based on a valid curriculum or intervention program in a group or embedded format, as are interventions with specific, troublesome classroom activities such as transitions. Tier 3 is based on intensified and individualized plans related to social behaviors. RTI and PBS are integrated in some RTI models and have many commonalities (Batsche et al., 2005).

RTI and Target Variable Selection

Universal Screening

The success of RTI is dependent on the early and accurate identification of students at risk (Compton, Fuchs, Fuchs, & Bryant, 2006). Universal screening defines the initial variables that will be used for intervention decisions in RTI. Variables may include instruction in and mastering of key early literacy skills, rate and level of improvement in skills, and variables related to instructing and supporting social competence in schools.

As an example, teams conduct universal screening for academic performance three times a year using norm- and/or criterion-referenced (derived locally and/or nationally) cut points to identify students who need intervention (Ardoin & Christ, 2008; Good, Gruba, & Kaminski, 2002). Typically, a CBM probe or a median score from three CBM probes administered at one time in key areas (e.g., reading and math) is used, and students scoring below the cut point are considered for Tier 2 intervention (e.g., Ardoin et al., 2004). Other RTI models include universal screening only at the start of the school year to identify a group of students who show potential at-risk indicators. Students in this group are then closely monitored to determine need for preventive intervention (Fuchs & Fuchs, 2007). To determine response to Tier 1 instruction and need for Tier 2 intervention, Fuchs and Fuchs (2007) recommend using a "dual discrepancy" criterion based on both (1) student growth defined as differences in performance over time that show up as a *slope* on a graph (i.e., words read per minute plotted every week showing changes in reading fluency over time); and (2) the level of performance (e.g., mean level of a target student compared with peers or other norms). In this model, a student is selected for Tier 2 intervention if, after at least 5 weeks of progress monitoring in the general curriculum, his or her slope of improvement and final level of performance are both at least 1 standard deviation below those of peers. As a different example, VanDerHeyden, Witt, and Gilbertson (2007) use class CBM data to decide various next steps that may include a brief (10-minute) classwide academic intervention carried out for 10 days to help with screening decisions if the class performance is low. As the preceding examples suggest, there is not one RTI model at present, but there is a strong consensus on early universal screening for key instructional, curricular, and social variables and use of the measures of these variables for monitoring progress.

Tiered Variables

Although there are variations in RTI models, target variables and students are selected and analyzed by teams using specific procedures described by the RTI model for each of the aforementioned tiers. As introduced, RTI and PBS are characterized by structural components, or tiers, that organize school, classwide, group, and individual target variables and sequential decision points that are

analyzed by looking at student outcomes (Gresham, 2007; Sugai et al., 2002). Thus school teams analyze school, class, group, and individual contexts based on research on improving reading and social behaviors and reducing challenging behaviors. Table 2.3 shows RTI tiers and common target variables that may be used by schools or teams at each tier. Within RTI, in addition to targeted variables related to direct measures of students' academic skills and behavior, instructional and classroom variables (curriculum, adherence to the curriculum, qualities and prevalence of instruction, classroom management, discipline programs, etc.) may be targets of intervention. Tier 1 variables include those related to scientifically based instruction for academic skills and social behaviors (Kame'enui et al., 2005; Sugai et al., 2002; Vaughn et al., 2007). Similar to Tier 1, selection of Tier 2 target variables would yield measures related to the specific academic or social concern. Furthermore, accompanying the increasing intensity of interventions from Tier 1 to Tier 2 would be an increase in the intensity of progress monitoring (e.g., more frequent assessment of target variables, more refined measures of academic progress in early literacy skills or social behavior, more frequent reliability and intervention adherence checks). At Tier 3, the collection of data on target variables would intensify further as teams try to use resources efficiently while still promoting positive student outcomes. Other important Tier 2 and 3 variables are included in plans for generalization and maintenance of skills and performance of skills in typical educational settings (Tier 1). For example, when implementing a reading intervention, teams may assess for generalization by monitoring reading fluency on both practiced and unpracticed reading passages and may plan to improve generalization in other instructional contexts, such as math word problems. Social behavior targets taught in Tier 2 groups would be progress-monitored in classroom and other school settings. Across all tiers, data on the degree to which RTI procedures are implemented as intended and that show the quality of outcomes are required; these are characteristics of services not typically applied to traditional referral decisions.

Problem solving related to functional and testable hypotheses about student academic

TABLE 2.3. Examples of Target Variables and Measures across Tiers

	Academic		Behavior	
Tier	Variables	Measures	Target variables	Measures
1	• Reading • Math • Content-area achievement • Instruction	• DIBELS triannual benchmark data • Math and reading triannual CBM benchmark data • Achievement test scores • Opportunities to respond to academic stimuli • Adherence to the curriculum	• Disruptive behavior • Instruction	• Office discipline referrals • Teacher referrals • Opportunities to practice appropriate social behavior • Adherence to classroom management procedures
2	• Reading • Math • Content-area achievement • Instruction	• Weekly DIBELS, math and reading CBM progress-monitoring data • Homework and classwork completion & accuracy • Test scores • Opportunities to respond to academic stimuli	• Disruptive behavior • Engagement • Compliance • Peer interactions • Instruction	• Weekly direct observations of engagement, compliance, peer interactions • Weekly teacher report of behavior • Opportunities to practice appropriate social behavior
3	• Reading • Math • Content-area achievement • Instruction	• Twice weekly DIBELS, reading CBM progress-monitoring data • Homework and classwork completion and accuracy • Test scores • Opportunities to respond to academic stimuli	• Disruptive behavior • Engagement • Compliance • Peer interactions • Instruction	• Twice weekly direct observations of engagement, compliance, peer interactions • Daily teacher report of behavior • Opportunities to practice appropriate social behavior

and social learning and performance, which may be useful at all RTI tiers, are critical at Tier 3 (individualized and intensive), with more challenging and complex academic and social problem behavior. In other words, beyond increasing specific practice, when previous intervention attempts have failed and the environmental variables contributing to the problem behavior are unclear, problem solving and FBA methods described in the chapter may provide information that can lead to the efficient identification of effective interventions.

Conclusions: Achieving Confidence in Decisions

Target "behavior" selection is in keeping with traditional discussions of problem solving for students with concerning behavior. However, with the number of challenges faced by schools and in line with academic and social interventions that are based on systematic changes in instruction and envi-

ronment, we use the broader term of *target variable selection*. Target variable selection, measurement, and schedules of measurement create the data for intervention decisions. Students may come to the attention of professionals because of concerning behaviors or performance, after which target variables are selected; and target variables may be selected in advance by schools, with measures then used for screening and decision making. Target variables organized by RTI enable progress monitoring at various levels to address specific questions: at the school (what's working, what isn't); classroom (more or less teacher support, quality of instruction); and for students (change intervention or tier, quality of needed interventions and supports). Technical adequacy was stressed as a way to improve the validity and reliability of the decision-making process. The basic reason for technical adequacy is to get a "handle" on the overall confidence that teams can have in a complex process of decision making.

References

Ardoin, S. P., & Christ, T. J. (2008). Evaluating curriculum-based measurement slope estimates using data from tri-annual universal screenings. *School Psychology Review, 37,* 109–125.

Ardoin, S. P., Witt, J. C., Suldo, S. M., Connell, J. E., Koenig, J. L., Resetar, J. L., et al. (2004). Examining the incremental benefits of administering a maze and three versus one curriculum-based measurement reading probes when conducting universal screening. *School Psychology Review, 33,* 218–233.

Barnett, D. W., Bauer, A., Ehrhardt, K., Lentz, F. E., & Stollar, S. (1997). Keystone targets for change: Planning for widespread positive consequences. *School Psychology Quarterly, 11,* 95–117.

Barnett, D. W., Hawkins, R. O., Prasse, D., Macmann, G., Graden, J. L., Nantais, M., et al. (2007). Decision making validity in response to intervention. In S. Jimerson, M. Burns, & A. VanDerHeyden (Eds.), *The handbook of response to intervention: The science and practice of assessment and intervention* (pp. 106–116). New York: Springer Science.

Batsche, G., Elliott, J., Graden, J. L., Grimes, J., Kovaleski, J. F., Prasse, D., et al. (2005). *Response to intervention: Policy considerations and implementation.* Alexandria, VA: National Association of State Directors of Special Education.

Bell, S. H., & Barnett, D. W. (1999). Peer micronorms in the assessment of young children: Methodological reviews and examples. *Topics in Early Childhood Special Education, 19,* 112–122.

Compton, D. L., Fuchs, D., Fuchs, L. S., & Bryant, J. D. (2006). Selecting at-risk readers in first grade for early intervention: A two-year longitudinal study of decision rules and procedures. *Journal of Educational Psychology, 98,* 394–409.

Cooper, J. O., Heron, T. E., & Heward, W. L. (2007). *Applied behavior analysis* (2nd ed.). Upper Saddle River, NJ: Pearson.

Daly, E. J., Martens, B. K., Barnett, D. W., Witt, J. C., & Olson, S. C. (2007). Varying intervention delivery in response to intervention: Confronting and resolving challenges with measurement, instruction, and intensity. *School Psychology Review, 36,* 562–581.

Deno, S. L., Marston, D., & Tindal, G. (1985–1986). Direct and frequent curriculum-based measurement: An alternative for educational decision making. *Special Services in the Schools, 2,* 5–27.

Feinberg, A. B., & Shapiro, E. S. (2003). Accuracy of teacher judgments in predicting oral reading fluency. *School Psychology Quarterly, 18,* 52–65.

Fuchs, L. S., & Fuchs, D. (1986). Effects of systematic formative evaluation: A meta-analysis. *Exceptional Children, 53,* 199–208.

Fuchs, L. S., & Fuchs, D. (2007). A model for implementing responsiveness to intervention. *Teaching Exceptional Children, 39,* 14–20.

Glover, T. A., & Albers, C. A. (2007). Considerations for evaluating universal screening assessments. *Journal of School Psychology, 45,* 117–135.

Good, R. H., Gruba, J., & Kaminski, R. A. (2002). Best practices in using dynamic indicators of basic early literacy skills (DIBELS) in an outcomes-driven model. In A. Thomas & J. Grimes (Eds.), *Best practices in school psychology* (4th ed., pp. 699–720). Bethesda, MD: National Association of School Psychologists.

Good, R. H., Wallin, J. U., Simmons, D. C., Kame'enui, E. J., & Kaminski, R. A. (2002). *System-wide percentile ranks for DIBELS benchmark assessment* (Technical Report No. 9). Eugene, OR: University of Oregon.

Greenwood, C. R. (1991). A longitudinal analysis of time, engagement, and achievement in at-risk versus non-risk students. *Exceptional Children, 57,* 521–535.

Gresham, F. M. (2007). Evolution of the response-to-intervention concept: Empirical foundations and recent developments. In S. Jimerson, M. Burns, & A. VanDerHeyden (Eds.), *The handbook of response to intervention: The science and practice of assessment and intervention* (pp. 10–24). New York: Springer Science.

Gresham, F. M., Reschly, D. J., & Carey, M. (1987). Teachers as "tests": Classification accuracy and concurrent validation in the identification of learning disabled children. *School Psychology Review, 16,* 543–563.

Gresham, F. M., Watson, T. S., & Skinner, C. H. (2001). Functional behavioral assessment: Principles, procedures, and future directions. *School Psychology Review, 30,* 156–172.

Habedank, L. (1995). Best practices in developing local norms for problem solving in the schools. In A. Thomas & J. Grimes (Eds.), *Best practice in school psychology* (3rd ed., pp. 701–715). Washington, DC: National Association of School Psychologists.

Hawkins, R. P. (1986). Selection of target behaviors. In R. O. Nelson & S. C. Hayes (Eds.), *Conceptual foundations of behavioral assessment* (pp. 331–385). New York: Guilford Press.

Hawkins, R. P., & Dobes, R. W. (1975). Behavioral definitions in applied behavior analysis: Explicit or implicit. In B. C. Etzel, J. M. LeBlanc, & D. M. Baer (Eds.), *New developments in behavioral research: Theory, methods, and applications. In honor of Sidney W. Bijou* (pp. 167–188). Hillsdale, NJ: Erlbaum.

Heller, K. A., Holtzman, W. H., & Messick, S. (Eds.). (1982). *Placing children in special education: A strategy for equity.* Washington, DC: National Academy Press.

Horner, R. (1994). Functional assessment contributions and future directions. *Journal of Applied Behavior Analysis, 27,* 401–404.

Hosp, J. L., & Reschly, D. J. (2004). Disproportionate representation of minority students in special education: Academic, demographic, and economic predictors. *Exceptional Children, 70,* 185–199.

Kame'enui, E. J., Good, R. H., III, & Harn, B. A. (2005). Beginning reading failure and the quantification of risk: Reading behavior as the supreme index. In W. L. Heward, T. E. Heron, N. E. Neef, S. M. Peterson, D. M. Sainato, G. Cartledge, et al. (Eds.), *Focus on behavioral analysis in education: Achievements, challenges, and opportunities* (pp. 68–88). Upper Saddle River, NJ: Pearson.

Kanfer, F. H. (1985). Target selection for clinical change programs. *Behavioral Assessment, 7,* 7–20.

Kazdin, A. E. (1985). Selection of target behaviors: The relationship of treatment focus to clinical dysfunction. *Behavioral Assessment, 7,* 33–47.

Kennedy, C. H. (2005). *Single-case designs for educational research.* Boston: Allyn & Bacon.

Kratochwill, T. R. (1985). Selection of target behaviors in behavioral consultation. *Behavioral Assessment, 7,* 49–61.

Kratochwill, T. R., & Bergin, J. R. (1990). *Behavioral consultation in applied settings: An individual guide.* New York: Plenum.

Macmann, G. M., & Barnett, D. W. (1999). Diagnostic decision making in school psychology: Understanding and coping with uncertainty. In C. R. Reynolds & T. B. Gutkin (Eds.), *Handbook of school psychology* (3rd ed., pp. 519–548). New York: Wiley.

Macmann, G. M., Barnett, D. W., Allen, S. J., Bramlett, R. K., Hall, J. D., & Ehrhardt, K. E. (1996). Problem solving and intervention design: Guidelines for the evaluation of technical adequacy. *School Psychology Quarterly, 11,* 137–148.

Meehl, P. E., & Rosen, A. (1955). Antecedent probability and the efficiency of psychometric signs, patterns, or cutting scores. *Psychological Bulletin, 52,* 194–215.

Newell, M., & Kratochwill, T. R. (2007). The integration of response to intervention and critical race theory-disability studies: A robust approach to reducing racial discrimina-

tion in evaluation decisions. In S. Jimerson, M. Burns, & A. VanDerHeyden (Eds.), *The handbook of response to intervention: The science and practice of assessment and intervention* (pp. 65–79). New York: Springer Science.

Shapiro, E. S. (2004). *Academic skills problems: Direct assessment and intervention* (3rd ed.). New York: Guilford Press.

Shinn, M. R., Walker, H. M., & Stoner, G. (Eds.). (2002). *Interventions for academic and behavior problems: II. Preventive and remedial approaches.* Washington DC: National Association of School Psychologists.

Skiba, R. J., Simmons, A. B., Ritter, S., Gibb, A. C., Rausch, M. K., Cuadrado, J., et al. (2008). Achieving equity in special education: History, status, and current challenges. *Exceptional Children, 74,* 264–288.

Sugai, G., Horner, R. H., & Gresham, F. M. (2002). Behaviorally effective school environments. In M. Shinn, H. Walker, & G. Stoner (Eds.), *Interventions for academic and behavior problems: II. Preventive and remedial approaches* (pp. 315–350). Bethesda, MD: National Association of School Psychologists.

VanDerHeyden, A. M., & Witt, J. C. (2005). Quantifying context in assessment: Capturing the effect of base rates on teacher referral and a problem-solving model for identification. *School Psychology Review, 34*(2), 161–183.

VanDerHeyden, A. M., Witt, J. C., & Gilbertson, D. (2007). A multi-year evaluation of the effects of a response to intervention (RTI) model on identification of children for special education. *Journal of School Psychology, 45,* 225–256.

VanDerHeyden, A. M., Witt, J. C., & Naquin, G. (2003). Development and validation of a process for screening referrals to special education. *School Psychology Review, 32,* 204–227.

Vaughn, S., Wanzek, J., Woodruff, A. L., & Linan-Thompson, S. (2007). Prevention and early identification of students with reading disabilities. In D. Haagar, J. Klingner, & S. Vaughn (Eds.), *Evidence-based reading practices for response to intervention* (pp. 11–27). Baltimore: Brookes.

Watson, T. S., & Steege, M. W. (2003) *Conducting school-based functional behavior assessments: A practitioner's guide.* New York: Guilford Press.

Wilson, F. E., & Evans, I. A. (1983). The reliability of target-behavior selection in behavioral assessment. *Behavioral Assessment, 5,* 15–32.

Wolf, M. M. (1978). Social validity: The case for subjective measurement, or how applied behavior analysis is finding its heart. *Journal of Applied Behavior Analysis, 11,* 203–214.

PART II

ASSESSMENT AND ANALYSIS
Focus on Academic Outcomes

Chapter 3

Analysis of Universal Academic Data to Plan, Implement, and Evaluate Schoolwide Improvement

Amanda M. VanDerHeyden

Scientific findings and keystone legislative events have created a climate in which students' learning outcomes are increasingly attended to, evaluated, and prioritized in public education. This movement toward accountability is an exciting development for researchers, practitioners, and consumers who care deeply about the consequences of their professional actions on children (Messick, 1995). Although such an idea may seem self-evident or intuitive in public education, the idea of examining the consequences of educational services for children is rather radical (Macmann & Barnett, 1999). There has been tremendous debate about how best to bring scientific findings to bear on educational practices (Feuer, Towne, & Shavelson, 2002; Odom et al., 2005). Schools are now demanding that research findings deliver pragmatic information about how to implement practices that produce measurable and meaningful outcomes.

The School Psychologist as Change Agent

In this context, data-driven practices in education have become highly sought after by schools. School systems are becoming savvy data consumers, and school psychologists

are experiencing a changing role first forecast by Deno (1986) and by Lentz and Shapiro (1986) and recently codified through practice guidelines (see Volume 33 of *School Psychology Review*; Dawson et al., 2004; Kratochwill & Shernoff, 2004; Thomas & Grimes, 2008). A cornerstone of current best practices in school psychology is data-based decision making within response-to-intervention service (RTI) models (Hojnoski & Missall, 2006). School psychologists have an opportunity to serve as data and decision-making consultants for schools and school systems.

The school psychologist and special education team at a site are well situated to serve in the role of data consultants. Someone must serve in this role, or the system is likely to overassess and underintervene. Given that all time spent in assessment is time lost to instruction, systems must emphasize efficiency in assessment—seeking to attain the most relevant information in the shortest possible period of time toward the greatest end for the greatest number (Shinn & Bamonto, 1998). Consultants acting as system change agents must recognize that resources are finite and therefore work to guide decision makers to maximize resources and outcomes (VanDerHeyden & Witt, 2007). The effective consultant is one who can deliver results for a system. In the following section, a model is described for using universal academic data to identify system targets and to implement change strategies to enhance system outcomes.

Focus on Academic Outcomes

Although students may gain many important skills throughout their schooling experience (e.g., social development, peer relationships, communication, and personal organization skills), teachers, parents, and students can generally embrace the idea that the primary purpose of academic instruction is student learning. If instruction is intended to meaningfully accelerate learning and to help students build an adaptive and useful skill set and knowledge base, then evaluating the degree to which that goal is being met requires a focus on academic outcomes. Persuasive arguments for focusing on key academic outcomes can be found in recent policy statements, including the National Reading Panel Report (National Institute of Child Health and Human Development, 2000) and the National Mathematics Advisory Panel Report (U.S. Department of Education, 2008). Key skills have been identified that should emerge at particular stages of instruction to forecast continued growth toward functional skill competence for students. These skills and their expected time of development provide benchmarks against which child learning can be evaluated to ensure that instruction is advancing child mastery of fundamental skills and concepts and is doing so at the right pace. Child learning outcomes can be evaluated in two ways: (1) Static performance can be evaluated relative to established expectations for performance at that point in the program of instruction, and (2) the learning trajectory can be evaluated relative to the trajectory that is needed to reach key benchmarks over time or relative to trajectories of students who are not at risk for poor learning outcomes.

Critical skills are skills that are generative, meaning that if they are mastered child functioning is improved in a robust way across a variety of contexts (Slentz & Hyatt, 2008). Early reading skills, including the ability to identify and manipulate phonemes

(sounds) to decode words and ultimately to fluently read words and connected text, are essential to deriving meaning from what is read. The ability to independently comprehend printed material provides the foundation for students to read for information as schooling progresses and facilitates learning of content in topical areas such as history or science. Hence phonemic awareness is an example of a critical outcome of early literacy instruction that should be monitored to ensure that instruction successfully establishes that outcome. Once a child can read text, fluent reading of grade-level text and comprehension are functional and generative outcomes that can be assessed at regular intervals to ensure that students are on track to attain the goals of reading instruction. In the area of mathematics, a logical sequence of computational skills can be identified that reflects functional and generative learning outcomes of early mathematics instruction (e.g., addition, subtraction, and multiplication facts and procedures). These skills are generative skills because a child's ability to fluently handle multiplication with regrouping will be highly related to the child's ability to master skills that will be introduced later in the program of instruction, such as converting fractions or computing percentages. Further, a child's ability to fluently complete multiplication problems enhances the child's ability to benefit from instruction that will take place in mathematics in the future to establish understanding of mathematical concepts such as factors. Hence computational skills offer logical targets for evaluating learning outcomes in mathematics (see Burns & Klingbeil, Chapter 6, this volume, for more on this issue).

States have established performance standards for learning to guide instructional efforts. These performance standards can be accessed online via state department of education websites. For many schools and districts, the performance standards offer a logical way to identify key learning outcomes across grade levels that can be monitored to ensure that instruction is reaching the intended goal of accelerating student learning and building useful skill sets for the future (e.g., see *www.ade.az.gov/standards/*). Use of early and regular universal screening can prevent the occurrence of more complex and intractable learning problems later in the schooling process (Torgesen, 2002). Schooling may be compared to running a marathon. Early in the schooling process there seems to be such a long way to go and such a lot of time to get there that a slow pace may not seem particularly problematic or alarming. As such, it may be easy to fall behind. Runners who fall only slightly behind on each mile during the first half of a marathon will find themselves having to attain impossible paces in the later miles to meet their end goal. Similarly, instruction builds across the years of schooling, and failing to meet expected learning outcome goals and to grow at the expected pace signals the need for intervention early, before the deficits accumulate and create insurmountable obstacles to the final goal.

In the next section, a model for using data to accelerate learning outcomes systemwide is presented. The first part of the model involves examining schoolwide or systemwide data. The second stage involves selecting and implementing interventions. The third stage is evaluating the change effort(s). The final stage is engaging in results-driven revisions or iterations to ensure that the desired outcomes maintain over time.

Obtaining and Examining Universal Screening Data

The purpose of screening is to provide information to identify areas of needed instruction and direct instructional efforts in multitiered intervention models so as to meet the needs of all students. As discussed in detail by Hawkins, Barnett, Morrison, and Musti-Rao in Chapter 2, this volume, generally multitiered intervention models describe three tiers of service delivery. Tier 1 refers to assessment and instructional activities directed to all students. Tier 1 is sometimes referred to as core instruction because it is the instruction that all students experience. Tier 2 refers to assessment and instructional activities directed to a subset of students who are not responding successfully to Tier 1 instruction. Tier 2 activities are distinguished from Tier 1 in that instruction is more intense and assessment is more frequent and in that these services are generally delivered in small-group settings as a supplement to Tier 1 instruction. Tier 3 refers to assessment and intervention activities directed to the small

number of students who do not respond successfully to Tier 1 and Tier 2 instruction. Generally, Tier 3 activities are conducted individually and tailored to the individual student's needs; they represent the most intensive level of intervention support available in the school setting. Screening is an opportunity to introduce student learning as the arbiter of instructional efforts, to engage teams to seek answers to questions that will help them know how best to help students learn, and to initiate (or maintain) a focus on the variables of effective instruction that can be altered to improve student learning outcomes (Gettinger & Seibert, 2002).

Step 1: Select a Valid Screening Measure

Screening measures must be (1) matched to performance expectations in the classroom at that point in the program of instruction and (2) of appropriate difficulty to allow accurate identification of the individual students who are at particular risk for learning difficulties relative to their peers. In my experience (VanDerHeyden & Witt, 2005), effective screening cannot be accomplished with a single screening measure if there are pervasive learning problems in the system. Hence, the first step is to select measures that reflect what students ought to be able to do at that point in the program of instruction. Examining state-specified performance standards and talking with teachers about the ongoing program of instruction is an efficient way to identify skills that students are expected to have mastered at that point in the instructional program. Use of this single measure will be sufficient to reach a screening decision if the students' scores are normally distributed (i.e., if there is not a classwide learning problem). So, for example, in the winter of first grade, a teacher may explain that, although mathematics instruction has focused on a broad array of concepts such as measurement, time, and money, children are expected to have mastered rapid computation of sums to 10 in order to best benefit from mathematics instruction that will follow (e.g., sums to 20, subtraction, fact-family tasks, solving measurement problems that involve addition computations). If the median score for the class is above criterion on a sums-to-10 probe, then the lowest performing students can be readily identified as needing further assessment and potentially intervention to enhance mathematics learning.

The intervention/RTI team (data consultant, principal, grade-level teachers) should examine performance standards for each grade level by topic area (reading, math, and language arts). The role of the data consultant is to guide the team in selecting screening measures from a bank of available measures that are well matched to key performance standards at that time in the year. These data will allow the team to identify where student performance does not meet expectations (defining a learning problem), and the team can then set about developing the most efficient solution to resolve that learning problem. Some teachers may voice concern that their students will not be able to successfully perform the task even though it reflects expected learning at that point in the year. Whereas some teams may be tempted to select an easier task, leaders in the change process (e.g., the principal, grade-level team leader, data consultant) should guide the team to select the screening measures that will answer the questions that allow the team to get the students back on track. These questions include "What is expected of students currently?" and "Are most students able to perform the skill that is currently expected?" Asking these two questions allows the team to identify whether intervention efforts could most efficiently occur at Tier 1 (targeting all students), Tier 2 (targeting small groups of students who are not performing as expected), or Tier 3 (targeting individual students who are not performing as expected). Whereas an easier screening task might better identify individual children who are most at risk relative to their peers, it can also cause the team to incorrectly conclude that the majority of students are not at risk for negative learning outcomes. Thus the first screening task should be a skill that reflects expected performance for children at that grade level at that point in the instructional program.

With the emphasis on data-based decision making in RTI, quantifying the accuracy of decisions about student progress and response to interventions for screening tasks is very important. Estimates such as sensitivity, specificity, positive predictive power, and negative predictive power are being examined by teams in their quest to identify screening tasks that are valid for RTI decision making. Sensitivity and specificity refer to the power of the test to detect true positives and negatives, respectively.[1] In the case of screening decisions to reach RTI judgments, true positives would be students who are predicted to fail without intervention who actually did fail. True negatives would be students who are predicted to not fail without intervention and who did not fail. Positive predictive power is the probability that a positive screening decision (e.g., a failed screening) correctly signified failing the year-end accountability measure. Negative predictive power is the probability that a negative screening decision (i.e., a passed screening) correctly signified passing the year-end accountability measure.[2] Indeed, quantifying predictive power estimates such as sensitivity, specificity, and positive and negative predictive power is essential to understanding the effect cut scores have on the accuracy of screening decisions. A cut score is a score used for decision-making purposes. Scores above the cut score lead to a different decision than do scores below a cut score. For example, if a cut score of 105 correctly read words per minute is used to determine who receives supplemental assistance, students with scores at or above 105 will not receive services, whereas students with scores below 105 will receive services. The screening tool will be used to make a dichotomous judgment that a student is or is not at risk (i.e., fails or passes the screening). A criterion can be identified that is meaningful to the system, such as meeting or not meeting the proficiency criterion on the state year-end accountability measure. The accuracy of the decisions made based on the screening task can be quantified by computing percentage match with the criterion and sensitivity, specificity, and positive and negative predictive power. The screening task must be well matched to performance expectations in the classroom *and* the resulting distribution must be evaluated prior to reaching conclusions about which students need intervention. A screening task that is well matched to performance expectations and that yields a normal distribution of scores ensures the meaning of predictive power estimates in characterizing the value of a screening tool.

Step 2: Specify Comparison Criteria

The school-level team overseeing screening should compare the general performance of the class or grade with some level of performance that reflects the desired outcome or learning goal. Two approaches to establishing an external criterion are possible. In the first approach, districts or schools can use their own data to establish a criterion that is related to an outcome that is meaningful to their system. Using local curriculum-based measurement (CBM) and year-end accountability scores, a statistical analysis can be performed to identify a score that is associated with a high probability of passing the year-end accountability measure. For example, by investigating the relationship between screening results and state proficiency test scores, district personnel may find that 99% of children who read 105 words correctly per minute in a fourth-grade-level passage actually passed the high-stakes test of reading in the spring. District personnel might then establish a criterion of 105 words read correctly (WRC) per minute as the criterion against which student performances will be compared at screening. Thus any child who reads fewer than 105 words correctly per minute at screening is considered to be in need of some type of intervention in reading.

The second approach to establishing an external performance criterion is to adopt one that has been reported in the literature. For example, the frustrational, instructional, and mastery criteria set forth by Deno and Mirkin (1977) and replicated more recently (Burns, VanDerHeyden, & Jiban, 2006; Deno, Fuchs, Marston, & Shin, 2001; Fuchs, Fuchs, Hamlett, Walz, & Germann, 1993) may be used to evaluate whether the class is on track for successful learning in that classroom without an instructional change.

Step 3: Interpret Screening Data

Recall that resulting screening data will be used to identify the need for wide-scale intervention (at Tier 1 or 2) and then to identify which students are in need of individualized intervention at Tier 3. Hence the screening data are being used to make two judgments: whether or not the performance of most students in a class, grade, and school are meeting expected learning standards and which individual students are in need of intervention. To reach valid conclusions, the screening task must reflect the learning goals that are expected in the classroom and be of approximate difficulty to result in an approximately normal distribution of scores. Use of a single screening task to accomplish both decisions is sometimes possible (e.g., when most students are thriving and meeting learning expectations). Sometimes, however, screening decisions will need to be made in stages. Consider the following case example.

The graph that appears in Figure 3.1 shows the performance of a fourth-grade class on multiplication facts 0–9 administered during the fall schoolwide screening. All of the students performing in the lower shaded area of the figure (below 40 digits correct per 2 minutes) are performing in the frustrational range (Deno & Mirkin, 1977), indicating that many children in this class are at risk for poor learning outcomes in mathematics without intervention. Multiplication facts 0–9 is a foundational skill that students should have mastered before leaving third grade (Shapiro, 2004). If students cannot fluently multiply basic facts, then they are likely to make errors and fail to master more complex but related skills (e.g., multidigit multiplication with regrouping, solving word problems that require multiplication, multiplication of decimals, finding the least common denominator). Because the median score falls in the frustrational range, this class can be characterized as needing supplemental instruction to improve math computation. Further, poor classwide performance with computational fluency tasks may signal that other learning deficits (e.g., fluent performance of other computation tasks, understanding of related mathematics concepts) are present in mathematics. Gradewide performance should be examined next.

The graph in Figure 3.2 shows the performance of all students in the fourth grade on the multiplication facts 0–9 probe administered during the fall screening. Only six students in the entire grade are performing in the mastery range (Deno & Mirkin, 1977), and the majority of students are performing in the frustrational range, with fewer than 40 digits correct per 2 minutes (Deno &

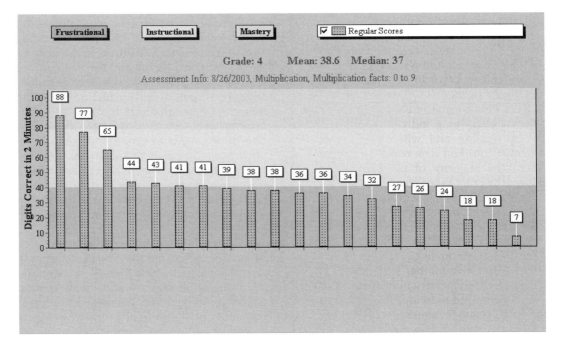

FIGURE 3.1. Universal screening data indicate that this class has a classwide learning problem in mathematics.

Mirkin, 1977). These data should serve as an urgent signal that supplemental instruction is needed throughout the entire grade level. Grade-level data for all grades should next be examined to determine when the deficits first appear and whether they continue across all subsequent grades.

Recall that the first comparison is a comparison of student performance with some external criterion that reflects the intended learning outcome (the right skill at the right level of performance). If many children in a class are performing in the risk range, then additional data (i.e., classwide intervention data or assessment on an easier, prerequisite task) will be required before the second type of comparison may be made. The second comparison is a normative comparison in which student performance is compared with that of others within a class, grade, or district to determine who is most at risk academically in a classroom, grade, or district. Classes in which many children perform below expectations for learning will produce

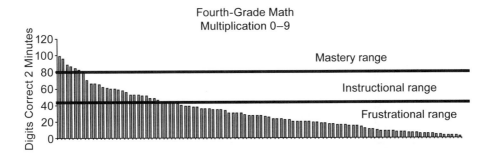

FIGURE 3.2. Universal screening data indicate that multiple classwide learning problems are present in mathematics at fourth grade. In this fourth grade, there is a gradewide learning problem in mathematics.

a positively skewed dataset (in which most of the student scores occur in the low end of the score range). Accurate discrimination of individual children's learning problems is difficult in cases in which the dataset is positively skewed (VanDerHeyden & Witt, 2005). This normative comparison is important in identifying individual children who are struggling and who require intensive intervention, and it is readily accomplished when the majority of the class scores fall above the external criterion at screening but below a ceiling (i.e., a score at which learning improvements or higher scores cannot be detected) for the measure. In cases in which the class median score, for example, exceeds the external criterion (e.g., instructional criterion), normative comparisons may be undertaken to identify particular children in need of intensive and individualized intervention. When the class median score falls below that external criterion, however, additional data will be needed (e.g., classwide intervention data) to identify individual students who are most at risk. When many children perform below expectations, it is logical and most effective to address the learning problem through Tier 1 or 2 intervention strategies and to use the resulting trend data or follow-up screening data to evaluate (1) the degree to which the classwide learning problem has been repaired and (2) which children have not responded successfully and require additional assessment and/or intervention (Fuchs & Fuchs, 1998; VanDerHeyden & Witt, 2005).

Following classwide or gradewide intervention, the screening may simply be repeated to determine whether the planned intervention is having the desired effect on the

intervention target. In this case, a follow-up probe of multiplication facts 0–9 indicated that most students performed in the instructional or mastery range following only a few weeks of supplemental intervention. Results are displayed in Figure 3.3. Follow-up probes of more challenging computation or applied skills that students are expected to master can be administered to ensure that adequate progress continues to be made and that learning that occurs during intervention is followed by adequate learning of more challenging skills as instruction progresses (e.g., decimal work with multiplication after students have been instructed in decimals in multiplication). Further, each class may be examined to ensure that adequate growth is occurring on targeted skills, as in Figure 3.4. Efficient assessment can be planned to ensure that modifications made to Tier 1 or to the core instructional program in mathematics is having the desired effect on learning in mathematics and reading.

As another example, consider the case of a first-grade classroom for which a classwide reading assessment was conducted. The top graph in Figure 3.5 shows the performances of all students in the class at screening, reflected as WRC per minute on a first-grade passage selected by the first-grade team of teachers from a bank of standard reading passages. The second panel shows the performances of the same students following several weeks of classwide peer tutoring reflected as WRC per minute (intervention protocol available at www.gosbr.net). Each assessment occasion used a probe or passage on which students had not been instructed, and all data contained in the graphs were collected by the school psychologist and

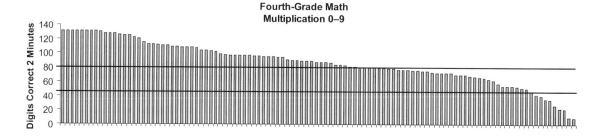

FIGURE 3.3. Gradewide performance on the screening probe following systematic classwide intervention in all fourth-grade classrooms.

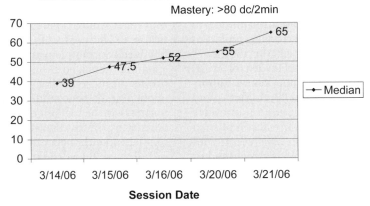

FIGURE 3.4. Growth during classwide intervention for mathematics on a single skill.

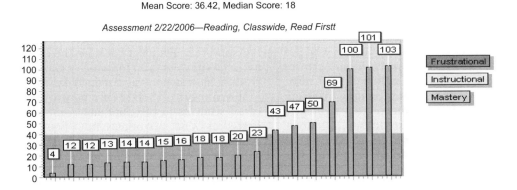

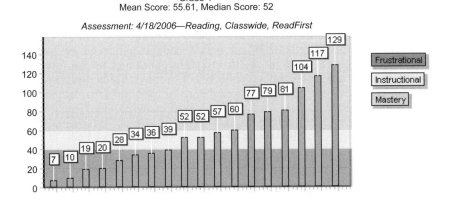

FIGURE 3.5. The top panel of the figure shows performance of a first-grade class during screening in reading. The bottom panel shows performance of the same class following 2 weeks of classwide reading intervention.

teacher. The median score increased from 18 to 56 WRC per minute. These data indicated that most children rapidly responded to the intervention. They also made apparent which students were in need of additional intervention at Tier 2, which involved 30 minutes of daily, small-group instruction by the reading resource teacher.

As the team works together to interpret the screening data for every child, the data consultant can highlight how the data obtained during such a screening are linked to variables of effective instruction that could be modified intentionally. For example, the consultant can point out that students began the school year with deficient skills while noting that without some supplemental instruction they are unlikely to catch up *and* master all the new skills that must be introduced during the school year. For example, the consultant might say, "Given routine instruction, most children will gain about 1.5 words correct per minute per week of instruction. On average, the students in your class need to gain about 2.3 words correct per minute per week to catch up by the end of the year. Hence, these students will need supplemental instruction to catch up." The variables of effective instructional pacing of new content or skills, review of old skills to ensure maintenance, and ensuring adequate instructional time to master key skills are not likely to be new concepts to teachers, but this grade-level team meeting is an opportunity to emphasize how such activities are the most important responsibilities of the teacher that, if consistently attended to, will produce strong learning outcomes over time.

When screening data are collected and evaluated, intervention planning may begin. Up to this point, the data consultant, principal, and other members of the school's RTI team have worked together to (1) introduce data-based problem solving to grade-level teams, (2) specify learning goals for grades tied to the performance standards, and (3) organize screening data that will serve as baseline data for the school. Because the data consultant, principal, and other members of the team have worked together with teachers to select and administer the screening task and score the screening data, the basis for future decisions is transparent to teachers, and the process should be gaining

some credibility and momentum. A critical function of the data consultant is to rapidly move the school through screening to intervention. The goal is to obtain intervention results as quickly as possible, because teachers and others who are being asked to engage in the problem-solving efforts will be wary of the change process until they begin to see results. Following screening, the data consultant should distribute graphs to teachers with direct feedback, organize the screening data, and present them to the principal and other members of the school's RTI team with suggested targets for intervention.

Step 4: Organize and Present Screening Data

The data consultant should prepare grade-level graphs of student performance relative to a meaningful external criterion or benchmark. The consultant should be prepared to present typical growth rates in a given skill relative to the growth that students at his or her school will have to make to attain expected performance outcomes. He or she should be prepared to present student data by gender, race, poverty, and language status. Generally, the best approach is to provide grade-level performance graphs, followed by median scores (i.e., middle score) for each teacher's class, followed by individual-child graphs in key topic areas (e.g., reading and math). As these data are presented, the data consultant should highlight areas in which many children are performing below expectations and stimulate discussion about how intervention can most efficiently be provided to those students (e.g., via Tier 1 or Tier 2 efforts). Patterns should be described for the team. For example, are performance problems clustered by topic area, by grade level, or by student demographics? If so, a pattern exists. Figure 3.6 provides an example of a troubleshooting list that a team might use to organize data to identify causes of systemic problems and to plan actions to resolve and prevent those problems.

If, for example, class median scores on the reading screening are below the external criterion for performance only at grade 1 in the fall and never at the higher grades in consecutive years, then this finding may indicate that Tier 1 reading instruction is functioning well at the school. If students in one teacher's class are performing much

Gradewide problem?

If yes:	Actions to resolve current problem	Examine patterns	Actions to prevent recurrence
	• Check curriculum • Calendar of instruction (are all skills introduced with sufficient time for mastery? are mastered skills adequately reviewed?) • Mastery of prerequisite skills • Increase progress monitoring with weekly graphed feedback to teachers • Check instructional basics (e.g., student engagement, materials of appropriate difficulty, frequency of feedback, adequate explanation of new skills with feedback matched to skill proficiency) during core instruction	• Is it isolated to one grade or pervasive? • Affecting students disproportionately by demographics (e.g., SES, language status, gender)? • Related to flexible grouping or inadvertent tracking? • Deficient skills from previous year?	• How can students be identified earlier (what predictors discriminated those who would perform below criterion at this grade level)? • Can supplemental intervention be efficiently provided to all or to subgroups of students in the preceding year or semester to prevent future deficit? • Does the calendar of instruction need revision? Should more instructional time be allocated to this skill in the preceding or current year? • Are the instructional materials and program of instruction adequate, or can they be modified or changed to maximize results? • Professional development activities to facilitate active student engagement, increase instructional time. • Maintain more frequent progress monitoring to ensure that the solution continues to be implemented consistently and to detect recurrence earlier. • Restructure planning periods to function as data-based problem-solving teams and mentor school- and grade-level leadership.

If no:	Consider classwide problem		

Classwide problem?

If yes:	Actions to resolve current problem	Examine patterns	Actions to prevent recurrence
	• Check adherence to curriculum • Check adherence to calendar of instruction (are all skills introduced with sufficient time for mastery? are mastered skills adequately reviewed?) • Mastery of prerequisite skills • Increase progress monitoring with weekly graphed feedback to teachers • Check instructional basics during core instruction • Provide classwide intervention that is protocol based and monitored for integrity until student learning improves to benchmark performance.	• Characteristics of the teacher or teaching environment (first-year teacher, teacher out sick) • Is it isolated to one class or are there multiple classes in the school (if multiple classes, what common features)? • Affecting students disproportionately by demographics (e.g., SES, language status, gender)? • Related to flexible grouping or inadvertent tracking? • Deficient skills from previous year?	• More frequent monitoring • If problem is unique to first-year teachers, increase support and coaching to first-year teachers. Integrate personnel review with student outcome data collection and intervention or instruction integrity checks. • If many teachers show weak instructional basics, gear professional development activities to remediate with prescriptive actions that are monitored for implementation integrity. Consider schoolwide positive behavior support program. • Continue increased progress monitoring for the class to detect recurrence of the problem more quickly and evaluate ongoing implementation. • Ensure adequate resources allocated to instruction in problem classrooms. • Restructure planning periods to function as data-based problem-solving teams and mentor grade-level leadership.

If no:	Consider small-group and individual interventions.		

FIGURE 3.6. Checklist to summarize and prioritize targets. See VanDerHeyden and Burns (2005) for an overview of characteristics of instruction relevant to enhancing learning outcomes for all students.

lower than students in other teachers' classes at a particular grade level, then the team should troubleshoot why that may be the case (e.g., students are deliberately grouped by ability level; teacher could benefit from support or additional resources) and identify actions that can help students improve in that class (e.g., ensure that tracked students in a low-performing group are getting supplemental, sustained instruction that accelerates their learning relative to typically developing peers; provide teacher with an onsite mentor or coach for math instruction). Critically, the outcome of this meeting is an action plan. Ideally, a single person on the team takes responsibility for drafting the action plan and pulling together needed materials and resources to implement the action plan. The data consultant may be the most logical choice for this role. As the meeting concludes, the data consultant should summarize potential targets, describe costs of proposed solutions, and ask the team to prioritize the targets.

The data consultant now must organize the school's intervention plan, specifying what intervention will be implemented with which students and what data will be collected to know whether that intervention is working. Where problems were detected, more frequent progress monitoring must be part of the corrective plan. The data consultant should list existing resources that can be used for intervention. If students are being identified for supplemental intervention provided by the school (e.g., tutoring, special reading instruction), the screening data can now be considered as the basis for selecting which students should receive specialized interventions. The data consultant or other members of the school's RTI team should meet with grade-level teams of teachers with a working plan and brainstorm ways to deliver intervention to children who performed poorly during the screening. Often the morning period during which organizational routines are completed for the school day (e.g., roll is taken, lunch money is collected, homework is turned in), student free time, and flexible grouping provide opportunities to shift additional instruction to students who need it. Individual peer tutoring and classwide peer tutoring are highly efficient ways to bring additional intervention into the classroom. Computer resources are available and can be very helpful to students who are struggling in core content areas according to the screening data (e.g., Headsprout early reading program: *www.headsprout.com/*; Accelerated Math: *www.renlearn.com/am/*). Finally, the school may provide tutoring services or other specialized reading interventions that can be refined to enhance their effectiveness and more effectively target at-risk students (see Linan-Thompson, Chapter 16, this volume).

Step 5: Plan for Implementation

Guiding principles of effective implementation include (1) recognizing the role of the principal as the instructional leader of the school, (2) ensuring that the intervention plan reflects the identified problem *and* the priorities of the system or school, (3) ensuring that the plan set forth is one that will be effective if properly implemented, (4) ensuring that an agreed-upon progress monitoring system has been identified to evaluate the effects of the intervention, and (5) ensuring that a single person has been identified to manage day-to-day logistics of implementation. The person selected to manage the logistics of implementation should be someone who has complete access to the lead decision maker in the school (the principal) and who has the time, resources, and skills to troubleshoot implementation on a continuous basis. Because no plan can be perfect, it is sensible to start on a small scale and expand once those responsible for implementation are fluent with all necessary tasks (Neef, 1995).

• *The principal is the lead change agent as the instructional leader of the school.* Intervention and instruction plans are futile without principal support. If one thinks of the change effort as software being installed onto an operating system, one can imagine that for some operating systems the change effort will be nearly seamless. Other systems, however, might require substantial patching, patience, rebooting, and near constant follow-up to ensure that a change effort gets off—and stays off—the ground. Failure to attend to minor problems can lead to major derailment and system failure. Key to implementing an effective system intervention is principal leadership. The principal must be willing to stand before the faculty and endorse the effort, to provide a rationale for the intervention or interventions, and to describe which data will be collected and attended to for what purpose. It is important that once a rationale for the effort has been provided, teachers understand as specifically as possible what actions will be required of them and when implementation will begin. Most critically, the principal should indicate that outcome data will be tracked and should provide the specifics of how this will be done, what success will look like, and what failure will look like. The principal should also indicate that implementation accuracy will be monitored to ensure that the best effort at implementation has been given. Most critically, the principal must provide sufficient resources and time for intervention to occur and must attend to two types of data: student learning and implementation integrity data.

The data consultant must hand the RTI team the data that are needed to reach the decisions that move the system forward toward the desired outcomes. Periodically, the principal or other members of the RTI team should stand before the faculty and present student learning outcome data and implementation data and actively guide discussion about what is working and what needs to be revised. Feedback should be solicited at grade-level team meetings but also at whole-faculty meetings. Not just soliciting but, most important, responding to or using feedback to improve the RTI effort will ensure its success and sustainability over time. Even in cases in which all efforts to establish a foundation for problem solving have occurred (e.g., teachers have been involved in selecting and administering screening tasks, screening data have been linked to interventions via collaboration with grade-level planning teams, and frequent communication and feedback about student learning has been provided to teachers individually via grade-level teams and faculty-wide presentations), the change process can still be challenging for some systems. In some systems, considerable efforts may be required to contend with any behaviors or events that could cause failure of the interventions and to reinforce correct implementation and improved learning at the site. If the principal is viewed as the instructional leader of a school, then principal support is essential to effective implementation. Large-scale imple-

mentation efforts are likely to suffer without principal support. Hence, in cases in which principals are not supportive of implementation, teams should consider starting on a very small scale (e.g., a single classroom) and treating the implementation as a pilot effort that might be used to bring about more sustained support for broader implementation.

• *The intervention plan targets the data-based problem definition and reflects the priorities of the school.* The intervention plan should target one or two key adaptive behaviors (e.g., mathematics performance at second grade, reading trajectories of first-grade students) identified by the principal and teachers as key objectives for the school. The data consultant can help to focus and reframe the goal to reflect a learning goal that is inclusive of all students and linked to meaningful student outcomes (e.g., reading performance, mathematics problem solving).

• *The intervention plan can work if properly implemented.* Research on implementation integrity has identified several effective methods for enhancing integrity (see Noell, Chapter 30, this volume, for a discussion of this issue). First, the intervention should be made as simple as possible. Given prioritized learning outcomes, teams should identify the top priorities for intervention, determine where existing intervention services or programs can be revised and utilized, and pilot the intervention on a small scale to start. Once a research-backed intervention has been selected, the RTI team should guide the school to focus on mastering the implementation of that intervention on a large scale, integrating the intervention with ongoing instructional efforts, and monitoring progress. Choosing and implementing a single intervention on a large scale is a significant accomplishment and one that should bring results assuming the right intervention has been selected. There can be a tendency for instructional leaders and decision makers to commit to a variety of intervention programs. This approach may be counterproductive to attaining system change. Increasing the number of interventions increases the likelihood that none will be implemented well. Hence selecting and committing to correctly implementing one intervention is preferred. There is obvious value in carefully selecting an intervention for use in a system, and there are a variety of ways to identify interventions that are likely to be effective (see Daly, Hofstadter, Martinez, & Andersen, Chapter 8, this volume); yet adequate selection is not enough to ensure effective implementation.

Many systems function well through universal screening, problem identification and definition, and intervention selection. In many systems, there is an overemphasis on these activities that occur before intervention is implemented. The intervention implementation stage is often poorly planned and managed for optimal effects. Effective implementation requires active management of training, progress monitoring of student outcomes, and contingency management for correct implementation. There must be a single person responsible for the logistics of intervention implementation. This person's role is to troubleshoot obstacles that arise as implementation begins. No amount of planning can foresee all possible implementation challenges, so this person must actively troubleshoot to ensure that correct implementation is established and maintained. With the right data and commitment, the question becomes not "whether" a system intervention will be effective but "how." The RTI team and teacher implementers should actively guide revisions to the intervention based on system data to ensure that learning gains are accelerated and maintained with the intervention.

• *A progress monitoring system has been identified.* As implementation occurs, progress monitoring data are needed to evaluate whether the intervention is having the de-

sired effect. At a minimum, the data consultant may use universal screening data to track effects of intervention efforts on student learning. Collected student outcome data will serve as the basis for evaluating intervention effects and for informing future revisions to the intervention process to ensure continued success. These data can be used to form, test, and evaluate hypotheses about student learning at the school. Principals and teachers can formulate goals and identify targets for their efforts. For example, the system may decide to target children who frequently fail the universal screening with a more sustained intervention effort or to target children already receiving special education, English language learners, or students who come from low socioeconomic environments. Consider, for example, the data in Figure 3.7, which come from a school that decided to use specialized reading resources to provide small-group reading intervention to groups of first- and second-grade students who performed below the benchmark at the fall screening. These students were provided with 45 minutes of instruction in groups of three to four students. The reading resource teacher chose the intervention. Students were administered a timed-reading passage each week to chart their growth in reading performance. These data could be compared with the growth that would be needed for each individual student to "catch up" during the period of time over which the intervention was allotted to continue. Figure 3.7 shows the percentage of students at this school who were on track to meet the end of

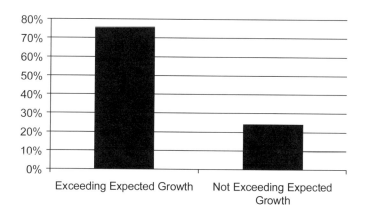

FIGURE 3.7. About 80% of students receiving specialized Tier 2 intervention services at this school are on track to achieve the end-of-intervention goal of grade-level reading performance.

intervention goal of on-grade-level reading performance. In this case, the majority of students were adequately responding to this system intervention. Problem solving can now take place for the small percentage of students for whom the intervention program is not sufficient to remediate their reading deficit by the program's conclusion. If an opposite pattern had been detected, then the team would have examined implementation integrity data; if the intervention was being properly implemented, the team would suggest that the intervention be changed.

Conclusion

Education has experienced an exciting shift toward scrutinizing the degree to which our professional activities positively affect the experiences and outcomes of those students and families they are intended to benefit (a concept referred to in the psychometrics literature as "consequential validity"). School psychologists are uniquely positioned to bring data to bear on everyday instructional practices in classrooms and to help instructional leaders chart system change plans to improve student learning outcomes. This evolved role requires school psychologists to gain new skills in academic assessment and intervention, effective instruction, and system change and requires the adaptation of old skills (e.g., assessment) to address new problems. School psychologists have an opportunity to use their skills to advance learning outcomes for all students and particularly for students at risk. This chapter described how to obtain and analyze universal screening data to identify system targets, collaborate with the instructional leader of a school or district to prioritize system targets and develop an implementation plan, implement the plan for maximal effects, and evaluate the plan in ways that communicate to all stakeholders (parents, teachers, administrators) whether or not the system solutions were effective for that system.

Notes

1. Using the year-end accountability measure as the standard of comparison, sensitivity is computed as the number of students who failed both the screening and the year-end accountability measure divided by the total number of students who failed the year-end accountability measure. Thus sensitivity is the proportion of true positives (students who will fail the year-end accountability measure) correctly detected by the screening. Specificity is computed as the number of students who passed both the screening and the year-end accountability measure divided by the total number of students who passed the year-end accountability measure. Specificity is the proportion of true negatives correctly detected by the screening. Functionally, sensitivity and specificity are thought to be more static variables tied to a particular test (less likely to change across different contexts) and are useful for selecting tests.

2. Positive predictive power is computed as the number of students who failed both the screening and the year-end accountability test divided by the total number of students who failed the screening. Functionally, positive predictive power is useful in interpreting individual failed screening results, as it represents the probability that a student who failed the screening will fail the year-end accountability measure. Negative predictive power is computed as the number of students who passed the screening and passed the year-end accountability test divided by the total number of students who passed the screening. Each of these values is interdependent, with sensitivity and negative predictive power being highly related and generally coming at a cost to specificity and positive predictive power, which are also highly related. When reaching a screening decision, it is logically desirable to maximize the identification of true positives, and so sensitivity is prioritized over specificity in selecting a screening device. For screening, the idea is to minimize false negative errors (or failing to identify students who will not pass the year-end accountability measure without intervention) in the most efficient way possible (i.e., with the least cost to specificity).

References

Burns, M. K., VanDerHeyden, A. M., & Jiban, C. (2006). Assessing the instructional level for mathematics: A comparison of methods. *School Psychology Review, 35*, 401–418.

Dawson, M., Cummings, J. A., Harrison, P. L., Short, R. J., Gorin, S., & Polomares, R. (2004). The 2002 multi-site conference on the future of school psychology: Next steps. *School Psychology Review, 33*, 115–125.

Deno, S. L. (1986). Formative evaluation of individual student programs: A new role for school psychologists. *School Psychology Review, 15,* 358–374.

Deno, S. L., Fuchs, L. S., Marston, D., & Shin, J. (2001). Using curriculum-based measurement to establish growth standards for students with learning disabilities. *School Psychology Review, 30,* 507–524.

Deno, S. L., & Mirkin, P. K. (1977). *Data-based program modification: A manual.* Reston, VA: Council for Exceptional Children.

Feuer, M. J., Towne, L., & Shavelson, R. J. (2002). Scientific culture and educational research. *Educational Researcher, 31,* 4–14.

Fuchs, L. S., & Fuchs, D. (1998). Treatment validity: A unifying concept for reconceptualizing the identification of learning disabilities. *Learning Disabilities Research and Practice, 13,* 204–219.

Fuchs, L. S., Fuchs, D., Hamlett, C. L., Walz, L., & Germann, G. (1993). Formative evaluation of academic progress: How much growth can we expect? *School Psychology Review, 22,* 27–48.

Gettinger, M., & Seibert, J. K. (2002). Best practices in increasing academic learning time. In A. Thomas & J. Grimes (Eds.), *Best practices in school psychology* (4th ed., pp. 773–788). Bethesda, MD: National Association of School Psychologists.

Hojnoski, R. L., & Missall, K. N. (2006). Addressing school readiness: Expanding school psychology in early education. *School Psychology Review, 35,* 602–613.

Hojnoski, R. L., & Missall, K. N. (2006). Addressing school readiness: Expanding school psychology in early education. *School Psychology Review, 35,* 602–614.

Kratochwill, T. R., & Shernoff, E. S. (2004). Evidence-based practice: Promoting evidence-based interventions in school psychology. *School Psychology Review, 33,* 34–48.

Lentz, F. E., & Shapiro, E. S. (1986). Functional assessment of the academic environment. *School Psychology Review, 15,* 346–357.

Macmann, G. M., & Barnett, D. W. (1999). Diagnostic decision making in school psychology: Understanding and coping with uncertainty. In C. R. Reynolds & T. B. Gutkin (Eds.), *The handbook of school psychology* (3rd ed., pp. 519–548). New York: Wiley.

Messick, S. (1995). Validity of psychological assessment: Validation of inferences from persons' responses and performances as scientific inquiry into score meaning. *American Psychologist, 50,* 741–749.

National Institute of Child Health and Human Development. (2000). *Teaching children to read: An evidence-based assessment of the scientific literature on reading and its implications for reading instruction* (NIH Publication No. 00-4769). Washington, DC: U.S. Government Printing Office.

Neef, N. A. (1995). Research on training trainers in program implementation: An introduction and future directions. *Journal of Applied Behavior Analysis, 28,* 297–299.

Odom, S. L., Brantlinger, E., Gersten, R., Horner, R. H., Thompson, B., & Harris, K. R. (2005). Research in special education: Scientific methods and evidence-based practices. *Exceptional Children, 71,* 137–148.

Shapiro, E. S. (2004). *Academic skills problems: Direct assessment and intervention* (3rd ed.). New York: Guilford Press.

Shinn, M. R., & Bamonto, S. (1998). Advanced applications of curriculum-based measurement: "Big ideas" and avoiding confusion. In M. R. Shinn (Ed.), *Advanced applications of curriculum-based measurement* (pp. 1–31). New York: Guilford Press.

Slentz, K. L., & Hyatt, K. J. (2008). Best practices in applying curriculum-based assessment in early childhood. In A. Thomas & J. Grimes (Eds.), *Best practices in school psychology* (5th ed., Vol. 2, pp. 519–534). Bethesda, MD: National Association of School Psychologists.

Thomas, A., & Grimes, J. (2008). *Best practices in school psychology* (5th ed.). Bethesda, MD: National Association of School Psychologists.

Torgesen, J. K. (2002). The prevention of reading difficulties. *Journal of School Psychology, 40,* 7–26.

U.S. Department of Education. (2008). *Foundations for success: The final report of the National Mathematics Advisory Panel.* Washington, DC: U.S. Government Printing Office.

VanDerHeyden, A. M., & Burns, M. K. (2005). Effective instruction for at-risk minority populations. In C. L. Frisby & C. R. Reynolds (Eds.), *Comprehensive handbook of multicultural school psychology* (pp. 483–513). Hoboken, NJ: Wiley.

VanDerHeyden, A. M., & Witt, J. C. (2005). Quantifying context in assessment: Capturing the effect of base rates on teacher referral and a problem-solving model of identification. *School Psychology Review, 34,* 161–183.

VanDerHeyden, A. M., & Witt, J. C. (2007). Section commentary on effective consultation. In W. Erchul & S. Sheridan (Eds.), *Handbook of research in school consultation: Empirical foundations for the field* (pp. 115–124). London, UK: Routledge.

Chapter 4

Assessment of Cognitive Abilities and Cognitive Processes

Issues, Applications, and Fit within a Problem-Solving Model

Randy G. Floyd

Nothing seems to stir the passion of a school psychologist more than the publication of a new test. The brightly colored images with more realistic depictions of people and things, the more durable, precise, and carefully engineered blocks, the utilitarian aspects of the folding manual, the precision sheen of the protocol, and, of course, the crisp smell of those current norms, are enough to send the pulse of the average school psychologist racing into orbit. Tests, it seems, have become an indelible part of the character of school psychologists and a nearly indispensable tool within their intellectual assessment repertoire.

—FLANAGAN AND ORTIZ (2002, p. 1352)

School psychology was born in the prison of a test and, although the cell has been enlarged somewhat, it is still a prison. Alfred Binet would have been aghast, I think, to find that he gave impetus to a role which became technical and narrow, a role in which one came up with analyses, numbers, and classifications which had little or no bearing on what happened to children in classrooms.

—SARASON (1976, p. 587)

School psychologists have historically been assessment specialists, and their assessments have most often included cognitive ability test batteries, such as the Stanford–Binet and the Wechsler Intelligence Scale for Children (WISC; Fagan & Wise, 2007). As Sarason's quote conveys, this role of tester has long been one that has defined—as well as restricted—the field of school psychology (see Reschly & Grimes, 2002). Despite the increased emphasis on the use of alternate assessment methods and tools (e.g., Shapiro & Kratochwill, 2000), as well as abundant criticisms of norm-referenced tests (Brown-Chidsey, 2005; Shapiro, 2005; Shinn, 1998, 2002), there is no doubt that the history of school psychologist as tester continues to influence current practice in substantial ways. For example, the most recent surveys of school psychologists reveal that testing activities continue to fill, on average, a little more than half of the work week (e.g., Hosp & Reschly, 2002). As evident from social psychology research, familiarity leads to feelings of affection and attraction. It is no wonder that tests often stir the passion of school psychologists.

Cognitive ability testing via norm-referenced tests has seemed to offer useful information to school psychologists. First, cognitive ability tests, since their inception (Binet & Simon, 1905), have been designed to produce objective measures. Thus, rather than relying on teacher ratings of student performance in the classroom, which were seen as having great potential for bias by Binet and others, the cognitive ability test could determine who was in greatest need of aid and who demonstrated the greatest potential—in an objective manner. Second, cognitive ability tests allowed for normative and developmental comparisons to be made, for example, by situating a child's total score within the distribution of those expected based on age. Just as growth curves used by pediatricians to track height and weight over time provide indications about children's size, cognitive ability tests allowed school psychologists to make inferences about how a child "stacked up" relative to others of the same age at single points in time and across time on relatively novel tasks. Thus cognitive ability tests allowed the school psychologist to move from idiographic interpretation (e.g., "John knows the definition of the word *window* but not the definition of the word *putative*") to normative interpretation ("John is scoring well below what we would expect for a child his age").

Third, cognitive ability tests provided school psychologists with a standard method to capture behaviors indicating knowledge and skills under controlled circumstances. Thus cognitive ability tests approximated a well-controlled experiment in which variables extraneous to the simple display of knowledge and skills in classroom settings (e.g., peer or teacher influences) were removed, so that the independent variables (i.e., test items) could be carefully presented to evoke responses in the examinee. Fourth, accumulating evidence revealed that the scores from cognitive ability tests, especially IQs, allowed school psychologists and other test users to predict, with confidence, many outcomes. For example, across a large body of research, IQs have been shown to predict a number of socially important variables, including academic attainments (e.g., achievement test scores, grades, and years of schooling), job performance, occupational and social status, and income (Jensen, 1998; Neisser et al., 1996; Schmidt, 2002). Thus cognitive ability tests allowed school psychologists to develop hypotheses to explain reasons for learning problems. Some have asserted that this practice was enhanced when cognitive ability tests, such as the Wechsler–Bellevue (Wechsler, 1939), began yielding subtest or composite scores in addition to a single IQ. Finally, in recent years, cognitive ability tests allowed school psychologists to provide information that was central to

identification of individuals with learning disabilities, mental retardation, or intellectual giftedness.

Some of the reasons that school psychologists have used cognitive ability tests have been shown by relatively recent research to be poorly supported. For example, despite the promise of tailoring treatments to the results of testing that emerged in the 1960s, much of this promise has been unfulfilled (see Kavale & Forness, 1999; cf. Naglieri, 2002). In addition, the use of IQs to predict achievement in the identification of learning disabilities appears to be problematic for a number of reasons. A sizable body of research by Fletcher, Francis, and others has indicated that this practice of identification is unreliable across time and across instruments and that it fails to differentiate children with learning disabilities from children with only low achievement across key reading aptitudes (Fletcher, Denton, & Francis, 2005; Fletcher, Lyon, Fuchs, & Barnes, 2006; Francis et al., 2005; Hoskyn & Swanson, 2000). Based on the problems with this method of identifying learning disabilities, school psychologists appear to be moving toward a model of identifying learning disabilities based on children's failure to respond to empirically based interventions (Fletcher, Coulter, Reschly, & Vaughn, 2004; Fletcher et al., 2006).

Despite the increasing evidence for the restrained usage of cognitive ability tests, school psychologists now, more than at any other point in history, have access to many well-developed cognitive ability tests that produce reliable and well-validated scores. It appears that these cognitive ability tests have benefited from the incorporation of a larger body of research, as well as prominent models of cognitive abilities (Flanagan & Ortiz, 2002). In light of these advances, the overarching goal of this chapter is to illuminate a tentative answer to the following question: Do the exceptionally well-developed and substantiated cognitive ability tests aid school psychologists in applying the problem-solving model to improve the reading, mathematics, and writing skills of children with whom they work? One purpose of this chapter is to provide a review of and to highlight distinctions between the constructs commonly measured by cognitive ability tests. In doing so, the chapter provides an overview of the Cattell–Horn–Carroll theory, which is perhaps the most prominent model forming the foundation of contemporary cognitive ability testing. The second goal is to provide reflections about the applications of school psychologists' focus on cognitive constructs when engaging in problem solving to address student difficulties in reading, mathematics, and writing.

Defining the Subject Area

This section of the chapter presents several key terms that are prominent in the discussions about the application of the results of cognitive ability testing to school psychology. Many of these terms often seem to be used incorrectly or poorly in the school psychology and related literature.

Individual differences are defined as "deviations or variations along a variable or dimension that occur among members of any particular group" (Corsini, 1999, p. 481) or as "all the ways in which people differ from one another" (Colman, 2001, p. 389). These differences across persons typically can be conceptualized by a normal, Gaussian, or bell curve, in which most persons fall under the center of the curve (i.e., the "hump") and those with more extreme values on the variable of interest are included in its tails. These differences are thought to surface "naturally" as individuals mature and interact with their environment over time; thus they are not manipulated, per se, as in experimental research. Examples of individual differences from the physical sciences include weight, head circumference, foot size, heart rate, and blood pressure (see Kranzler, 1999). In addition, most variables that school psychologists use to represent knowledge and skills in performing academic tasks and other "intelligent" behaviors represent individual differences.

Intelligence is a general term used to describe a within-person construct and an individual-difference variable underlying adaptive functioning. However, from the survey conducted by Thorndike (1921) to the more recent survey by Sternberg and Detterman (1986), experts' definitions of intelligence have varied greatly. The recent *APA Dictionary of Psychology* (VandenBos, 2006) defines intelligence as the following

string of general properties: "the ability to derive information, learn from experience, adapt to the environment, understand, and correctly utilize thought and reason" (p. 488). Not only is intelligence difficult to define with great detail, but there also is excess baggage in use of the term, such as value judgments about the worth or potential of a person, as well as questions about bias against minority racial groups (Jensen, 1998). School psychologists are probably better served by using other vocabulary.

An *ability* is defined as a "developed skill, competence, or power to do something, especially … existing capacity to perform some function, whether physical, mental, or a combination of the two, without further education or training"(Colman, 2001, p. 1). Jensen (1998) defined ability as a directly observable behavior that can be judged in terms of level of proficiency, that is stable over time, and that is consistently displayed across varying opportunities to perform the behavior (see Jensen, 1998, pp. 51–52). At its most basic level, an ability may be viewed as the consistent performance of a discrete behavior in appropriate contexts (e.g., saying the word "No" in response to a question or writing the letter "X" when asked to do so). However, abilities typically reflect individual differences in the performance of these behaviors under different conditions of task difficulty (Carroll, 1993, p. 8).

Cognitive ability is defined as "any ability that concerns some … class of tasks in which correct or appropriate processing of mental information is critical to successful performance" (Carroll, 1993, p. 10). In contrast, *mental ability* is defined as a cognitive ability that (1) is not intricately linked to a singular sensory input mechanism or to a singular output mechanism and (2) does not demonstrate significant correlations with measures of related sensory or physical abilities, such as sensory acuity and dexterity (Jensen, 1998). Thus mental abilities reflect a subset of cognitive abilities, and tests targeting Visual Processing and Auditory Processing abilities would likely be considered tests of cognitive abilities, not of mental abilities.

There are many challenges in distinguishing between cognitive abilities and *achievement*. Carroll (1993) stated that the argument that all cognitive abilities are, in fact, learned achievement is difficult to refute—especially when achievement is considered in terms of declarative knowledge and procedural knowledge. Declarative knowledge can be conceptualized as knowing what to do, and it comprises memories and language-based knowledge, such as facts. Procedural knowledge can be conceptualized as knowing how to perform a behavior, and it comprises if–then rules or strategies used to achieve goals. Thus most all tests of cognitive abilities require application of both declarative knowledge and procedural knowledge in varying degrees. Carroll added that the distinction between cognitive abilities and achievement may be one of degree rather than type. This variation in degree may be in how general or specialized the ability is. For example, a measure of Fluid Reasoning may reflect the ability to reason, to form concepts, and to solve problems across a number of different types of tasks. This ability measure appears to be more cognitive in nature because it is not tied to specific types of concepts or problems within items. In contrast, a measure of mathematics would require specialized knowledge of terminology, symbols, and algorithms across a more narrow range of items, and this specialized knowledge would likely stem from formal learning experiences. Measures of cognitive ability that target the specialized knowledge produced by instruction or self-study can be considered measures of achievement.

Most cognitive abilities are deemed important because they are viewed as *aptitudes*. Aptitudes may be defined as "any characteristic of the person that affects his response to the treatment" (Cronbach, 1975, p. 116), but Carroll (1993) defines aptitudes more restrictively as "a cognitive ability that is possibly predictive of certain kinds of future learning success ... beyond a prediction from degree of prior learning" (pp. 16–17). Thus the term *aptitude* implies consideration of the future, whereas *achievement* implies consideration of prior learning (Corno et al., 2002). Although *aptitude*, *intelligence*, *cognitive ability*, and *mental ability* are often considered equivalent terms, aptitudes include characteristics of persons that are not limited to intelligent behaviors, and they include personality facets, motivation, gender, physical size, and, in some cases, prior achievement.

Cognitive processes can be defined as "hypothetical constructs used by cognitive theorists to describe how persons apprehend, discriminate, select, and attend to certain aspects of the vast welter of stimuli that impinge on the sensorium to form internal representations that can be mentally manipulated, transformed, related to previous internal representations, stored in memory ... and later retrieved from storage to govern the person's decision and behavior in a particular situation" (Jensen, 1998, pp. 205–206). Thus a cognitive process can be considered the fundamental mental event in which information is operated on to produce a response (Carroll, 1993). All voluntary behaviors are the results of some sequence of cognitive processes; consequentially, all measures of cognitive abilities (including those measuring achievement) can be said to be the result of cognitive processes. Although abilities typically represent individual differences and can be identified only via comparison of an individual's performance to those of others, cognitive processes can be inferred based on the performance of a single individual (Jensen, 1998).

Clarification in Use of Terms

School psychologists and other professionals seem to use many of the terms described in the previous subsection interchangeably. In addition, some of the general terms do subsume more specific ones. For instance, the term *cognitive abilities* can subsume the term *achievement*, and the term *aptitude* overlaps substantially with these terms, but it also includes other constructs. Perhaps the most commonly occurring deviation from the definitions provided earlier is in the use of the term *cognitive processes* (see Floyd, 2005). For example, many contemporary cognitive ability tests yield scores with titles such as "Visual Processing," "Auditory Processing," "Simultaneous Processing," and the like. It is probably best to avoid the interpretation of most norm-referenced scores from cognitive ability tests as indicating, with any meaningfulness, a cognitive process (Jensen, 2006). Most of these scores are probably best seen as measures of cognitive ability. These measures of cognitive ability represent individual differences in the complete series of cognitive processes used when completing items, which are typically summed into a subtest score, a composite score, or both and compared with some norm group. Because of this aggregation and subsequent relative comparisons, ability scores should not be viewed as pure measures of distinct cognitive processes. Perhaps continued misuse of the terms associated with cognitive processes stems from a number of influences: (1) the excess baggage associated with intelligence testing, (2) a tendency to soft-pedal our measurement of individual differences (i.e., an ability), (3) a desire to appear that we are measuring something different from the cognitive abilities and mental abilities that we have been measuring through testing for at least 100 years. We should probably use the terms *process* or *processing* to refer to the many unseen steps in completing a task rather than to the sum or outcome of those steps.

CHC Theory, Achievement, and Cognitive Processes

Research stemming from the Cattell–Horn–Carroll (CHC) theory (McGrew, 2005, 2009; McGrew & Woodcock, 2001) likely provides the most well-supported model of human cognitive abilities. The theory is grounded in factor-analytic evidence, as well as supported by developmental, neurocognitive, genetic, and external validity evidence. It has the potential to offer a common nomenclature and taxonomy for describing and understanding the relations between cognitive abilities per se and measures of cognitive abilities (Carroll, 1993; McGrew, 2009).

CHC theory describes a hierarchical model of cognitive abilities that vary according to level of generality: narrow abilities (stratum I), broad abilities (stratum II), and, in the minds of many, general intelligence (*g*; stratum III). Narrow abilities include approximately 70 highly specialized abilities. Perhaps the most often-cited CHC narrow ability described is Phonetic Coding, the ability to break apart and blend speech sounds. This narrow ability has been implicated in early reading success and is likely the ability measured by most tasks targeting phonological awareness, phonological processing, and the like (Floyd, Keith, Taub, & McGrew, 2007). A pair of other narrow abilities, Memory Span and Working Memory, provides evidence of the key link between

specific types of tasks and the narrow abilities they measure. By requiring examinees to repeat orally presented numbers, Memory Span tasks target the ability to retain information in immediate memory for brief periods. In contrast, Working Memory tasks, which require examinees to repeat orally presented numbers in reversed order, target the transformation or manipulation of information held in immediate memory for brief periods. Thus the narrow abilities do not appear as a result of the use of different stimuli (e.g., numbers) or different input (e.g., orally presented information) or output (e.g., oral responses) mechanisms; rather, they appear to differ only in terms of the cognitive processes required.

Measures representing CHC broad abilities have received much greater research attention than those representing narrow abilities. Broad abilities include the following (McGrew, 2009). Fluid Reasoning refers to the ability to reason abstractly, form concepts, and solve problems using unfamiliar information. Two memory-related abilities at this stratum include Short-Term Memory, which refers to the ability to hold and manipulate information in immediate memory, and Long-Term Storage and Retrieval, which refers to the ability to store information in and retrieve information from long-term stores. Two abilities associated with sensory modalities include Visual Processing, which refers to the ability to perceive, analyze, and synthesize visually presented information and patterns, and Auditory Processing, which refers to the ability to perceive, analyze, and synthesize sounds and their patterns. Two broad abilities reflect variations in the speed with which cognitive tasks are completed. Cognitive Processing Speed refers to the ability to perform repeatedly and rapidly a series of simple tasks, whereas Decision and Reaction Time refers to the ability to respond quickly to environmental cues across multiple independent trials. Three broad abilities reflect, in large part, accumulation of declarative knowledge. Comprehension–Knowledge refers to the ability associated with comprehensiveness of acquired knowledge, the ability to communicate knowledge verbally, and the ability to reason by drawing on previous experiences. Quantitative Knowledge refers to the ability to complete mathematics operations and "story problems" and to reason with numbers. Reading and Writing refers to the ability associated with general literacy skills; it subsumes more narrow abilities such as Reading Decoding, Spelling, and Written Expression. Note that these last two broad abilities reflect what most would consider achievement, because literacy and mathematics are the primary targets of instruction and study in school settings.

In contrast to the broad abilities, the existence of a single, higher order general factor (psychometric g) has been the focus of much debate (see McGrew, 2005). Some researchers, such as Carroll (1993, 2003) and Jensen (1998), assert (1) that this general factor represents well what is shared among the broad abilities and (2) that it is the only cognitive ability tapped by all ability measures. Despite some logical arguments and some empirical evidence offered by Horn (1991) and others, it appears that, after more than 100 years of study and debate, this common variance demonstrated across broad abilities and individual tests is best conceptualized as the general factor (see Floyd, McGrew, Barry, Rafael, & Rogers, in press). Thus the general factor is the least specialized ability in CHC theory, and because it is the most general and most pervasive, it may dictate, at least in part, how much declarative and procedural knowledge individuals accumulate across development (Jensen, 2006).

Cognitive processes per se are not included in CHC theory, but suggestions regarding their fit into the CHC theory have been presented in a previous publication (Floyd, 2005). Many cognitive processes fit well into a hierarchical model of cognitive abilities such as CHC theory. Although cognitive abilities are not necessarily processes, abilities likely stem from combinations of like processes. As the cognitive ability testing field moves toward a standard taxonomy, such as CHC theory, cognitive processes will likely provide a clearer link to narrow (stratum I) cognitive abilities (Carroll, 1993; Sternberg, 1977). For example, a model by Sternberg (1977) has been adapted to indicate the importance of tasks and components below the level of general, broad, and narrow ability factors of CHC theory (Floyd, 2005). Cognitive processes facilitating analogical reasoning were labeled *encoding*, *inferring*, *mapping*, *justification*,

and *preparing–responding*. Analogical reasoning has been shown to measure the CHC narrow ability Induction, which is subsumed by the broad ability Fluid Reasoning. Measures of Fluid Reasoning tend to be highly correlated with the general factor. Despite this potential of linking cognitive processes to cognitive abilities, a number of criticisms have been offered concerning the inferences made about cognitive processes. Most notably, due to the inference required in delineating cognitive processes, their identification and labeling seem somewhat arbitrary and idiosyncratic.

Cognitive Abilities and Cognitive Processes and Potential Application to School Psychology Practice

At least since the Education for All Handicapped Children Act was passed in 1975, school psychologists have engaged in testing to identify cognitive abilities in order to follow the rule of the law in identifying children as eligible for special education services. For example, measures of the general factor (i.e., IQs) have been required for identification of learning disabilities and mental retardation. Although the requirements to identify learning disabilities were unconstrained to allow for response-to-intervention (RTI) methods in the revision of the Individuals with Disabilities Education Act in 2004, the definition of a learning disability has remained unchanged since 1975. It begins with the following sentence:

> *Specific learning disability* means a disorder in one or more of the *basic psychological processes* [italics added] involved in understanding or in using language, spoken or written, which may manifest itself in the imperfect ability to listen, think, speak, read, write, spell, or do mathematical calculations.

Although the pathognomonic indicator of a learning disability was considered to be the IQ–achievement discrepancy, this indicator has fallen out of favor for good reason, as described earlier. However, the definition continues to make reference to basic psychological processes, which seems to implore school psychologists to complete assessments designed to target these processes. In a manner largely consistent with the federal definition of a learning disability, the National Association of School Psychologists (NASP; 2007) issued a position statement that conveys the following:

> There is general agreement that: specific learning disabilities are endogenous in nature, and are characterized by neurologically-based deficits in *cognitive processes* [italics added] [and that] these deficits are specific, that is, they impact particular cognitive processes that interfere with the acquisition of formal learning skills. (pp. 4–5)

This position statement also recommends utilization of a multitiered model of identification of students with learning disabilities—with Tier 3 involving cognitive ability testing. Tier 1 includes instructional and behavioral supports provided in the general education setting. Tier 2 includes interventions, such as remedial programs, for children who fail to respond to the supports provided in the general education setting. Tier 3 includes both a comprehensive assessment and resulting intensive interventions. The position statement continues as follows:

> The purpose of comprehensive Tier 3 assessment is to provide information about the instructional interventions that are likely to be effective for the student. ... NASP recommends that initial evaluation of a student with a suspected specific learning disability includes an individual comprehensive assessment, as prescribed by the evaluation team. This evaluation may include measures of academic skills (norm-referenced and criterion-referenced); *cognitive abilities and processes* [italics added], and mental health status (social-emotional development); measures of academic and oral language proficiency as appropriate; classroom observations; and indirect sources of data (e.g., teacher and parent reports). (pp. 4–5)

It appears that the increased emphasis on children's responsiveness to empirically based treatments (also known as RTI) in Tiers 1 and 2 is not necessarily the end of cognitive ability testing. In fact, as indicated in the NASP position statement, numerous proponents of cognitive ability testing have advocated a complementary approach (Mather & Kaufman, 2006; Willis & Dumont, 2006). Regardless, those who advocate use of and those who use cognitive ability tests should

not continue to confuse specific cognitive abilities with cognitive processes. As stated earlier, cognitive processes contribute to cognitive abilities, but ability measures are typically too complex to infer processes with any degree of reliability. They are related but distinct concepts.

Application of Understanding of Cognitive Abilities and Cognitive Processes to the Problem-Solving Model Focusing on Academic Achievement

In this section, the potential contributions of (1) interpretation of measures of cognitive abilities and (2) inferences about cognitive processes from task performance to problem solving are addressed. Although a number of descriptions of problem-solving models exist (e.g., Bransford & Stein, 1984; Brown-Chidsey, 2005; Deno, 2002, 2005; Shinn, 2002), the steps included in Tilly's (2002, 2008) problem-solving model will be used to be consistent with this book's companion text (Merrell, Ervin, & Gimpel Peacock, 2006) and with Ervin, Gimpel Peacock, and Merrell, Chapter 1, this volume. Measures of some cognitive abilities—primarily at the most general level (i.e., IQs)—are seen as important to the identification of children as being eligible for special education services, as well as to the diagnosis of some psychiatric disorders, but very few sources appear to have incorporated measures of cognitive abilities and consideration of cognitive processes into all steps of the problem-solving model (cf. Hale & Fiorello, 2004; Reschly, 2008). I believe that school psychologists would benefit from consideration of the potential fit of measures of cognitive ability and related constructs to the problem-solving process, as well as from consideration of many of the reasons that these measures do not fit well, at present, into such a process.

Is There a Problem?

Tilly (2002, 2008) proposed four general questions to guide school psychologists' problem-solving: (1) Is there a problem, and what is it? (2) Why is the problem happening? (3) What should be done about the problem? (4) Did the intervention work? The first question guides problem solvers to determine the existence of a perceived problem and to clarify the nature of the difference between "what is" and "what should be" (Deno, 2002).

Areas of Fit

Traditional models used to identify high-incidence disabling conditions, such as learning disability and mental retardation, and to determine the need for special education services have often required (1) deficits in performance based on norm-reference measures and (2) cut scores to determine the degree of normative deviancy necessary for such deficits to be identified (e.g., an IQ of 70 or below). Few would argue that scores from norm-referenced achievement tests fail to provide useful information in identifying the existence of a problem during the problem-solving process. Results from such tests are snapshots reflecting relative levels of performance in reading, mathematics, and writing. In particular, norm-referenced scores from such tests provide insights about the relation between the child's performance during the test sessions (i.e., a sample of "what is") and general, relative expectations for achievement (i.e., "what should be").

It is logical that some tests of specific cognitive abilities distal to reading, mathematics, and writing measures may be useful in identifying a problem or a potential problem during the developmental period before reading, mathematics, and writing develop. For example, expressive and receptive language abilities and knowledge of basic concepts are important aptitudes for success in school and can be targeted for assessment and intervention during the toddler and preschool years. If a young child demonstrates low levels of performance on measures of these abilities when compared with peers, a problem is apparent. In addition, because most toddlers and preschool-age children cannot yet read words, measures of abilities related to phonological or phonemic awareness, such as the ability to identify phonemes in spoken words, can be targeted to identify those children displaying a large enough problem to warrant early intervention (see Good & Kaminski, 2002).

Tests that yield measures of the general factor seem to allow school psychologists to identify global failure to meet environmental expectations. For example, a child who obtains an IQ below 70 and who displays significant impairment in adaptive functioning when compared with same-age peers will likely be said to have the disability of mental retardation (American Psychiatric Association, 2000). The low IQ can provide one substantial piece of evidence that the child has not likely been accumulating declarative and procedural knowledge at the rate of others the same age. Thus when asking the question, Is there a problem, and what is it? cognitive ability measures can reveal legitimate answers.

Challenges to Fit

Although some potential applications of cognitive ability measures to the first step of the problem-solving process exist, in many cases, these applications are tied closely to eligibility for services, which is not a goal of problem solving as a whole (Shinn, 2008). In contrast to these applications, there are a number of challenges to the fit of traditional norm-referenced measures of cognitive abilities with this step in the problem-solving model. One challenge to the use of traditional cognitive ability measures is that the content of cognitive ability tests, be they measures of reading decoding, mathematics reasoning, or visual processing, do not well represent what has been taught in classrooms or in other school settings. For example, item content from norm-referenced tests of the achievement domains is often poorly matched with school and classroom curricula (Shapiro & Elliott, 1999). In addition, tests of cognitive abilities distal to achievement, such as tests of Visual Processing that often require the construction of patterns using blocks, may not reflect well map-reading assignments or geometry assignments required in the classroom, despite their apparent similarities. Thus, when such measures are obtained from nationally normed tests, lack of alignment probably exists between measurement of the domains of interest, the students' instruction, and the curriculum from which instruction emerges (Ikeda, Neesen, & Witt, 2008).

Another challenge is that the norm-referenced comparisons (based on national norms) reflected in the cognitive ability scores may not reflect validly the relative comparisons within a classroom, a school, or a district. For example, a standard score in the average range on a word identification test based on national norms may not well represent a child's very low performance in reading when compared with her classmates. On the other hand, using a cut score of 85, which is 1 standard deviation below the mean, on a test of reading decoding skills based on national, age-based norms may identify the majority of children in a class or grade that contains a lot of struggling readers. Overall, with respect to norm-referenced tests of cognitive abilities, what is unclear is whether an observed normative weakness in test scores indicates that there are real problems across settings, such as the classroom. Real-world problems are inferred from performance on a test or battery of tests—sometimes without collecting information to validate that a problem exists beyond the perceptions of those reporting it and these test scores (Ikeda et al., 2008).

A third challenge to the use of traditional cognitive ability measures is that they are yielded from assessments conducted at single points in time. This practice is often problematic—in fact, often rife with error— and this problem is exacerbated by use of cut scores (Macmann & Barnett, 1999). According to Francis et al. (2005):

> When any test is used, there is still measurement error. … Because of this error in measurement, any attempt to set a cut-point will lead to instability in classification, as scores fluctuate around the cut-point with repeated testing, even for a decision as straightforward as demarcating low achievement or mental deficiency. This fluctuation is not a problem of repeated testing, nor is it a matter of selecting the ideal cut-point, or one that is intrinsically meaningful. The problem stems from the fact that no single score can perfectly capture a student's ability in a single domain. (pp. 99–100)

Such conclusions are evident from studies of score exchangeability targeting IQs and score composites measuring CHC broad cognitive abilities (Floyd, Bergeron, McCormack, Anderson, & Hargrove-Owens, 2005; Floyd, Clark, & Shadish, 2008). In contrast, progress monitoring and its operationalization of achievement by measures from the curriculum-based measurement (CBM) and general outcome measurement traditions appears to overcome these limitations by facilitating ef-

ficient, repeated measurement of constructs of interest to compare the same ability over time. In a sense, such serial measurements accomplish more than one-shot tests and summative assessment because they borrow precision from repeated measurement (Fletcher et al., 2006, p. 54).

The final challenge to the use of traditional cognitive ability measures is that norm-reference tests of cognitive abilities employed by school psychologists do not appear to be time and cost-effective (Gresham & Witt, 1997; Yates & Taub, 2003). These tests are individually administered and lengthy, and they often seem to provide information that is already known by educators. Although IQs have been shown to predict a number of socially important variables, including academic achievement, job performance, and income (as noted earlier in this chapter), it is important to remember that children typically spend 5 days a week across 9 or 10 months in the school setting demonstrating these achievement outcomes. So, if actual achievement is known, some may ask, Why do we want to predict achievement when it is already known? Perhaps such aptitude measures have outlived their usefulness in school settings in which benchmarking and progress monitoring using CBM probes can be implemented. However, such aptitude measures may be better employed in other settings, such as clinics and business organizations during diagnostic and selection processes. It appears that group-administered and individually administered CBM probes allow for rapid screening, benchmarking, and progress monitoring and that they represent a more economical method than the traditional cognitive ability test battery.

Why Is the Problem Happening?

The second step in problem solving, designed to answer the question, Why is the problem happening? prompts the problem solver to develop hypotheses based on data to explain the reason for the problem identified in the previous step.

Areas of Fit

Interpretations based on consideration of cognitive processes may offer their greatest benefit at this stage of problem solving, and measures representing some cognitive abilities may be useful in understanding the problems of some children—especially after other methods, such as direct observations and CBM probes, have been completed (Brown-Chidsey, 2005).

Most school psychologists engaged in problem solving, in special education eligibility determination, or in diagnosis of learning disabilities probably infer the presence or absence of cognitive processes based on their observation of children's task performance (e.g., on items) or from the reports of others, such as teachers, who have observed the children during task completion (Floyd, 2005). These observations of behavior target cognitive processes and related behaviors. Be it called a *subskill analysis*, *task analysis*, or *error analysis*, this criterion-referenced approach to examining task performance and underlying cognitive processes most likely enhances understanding of why individuals display problems with reading, mathematics, and writing (Busse, 2005; Howell, Hosp, & Kurns, 2008; Howell & Nolet, 2000). For example, it makes sense to examine item-level performance in terms of influences associated with *input* into the cognitive system and *output* via responses. For example, a child with visual acuity problems would be expected to read words slowly and inaccurately, and a child with fine motor control problems would be expected to struggle to write letters correctly. Labeling of the variations in the input and output steps from tests of cognitive abilities is modeled well in recent publications (e.g., Hale & Fiorello, 2004; Kaufman, 1994; Kaufman & Kaufman, 2004).

It appears that the standard set of cognitive processes and related behaviors used to complete reading, mathematics, and writing tasks are relatively easy to identify and relatively uniform across persons. The range of processes needed to complete items from most tasks measuring these domains is much narrower than the range of processes needed for tasks measuring most cognitive abilities. Many achievement tests that focus on basic or functional levels of performance target procedural knowledge associated with the domain of interest and limit the number of operations or strategies to be used. The task stimuli (i.e., input) also are generally uniform within the domain of interest (e.g.,

with reading, words or sentences), and response modalities (i.e., output) are similar across related tasks. For example, responses to mathematics calculation items often require writing or written responses. The common processes required for tasks within each of these achievement domains make them viable targets for interpretative approaches based on consideration of cognitive processes (Floyd, 2005).

Rather than focusing on why a child constructs block designs slowly or inaccurately and attempting to generalizing those findings to performance during completion of academic tasks (in the test session and in the classroom), it seems prudent to focus first on actual performance during the academic tasks and the processes that lead to successful performance on them. For example, problems with visual–spatial orientation (relative to peers) identified during a test of Spatial Relations could be hypothesized to affect performance on a test of mathematics calculations that requires such visual–spatial orientation, such as when adding down columns. However, a similar conclusion could have been drawn from a more authentic assessment of mathematics calculation. Thus, if a child consistently makes errors in mathematics calculations when adding down columns but appears to have mastered the recall of addition facts, that child may be seen as having a problem with visual–spatial orientation during mathematics calculation tasks. Because this conclusion is grounded in processes of the achievement task (i.e., it is "close to the task"), it will probably lead to tangible benefits. Overall, it would appear that an analysis of processes stemming from performance on achievement tasks, like the example provided earlier, may best reflect the diagnostic criteria for learning disabilities that call for identification of the deficits or disorders in processes.

In contrast to the focus on cognitive processes that underlie reading, mathematics, and writing tests, as well as cognitive processing that underlies more distal abilities, many test authors and other professionals in school psychology promote measurement of *cognitive components* during assessments designed to answer the question, Why is the problem happening? Using the cognitive-components approach, (1) cognitive ability measures thought to represent the cognitive processes required to complete reading, mathematics, and writing tasks, (2) cognitive ability measures that statistically relate substantially with scores from the academic tasks, or (3) both (1) and (2), are included in the assessment battery to develop hypotheses regarding the reason for the problem. An example of the cognitive-components approach can be found in the work of Berninger (2001, 2006). When Berninger's *component-skills approach* is applied, children are asked to complete relatively narrow cognitive ability tasks that likely involve some of the same cognitive processes or task stimuli that are included in achievement tasks. For example, children in second grade may be screened using reading tasks that require them to read real words, pseudowords, and connected text. Those with the greatest deficits on these tasks are administered additional assessment tasks to pinpoint some of the specific cognitive abilities that are linked to the weaknesses in these achievement domains. These tasks may include those that require children to identify whether two words are spelled the same; to identify the syllables, phonemes, and rimes in orally presented words; to name letters and words quickly; and to answer questions about word meanings. Following this component-skills approach, from the perspective of CHC theory (Floyd et al., 2007), it could be hypothesized that an elementary school-age child who demonstrates a normatively low score on a measure of Reading Decoding and a commensurately low score on a measure of Phonetic Coding has an ability deficit in Phonetic Coding that leads to the problem with Reading Decoding.

Challenges to Fit

Interpretation of item-level performance as indicating cognitive processes and interpretation of cognitive ability test scores are typically based on substantial inference. Christ (2008) explained well that all hypotheses generated during assessment (and during problem solving in general) are inferences because little is actually known about the causes of "the problem." Whereas high-inference hypotheses tend to stem from consideration of constructs not visible to the eye (e.g., cognitive abilities and cognitive processes), low-inference hypotheses stem from consideration of overt behaviors and antecedents and consequences in the environment that influence them. Thus a conservative approach to problem solving would be to exhaust low-inference hypotheses related to directly observable behaviors before turning to high-inference hypotheses to explain the problem. This approach is prudent considering that inferences generated by psychologists and other clinicians often fall prey to heuristics, biases, and decision-making errors that vary widely across those generating the inferences (see Macmann & Barnett, 1999; Watkins, 2008). Therefore, it may be most prudent and efficient to assume that a student who has difficulties with correct placement of digits in columns when adding numbers simply needs to be taught how to do it correctly through explanations, modeling, and guided practice.

It is possible that the increasing recognition that almost every cognitive ability test score is reflective of some part general factor, some part broad ability or abilities, and some part narrow ability or abilities (in addition to random error) will lead school psychologists away from the cognitive-components and related approaches (Floyd et al., in press). The viability of such approaches seems to be weakened notably because the targeted cognitive abilities may not be measured accurately because of construct-irrelevant variance stemming from the measurement of cognitive abilities at other strata (Watkins, Wilson, Kotz, Carbone, & Babula, 2006). For example, measures of Comprehension–Knowledge, such as those stemming from a vocabulary test, typically relate strongly to the general factor. Measures of Comprehension–Knowledge may also relate substantially to the broad ability of the same name or to narrow abilities subsumed by the broad ability, but the relations between the obtained score and these broad or narrow factors are often much weaker than those relations between the obtained score and the general factor. Even the most highly touted measures of the general factor, IQs, are only about 50–90% attributable to the general factor on average—with 10–50% of variance due to (1) the specific way in which the IQ is formed and (2) error (Jensen, 1998). Although the body of evidence indicating that a test score is due in part to different sources of cognitive abilities may be theoretically interesting, the sources of variance across multiple strata of abilities muddies the waters of clinical interpretation of test and composite scores (Floyd et al., in press). More sophisticated methods are needed to determine the effects of cognitive abilities at each stratum of the CHC theory model.

Perhaps the most deleterious effects of focusing on cognitive abilities and cognitive processes are that viable alternative hypotheses for explaining the reasons for academic troubles are not typically considered. As a result, assessors may attribute causality to within-child deficits that are not seen as malleable. In addition, it is unlikely that most school psychologists engage in assessment of the learner plus assessment of their instruction, their curriculum, and their educational environment during assessment (Howell et al., 2008). For example, some school psychologists probably consider only minimally the child's ecology (e.g., in the classroom) and his or her interaction with it (Ysseldyke & Elliott, 1999). For example, the following may be causes of poor performance in mathematics in the classroom: (1) the child does not want to complete the math problems, (2) external motivators for performing the math problem are absent, or (3) math problem worksheets are aversive to the child, so that the child avoids or escapes from them (Witt, Daly, & Noell, 2000). In a similar vein, the problem may be happening because of variables at the broader classroom or system levels (Shapiro, 2000). It may be that a focus on immediate and more distal environmental influences on behavior promotes more efficient and more effective solutions to the achievement problems than does cognitive ability testing or any other type of individual assessment that leads to a preponderance of within-child attributions and away from a focus on alterable variables (Howell et al., 2008).

What Should Be Done about the Problem?

The third question, What should be done about the problem? addresses intervention development and implementation and logically follows from the conclusions drawn at the previous step of problem solving. As noted earlier, despite the promise of tailoring treatments to the results of cognitive ability testing, much of this promise has been unfulfilled, and there is little doubt that this step in problem solving reveals an Achilles' heel for those advocating the importance of cognitive ability tests and their scores. At present, there is no sizable body of evidence revealing that scores from tests measuring cognitive abilities distal to achievement provide direct links to effective academic interventions (also known as treatment utility; Braden & Kratochwill, 1997; Gresham & Witt, 1997). Although valid arguments are made that school psychologists and other professionals are the ones who link results to interventions (i.e., not the tests or test results per se), (1) it is expected that results from these tests should inform such decisions and (2) there are research designs that can test assumptions of the treatment utility of cognitive ability test scores (Hayes, Nelson, & Jarrett, 1987; Nelson-Gray, 2003). It does appear that Naglieri and colleagues have demonstrated significant efforts in recent years to protect or overcome this limitation by demonstrating that the results of the Cognitive Assessment System (Naglieri & Das, 1997; Naglieri & Johnson, 2000) produce decisions leading to positive treatment outcomes for some children. Berninger's (2001, 2006) component-skills approach (mentioned earlier) also appears to have accumulated empirical evidence supporting a process of universal screening, in-depth assessment, and intervention. Advocates of the application of CHC theory (e.g., Mather & Wendling, 2005) have offered useful suggestions for linking test scores that measure the CHC broad and narrow abilities to interventions, but, to my knowledge, new empirical evidence is not offered.

There are many school psychologists and other experts—shackled by limitations in measurement and asked to develop high-inference hypotheses—who possess the skills to interpret a large number of cognitive ability test scores in order to develop sound interventions to treat reading, mathematics, and writing problems. Perhaps they complete an analysis of task performance, consider carefully the patterns of key cognitive processes relevant to the academic domains, and integrate information from a variety of sources and instruments. These experts may even recommend interventions that (1) capitalize on relative or normative strengths evidenced from test scores, (2) allow for compensation for relative or normative weaknesses, and (3) remediate relative or normative weaknesses. On the other hand, they may simply recommend interventions that yield positive gains for most everyone who engages in them. Although there is little empirical support for the practice (and some evidence that indicates that it is not an effective practice, as described later), the selection of interventions based on consideration of cognitive abilities and processes is not necessarily problematic during this stage of problem solving, as long as evidence is collected to determine the effects of these interventions during the next step of problem solving (Hale & Fiorello, 2004). Regardless of the source of evidence informing intervention selection, those interventions that are based on principles of learning and that have solid empirical support will most likely be the most effective.

The treatment utility of cognitive ability scores is intertwined with prominent criticisms of *aptitude × treatment interactions* (ATIs; Cronbach, 1957, 1975; Corno et al., 2002; Reschly, 2008; Reschly & Ysseldyke, 2002; Whitener, 1989). ATIs reflect differential RTIs due to the aptitudes displayed by those experiencing the intervention, and they are at the heart of differentiated instruction. Some advocates of differentiated instruction within school settings have been encouraged by results from ATI research, and they have sought and applied cognitive ability aptitude measures that they believed would be lawfully related to intervention outcomes (see Kavale & Forness, 1999; Mann, 1979). School psychologists and special educators historically have been some of their strongest advocates in school settings. Despite the historical use of these cognitive ability aptitude measures, there are at least four serious challenges associated with applying to practice ATIs identified in research. These challenges relate to (1) the measurement of the aptitude constructs and use of these measures, (2) the sheer number of possible aptitudes, (3) the existing evidence for using cognitive ability measures to guide differentiated instruction, and (4) the availability of a better method to determine whether differentiated instruction is needed. The first three challenges are addressed in this subsection, and the final challenge is addressed in the subsection titled "Did the Intervention Work?"

First, as noted earlier, interpretation of measures of cognitive abilities has its limitations, and inferences drawn about related cognitive processes may be idiosyncratic and are most likely error prone. In addition, whereas most cognitive ability aptitude measures are continuous variables and most likely normally distributed in the population, cognitive ability aptitudes in practice have been conceptualized as categorical variables (e.g., high aptitude and low aptitude). This process of converting a continuous variable to a categorical variable focuses on the extremes of the distribution and fails to inform practices regarding what to do with those individuals without either high or low aptitude (who would be the largest group because they lie below the hump of the normal curve). In addition, no sound method seems to have been offered to guide decision making regarding identifying the appropriate categories to represent aptitude levels.

Second, all of the possible aptitudes for learning multiplied by all viable interventions is countless. To demonstrate this point, Cronbach and Snow (Cronbach, 1975; Cronbach & Snow, 1977) made references to entering a hall of mirrors when attending to interactions, coping with a swarm of ATI hypotheses, and struggling to track down fourth-order interactions with any aptitude. The taxonomy of CHC theory—with its 10 or so broad abilities and 70 or so narrow abilities—may only complicate the selection of the cognitive ability aptitudes. Compounding this issue of the multitude of aptitudes is (1) that generalizations about ATIs from basic research studies may not apply to classrooms and (2) that generalizations about ATIs from more applied research may not apply to other schools or classrooms—with this limited generalization most likely being due to additional, uncontrolled interactions. The search for the grand aptitude is ongoing; however, even if a grand aptitude is reliably identified across research studies, in classroom settings this grand aptitude would compete with a host of other variables (e.g., prerequisite academic skills, the clarity with which instructional exercises are presented, and the amount of time devoted to instructional tasks) that are more likely to affect the child's performance.

Third, when research employing cognitive ability tests commonly used by school psychologists has been conducted to identify aptitudes, the series of results have not typically supported the practice of differentiated instruction based on cognitive ability aptitudes. Thus, although there is evidence of ATIs from many studies with aptitudes and aptitude complexes broadly conceived (Corno et al., 2002; Cronbach & Snow, 1977), widespread use of differentiated instruction based on cognitive ability aptitudes does not appear to be an empirically supported practice (Good, Vollmer, Katz, Creek, & Chowdhri, 1993; Gresham & Witt, 1997; Kavale & Forness, 1999). Although it is possible that advances in understanding cognitive ability aptitudes (e.g., based on CHC theory) or aptitude complexes could yield research results more supportive of such differentiated instruction, at present consideration of ATIs based on most cognitive ability aptitudes does not appear fruitful for those engaged in problem solving.

Did the Intervention Work?

The final question, Did the intervention work? focuses problem solvers on collecting data to determine whether the interventions implemented based on the most viable hypotheses led to reductions in the problem. This step requires repeated measurement of some representation of the problem across relatively brief periods, and it is this step that best represents Cronbach's (1975) recommendations for practice. His recommendation was to focus on implementing interventions that produce the greatest effects for the greatest numbers, as well as considering the idiosyncratic characteristics of individuals involved in the interventions, through the use of frequent data collection consistent with progress monitoring (Reschly, 2008; Reschly & Ysseldyke, 2002). As indicated earlier, it may not be fruitful to identify specific aptitudes for learning *before* beginning interventions (i.e., ATIs), but it is vital to consider an individual's response to the intervention *after* it has been implemented because interventions may not always demonstrate their intended effects.

Most cognitive ability measures have not been developed for multiple, repeated administrations over brief periods. It is at this step that traditional cognitive ability tests completely fail to meet the needs of the problem solver—at least at present. CBM measures better address the assessment needs of the problem solver in this step and across the varying steps of the problem-solving model (Shapiro & Lentz, 1985).

Conclusions

School psychologists as a whole know assessment and measurement better than any other group in the schools—and, arguably, better than any other large group in the broader fields of psychology and education. Furthermore, we have historically defined ourselves by our role as testers, in which our great knowledge of assessment and measurement has been apparent. Now, the paradigm shift from "traditional assessment" and resulting consideration of eligibility for special education to use of assessment in a problem-solving context is well under way (Reschly, 2008; Reschly & Ysseldyke, 2002). This paradigm shift is currently being fueled by the recent revisions to the Individuals with Disabilities Education Act that allow for consideration of RTI, in the absence of an IQ–achievement discrepancy, when examining eligibility for special education services as a student with a learning disability.

Although these changes are not the death knell of cognitive ability testing, the field's collective reliance on cognitive ability tests as the focal point of our psychoeducational assessments will come to an end. Even research supporting and recommendations for consideration of three levels of cognitive abilities (i.e., general, broad, and narrow) in well-supported models such as CHC theory do not seem to meet our needs as school psychologists. There is excessive baggage, such as continued accusations of bias associated with IQs, and there remains the belief that individual differences cannot be altered with interventions. Perhaps we have held cognitive ability tests to too high a standard or applied their scores inappropriately in school settings, but it seems obvious that more engagement of school psychologists in observing instructional practices and classroom performance, as well as participation in progress monitoring, will allow us to overcome the reliance on measures of cognitive abilities and inferences about cognitive processes obtained from one-on-one test sessions.

I asked at the beginning of the chapter, Do the exceptionally well-developed and substantiated cognitive ability tests aid school psychologists in applying the problem-solving model to improve the reading, mathematics, and writing skills of children with whom they work? In reply, I can say with confidence that, when more ecologically valid and efficiently administered assessment techniques are available to school psychologists, such as well-developed interviews and CBM probes, these cognitive ability tests should not be given top priority in our assessment batteries. Instead, many advocate the use of CBM across stages of problem solving (e.g., Shinn, 2002, 2008) for good reasons. Brief screening probes from the CBM perspective can be administered repeatedly (rather than at a single point in time) to determine children's level of progress in response to interventions. They tend to match the school or classroom curriculum better than nationally normed achievement tests (Shapiro & Elliott, 1999). CBM probes yield evidence of individual differences that are frequently based on national and sometimes local comparison groups. CBM probes take only a few minutes to administer and score, whereas norm-referenced achievement tests often include a wider variety of tasks but few items of each type, and they take longer to administer and score. Finally, CBM data are often used to link results directly to interventions, whereas cognitive abilities tests are often used in eligibility decision making, and recommendations stemming from them often lay dormant in psychoeducational assessment reports.

I believe that most school psychologists accustomed to norm-referenced testing of cognitive abilities would benefit from the recent provision of CBM benchmarking and progress monitoring probes available commercially through well-designed websites, such as those for the AIMSweb, the Dynamic Indicators of Basic Early Literacy Skills (DIBELS), and Edcheckup (see *www. studentprogress.org* and, in this volume, Marcotte & Hintze, Chapter 5; Burns & Klingbeil, Chapter 6; and Gansle & Noell, Chapter 7). These assessment materials are likely congruent with expectations for instruments found in traditional test kits. In addition, school psychologists who revel in their prowess in integrating assessment results may enjoy learning more about curriculum-based evaluation, which requires such skills and has an individual focus (see Howell & Schumann, Chapter 14, this volume). School psychologists should also not forget that there are limitations to assessing only the learner and that assessment technologies have advanced in a way that allows for a relatively clear picture of the child's ecology (Ysseldyke & Elliott, 1999). School psychologists would benefit greatly from further considering academic achievement as well as the classroom context in which instruction and academic performance occurs (see Howell & Schumann, Chapter 14; Linan-Thompson & Vaughn, Chapter 16; Chard, Ketterlin-Geller, Jungjohann, & Baker, Chapter 17; and McCurdy, Schmitz, & Albertson, Chapter 18, all in this volume).

Although interpretations based on consideration of cognitive process and cognitive ability measures may not have great relevance to problem solving based on academic concerns, school psychologists and other educational professionals should not abandon cognitive theories or those with strong cognitive mechanisms, such as general theories like social–cognitive theory (Bandura, 2001) and its extensions that focus on self-regulated learning (Zimmerman, Bonner, & Kovach, 1996), as well as specific models of the key processes involved in completion of academic tasks (e.g., Kintsch, 1998). Thus they should not fall prey to anticognitive bias or anti-intellectualism (see commentary by Haywood & Switzky, 1986) by ignoring entire fields of study, such as cognitive science (Betchel, Abrahamson, & Graham, 1998; Sobel, 2001). Instead, they should carefully consider the application of such cognitive research findings to practice.

Finally, after more than a year of consideration of the content of this chapter and several revisions, I ask myself with humility, If my daughter begins struggling with reading, mathematics, or writing when she begins first grade in 2009, what questions would I want a school psychologist to ask about her? Would I like for him or her to be focused primarily on cognitive abilities and cognitive processes and to ask, What is her IQ? What does her profile of CHC broad cognitive ability strengths and weaknesses look like? Does she have discrepancies between IQ and achievement? Where does she rank compared with age-based peers on a measure of Comprehension–Knowledge and Fluid Reasoning? Does she have auditory processing problems or visual processing problems? Does she have weak working memory? Or would I prefer that the school psychologist determine the existence of a perceived problem, complete an ecologically minded assessment and develop low-inference hypotheses to explain the reason for the problem, draw on empirically based interventions to remedy the problem, and collect data to determine whether the interventions led to reductions in the problem? There is no doubt that I would prefer the second option, which represents the problem-solving process. I expect that, in the near future, the passion for cognitive ability tests felt by many school psychologists in the past will be transferred to a passion for the problem-solving model applied to academic problems.

References

American Psychiatric Association. (2000). *Diagnostic and statistical manual of mental disorders* (4th ed., text rev.). Washington, DC: Author.

Bandura, A. (2001). Social cognitive theory: An agentic perspective. *Annual Review of Psychology, 52,* 1–29.

Berninger, V. (2001). *Process Assessment of the Learner (PAL) Test Battery for Reading and Writing.* San Antonio, TX: Psychological Corporation.

Berninger, V. (2006). Research-supported ideas for implementing reauthorized IDEA with intelligent professional psychological services. *Psychology in the Schools, 43,* 781–797.

Betchel, W., Abrahamson, A., & Graham, G. (Eds.). (1998). *Companion to cognitive science.* New York: Blackwell.

Binet, A., & Simon, T. (1905). The development of intelligence in the child. *L'anée Psychologique, 14,* 1–90.

Braden, J. P., & Kratochwill, T. R. (1997). Treatment utility of assessment: Myths and realities. *School Psychology Review, 26,* 467–474.

Bransford, J. D., & Stein, B. S. (1984). *The IDEAL problem solver.* New York: Freeman.

Brown-Chidsey, R. (2005). The role of published norm-referenced tests in problem-solving-based assessment. In R. Brown-Chidsey (Ed.), *Assessment for intervention: A problem-solving approach* (pp. 247–266). New York: Guilford Press.

Busse, R. T. (2005). Rating scale applications within the problem-solving model. In R. Brown-Chidsey (Ed.), *Assessment for intervention: A problem-solving approach* (pp. 200–218). New York: Guilford Press.

Carroll, J. B. (1993). *Human cognitive abilities: A survey of factor analytic studies.* New York: Cambridge University Press.

Carroll, J. B. (2003). The higher stratum structure of cognitive abilities: Current evidence supports g and about ten broad factors. In H. Nyborg (Ed.), *The scientific study of general intelligence: Tribute to Arthur R. Jensen* (pp. 5–21). New York: Pergamon.

Christ, T. J. (2008). Best practices in problem analysis. In A. Thomas & J. Grimes (Eds.), *Best practices in school psychology* (5th ed., Vol. 2, pp. 159–176). Bethesda, MD: National Association of School Psychologists.

Colman, A. M. (2001). *A dictionary of psychology.* New York: Oxford University Press.

Corno, L., Cronbach, L. J., Kupermintz, H., Lohman, D. F., Mandinach, E. B., Porteus, A. W., et al. (2002). *Remaking the concept of aptitude: Extending the legacy of Richard E. Snow.* Mahwah, NJ: Erlbaum.

Corsini, R. J. (1999). *The dictionary of psychology.* Philadelphia: Brunner/Mazel.

Cronbach, L. J. (1957). The two disciplines of scientific psychology. *American Psychologist, 12,* 671–684.

Cronbach, L. J. (1975). Beyond the two disciplines of scientific psychology. *American Psychologist, 30,* 116–127.

Cronbach, L. J., & Snow, R. E. (1977). *Aptitudes and instructional methods: A handbook for research on interaction.* New York: Irvington.

Deno, S. L. (2002). Problem-solving as "best practice." In A. Thomas & J. Grimes (Eds.), *Best practices in school psychology* (4th ed., Vol. 1, pp. 37–55). Bethesda, MD: National Association of School Psychologists.

Deno, S. L. (2005). Problem-solving assessment. In R. Brown-Chidsey (Ed.), *Assessment for intervention: A problem-solving approach* (pp. 10–40). New York: Guilford Press.

Fagan, T. K., & Wise, P. S. (2007). *School psychology: Past, present, and future* (3rd ed.). Bethesda, MD: National Association of School Psychologists.

Flanagan, D. P., & Ortiz, S. O. (2002). Best practices in intellectual assessment: Future directions. In A. Thomas & J. Grimes (Eds.), *Best practices in school psychology* (4th ed., Vol. 2, pp. 1352–1372). Bethesda, MD: National Association of School Psychologists.

Fletcher, J. M., Coulter, W. A., Reschly, D. J., & Vaughn, S. (2004). Alternative approaches to the definition and identification of learning disabilities: Some questions and answers. *Annals of Dyslexia, 54,* 304–331.

Fletcher, J. M., Denton, C., & Francis, D. J. (2005). Validity of alternate approaches for the identification of learning disabilities: Operationalizing unexpected underachievement. *Journal of Learning Disabilities, 38,* 545–552.

Fletcher, J. M., Lyon, G. R., Fuchs, L. S., & Barnes, M. A. (2006). *Learning disabilities: From identification to intervention.* New York: Guilford Press.

Floyd, R. G. (2005). Information-processing approaches to interpretation of contemporary intellectual assessment instruments. In D. P. Flanagan & P. Harrison (Eds.), *Contemporary intellectual assessment* (2nd ed., pp. 203–233). New York: Guilford Press.

Floyd, R. G., Bergeron, R., McCormack, A. C., Anderson, J. L., & Hargrove-Owens, G. L. (2005). Are Cattell–Horn–Carroll (CHC) broad ability composite scores exchangeable across batteries? *School Psychology Review, 34,* 386–414.

Floyd, R. G., Clark, M. H., & Shadish, W. R. (2008). The exchangeability of IQs: Implications for professional psychology. *Professional Psychology: Research and Practice, 39,* 414–423.

Floyd, R. G., Keith, T. Z., Taub, G. E., & McGrew, K. S. (2007). Cattell–Horn–Carroll cognitive abilities and their effects on reading decoding skills: *g* has indirect effects, more specific abilities have direct effects. *School Psychology Quarterly, 22,* 200–233.

Floyd, R. G., McGrew, K. S., Barry, A., Rafael, F. A., & Rogers, J. (in press). General and specific effects on Cattell–Horn–Carroll broad ability composites: Analysis of the Woodcock–Johnson III Normative Update CHC factor clusters across development. *School Psychology Review.*

Francis, D. J., Fletcher, J. M., Stuebing, K. K., Lyon, R. L., Shaywitz, B. A., & Shaywitz, S. E. (2005). Psychometric approaches to the identification of LD: IQ and Achievement scores are not sufficient. *Journal of Learning Disabilities, 38,* 98–108.

Good, R. H., III, & Kaminski, R. A. (Eds.). (2002). *Dynamic indicators of basic early literacy skills* (6th ed.). Eugene, OR: Institute for the Development of Educational Achievement.

Good, R. H., III, Vollmer, M., Katz, L., Creek, R. J., & Chowdhri, S. (1993). Treatment utility of the Kaufman Assessment Battery for Children: Effects of matching instruction and student processing strength. *School Psychology Review, 22,* 8–26.

Gresham, F. M., & Witt, J. C. (1997). Utility of intelligence tests for treatment planning, classification, and placement decisions: Recent empirical findings and future directions. *School Psychology Quarterly, 12,* 249–267.

Hale, J. B., & Fiorello, C. A. (2004). *School neuropsychology: A practitioner's handbook.* New York: Guilford Press.

Hayes, S. C., Nelson, R. O., & Jarrett, R. B. (1987). The treatment utility of assessment: A functional approach to evaluating assessment quality. *American Psychologist, 42,* 963–974.

Haywood, H. C., & Switzky, H. N. (1986). Transactionalism and cognitive processes: Reply to Reynolds and Gresham. *School Psychology Review, 15,* 264–267.

Horn, J. L. (1991). Measurement of intellectual capabilities: A review of theory. In K. S. McGrew, J. K. Werder, & R. W. Woodcock, *WJ–R technical manual* (pp. 197–232). Itasca, IL: Riverside.

Hoskyn, M., & Swanson, H. L. (2000). Cognitive processing of low achievers and children with reading disabilities: A selective meta-analytic review of the published literature. *School Psychology Review, 29,* 102–119.

Hosp, J. L., & Reschly, D. J. (2002). Regional differences in school psychology practice. *School Psychology Review, 31,* 11–29.

Howell, K. W., Hosp, J. L., & Kurns, S. (2008). Best practices in curriculum-based evaluation. In A. Thomas & J. Grimes (Eds.), *Best practices in school psychology* (5th ed., Vol. 2, pp. 349–362). Bethesda, MD: National Association of School Psychologists.

Howell, K. W., & Nolet, V. (2000). *Curriculum-based evaluation: Teaching and decision making* (3rd ed.). Scarborough, Ontario, Canada: Wadsworth.

Ikeda, M. J., Neesen, E., & Witt, J. C. (2008). Best practices in universal screening. In A. Thomas & J. Grimes (Eds.), *Best practices in school psychology* (5th ed., Vol. 2, pp. 103–114). Bethesda, MD: National Association of School Psychologists.

Jensen, A. R. (1998). *The g factor: The science of mental ability.* Westport, CT: Praeger.

Jensen, A. R. (2006). *Clocking the mind: Mental chronometry and individual differences.* Amsterdam, Netherlands: Elsevier.

Kaufman, A. S. (1994). *Intelligent testing with the WISC-III.* New York: Wiley.

Kaufman, A. S., & Kaufman, N. L. (2004). *Kaufman Test of Educational Achievement, Second Edition manual.* Circle Pines, MN: American Guidance Service.

Kavale, K. A., & Forness, S. R. (1999). Effectiveness of special education. In C. R. Reynolds & T. B. Gutkin (Eds.), *The handbook of school psychology* (3rd ed., pp. 984–1024). New York: Wiley.

Kintsch, W. (1998). *Comprehension: A paradigm for cognition.* Cambridge, UK: Cambridge University Press.

Kranzler, J. (1999). Current contributions of the psychology of individual differences to school psychology. In C. R. Reynolds & T. B. Gutkin (Eds.), *The handbook of school psychology* (3rd ed., pp. 223–246). New York: Wiley.

Macmann, G. M., & Barnett, D. W. (1999). Diagnostic decision making in school psychology: Understanding and coping with uncertainty. In C. R. Reynolds & T. B. Gutkin (Eds.), *The handbook of school psychology* (3rd ed., pp. 519–548). New York: Wiley.

Mann, L. (1979). *On the trail of process: A historical perspective on cognitive processes and their training.* New York: Grune & Stratton.

Mather, N., & Kaufman, N. (2006). Introduction to the special issue, part one: It's about the *what,* the *how well,* and the *why. Psychology in the Schools, 43,* 747–752.

Mather, N., & Wendling, B. J. (2005). Linking cognitive assessment results to academic interventions for students with learning disabilities. In D. P. Flanagan & P. L. Harrison (Eds.), *Contemporary intellectual assessment: Theories, tests, and issues* (2nd ed., pp. 269–294). New York: Guilford Press.

McGrew, K. S. (2005). The Cattell–Horn–Carroll theory of cognitive abilities: Past, present, and future. In D. P. Flanagan & P. L. Harrison (Eds.), *Contemporary intellectual assessment: Theories, tests, and issues* (2nd ed., pp. 136–181). New York: Guilford Press.

McGrew, K. S. (2009). CHC theory and the human cognitive abilities project: Standing on the shoulders of the giants of psychometric intelligence research. *Intelligence, 37,* 1–10.

McGrew, K. S., & Woodcock, R. W. (2001). *Woodcock–Johnson III technical manual.* Itasca, IL: Riverside.

Merrell, K., Ervin, R. A., & Gimpel Peacock, G. (2006). *School psychology for the 21st century: Foundations and practices.* New York: Guilford Press.

Naglieri, J. A. (2002). Best practices in interventions for school psychologists: A cognitive approach. In A. Thomas & J. Grimes (Eds.), *Best practices in school psychology* (4th ed., Vol. 2, pp. 1373–1393). Bethesda, MD: National Association of School Psychologists.

Naglieri, J. A., & Das, J. P. (1997). *Cognitive Assessment System.* Itasca, IL: Riverside.

Naglieri, J. A., & Johnson, D. (2000). Effectiveness of a cognitive strategy intervention to improve math calculation based on the PASS theory. *Journal of Learning Disabilities, 33,* 591–597.

National Association of School Psychologists.

(2007). *NASP position statement on identification of students with specific learning disabilities.* Retrieved October 7, 2007 *www. nasponline.org/about_nasp/positionpapers/ StudentsLearningDisabilities.pdf*

Neisser, U., Boodoo, G., Bouchard, T. J., Boykin, A. W., Brody, N., Ceci, S. J., et al. (1996). Intelligence: Knowns and unknowns. *American Psychologist, 51,* 77–101.

Nelson-Gray, R. O. (2003). Treatment utility of psychological assessment. *Psychological Assessment, 15,* 521–531.

Reschly, D. J. (2008). School psychology paradigm shift and beyond. In A. Thomas & J. Grimes (Eds.), *Best practices in school psychology* (5th ed., Vol. 1, pp. 3–16). Bethesda, MD: National Association of School Psychologists.

Reschly, D. J., & Grimes, J. P. (2002). Best practices in intellectual assessment. In A. Thomas & J. Grimes (Eds.), *Best practices in school psychology* (4th ed., Vol. 2, pp. 1337–1351). Bethesda, MD: National Association of School Psychologists

Reschly, D. J., & Ysseldyke, J. E. (2002). Paradigm shift: The past is not the future. In A. Thomas & J. Grimes (Eds.), *Best practices in school psychology* (4th ed., Vol. 1, pp. 3–20). Bethesda, MD: National Association of School Psychologists.

Sarason, S. B. (1976). The unfortunate fate of Alfred Binet and school psychology. *Teacher College Record, 11,* 579–592.

Schmidt, F. L. (2002). The role of general cognitive ability and job performance: Why there cannot be a debate. *Human Performance, 15,* 187–211.

Shapiro, E. S. (2000). School psychology from an instructional perspective: Solving big, not little problems. *School Psychology Review, 29,* 560–572.

Shapiro, E. S. (2005). *Academic skills problems: Direct assessment and intervention* (3rd ed.). New York: Guilford Press.

Shapiro, E. S., & Elliott, E. S. (1999). Curriculum-based assessment and other performance-based assessment strategies. In C. R. Reynolds & T. B. Gutkin (Eds.), *The handbook of school psychology* (3rd ed., pp. 383–408). New York: Wiley.

Shapiro, E. S., & Kratochwill, T. R. (Eds.). (2000). *Behavioral assessment in schools: Theory, research, and clinical foundations* (2nd ed.). New York: Guilford Press.

Shapiro, E. S., & Lentz, F. E. (1985). Assessing academic behavior: A behavioral approach. *School Psychology Review, 14,* 325–338.

Shinn, M. R. (1998). *Advanced applications of curriculum-based measurement.* New York: Guilford Press.

Shinn, M. R. (2002). Best practices in using curriculum-based measurement in a problem-solving model. In A. Thomas & J. Grimes (Eds.), *Best practices in school psychology* (4th ed., pp. 671–697). Bethesda, MD: National Association of School Psychologists.

Shinn, M. R. (2008). Best practices in using curriculum-based measurement in a problem-solving model. In A. Thomas & J. Grimes (Eds.), *Best practices in school psychology* (5th ed., Vol. 2, pp. 243–262). Bethesda, MD: National Association of School Psychologists.

Sobel, C. P. (2001). *The cognitive sciences: An interdisciplinary approach.* Mountain View, CA: Mayfield.

Sternberg, R. (1977). *Intelligence, information processing, and analogical reasoning.* Hillsdale, NJ: Erlbaum.

Sternberg, R. J., & Detterman, D. K. (Eds.). (1986). *What is intelligence? Contemporary viewpoints on its nature and definition.* Norwood, NJ: Ablex.

Thorndike, E. L. (1921). Intelligence and its measurement: A symposium. *Journal of Educational Psychology, 12,* 123–147.

Tilly, W. D. III. (2002). Best practices in school psychology as a problem-solving enterprise. In A. Thomas & J. Grimes (Eds.), *Best practices in school psychology* (4th ed., Vol. 1, pp. 21–36). Bethesda, MD: National Association of School Psychologists.

Tilly, W. D. III. (2008). The evolution of school psychology to science-based practice: Problem-solving and the three-tiered model. In A. Thomas & J. Grimes (Eds.), *Best practices in school psychology* (5th ed., Vol. 1, pp. 17–36). Bethesda, MD: National Association of School Psychologists.

VandenBos, G. R. (2006). *APA dictionary of psychology.* New York: American Psychological Association.

Watkins, M. W. (2008). Errors in diagnostic decision making and clinical judgment. In T. B. Gutkin & C. R. Reynolds (Eds.), *The handbook of school psychology* (4th ed., pp. 210–229). New York: Wiley.

Watkins, M. W., Wilson, S. M., Kotz, K. M., Carbone, M. C., & Babula, T. (2006). Factor structure of the Wechsler Intelligence Scale for Children-Fourth Edition among referred students. *Educational and Psychological Measurement, 66,* 975–983.

Wechsler, D. (1939). *The measurement of adult intelligence.* Baltimore: Williams & Wilkins.

Whitener, E. M. (1989). A meta-analytic review of the effect on learning of the interaction between prior achievement and instructional support. *Review of Educational Research, 59,* 65–86.

Willis, J., & Dumont, R. (2006). And never the twain shall meet: Can response to intervention and cognitive assessment be reconciled? *Psychology in the Schools, 43,* 901–908.

Witt, J. C., Daly, E. M., & Noell, G. (2000). *Functional assessments: A step-by-step guide to solving academic and behavior problems.* Longmont, CO: Sopris West.

Yates, B. T., & Taub, J. (2003). Assessing the costs, cost-effectiveness, and cost-benefit of psychological assessment: We should, we can, here's how. *Psychological Assessment, 15,* 478–495.

Ysseldyke, J., & Elliott, J. (1999). Effective instructional practices: Implications for assessing educational environments. In C. R. Reynolds & T. B. Gutkin (Eds.), *The handbook of school psychology* (3rd ed., pp. 497–518). New York: Wiley.

Zimmerman, B. J., Bonner, S., & Kovach, R. (1996). *Developing self-regulated learners: Beyond achievement to self-efficacy.* Washington, DC: American Psychological Association.

Chapter 5

Assessment of Academic Skills in Reading within a Problem-Solving Model

Amanda M. Marcotte
John M. Hintze

For problem solvers, assessment is inextricably linked to instructional decisions. Assessment involves testing students in order to arrive at quantifiable scores that reflect student performance on a set of test questions. However, the process of assessment is much broader than simply administering tests. Assessment is a process of gathering data, examining student performance, and making decisions in the broader context of curriculum and instruction. Effective evaluators have an understanding of the domain in which the evaluation is taking place, the range of task difficulty in that domain, and the varieties of tasks students are able and unable to do. They also know what typical student performance looks like so as to compare performance of struggling students. With a comprehensive understanding of the factors that contribute to learning problems, evaluators are able to develop hypotheses about the reasons students continue to struggle.

This chapter is designed to examine the developmental reading process in the context of a problem-solving approach. In doing so, it presents problem solving as a dynamic, multistepped approach to evaluation. Because such comprehensive evaluations require a broad understanding of the skills

and deficits related to reading problems, this chapter presents an overview of the five essential components of literacy instruction. Through a deeper understanding of early literacy development, problem-solving assessors should be able to better identify specific skill deficits and instructional priorities for struggling readers. Additionally, this chapter presents a variety of assessment tools that can assist the evaluator in quantifying reading problems and examining student performance as a function of instructional changes. For problem-solving educators, formative assessment serves as a conduit to effective decision making, in which evaluation requires a comprehensive understanding of every dimension of curriculum, what is intended to be taught, what is taught, and what is learned.

Problem Solving as a Dynamic, Multistep Evaluation Process

There are five related purposes for which educators assess students in a problem-solving model: (1) problem identification, (2) problem certification, (3) exploring solutions, (4) goal setting, and (5) monitoring student progress (Deno, 2002; Shinn, Nolet, &

Knutson, 1990). For the purpose of identifying problems, educators gather data to identify whether a problem exists by examining the difference between the student's current performance level and what is expected of the student. Expectations can be based on the performances of typical peers or on important learning objectives students are expected to meet. Using these data, problem solvers examine the magnitude of the observed discrepancy to draw conclusions about the extent of the observed problem. As such, the magnitude of the problem can be described in terms of the discrepancy observed between the target student as compared with same-grade peers or in terms of their failure to achieve important academic criteria. These latter activities are part of problem certification, in which the magnitude, for the purpose of certifying the discrepancy, is indeed a problem that needs to be resolved.

Problem solvers engage in assessment for the purpose of setting meaningful goals for students through a process of examining the current performance and the presenting discrepancy. From this analysis the evaluator can determine the amount of growth in learning a student would need to achieve to close the gap. The best goals are written so that they are ambitious enough to reduce the observed discrepancy in a meaningful way and yet realistic enough so as to be attainable with strategic instructional planning. Valid and reliable assessments are essential for problem solvers to gather data that provide a baseline of the current skill estimates from which they set meaningful goals for students. Effective goals must be measureable and should be set as outcome criteria on an assessment validated for the specific skill for which the problem is observed. Therefore, the most useful tests for goal setting are the same tests used to help define the magnitude of the problem during the first two steps of problem-solving evaluation. An additional consideration in selecting tests for initial data collection is that assessment tools used for progress monitoring must have multiple, equivalent forms so as to be given repeatedly to measure student growth toward the goal.

Rather than focus on the assessment process to identify underlying disabilities for struggling students, problem solvers engage in assessment for the purpose of identifying specific skill deficits. In doing so, data is collected that can be used to design instructional programming to target foundational skills the student is lacking. Assessments useful for evaluating students' reading acquisition help us to observe students' performance on the essential components of literacy development, including phonological processing skills, phonics acquisition, reading fluency, vocabulary, and comprehension outcomes.

Once an instructional plan is in place to address the identified skill deficits, the progress of struggling students warrants close supervision so as to ensure that meaningful progress is gained. The purpose of progress monitoring assessment activities is to closely examine student progress in relation to the instruction they receive. Progress monitoring is a strategy for monitoring student achievement toward the goals set for them through the use of continuous assessment. Regularly, students are tested using brief assessments—all of equivalent form and content—to evaluate important general indicators of a broader academic domain. This method of continuous assessment results in a set of data that reflects a learning trend that can be evaluated for program effectiveness. When students are making gains toward the goals set for them, their academic programming can be judged effective. For those who are not making expected gains, their programs should be reconsidered and redesigned.

Effective problem-solving evaluation requires the use of a unique set of testing tools for formative evaluation, in which assessment can occur amid instruction, providing educators frequent feedback on the effectiveness of their instructional programming. With the goal of developing a valid and reliable data-gathering system that married teacher observations of student learning to the reliability and validity of testing procedures, researchers created the technology of curriculum-based measurement (CBM; Deno & Mirkin, 1977). CBM can be broadly defined as a process of testing through which data are collected frequently so as to gather a dataset of the academic performance of an individual student in a target skill area (Deno, 1985). More specifically, a brief assessment is given in an academic domain of interest. The score from this initial test is plotted on a line graph and compared with criteria for problem identification decisions.

From this initial score, a goal is determined based on the expected rate of learning and a time line for judging progress. The goal is plotted on the line graph. At set intervals (i.e., each week or each month), the student is assessed using equivalent forms of the same test so that any variability in the scores reflects student learning in the specific skill area. Each test score is plotted on the line graph so as to examine the student's rate of learning in comparison with the expected rate of learning. As this dataset grows, it reflects the dynamic interaction between instruction and learning that is necessary for problem-solving evaluation. Researchers have described CBM as providing the measurement technology necessary for operationalizing the decisions made throughout the problem-solving process (Kaminski & Good, 1998).

Tests useful for the decision-making process of CBM must be standardized and reliable testing procedures and must exist in multiple equivalent forms. That is, each form of the test must elicit reliable scores for which differences in test scores can be attributed to student learning. The test must elicit valid scores that reflect vital indicators of a specific academic domain so that any improvement in test scores can reliably be interpreted as meaningful learning. When tests reflect the essential skills of curricular content, results from CBM are useful across the broad range of instructional decisions. Because CBM requires that tests be given frequently, tests useful for CBM must be brief and efficient to administer and score. Finally, when given frequently over time, the tests must elicit scores that reflect student learning as a function of instructional programming so as to make timely educational decisions.

CBM effectively allows educators to draw conclusions at each step of a problem-solving evaluation, and two additional types of tests may also prove useful when examining persistent reading problems. Standardized norm-referenced tests (NRTs) and criterion-referenced tests (CRTs) are typically designed to examine the broad range of skills that subsume a larger academic domain. NRTs tend to include a vast range of test items, of which only a few of the items represent each subset skill. For example, an NRT designed to evaluate reading might include items rep-resenting nonword decoding and real-word reading, vocabulary, sentence- level comprehension, and passage comprehension, and the score of the test would be an estimate of overall reading ability. CRTs tend to sample a less broad academic domain and to provide more items to estimate each subskill. For example, a CRT might be designed to evaluate phonics skills and to provide an array of items in which students are asked to read and spell a variety of words with varying spelling patterns so as to help identify phonics skills that have been mastered and areas of weakness.

NRTs and CRTs differ in how their scores are interpreted. NRTs are used to make comparisons between an individual student's performance and a typical peer group. CRTs are used to examine a student's level of skill acquisition compared with the expectation of content mastery. Both tests elicit scores that can be interpreted for the moment in time at which the test was given. CBM can also be used to make between-student comparisons, similar to other NRTs, and can be used to examine the mastery of essential skills necessary to achievement in a broader academic domain, similar to CRTs. However, the most useful characteristic of CBM is that it allows educators to examine within-student comparisons. That is, CBM allows educators to determine rates of learning for an individual student amid varying contextual factors, such as the content and delivery of instruction. Whereas NRTs and CRTs are typically time-consuming to administer and do not exist in multiple equivalent formats that can be given frequently, CBM is designed to be given often for constant feedback on an individual student's performance.

Although NRTs and CRTs are not useful for answering each question of a dynamic problem-solving assessment, there are enabling skills to reading that are difficult to observe and measure for which these tests might be useful. For example, there are limits to the CBM technology when measuring vocabulary skills. For problem-solving evaluators who suspect that vocabulary deficits are a contributing factor to reading problems, NRTs are useful for quantifying this area of discrepancy. Some NRTs are useful for identifying the magnitude of a problem when a student's performance can be compared with those of a normative peer group. Some

CRTs can also be useful for problem identification when conclusions can be drawn regarding students' levels of skill acquisition when compared with a criterion of mastery. Additionally, some CRTs can be useful for gathering information about skill deficits with which to design targeted instructional programming. Therefore, problem-solving evaluators must develop a battery of assessments useful for CBM so as to address each step of a problem-solving assessment, as well as to develop expertise in the purposeful selection and use of other available testing tools.

Originally, two CBM tests existed for the evaluation of reading—Oral Reading Fluency (CBM-R or ORF) and CBM Spelling (CBM-S)—and provided an estimate of student literacy achievement. As with all CBM measures, these were designed to assess students in limited time so as to get a fluency estimate that should increase as a function of learning. For ORF, students are asked to read a standard grade-level reading passage for 1-minute, and the words read correctly represent the score elicited by the test. For CBM-S, students are asked to spell a series of standard grade-level words and given 7–10 seconds to spell each word, depending on the grade level of the students. The test score is derived from counting the correct letter sequences in each word. Both ORF and CBM-S are useful for observing student performance on important indicators of overall literacy development to identify whether there is a problem, to establish measurable goals, to guide instructional decisions, and to monitor student progress. However, both measures can be used only to evaluate students who have already achieved a relatively advanced level of literacy skills. Although useful for students with emergent reading behaviors, ORF and CBM-S are less useful for examining students with preliterate skills or for students with underlying skill deficits that may contribute to learning failure.

Researchers developed a set of measures based on the CBM technology that reflect the developmental nature of the reading process. The Dynamic Indicators of Basic Early Literacy Skills (DIBELS; Kaminski & Good, 1998) and assessments similar to the DIBELS can be used to evaluate the progress of students who are in the initial stages of learning to read. These tests of early literacy skills are also fluency measures in which students are given a limited time to respond; thus the scores provide evaluators with estimates of a student's level of acquisition and fluency for each skill. The tests from the DIBELS that are useful for measuring early phonics skills include a letter-naming fluency task (LNF) and a nonsense-words fluency task (NWF). To administer LNF, a student is given a testing probe of randomly presented upper- and lower-case letters and asked to name as many letters as they know for one minute. NWF was designed to examine the agility with which students can decode simple words. Similar to LNF, students are presented with a testing probe and asked to respond for 1 minute. During the minute's time, the test administrator counts the number of letter sounds the students read correctly within each nonsense word.

DIBELS also include two tests of phonological awareness, Initial Sound Fluency (ISF) and Phoneme Segmentation Fluency (PSF). In ISF, students are presented with a testing plate of four pictures and told the names of each one. Students are asked to point to the picture that begins with the sound the tester presents. For example, they are presented with a probe and the tester says, "This is mouse, flowers, pillow, letters. Which picture begins with /m/?" The PSF test is administered using standard test procedures through which students are orally presented words and asked to segment each sound component in each word. For example, students are asked, "Tell me the sounds in /that/," and the student is expected to answer /th/, /a/, /t/ as three distinct sounds. Students are given credit for every partial and unique sound unit they say.

In addition to those included with DIBELS, other tests of early literacy skills are useful for CBM. For example, the letter-sound fluency test is administered similarly to LNF; however, students are asked to say the sounds of each letter rather than the names. Another test is the Word Identification Fluency Test, in which students are asked to read lists of real words for 1 minute (WIF; Deno, Mirkin, & Chang, 1982). Each test of early literacy that is useful for problem-solving evaluation is designed to help evaluate vital indicators of developing reading skills. Each measure makes use of a relatively brief response time, which allows evaluators to examine the degree of skill acquisition and results in dynamic test scores. As children acquire a level of fluency with each skill, they are able to answer more items quickly and accurately, resulting in sensitive indicators of learning.

Although problem solvers must know how to administer and score these tests, the scores they elicit can be interpreted only within the context of instructional content and delivery, with a deep understanding of the developmental nature of reading. An effective evaluator must have access to an array of assessments that allow him or her to address the dynamic questions of a problem-solving assessment, but he or she also must be able to interpret them within the context of reading as a broad developmental construct. Thus problem-solving evaluation requires an understanding of effective instruction so as to draw conclusions about student performance in the context of the instruction they have received. Knowing best practices in teaching allows the problem solver to consider the quality, appropriateness, and effectiveness of the instruction delivered and to design alternative programming for struggling students.

The Relationship of Essential Skills for Literacy Development to Reading Assessment

Effective reading instruction is designed on a deep understanding of the interaction between our spoken language and how it is represented in print, from the smallest units of sound to the semantic and grammatical mechanics of spoken and printed words. Sounds in spoken language are represented in print by letters and letter combinations. Letters are put together in predictable ways so as to form words, and words are put together in meaningful ways so as to create sentences. Print is our spoken language coded on paper. This simple concept is confounded by the abstract and important interactions between linguistic understanding, vocabulary development, phonemic awareness, and mechanical phonics. At any point, a student may fail to make these connections. Therefore, problem-solving evaluators must understand the development of reading so as to identify the specific points on which students may fail to make adequate progress.

Additionally, they must know effective reading instruction so that they can critically examine that which is delivered to struggling students and identify environmental factors that may contribute to the failure.

Although learning to read may appear a natural process for some, it is in fact a purposeful process through which children learn the mechanics of how spoken language is represented in print (Moats, 2000). Effective literacy instruction takes into account the complex interaction between speech and print and addresses both. It includes immersion in rich spoken language, robust vocabulary development, and listening comprehension strategies. It also includes direct and systematic instruction in phonics for automatic word reading and fluency. The best literacy instruction is designed to strategically incorporate both by addressing the essential components of decoding through phonics and robust oral language development. Large-scale meta-analyses have identified the most essential components of effective early literacy instruction (National Reading Panel [NRP], 2000; National Research Council [NRC], 1998; see also Linan-Thompson & Vaughn, Chapter 16, this volume). Minimally, it is essential to ensure that instruction in phonemic awareness, phonics, fluency, vocabulary, and comprehension are part of all early reading curricula. Assessment of these skills plays an essential role in ensuring that the instruction that is delivered is appropriate to students' instructional needs.

Phonemic Awareness

Phonemic awareness is an essential reading readiness skill that enables the learning of the alphabetic code that connects our spoken language to our written language (Adams, 1990; Brady, 1997; NRC, 1998). Phonemic awareness is the conscious ability to perceive individual sound units in spoken language (Moats, 2000; NRP, 2000). It is a complex cognitive process that rests within a larger domain of phonological awareness (Goldsworthy, 2003). Phonological awareness can be defined as recognition of all the ways spoken language can be broken down into smaller sound units (Goldsworthy, 2003; NRP, 2000). Within spoken language are smaller sound units. For example, sentences can be broken down into words, words into syllables, and syllables into the isolated sound units (Goldsworthy, 2003). Phonemic awareness is the ability to perceive these smallest units of sound, called phonemes.

Reading involves a sound processing system in which students recognize strings of letters, translate those letters into the individual sounds they represent, and blend those sounds into larger units of word sounds (Moats, 2000). Instruction in phonemic awareness facilitates the word reading process by making sense of the elusive sound–symbol relationships of the alphabetic code (Adams, 1990; NRC, 1998). Repeatedly, studies demonstrate that when young children can perceive and manipulate the sounds in language, they are better able to learn letter–sound correspondences, better able to blend sounds to make words, and better able to spell words in their writing (Ball & Blachman, 1988; Bradley & Bryant, 1983; Ehri, 2004; Lundberg, Frost, & Peterson, 1988; Nation & Hulme, 1997). For many children, phonemic awareness develops through exposure to language and reading instruction; however, without explicit instruction in phonemic awareness, this abstract concept of sound perception will elude many children (Adams, 1990; Juel, Griffith, & Gough, 1986). Lack of phonemic awareness is strongly correlated with reading disability; however, research suggests that such a skill deficit does not always result in a reading disability, as phonemic awareness can be taught to all children (Ball & Blachman, 1988, 1991).

The goal of phonemic awareness instruction is to ensure that children develop phonemic processing skills such that they can identify, isolate, and manipulate the sounds they hear. To get students to manipulate phonemes, comprehensive phonological awareness instruction begins with helping students become aware of the larger sound units of speech; students are taught to hear, identify, and manipulate words in sentences and syllables in words.

In preschool and the beginning months of kindergarten, phonological awareness instruction begins with teaching children to listen to sounds in the environment, to understand what it means to listen, to understand the concepts of same and different, and to increase their ability to remember sounds they hear (Adams, Foorman, Lundberg, & Beeler, 1998). Once students develop listening skills for learning, instruction should incorporate phonological awareness activities into their daily routines. Some phonological awareness activities are designed to help students become aware of words in sentences and syllables in words. Others help young children develop their sound manipulation skills through rhyming activities.

Phonological awareness activities give young children practice in manipulating sounds in language and prepare them for the most complex phonological of phonemic awareness, which includes identifying and manipulating individual sounds of speech. Phonemic awareness tasks consist of segmenting, blending, deleting, and making substitutions of individual sounds of spoken words. Segmenting is achieved when students are able to isolate and produce individual sounds from a spoken word. For example, the word *cat* is segmented as /c/, /a/, and /t/. Blending activities involve orally presenting individual sounds to students, which they then blend together to make the word. For example, students are orally presented the individual sounds /f/, /i/, /t/ and prompted to say the sounds together to generate the word *fit*. Sound manipulation activities may ask students to delete sounds from words and replace them with new sounds to make new words. An example of a manipulation routine is to orally present the word *can* and ask the students to say "can" without saying /c/. Then replace the /c/ with a /p/ to produce the word *pan*.

Importantly, findings of the meta-analysis conducted by the National Reading Panel (NRP, 2000) found blending and segmenting instruction to have the largest effects on preparing students to learn to read when compared with other phonemic awareness tasks (Ehri, 2004). The ability to segment phonemes helps young children develop a better understanding of the letters of the alphabet and the role they represent in spoken words and print and eventually supports strategic spelling skills. Blending, on the other hand, appears to support the decoding process. Students who can perceive individual sounds in speech and blend those sounds together to make words are better able to decode unknown words by recognizing the isolated sounds represented in the print and synthesizing them into the whole word they represent.

Assessing for Phonological Deficits

When a student is observed to struggle in the early decoding stage of reading development and it is suspected that phonemic awareness may be contributing to the problem, a problem-solving school psychologist will begin the evaluation process by selecting testing procedures to help identify the problem, examining the magnitude of the problem, and providing useful information for instructional planning. Additionally, the school psychologist will examine the delivery of phonemic awareness instruction. A thorough evaluation requires an examination of what phonological skills have been taught to students and how explicit and systematic the delivery of the instruction has been. Additionally, evaluators need to understand the logical order of phonological skill development so as to identify any skill deficits a student may have.

The DIBELS were specifically designed to help educators prevent reading problems from occurring by helping to identify students who fail to develop essential early literacy skills (Kaminski & Good, 1998). As phonemic awareness is critical to reading acquisition, the DIBELS include two tests that allow educators to identify students who fail to develop this foundational skill. The ISF (Good & Kaminski, 2002) can be used to identify problems in early phonological development by measuring children's ability to identify initial sound in words. Using ISF, problem-solving evaluators can compare students' performances with those of typical peers through local norms (Shinn, 1988, 1989). They can set a goal for improvement in identifying initial sounds in words, which has direct implications for instructional programming. The ISF test exists in multiple forms so educators can collect data frequently and evaluate student growth on this specific skill over time.

Whereas ISF is useful for measuring the early phonological awareness skill of initial sound identification, PSF (Good & Kaminski, 2002) allows educators to evaluate discrepant phonemic segmentation skills, set performance goals, and frequently monitor student progress toward those goals. Progress in phoneme segmentation proficiency is observed as students are better able to identify the individually phonemes in each word. As is true for CBM measures, the results of PSF can be compared with typical student performance, with benchmark performance criteria, and with normative growth rates.

There are a vast array of phonological awareness activities that students can be asked that represent the entire development continuum of phonological awareness development. The DIBELS provide two measures that can help quantify a student's awareness of initial sounds and their ability to segment sounds in words. However, often problem-solving evaluators seek more information about students' phonological awareness skills. Norm-referenced assessments are available to provide evidence identifying phonological awareness as a problem and may provide one vehicle for quantifying the discrepancy of the problem in relation to typically developing peers. Two examples of NRTs that allow school psychologists to make peer comparisons in the area of phonological awareness include the Comprehensive Test of Phonological Processing (CTOPP; Wagner, Torgesen & Rashotte, 1999) and the Test of Phonological Awareness (TOPA; Torgesen & Bryant, 1993). Criterion-referenced tests useful for making decisions about students' phonological awareness development include the Yopp–Singer Test of Phoneme Segmentation (Yopp, 1995) and the Emergent Literacy Tests of the Ekwall–Shanker Reading Inventory (Shanker & Ekwall, 2000). Another useful resource for examining student performance on a range of phonological tasks, from detecting rhymes to counting phonemes, is The Assessment Test from the phonemic awareness classroom curriculum Phonemic Awareness in Young Children (Adams, Foorman, Lundberg, & Beeler, 1998).

Phonics

Phonological awareness instruction is essential to helping students understand phonics and to increasing the efficiency of phonics instruction (NRP, 2000). Phonics is distinctly different from phonological or phonemic awareness. Whereas the latter are purely about the sounds in spoken language, phonics refers to the predictable association between printed symbols and the sounds we speak (Moats, 2000; NRP, 2000). The English language is represented in print through a rule-based alphabetic code. The benefit of such a speech–print system is that, by learning the rules of the alphabetic code, students are able to read and write any word in our language, known or unknown to them.

Effective phonics instruction provides students with the essential strategies for recognizing written words they encounter for the first time or those so rarely encountered that they remain unfamiliar by sight. When students are given strategies, they are armed with skills to independently solve novel problems. Thus for emerging readers phonics instruction is essential to provide them with the keys to unlock the code of the written language. For all readers phonics is essential for deciphering any word unfamiliar to us.

The initial objective of phonics instruction is to teach children strategies of decoding. Decoding is a word recognition process through which a reader translates letters into the sounds they represent and then merges those sounds together to form the word (Brady, 1997). The subcomponent skills essential for decoding include visual recognition and phonological translation of every letter in the alphabet, as well as various letter combinations and strategies for synthesizing the sounds represented in print into words. An equally important objective of phonics instruction is to provide students with enough practice in decoding common words and spelling patterns so that students no longer need to decode every word they see and are able to recognize words automatically (NRP, 2000; Ehri, 2004). Helping students to read words automatically requires ample opportunities to successfully apply the decoding strategies they have been taught.

The first step in teaching children to decode is to teach the letters of the alphabet and the sounds they represent. There are two important principles for teaching letter–sound correspondences to children. First, phonemic awareness activities should be explicitly linked to the teaching of letters; and, second, children should be shown the consistency of letter sounds in various positions within a word—first, ending, and medial positions (Beck, 2006). Many struggling readers are able to recognize the correct letter sounds

when the letter is presented as the initial sound but are unable to recognize letters at the end or in the middle of the word (McCandliss, Beck, Sandek, & Perfetti, 2003).

As soon as children are able to recognize and produce a few letter sounds by sight, with assistance they should be able to read simple words with consonant–vowel–consonant (CVC) patterns in which all letters are decoded using their most common sounds. Phonics instruction provides children with strategies to blend individual sounds together. The most common blending technique teaches children to articulate each sound in a word by pointing to each letter and then swooping their fingers under the whole word while coarticulating (blending) the sounds together to pronounce the sounds as a whole word (Beck, 2006).

Once students can decode the most common CVC word patterns, they have acquired important foundational skills for subsequent phonics instruction. Sounds in our language are not represented in one-to-one correspondence with the letters of the alphabet. If that were the case, there would be only 26 individual sounds in our language. There are, in fact, approximately 44 sounds in English speech patterns (Moats, 2000). Many letters represent multiple sounds, and many sounds are represented in multiple ways. Often two or more letters represent a single sound. It is estimated that there are more than 200 sound–spelling correspondences in the English language systems (Adams, 1990). Comprehensive phonics instruction is designed to teach these rules to children in a systematic way so that there is a continuous development in understanding the rules of the alphabetic system and an ability to recognize these correspondences automatically.

Automaticity is important to every aspect of phonics instruction. Automaticity is the ability to recognize something quickly and accurately while exerting little cognitive energy in the recognition process. For students to become accurate word readers, they must be able to recognize the sounds of every letter in the alphabet by sight with little conscious thought. Rapid word recognition is the primary goal of effective phonics instruction. When automaticity is observed, underlying word reading skills have been achieved, and reading instruction can progress to more complex skills.

Assessing for Phonics Deficits

Evaluating the performances of students who have not mastered phonics skills requires an analysis of the instructional content and delivery, including an examination of the scope and sequence of instruction, the pacing in relation to adequate skill acquisition, and the amount of practice afforded for mastery. Some students can learn to read with phonics patterns implicitly taught during reading experiences, whereas others need each skill presented in a systematic and purposeful way. For these students, knowing the sequence in which the skills were been taught allows an examination of their mastery of previous lessons. If they did not receive phonics instruction as systematically as was needed, the examiner must uncover each skill that they do not have for instructional planning. This knowledge can provide information about a struggling student's specific instructional needs so that more systematic phonics lessons can be redesigned.

A variety of CBM tools are available to help assess various areas of word reading development. Students with emergent decoding skills can be monitored using the NWF from the DIBELS (Good & Kaminski, 2002) or the WIF (Fuchs, Fuchs, & Compton, 2004). The progress of students with decoding problems who are able to read connected text can be monitored using CBM-ORF (Deno, 1985). For students who struggle to spell words using phonetic strategies, CBM-S (Deno, 1985) is an effective assessment for problem-solving evaluation.

The NWF test is designed to measure students' reading of nonsense words in the form of CVC words (e.g., *nom*, *yim*, *ot*). Through NWF, evaluators can observe students blending sounds together to read them as entire word units. Mastery of the NWF test indicates that students are able to decode words with simple CVC spelling patterns. As with other forms of CBM, the scores from NWF tests can be compared with normative samples and with criteria indicating achievement on these basic skills. The initial score can be used to determine a goal, and the test exists in multiple equivalent forms for purposes of progress monitoring.

WIF is a simple CBM measure that is designed to measure word reading automaticity. WIF is administered by presenting students with high-frequency word lists and having them read aloud (Deno et al., 1982). The number of words that students accurately read in 1 minute provides a score of their word reading automaticity. WIF also exists in multiple forms and can be a useful measurement tool for students who have mastered the most basic decoding skills of NWF but who continue to struggle learning to read. In fact, research indicates that WIF might be a more valid indicator of students' reading ability and might produce more reliable slopes for predicting improvement in reading skills for struggling readers than NWF (Fuchs et al., 2004).

If further analysis is necessary for convergent evidence that decoding is a problem, NRTs of word reading skills may be useful in quantifying the extent of the problem. Some tests include the Word Reading and Pseudoword Decoding subtests of the Weschler Individual Achievement Test–II (WIAT; Weschler, 2001) or the Word Identification and Word Attack subtests of the Woodcock–Johnson–III (WJ-III; Woodcock, McGrew, & Mather, 2001). The Test of Word Reading Efficiency (TOWRE; Torgesen, Wagner, & Rashotte, 1999) is an NRT that may be useful in assessing automatic word identification skills. Additionally, CRTs such as the Ekwall–Shanker Reading Inventory (Shanker & Ekwall, 2000) may provide more specific information regarding which phonics skills students do and do not know.

Fluency

Reading fluency has been determined to be the most salient characteristic of skillful reading (Adams, 1990) and is an essential and complex component of early literacy development. Theoretically, it encompasses all the subcomponents of reading, including lower order word recognition processes and higher order thinking skills. Because fluency relies on efficient processing of word reading skills, it is indicative of mastery of phonemic awareness and phonics skills (Fuchs, Fuchs, Hosp, & Jenkins, 2001), but fluent reading is also important indicator of overall reading comprehension (Fuchs, Fuchs, & Maxwell, 1988).

Fluency can be defined as the ability to read text quickly and accurately with proper expression. The three essential subcomponents of reading fluency that support the interaction between decoding, word-level reading, and understanding include automaticity, reading rate, and prosody (Hudson, Lane, & Pullen, 2005). *Automaticity* refers to the speed and accuracy of the word recognition process. Although automatic word recognition often results in a faster reading rate, many students need support in reading words in connected text at a reading rate sufficient to support understanding; thus *reading rate* reflects the agility with which students read connected text. *Prosody* is the intonation one uses when reading, referring to the degree to which one properly attends to the phrasing, punctuation, dialogues, and voice within a text. Students cannot become prosodic readers without achieving word-level automaticity in the text. Thus automaticity is a foundational component for both reading rate and prosody.

Automaticity is achieved when a reader sees a word and immediately recognizes it. As discussed earlier, automaticity develops word by word and spelling pattern by spelling pattern through repeated decoding of letter sequences. Most students develop automaticity with a few exposures to a word, especially those words that are common in their oral vocabulary. However, many struggling readers fail to achieve automaticity at the word level. For these students, reading remains an arduous task, consuming valuable cognitive energy at lower level word recognition processes, leaving little left to enjoy the meaning of the words they read and resulting in longer term negative effects on their reading achievement (LaBerge & Samuels, 1974; Cunningham & Stanovich, 1998; Stanovich, 1986).

Automaticity requires two important elements: accuracy and speed at the word level. Instruction designed to target reading fluency includes well-designed phonics instruction that teaches students accurate decoding skills and provides ample practice in reading words and texts that contain the new skills. Once students become accurate in their decoding, they are provided with enough practice and successful exposures until the process required to read the word becomes so fast that they reach word-level automaticity with their new phonics skill.

Some students may achieve automaticity at the word level and still require instructional support to improve the rate with which they read connected text. Classroom activities that improve students' reading rates include repeated reading activities and supported oral reading routines. Repeated reading allows children multiple exposures to the words and features of a text so as to develop fluency. Additionally, repeated reading builds habits of fluent reading rates for novel texts beyond the repeated-reading routines. Repeated reading has been found to be most effective when feedback and motivation are provided for improved reading rates (Morgan & Sideridis, 2006).

When students are able to recognize most of the words in a text automatically, they are able to read while attending to the prosodic features of text. Prosody refers to the expression with which a text is read. Some students will immediately read as if they are talking; others might require instruction and feedback when they read to develop prosody. Fluency is often regarded as the bridge between decoding and reading for meaning, particularly as students develop prosody as they read. For some prosody is viewed as evidence that readers understand what they read (Kuhn & Stahl, 2000).

Assessing for Fluency

Fluency can be observed by assessing students' oral reading rates and their accuracy when reading. Although other published NRTs are available to evaluate student reading rates, such as the Reading Fluency subtest of the WJ-III, the CBM-ORF (Deno, 1985) provides the most efficient and reliable vehicle for evaluating oral reading fluency at every step of the problem solving approach. ORF allows an evaluator to observe whether a student's oral reading rate on grade-level materials is significantly discrepant from that of same-grade peers. ORF is simple to administer. A student is asked to read aloud a standard grade-level text for 1 minute. At the end of the 1-minute period, the student's total words read correctly (WRC) is simply the score of the test. This score can be compared with normative data samples and with criteria that indicate expected fluency criteria at each grade level. As such, this simple test allows both peer comparisons and criterion-referenced comparisons to be made for problem identification.

Additionally, from a baseline ORF score, problem solvers can establish meaningful goals for their students using published normative growth rates (Deno, Fuchs, Marston, & Shin, 2001). These growth rates provide educators with information about rates of improvement for typical students. For example, typical first-graders may gain approximately 1.8 words per week in their ORF scores. This information can be used as a guideline for setting goals for struggling students. By determining a time line for evaluation (e.g., 10 weeks), an evaluator can know that typical first-grade students will gain approximately 18 words in their ORF rate in 10 weeks. By adding that growth to the baseline reading rate, one can set a goal for a student to increase his or her current reading rate by 18 words in a 10-week period. However, a goal of similar growth to that of peers means that a gap would persist between the struggling student and his or her peers. By setting a goal based on a more ambitious reading rate than that of typical peers, the evaluator sets the expectation that an ambitious instructional plan will be implemented to close the gap for the target student.

Importantly, ORF is an excellent overall measure for many of the subcomponent skills involved in the decoding process. Fuchs et al. (2001) describe ORF as "a direct measure of phonological segmentation and recoding as well as rapid word recognition" (p. 239), as they presented evidence identifying ORF as a reliable indicator of overall reading competence. Despite the simple nature of the test itself, ORF represents a valid assessment of phonemic awareness skills such as segmenting and decoding, the application of the alphabetic principle necessary for blending and recoding, and automatic word recognition. As such, ORF is also an effective assessment tool for monitoring students who are observed to have specific skill deficits in phonics and phonemic awareness.

Additionally, ORF has been found to be an excellent measure of reading comprehension. Researchers found that ORF more closely correlated with criterion measures of reading comprehension than did other tests specifically designed to measure comprehension. These other tests included a question-and-answer test, an oral-retell task, and a cloze assessment (Fuchs et al., 1988). Jen-kins, Fuchs, van den Broek, Espin, and Deno (2003) conducted another study supporting the hypothesis that ORF is a good indicator of overall reading competence. Here, the authors explored the relationship between list reading and context reading. Results suggested that comprehension skills play a role in oral reading fluency by demonstrating that context reading fluency is a stronger predictor of reading comprehension than list reading fluency. These researchers concluded that fluent text reading reflects both rapid decoding as manifested in facile word identification skills and comprehension processes.

Vocabulary

Although the ability to read text fluently is an essential enabling skill for independent reading comprehension, equally important is a student's vocabulary. On entering kindergarten, students' vocabulary has been identified as an important predictor of learning to read (National Research Council, 1998). The role that vocabulary plays in developing reading warrants a closer look, as vocabulary is likely to affect every component of reading acquisition, including phonemic awareness, decoding, word reading, word-level automaticity, and comprehension.

Phonological awareness and phonemic awareness instructional activities are designed to draw students' attention to sounds in our spoken language. In a typical activity, teachers orally present words and have students manipulate their sounds. If a word is that a student knows presented orally, the student's working memory is able to simply focus on the sound manipulation task. If the student is unable to recognize the word meaning, the vocabulary deficit forces working memory to conduct two challenging tasks. The first is to hold on to the sound representation of the unknown word; it is as if the student must remember a nonsense word while attending to the target task. The second is to manipulate the sounds in the word. The task is made significantly harder to accomplish because of the vocabulary deficit; thus the target skill is harder to learn. Even if developing awareness of sounds in speech might have come easily, a student with vocabulary deficits might fall behind in this important foundational skill.

Vocabulary deficits may also impede the development of basic decoding skills and automatic word reading. As students are taught to decode, they engage in word reading activities in which letters on a page are translated into individual sounds, individual sounds are blended into words, and the newly decoded words are read aloud as whole words. If the word meaning is not available, the student has no means to check the accuracy of his or her decoding skills. When word meanings are known to the student, the spelling patterns of the word will be more readily recognized, requiring less decoding rehearsal until it is recognized automatically.

Finally, vocabulary is essential for reading comprehension. The proportion of familiar words in a given text directly relates to students' ability to comprehend that text (Anderson & Freebody, 1981). Additionally, the more words in a text that are familiar to students, the more likely they will be able to decipher unknown words from the context and meanings of other words while they read, an important process in developing more vocabulary (Nagy, Anderson, & Herman, 1987). Therefore, students with more robust vocabularies are actually more likely to increase their vocabularies while reading than students with vocabulary deficits.

The vocabulary we know and use in our spoken language can be broken into two types. Oral receptive vocabulary is the first to develop and the largest in size. Our oral receptive vocabulary includes all the words for which we know the meaning when we hear them spoken aloud. Oral productive vocabulary is defined by the words in our spoken language that we are able to use in our own speech. Students enter school with varying degrees of oral receptive and oral productive language.

In their seminal longitudinal study, Hart and Risley (1995) observed and quantified the vocabulary development of American children, adding an important element to our understanding of the literacy achievement gap in the United States. Risley and Hart's research team observed babies and their interactions with their families each month from the babies' birth until age 3. The researchers found stark and compelling differences in the receptive vocabularies of children by the time they were 3 years old.

During 1-hour observations, some parents spoke a total of more than 3,000 words to their babies, whereas others spoke less than 200 words. This means that, over time, some children in the United States would have encountered more than 33 million words, whereas others would hear approximately only 10 million words.

These researchers also found that the more infants are spoken to, the more they themselves talk. Talk provides practice for the development of productive vocabularies. They found that average American children speak approximately 400 times in an hour but that infants who are spoken to the most express themselves more than 600 times an hour whereas those in less talkative families express themselves only about 200 times an hour. Young children in families that do not encourage spoken interactions have half the expressive language vocabularies of the average American child.

As students begin to encounter print, their vocabularies develop into written receptive and written productive vocabularies. Written receptive vocabulary is defined as the words a student is able to read and know the meaning of. Written receptive vocabulary develops as an interaction between decoding and word recognition processes, in which words never seen before are read for the first time and the student recognizes the sound of the newly read word from the oral vocabulary stored in his or her memory. The more quickly students acquire word reading skills, the more quickly their written receptive vocabularies develop. Last to develop, written productive vocabulary is the sum total of words we use when we write, those that we recall when selecting words for the page, and those we can spell.

As oral receptive and productive vocabularies develop through wide exposure to oral language, our print vocabularies develop with wide exposure to print. Most of our vocabulary develops through broad language opportunities; the more robust our mental dictionary (lexicon) is, the more we engage in language interactions, and the more our lexicon grows. Additionally, the larger our lexicon, the more readily we develop reading skills, engage in reading activities, and expand our mental dictionaries. Because of the reciprocal nature of vocabulary development, in which robust vocabulary begets further vocabulary development, strategic and targeted vocabulary instruction is essential for children with vocabulary deficits. For these children, their prior knowledge will not readily support the acquisition of new vocabulary and may hinder their ability to learn how to read; thus vocabulary instruction and support is a critical component of early reading instruction.

Many students will expand their vocabularies through wide exposure to reading. It is important to encourage reading opportunities for students who are able to derive meaning from independent reading. However, reading widely is not a vehicle for developing vocabulary for students who struggle to decode words and those for whom many words are unknown. For the latter, too many unknown words prevent the student from deducing word meaning. In fact, researchers estimate that of every 100 unknown words we encounter during reading, approximately 5 will be learned for their meaning (Nagy et al., 1987; Swanborn & deGlopper, 1999). Although this appears to be a small proportion, students who encounter 100 new words each day and read every day of the week could learn up to 35 words each week and almost 2,000 words each year. However, for students who struggle to read, reading experiences are less available to them as a vehicle for developing robust vocabularies that support literacy development at a level of proficiency.

Beck, McKeown, and Kucan (2002) presented a powerful instructional model for weaving direct and systematic instruction into broad language exposure via "text talk." They encourage teachers to present to their students new words chosen from stories read aloud via direct instructional strategies. They recommend that teachers select words that represent mature language useful across a variety of domains and words for which the underlying concept is clearly understood by their students. First, the selected word is revisited in the context of the story, then it is defined for students using student-friendly definitions. The teacher discusses the meaning of the word as it relates to the story so children can observe the interaction of the new word within a context. Next, the teacher describes the various ways that the word's meaning is used in common language by providing various examples of the word in different sentences across varying domains. The final step involves helping students relate to the new vocabulary word on a personal level. Teachers provide opportunities for students to use the word in interesting contexts through conversations, role play, and writing activities.

Assessing for Vocabulary Deficits

Oral language deficits are often a contributing factor in students' failure to acquire reading skills. Evaluating students' vocabulary can provide useful information regarding the oral language deficits that are contributing to the reading failure. To date, a wide variety of published NRTs is available to evaluate students' expressive and receptive vocabularies. Some of these tests include the Comprehensive Receptive and Expressive Vocabulary Test—Second Edition (CREVT-2; Wallace & Hammill, 2002), the Expressive One-Word Picture Vocabulary Test (EOWPVT; Gardner, 2000) and the Receptive One-Word Picture Vocabulary Test (ROWPVT; Brownell, 2000). The Peabody Picture Vocabulary Test (PPVT-III; Dunn & Dunn, 1997) is also available to measure receptive vocabulary.

Despite the many tests available for measuring vocabulary, tests for monitoring student progress on vocabulary acquisition have yet to become widely available, and expected rates of growth on vocabulary development are not yet known. In fact, it is yet to be determined whether meaningful gains in vocabulary development can be detected through existing tests for which a finite number of vocabulary questions can be asked. However, problem-solving evaluators who suspect oral language and vocabulary deficits can use NRTs to quantify the problem. Once the magnitude of the problem is identified, evaluators should consider the negative consequences that vocabulary deficits may have on the development of reading and should examine students' acquisition of critical enabling skills. They may examine performance on tests of phonemic awareness, word reading skills, and fluency to ensure that the vocabulary deficits do not inhibit reading development. Vocabulary deficits put students at risk for reading failure. By targeting at-risk students with excellent reading instruction and monitoring their development of the essential skills necessary for reading, educators provide these vulnerable students with an important weapon—the ability to read, which can have powerful effects on their subsequent vocabulary growth.

Comprehension

Comprehension is inarguably the reason for reading. Proficient readers are able to read text and understand the messages conveyed in print. Reading comprehension is a complex process involving the interaction between word identification processes, the integration of prior knowledge, vocabulary and general language knowledge, and cognitive monitoring strategies (Adams, 1990). The processes involved in successful reading comprehension can be organized into two categories: enabling skills that facilitate the process of comprehension and cognitive strategies that readers use to make sense of text as they read (Howell & Nolet, 2000).

Children bring with them enabling skills to access the print from the page. Both facile word recognition skills and access to word meanings play important roles in the task of text comprehension. Children approach text reading with a prior knowledge base that may facilitate understanding, and to every task of reading they bring with them different levels of motivation and persistence. As such, instruction that prepares students for comprehension of text includes providing students with word recognition strategies, robust vocabulary, and a depth of background knowledge. Equally important, instruction designed to ensure that students consistently have successful interactions with text is likely to ensure motivation for reading. Repeated failure with reading will decrease motivation to read and to endure through difficult reading tasks. Most children with reading problems do not maintain attention well when reading (McKinney, Osborne, & Schulte, 1993).

Most research regarding effective comprehension instruction has focused on cognitive strategies that best facilitate understanding (Lysynchuk, Pressley, d'Ailly, Smith, & Cake, 1989). The goals of cognitive strategy instruction are to provide students with a specific set of organized activities and to facilitate understanding and aid problem solving on intellectual tasks (Torgesen, 1982). The NRP (2000) found at least five strategies that can be taught to children that resulted in meaningful gains in comprehension. They include explicit instruction that teaches students to (1) monitor their own understanding while they are reading, (2) answer questions during and after reading, (3) generate questions, (4) summarize what they read, and (5) make use of multiple cognitive strategies while reading, all of which lead to positive gains in comprehension.

Comprehension monitoring is the awareness of one's own understanding and the cognitive activities one might engage in when actively searching for meaning. The goal of comprehension-monitoring strategy instruction is to help students develop self-awareness when they encounter an obstruction to effective understanding and to provide students with the means to fix the misunderstanding. Steps in such instruction often include teaching students to become aware of what they understand, to identify what they do not understand, and to repair confusions so as to create meaning (Baumann, Jones, & Seifert-Kessell, 1993; Paris, Lipson, & Wixon, 1983).

Comprehension monitoring has been reported as being a common skill deficit for many students with reading difficulties. Torgesen (1977) described students with learning disabilities as "inactive learners," passively perceiving new information without the purposeful integration of the information into their knowledge base. He and others (Tarver, Hallahan, Kauffman, & Ball, 1976; Wong, 1980) demonstrated that struggling learners did not employ goal-directed strategies to aid them in tasks of perception, attention, and memory. Importantly, much of the same research demonstrated that when students are taught specific strategies for active learning, they tend to use them.

Of all the strategies deemed effective by the NRP, teaching students to generate questions while they read showed the strongest empirical support. Singer and Donlan (1982) taught students specific story elements, including character, goal, obstacles, outcome, and theme, along with general corresponding questions. During each training session, students in the experimental condition were taught a new question framework, asked to write questions for a story they were going to hear, and then prompted to write more questions at the end of the story. Students in the control condition were asked teacher-generated questions. Each group took a 10-question test after each story. After the first two trials, there was an increase in performance for students in the experimental condition and a significant effect over all the testing sessions.

Teaching students to summarize what they read is also an effective strategy for engaging students in the meaning of text through instruction around main ideas and themes. The goal of summarization instruction is to teach children to detect the most important features of text by sifting through trivial details and redundancies so as to identify the central ideas. Instruction around summarization arises from a solid cognitive theoretical base that purports that a personal summary of a text naturally occurs as a result of understanding (Kintsch & van Dijk, 1978). An analysis of studies that examined summarization as an effective strategy to aid comprehension revealed that direct and explicit instruction in a specific set of steps resulted in the best outcomes, including better summarizations, memory of text details, and application of strategies to novel situations (Hare & Borchardt, 1984).

Being a purposeful and strategic reader requires actively seeking out meaning by any means available. Effective comprehension instruction provides students with multiple strategies to draw on to accommodate the various problem-solving situations they might encounter. Many studies on multiple strategy instruction incorporate peer interactions to increase student dialogue and scaffold "teacher talk" to "kid-talk" (Klingner & Vaughn, 1998; Klingner, Vaughn, & Schumm, 1998). Most commonly known as reciprocal teaching (Palincsar & Brown, 1984), this approach entails teaching students a set of cognitive strategies (i.e., making predictions, generating questions, using clarification strategies, and summarizing) through teacher modeling of each strategy and subsequently through student modeling for one another.

Assessing for Reading Comprehension Deficits

Assessing reading comprehension is less straightforward than measuring word read-

ing skill development, because comprehension is primarily a cognitive activity that cannot be directly observed. Tests of reading comprehension are likely to use formats in which students read a paragraph and answer questions about the text. Formats designed to evaluate sentence-level reading comprehension tend to use fill-in-the-blank formats. Published NRTs of reading comprehension include the Group Reading Assessment and Diagnostic Evaluation (GRA+DE; Williams, 2001) and the Test of Reading Comprehension—3 (TORC-3; Brown, Hammill, & Wiederholt, 1995). Unfortunately, the currently available tests of comprehension fail to adequately capture the complexity of this construct, and research is needed to identify tests that measure the underlying cognitive processes involved in comprehension (Snow, 2002).

Repeatedly, studies have shown ORF to be a robust indicator of performance on measures of reading comprehension (Fuchs et al., 1988; Hintze, Owen, Shapiro, & Daly, 2000; Hintze, Shapiro, Conte, & Basile, 1997; Hintze, Callahan, Matthews, Williams, & Tobin, 2002; Jenkins et al., 2003; Shinn, Good, Knutson, Tilly, & Collins, 1992). As such, ORF has been used as a measure to examine reading comprehension in developing readers. However, researchers have found that as decoding becomes efficient, ORF is a less valid measure of reading comprehension for students beyond third grade (Fuchs, Fuchs, Hamlett, Walz, & Germann, 1993; Shinn et al., 1992; Stage & Jacobsen, 2001). As such, problem-solving educators are in need of assessments that help quantify underlying skills subsumed in the comprehension process beyond that of text reading fluency.

The Maze is a curriculum-based measure that has been found to be useful for examining comprehension in a problem-solving evaluation process. The Maze can be give frequently to reliably assess student progress over time (Shin, Deno, & Espin, 2000). The maze task consists of a grade-level reading passage in which every nth word (e.g., every seventh word) is deleted and replaced by three word-choice options. Students must read the passages and circle the word that best fits the meaning of the sentence. Howell and Nolet (2000) have described this task as a measure of students' vocabulary knowledge and grammar skills, as well as of their ability to employ active reading strategies for meaning monitoring while they read (Howell & Nolet, 2000). Researchers have found that the maze task reflects student growth when the predictive utility of ORF begins to diminish and is more sensitive to differences in reading ability for students in upper grades than for students in lower grades (Jenkins & Jewell, 1993).

Fuchs et al. (1988) found a written retell a valid test of reading comprehension, second only to ORF, when they observed strong correlations ($r = .82$) between the written retell and the reading comprehension subtest of the Stanford Achievement Test—Seventh Edition (Gardner, Rudman, Karlsen, & Merwin, 1982). Additionally, Fuchs, Fuchs, and Hamlett (1989) demonstrated that a written retell assessment provided teachers useful feedback in an ongoing measurement system. Using a standardized written retell, teachers were able to use baseline assessment results to set ambitious goals for their students and adjust their instructional activities to support their students' needs.

Although these tests reflect some of the operations important in reading comprehension, there is clearly a lack of tests available to measure the complex reading comprehension construct. In addition to tests that reflect the components of reading comprehension, for effective problem solving evaluators need access to tests that are sensitive to learning, that are instructionally useful, and that can be used to evaluate learning as a function of instructional changes.

Conclusion

Most basically, problem-solving educators believe that every child can and will learn. The activities they engage in seek to resolve learning problems rather than to find reasons for failure. Problem solvers view every problem as multifaceted and dynamic, resulting from an interaction between the individual for whom the problem occurs and the environment in which it occurs.

Discovering solutions to problems depends on focusing on the essential skills of the problem domain. Problems are most often eliminated by shaping instructional content so as to ensure learning of the essential skills in a purposeful and strategic way. Through strategic assessment, problem solvers seek to understand deficits in essential skills that hinder student success and the instructional delivery that might address the observed deficits. Once identified, teacher-directed instructional approaches can be determined that are effective for students who are not meeting curricular objectives, with the goal of reestablishing rates of learning that are more typical of their peers (Howell & Nolet, 2000).

Finally, problem solvers view assessment as a data-gathering process that directly reflects the relationships between curriculum, instruction, and learning, in which these factors are inextricably linked. For problem solvers, assessment guides instructional decisions, and instructional decisions are evaluated through systematic assessment. This marriage between assessment and instruction is important for all students but essential to ensure progress for struggling students for whom a discrepancy exists between their performance and that of their peers.

References

Adams, M. J. (1990). *Beginning to read: Thinking and learning about print.* Cambridge, MA: MIT Press.

Adams, M. J., Foorman, B. R., Lundberg, I., & Beeler, T. (1998). *Phonemic awareness in young children.* Baltimore: Brookes.

Anderson, R. C., & Freebody, P. (1981). Vocabulary knowledge. In J. Guthrie (Ed.), *Comprehension and teaching: Research reviews* (pp. 11–177). Newark, DE: International Reading Association.

Ball, E. W., & Blachman, B. A. (1988). Phoneme segmentation training: Effect on reading readiness. *Annals of Dyslexia, 38,* 208–225.

Ball, E. W., & Blachman, B. A. (1991). Does phoneme awareness training in kindergarten make a difference in early word recognition and developmental spelling? *Reading Research Quarterly, 26*(1), 49–66.

Baumann, J. F., Jones, L. A., & Seifert-Kessell, N. (1993). Using think alouds to enhance children's comprehension monitoring abilities. *Reading Teacher, 47*(3), 184–193.

Beck, I. L. (2006). *Making sense of phonics: The hows and whys.* New York: Guilford Press.

Beck, I. L., McKeown, M. G., & Kucan, L.

(2002). *Bringing words to life: Robust vocabulary instruction*. New York: Guilford Press.

Bradley, L., & Bryant, P. (1983). Categorizing sounds and learning to read: A causal connection. *Nature, 30*, 419–421.

Brady, S. A. (1997). Ability to encode phonological representations: An underlying difficulty of poor readers. In B. Blachman (Ed.), *Foundations of reading acquisition and dyslexia: Implications for early intervention* (pp. 21–47). Mahwah, NJ: Erlbaum.

Brown, V., Hammill, D., & Wiederholt, J.L. (1995). *Test of Reading Comprehension—3*. Austin, TX: Pro-Ed.

Brownell, R. (2000). *Receptive one-word picture vocabulary test* (3rd ed.) Novato, CA: Academic Therapy Publications.

Cunningham, A. E., & Stanovich, K. E. (1998). What reading does for the mind. *American Educator, 22*, 8–15.

Deno, S. L. (1985). Curriculum-based measurement: The emerging alternative. *Exceptional Children, 52*, 219–232.

Deno, S. L. (2002). Problem-solving as "best practice." In A. Thomas & J. Grimes (Eds.), *Best practices in school psychology* (4th ed., Vol. 1, pp. 37–55) Bethesda, MD: National Association of School Psychologists.

Deno, S. L., Fuchs, L. S., Marston, D., & Shin, J. (2001). Using curriculum-based measurement to establish growth standards for students with learning disabilities. *School Psychology Review, 35*, 85–98.

Deno, S. L., & Mirkin, P. K. (1977). *Data-based program modification: A manual*. Reston, VA: Council for Exceptional Children.

Deno, S. L., Mirkin, P. K., & Chang, B. (1982). Identifying valid measures of reading. *Exceptional Children, 49*, 36–45.

Dunn, L., & Dunn, M. (1997). *Peabody Picture Vocabulary Test—III*. Circle Pines, MN: American Guidance Services.

Ehri, L. C. (2004). Teaching phonemic awareness and phonics: An explanation of the National Reading Panel meta-analyses. In P. McCardle & V. Chhabra (Eds.), *The voice of evidence in reading research* (pp. 153–186). Baltimore: Brookes.

Fuchs, L. S., Fuchs, D., & Compton, D. L. (2004). Monitoring early reading development in first grade: Word identification fluency versus nonsense word fluency. *Exceptional Children, 71*(1), 7–21.

Fuchs, L. S., Fuchs, D., & Hamlett, C. L. (1989). Monitoring reading growth using student recalls: Effects of two teacher feedback systems. *Journal of Educational Research, 83*(2), 103–110.

Fuchs, L. S., Fuchs, D., Hamlett, C. L., Walz, L., & Germann, G. (1993). Formative evaluation of academic progress: How much growth can we expect? *School Psychology Review, 22*, 27–48.

Fuchs, L. S., Fuchs, D., Hosp, M. K., & Jenkins, J. R. (2001). Oral reading fluency as an indicator of reading competence: A theoretical, empirical and historical analysis. *Scientific Studies of Reading, 5*(3), 239–257.

Fuchs, L. S., Fuchs, D., & Maxwell, L. (1988). The validity of informal reading comprehension measures. *Remedial and Special Education, 9*(2), 20–28.

Gardner, E. F., Rudman, H. C., Karlsen, B., & Merwin, J. C. (1982). *Stanford Achievement Test*. Iowa City, IO: Harcourt Brace Jovanovich.

Gardner, M. F. (2000). *Expressive One-Word Picture Vocabulary Test*. Novato, CA: Academic Therapy.

Goldsworthy, C. L. (2003). *Developmental reading disabilities: A language-based treatment approach* (2nd ed.). Clifton Park, NY: Delmar Learning.

Good, R. H., & Kaminski, R. A. (2002). *Dynamic Indicators of Basic Early Literacy Skills*. Eugene, OR: Institute for the Development of Educational Achievement.

Hare, V. C., & Borchardt, K. M. (1984). Direct instruction of summarization skills. *Reading Research Quarterly, 20*(1), 62–78.

Hart, B., & Risley, T. R. (1995). *Meaningful differences in the everyday experience of young American children*. Baltimore: Brookes.

Hintze, J. M., Callahan, J. E., Matthews, W. J., Williams, S. A., & Tobin, K. (2002). Oral reading fluency and the prediction of reading comprehension in African-American and Caucasian elementary school children. *School Psychology Review, 31*, 540–553.

Hintze, J. M., Owen, S. V., Shapiro, E. S., & Daly, E. J. (2000). Generalizability of oral reading fluency measures: Application of G theory to curriculum-based measurement. *School Psychology Quarterly, 15*, 52–68.

Hintze, J. M., Shapiro, E. S., Conte, K. L., & Basile, I. M. (1997). Oral reading fluency and authentic reading material: Criterion validity of the technical features of CBM survey-level assessment. *School Psychology Review, 26*, 535–553.

Howell, K., & Nolet, V. (2000). *Curriculum-based evaluation: Teaching and decision-making* (3rd ed.). Scarborough, Ontario, Canada: Wadsworth Thomson Learning.

Hudson, R. F., Lane, H. B., & Pullen, P. C. (2005). Reading fluency assessment and instruction: What, why and how? *Reading Teacher, 58*, 702–712.

Jenkins, J. R., Fuchs, L. S., van den Broek, P., Espin, C., & Deno, S. L. (2003). Sources of individual differences in reading comprehension and reading fluency. *Journal of Educational Psychology, 95,* 719–729.

Jenkins, J. R., & Jewell, M. (1993). Examining the validity of two measures of formative teaching: Reading aloud and maze. *Exceptional Children, 59,* 421–432.

Juel, C., Griffith, P., & Gough, P. (1986). Acquisition of literacy: A longitudinal study of children in first and second grade. *Journal of Educational Psychology, 78,* 243–255.

Kaminski, R. A., & Good, R. H. (1998). Assessing early literacy skills in a problem-solving model: Dynamic Indicators of Basic Early Literacy Skills. In M. R. Shinn (Ed.), *Advanced applications of curriculum based measurement* (pp. 113–142). New York: Guilford Press.

Kintsch, W., & van Dijk, T. A. (1978). Toward a model of text comprehension and production. *Psychological Review, 84*(5), 363–394.

Klingner, J. K., & Vaughn, S. (1998). Using collaborative strategic reading. *Teaching Exceptional Children, 30* (6), 32–37.

Klingner, J. K., Vaughn, S., & Schumm, J. S. (1998). Collaborative strategic reading during social studies in heterogeneous fourth-grade classrooms. *Elementary School Journal, 99*(1), 3–22.

Kuhn, M. R., & Stahl, S. A. (2000). *Fluency: A review of developmental and remedial practices.* Ann Arbor, MI: Center for the Improvement for Early Reading Achievement.

LaBerge, D., & Samuels, S. J. (1974). Toward a theory of automatic information processing in reading. *Cognitive Psychology, 6,* 293–323.

Lundberg, I., Frost, J., & Peterson, O. (1988). Effects of an extensive program for stimulating phonological awareness in preschool children. *Reading Research Quarterly, 23,* 263–284.

Lysynchuk, L. M., Pressley, M., d'Ailly, H., Smith, M., & Cake, H. (1989). A methodological analysis of experimental studies of comprehension strategy instruction. *Reading Research Quarterly, 24,* 458–470.

McCandliss, B., Beck, I. L., Sandek, R., & Perfetti, C. (2003). Focusing attention on decoding for children with poor reading skills: Design and preliminary tests of the word building intervention. *Scientific Studies of Reading, 7,* 75–104.

McKinney, J. D., Osborne, S. S., & Schulte, A. C. (1993). Academic consequences of learning disabilities: Longitudinal prediction of outcomes at eleven years of age. *Learning Disabilities Research and Practice, 8,* 19–27.

Moats, L. C. (2000). *Speech to print: Language essentials for teachers.* Baltimore: Brookes.

Morgan, P. L., & Sideridis, G. D. (2006). Contrasting the effectiveness of fluency interventions for students with or at risk for learning disabilities: A multilevel random coefficient modeling meta-analysis. *Learning Disabilities Research and Practice, 21,* 191–210.

Nagy, W., Anderson, R. C., & Herman, P. (1987). Learning word meanings from context during normal reading. *American Educational Research Journal, 24,* 237–270.

Nation, K., & Hulme, C. (1997). Phonemic segmentation, not onset–rime segmentation, predicts early reading and spelling skills. *Reading Research Quarterly, 32,* 154–167.

National Reading Panel. (2000). *Teaching children to read: An evidence-based assessment of the scientific research literature on reading and its implications for reading instruction.* Bethesda, MD: National Institute of Child Health and Human Development. Retrieved May 15, 2008, from *www.nationalreading panel.org/.*

National Research Council. (1998). *Preventing reading difficulties in young children.* Washington, DC: National Academy Press.

Palincsar, A. S., & Brown, A. L. (1984). Reciprocal teaching of comprehension-fostering and comprehension-monitoring activities. *Cognition and Instruction, 1,* 117–175.

Paris, S. G., Lipson, M. Y., & Wixon, K. D. (1983). Becoming a strategic reader. *Contemporary Educational Psychology, 8,* 293–316.

Rinehart, S. D., Stahl, S. A., & Erickson, L. G. (1986). Some effects of summarization training on reading and studying. *Reading Research Quarterly, 21,* 422–438.

Shanker, J. L., & Ekwall, E. E. (2000). *Ekwall/ Shanker Reading Inventory—Fourth Edition.* Needham Heights, MA: Allyn & Bacon.

Shin, J., Deno, S. L., & Espin, C. (2000). Technical adequacy of the maze task for curriculum-based measurement of reading growth. *Journal of Special Education, 34*(3), 164–172.

Shinn, M. R. (1988). Development of curriculum-based local norms for use in special education decision making. *School Psychology Review, 17,* 61–80.

Shinn, M. R. (1989). Identifying and defining academic problems: CBM screening and eligibility procedures. In M. R. Shinn (Ed.), *Curriculum-based measurement: Assessing special children* (pp. 90–129). New York: Guilford Press.

Shinn, M. R., Good, R. H., Knutson, N., Tilly, W. D., & Collins, V. L. (1992). Curriculum-based measurement of oral reading fluency: A confirmatory analysis of its relation to reading. *School Psychology Review, 21,* 459–479.

Shinn, M. R., Nolet, V., & Knutson, N. (1990). Best practices in curriculum-based measurement. In A. Thomas & J. Grimes (Eds.), *Best practices in school psychology* (2nd ed., pp. 287–307). Washington, DC: National Association of School Psychologists.

Singer, H., & Donlan, D. (1982). Active comprehension: Problem-solving schema with question generation for comprehension of complex short stories. *Reading Research Quarterly*, *17*(2), 166–186.

Snow, C. E. (2002). *Reading for understanding: Toward a R & D program in reading comprehension*. Santa Monica, CA: RAND.

Stage, S. A., & Jacobsen, M. D. (2001). Predicting student success on a state-mandated performance-based assessment using oral reading fluency. *School Psychology Review*, *30*, 407–420.

Stanovich, S. A. (1986). Matthew effects in reading: Some consequences of individual differences in the acquisition of literacy. *Reading Research Quarterly*, *21*(4), 360–407.

Swanborn, M. S., & deGlopper, K. (1999). Incidental word learning while reading: A meta-analysis. *Review of Educational Research*, *28*, 100–112.

Tarver, S. G., Hallahan, D. P., Kauffman, J. M., & Ball, D. W. (1976). Verbal rehearsal and selective attention in children with learning disabilities: A developmental lag. *Journal of Learning Disabilities*, *10*, 27–35.

Torgesen, J. K. (1977). The role of nonspecific factors in the task performance of learning disabled children: A theoretical assessment. *Journal of Learning Disabilities*, *10*(1), 27–34.

Torgesen, J. K. (1982). The learning disabled child as an inactive learner: Educational implications. *Topics in Learning and Learning Disabilities*, *2*, 45–52.

Torgesen, J. K., & Bryant, B. R. (1993). *Test of phonological awareness*. Austin, TX: Pro-Ed.

Torgesen, J. K., Wagner, R. K., & Rashotte, C. A. (1999). *Test of Word Reading Efficiency*. Austin, TX: Pro-Ed.

Wallace, G., & Hammill, D. D. (2002). *Comprehensive Receptive and Expressive Vocabulary Test* (2nd ed.). Dallas, TX: Pro-Ed.

Wagner, R. K., Torgesen, J. K., & Rashotte, C. A. (1999). *Comprehensive test of phonological processing*. Austin, TX: Pro-Ed.

Weschler, D. (2001). *Weschler Individual Achievement Test* (2nd ed.). San Antonio, TX: Psychological Corporation.

Williams, K. T. (2001). *The Group Reading Assessment and Diagnostic Evaluation*. Circle Pines, MN: AGS.

Wong, B. Y. L. (1980). Activating the inactive learner: Use of questions/prompts to enhance comprehension and retention of implied information in learning disabled children. *Learning Disability Quarterly*, *3*(1), 29–37.

Woodcock, R., McGrew, K., & Mather, N. (2001). *Woodcock–Johnson III Tests of Achievement*. Itasca, IL: Riverside.

Yopp, H. K. (1995). A test for assessing phonemic awareness in young children. *Reading Teacher*, *49*, 20–29.

Chapter 6

Assessment of Academic Skills in Math within a Problem-Solving Model

Matthew K. Burns
David A. Klingbeil

What are the goals and desired outcomes for education? This is a complex question with surprisingly controversial answers, but most would include some indication of preparing students for future career ambitions. Although reading is perhaps the keystone of academic skills, mathematics is becoming increasingly linked to successful employment in various occupations (Saffer, 1999). However, math research has been considerably less prominent in school psychology than reading research over the past decade (Badian, 1999; Daly & McCurdy, 2002), which is disconcerting given that less than one-third of the nation's fourth-grade students scored within a proficient range in math on the 2003 National Assessment of Educational Progress test (Manzo & Galley, 2003). Moreover, the achievement gap so frequently discussed in reading also seems to exist for math, with African American and Latino/a children demonstrating significantly lower achievement levels than their European American peers, though the gap is slowly closing (Lee, Grigg, & Dion, 2007).

 Math skills are directly linked to the quality of instruction that children receive in early grades (Fuchs, Fuchs, & Karns, 2001). What constitutes quality mathematics instruction is a matter of some debate (see Chard, Ketterlin-Geller, Jungjohann, & Baker, Chapter 17, this volume, for more information about math instruction), and this debate has been further fueled by the National Council of Teachers of Mathematics' (NCTM, 2000) standards that emphasize math as language, reasoning, and problem solving. Although some have questioned the research base for these standards (Hofmeister, 2004), there are some recommendations on which almost all would agree, including quality teacher preparation, well-designed curricula, and data-based instruction (NCTM, 2000). The latter recommendation is of great importance to school psychologists because data-based decision making is a foundation of the field (Ysseldyke et al., 2006). Therefore, the purpose of this chapter is to discuss types of data that can be used to better inform math instruction and intervention.

A chapter discussing academic skills in math would not be complete without a discussion of the process by which math is learned. Moreover, it is important to align assessment targets with appropriate interventions, and intervention decisions should consider the developmental functioning of the student. Accordingly, this chapter begins with a brief conceptualization of how students progress from a general number sense to the conceptual and procedural knowledge necessary for understanding complex mathematical tasks. Next, readers will find a description of commonly used types of math assessments and the respective procedures for conducting these assessments. Finally, we highlight how these assessments can be utilized in a tiered intervention system.

Learning Math

Learning math begins with the concept of number sense, which is difficult to define but easy to observe (Shapiro, 2004). Generally speaking, number sense involves the understanding of what numbers mean so that children can make accurate judgments about quantities and patterns in their surroundings; it is analogous to phonemic awareness in reading (Gersten & Chard, 1999). When children can successfully understand that 5 is more than 2, or when they count objects in their environment (e.g., counting steps while walking down a stairway), they are demonstrating number sense. Fortunately, most children come to school with some already established level of number sense, but those who do not, much as with phonemic awareness, require instruction in the basic concept of numbers before they can learn any other concepts or applications.

Once number sense is established, children can move into more advanced concepts regarding computation and problem solving. Although subsequent skills can and should build on one another, the learning process within a particular skill or domain also follows a predictable pattern, and instruction should follow that progression. Skills generally progress from a laborious process with frequent errors to more accurate but slow execution and eventually to proficient performance. Haring and Eaton's (1978) seminal writing conceptualized this process as an instructional hierarchy and suggested four phases. The first phase is called *acquisition* and represents the initial learning of the skill, which is marked by slow and highly inaccurate performance. Children in this phase require modeling, explicit instruction, and immediate feedback to improve the accuracy of responses. However, accurate responds are often completed slowly at first.

The goal of instruction at this point is to increase the rate of accurate skill production, otherwise known as *fluency*. *Generalization* of newly learned skills occurs when children can perform with accuracy and speed within the context in which the skill was learned and begin to apply the skill to a variety of material and contexts. Finally, in the adaption phase the student learns to apply the concept or the underlying principles to new situations without direction in order to solve problems.

The instructional progression just described could be interpreted to state that rote completion of items represents the onset of learning and that conceptual understanding is the final phase. However, successful completion of math procedures and conceptual understanding represent two related but distinct types of knowledge, and the relationship between them is somewhat complex. Conceptual knowledge is the understanding that math involves an interrelated hierarchical network that underlies all math-related tasks, and procedural knowledge is the organization of conceptual knowledge into action to actually perform a mathematical task (Hiebert & Lefevre, 1986). Although it may be somewhat unclear as to which type of knowledge develops first, and although the sequence may be specific to the domain or the individual (Rittle-Johnson & Siegler, 1998), the two are clearly interrelated, with conceptual understanding usually preceding successful application of operations and procedures (Boaler, 1998; Moss & Case, 1999). As shown in Figures 6.1 and 6.2, the instructional hierarchy applies to both conceptual and procedural knowledge to guide learning.

Types of Math Assessment

Assessment is critical to instruction (Linn & Gronlund, 2000), and math is no exception. Data used to drive and evaluate math instruction are gathered either with general outcome measures (GOM), which assess proficiency of global outcomes associated with an entire curriculum, or specific subskill mastery measures (SSMM), which assess smaller domains (e.g., double-digit addition) of learning based on predetermined criteria for mastery (Fuchs & Deno, 1991).

Instructional Hierarchy for Conceptual Knowledge

Phase of learning	Acquisition	Fluency	Generalization	Adaption
Examples of appropriate instructional activities	Explicit instruction in basic principles and concepts (e.g., time, larger than and less than, measurement). Demonstration and modeling with math manipulatives and concrete objects (e.g., using clocks, showing two objects and discussing which one is bigger, creating sets by placing a circle of string around objects). Immediate feedback on the accuracy of the student response.	Independent practice with manipulatives and objects (e.g., have the student count coins or practice with base 10 blocks). Immediate feedback on the speed of responding, but delayed feedback on the accuracy. However, all errors are corrected before additional practice occurs. Contingent reinforcement for speed of response.	Instructional games with different stimuli from what was used during instruction (e.g., telling time on different clocks, having them rewrite addition problems as sets: 4 + 4 + 4 + 4 +4 as 5 sets of 4, human number lines). Provide word problems for the concepts.	Use concepts to solve applied problems (e.g., asking the class whether something will fit inside of a smaller container or asking how many sets are needed to make enough for everyone in the class to have one).

FIGURE 6.1. Phases of learning for conceptual math knowledge and relevant instructional activities.

| Instructional Hierarchy for Procedural Knowledge | | | |

Phase of learning	Acquisition	Proficiency	Generalization	Adaption
Examples of appropriate instructional activities	Explicit instruction in task steps (e.g., explain how to add 5 + 5). Modeling with written problems in which the teacher does the first problem together with the class (e.g., demonstrates that 5+ 5 = 10), completes a second problem with the class, and then has each student complete a few sample problems with assistance from the teacher as needed. Immediate feedback on the accuracy of the work.	Independent practice with written skill (e.g., complete written problems faster than yesterday—often referred to as a "math minute" exercise). Immediate feedback on the speed of the response, but delayed feedback on the accuracy. However, all errors are corrected before additional practice occurs. Contingent reinforcement can be used for speed.	Apply number operations to applied problems (e.g., have the student write number equations for story problems). Complete real and contrived number problems in the classroom (e.g., "if I got 6 out of 10 correct on the assignment, how many more would I have to get right to get them all correct? 20 students earned their reward; how many more need to do so until the class gets its reward?").	Use numbers to solve problems in the classroom (e.g., "it is 10:30 and we go to lunch at 11:15; how many minutes until we go to lunch?").

FIGURE 6.2. Phase of learning for procedural math knowledge and relevant instructional activities.

Monitoring student progress with GOM data results in improved student learning (Fuchs, Fuchs, Hamlett, & Whinnery, 1991; Fuchs, Fuchs, Hamlett, & Stecker, 1991; Fuchs, Fuchs, & Maxwell, 1988), but SSMM seems to play an especially important role in math interventions because math curricula are composed of a series of standards, explicit objectives, and skills that build on those that precede them (NCTM, 2000). The narrow focus of SSMM allows teachers and school psychologists to use the data for diagnostic evaluation, to assess specific areas of concern, and to determine whether material should be taught (Burns, in press). However, SSMM has limited utility in monitoring student progress, whereas GOM data are particularly well suited for that role (Hosp, Hosp, & Howell, 2007).

Data obtained from SSMM have demonstrated sufficient psychometric properties (Burns, 2004; Burns, Tucker, Frame, Foley, & Hauser, 2000; Burns, VanDerHeyden, & Jiban, 2006), and data from one SSMM are dependable for criterion-referenced decisions regarding that skill (Hintze, Christ, & Keller, 2002). VanDerHeyden and Burns (2005) used SSMM measurement to identify objectives that students had mastered and those that required additional remediation. Students were instructed in each skill until the class demonstrated a median score on the SSMM that met or exceeded a criterion, at which time class instruction progressed to the next stage of the math curriculum. The results of this effort were increased math skills within the year and as compared with previous years.

Procedures for Math Assessments

Procedural Knowledge

Curriculum-based measurement (CBM; Deno, 1985) is a frequently used, research-based assessment procedure that allows the evaluator to gather standardized samples of academic behavior. CBM in math is accomplished by creating either multiskill (i.e., GOM) or single-skill (i.e., SSMM) samples, which are called probes. Educators can select published math CBM probes (e.g., AIMSweb, 2006; Edformation, 2005), use a Web-based system to create one (e.g., *www.mathfactscafe.com*), or create their own.

There is some debate over exactly how to build CBM math probes. Traditionally, math CBM probes contained at least 25 problems depending on the curriculum difficulty, and problems within a multiskill probe were randomly ordered (Fuchs & Fuchs, 1991; Hosp et al., 2007). However, recent research has suggested that creating a multiskill CBM for math should be done by arranging the items by skill and placing them in corresponding columns (Christ & Vining, 2006). For example, a multiskill probe may contain single-digit addition, single-digit subtraction, two-digit addition, and one-digit from two-digit subtraction without regrouping. All single-digit addition problems would be placed into the first column, single-digit subtraction into a second column, and so forth. Moreover, the number of items is not a hard-and-fast rule, and school psychologists should ensure that enough items are presented to adequately sample the skill given the individual student's proficiency.

After the probes are constructed, students are given 2–4 minutes to complete as many items as they can. Recent research has supported allowing 4 minutes to complete the task (Christ, Johnson-Gros, & Hintze, 2005), but some recommend allowing 2 minutes for students in grades 1–3 (AIMSweb, 2006). Most teachers find math CBM probes efficient and easy to administer (Hosp et al., 2007), and the probes can be used to test individuals or an entire class. Administration consists of providing the students the sheet to be completed and directing them to (1) write their answers to some problems, (2) look at each problem carefully before answering it, (3) start with the first problem and work across the page, (4) place an X over problems that they cannot complete, and (5) keep working until they complete the page or are told to stop (Shinn & Shinn, 2004). After 2–4 minutes the administration stops, and the probe is collected for scoring.

CBM math probes provide fluency scores measured in digits correct per minute (DCPM). DCPM is measured because it is more sensitive to change than is measuring the number of correct answers (Hosp et al., 2007). For example, if the answer to an addition problem is 1,185, the total possible digits correct is 4. If a child answered 1,180, the digits correct (DC) would equal 3; although this answer is incorrect, it shows

```
          1   2   5
      ×   2   1   7
          8   7   5
      1   2   5   0
  2   5   0   0   0
  2   7   1   2   5
```

= 17 digits correct

FIGURE 6.3. Example of digits correct in a multi-digit multiplication problem.

a greater understanding of addition than a response of, say, 500 (DC = 0). Digits correct are also scored in the critical processes of a problem, with placeholders counting as correct digits. The problem shown in Figure 6.3 has 17 possible digits correct rather than 5, with 3 in the first row, 4 in the second row, 5 in the third row, and 5 in the answer line. Thus the student would receive credit for 1 digit correct for the 0 placeholder in the second row and 2 digits correct for the double-0 placeholder in the third row.

In order to determine DCPM, the total number of digits correct in the probe is divided by the length of the administration (e.g., 80 digits correct in a 4-minute administration would result in 20 DCPM). Some interpretive criteria for math CBM are presented as DCPM (e.g., Shapiro, 2004), and some are presented as DC per 2 minutes (e.g., Edformation, 2005). Creating a DCPM metric allows data to be interpreted either way, because the score can simply be doubled to create a digits-correct-per-2-minutes score.

Conceptual Knowledge

The previously discussed math assessments are largely procedural and are designed to assess computational ability (Helwig, Anderson, & Tindal, 2002). Concept-oriented CBM directly assesses conceptual knowledge and applications of math procedures. Research on concept-oriented assessment is limited, but these data have been shown to be significant predictors of statewide assessment outcomes (Shapiro, Keller, Lutz, Santoro, & Hintze, 2006). Commercially prepared concept-oriented probes such as *Monitoring Basic Skills Progress: Basic Math Concepts and Applications* (Fuchs,

Hamlett, & Fuchs, 1999) are readily available to practitioners, but they can be developed as well.

Concept-oriented CBM probes should consist of 18 or more problems, depending on grade level, that assess mastery of concepts and applications (Shapiro et al., 2006). Concept-oriented probes cover a variety of math concepts beyond computation alone, such as measurement, charts and graphs, money, applied computation, and word problems (Shapiro et al., 2006; for example problems, see Helwig et al., 2002). The administration of concept-oriented assessments typically requires 6–8 minutes (Shapiro et al., 2006). Similar to the previously discussed assessments, the evaluator gives standardized directions regarding the nature of the task prior to administration. The data from a concept-oriented CBM are the number of correctly answered items.

In addition to concept-oriented CBM probes, asking students to judge whether or not items are correctly completed is an effective way to assess conceptual understanding (Bisanz & LeFevre, 1992; Briars & Siegler, 1984; Canobi, 2004; Canobi, Reeve, & Pattison, 1998, 2002, 2003; Cowan, Dowker, Christakis, & Bailey, 1996). For example, 10% of 5-year-old children who counted correctly did not identify counting errors made by others, such as omitting items, repeating numbers, or counting items twice (Briars & Siegler, 1984). An example of this approach to conceptual understanding assessment can be accomplished by providing three examples of the same mathematical equation and asking them to circle the correct one (e.g., 3 + 7 = 12, 4 + 7 = 10, and 3 + 7 = 10) or providing a list of randomly ordered correct and incorrect equations and asking them to write or circle "true" for the correct ones and "false" for the incorrect items (Beatty & Moss, 2007).

Math Assessment within Three Tiers

Tiered intervention systems, such as those used within response to intervention (RTI), are dependent on assessment data (Gresham, 2002). However, the type of assessment needed depends on the decisions being made. As student difficulties become more severe, the interventions needed to address those difficulties become more intense, and measurement becomes more frequent and more precise and results in more detailed problem analysis (Burns & Gibbons, 2008).

A problem-solving model, the underlying conceptual framework of RTI, typically involves problem identification, problem analysis, intervention implementation, and evaluation (Tilly, 2002). Problem analysis is the phase of the problem-solving model in which variables controlling the problem are identified as a basis for selecting an intervention (Kratochwill & Bergan, 1990; Tilly, 2002). This is best accomplished through a systematic analysis of instructional and motivational variables (Barnett, Daly, Jones, & Lentz, 2004; Howell, Hosp, & Kurns, 2008; Howell & Nolet, 2000; Upah & Tilly, 2002). As student needs become more intense, the specificity of the assessment data needed to design the intervention becomes greater (Burns & Gibbons, 2008). Thus, as shown in Table 6.1, assessment within Tier 1 (universal) of an RTI model usually involves collecting benchmark and universal screening data three times each year to determine whether a student's general skill level is discrepant from the norm group. Certainly teachers may collect additional data, but all collect at least benchmark assessments.

Math data in Tier 2 (selected) should identify the category of deficit (e.g., single-digit multiplication or three-digit-by-three-digit addition) among students experiencing difficulties. Those data are then used to identify intervention targets for small groups of students, and those interventions are then delivered within the general curriculum. Finally, math data in Tier 3 (targeted) should isolate the specific skill and the environmental variables that contribute to that deficit, which then suggest specific interventions for individual students. For example, data from Tier 1 could identify a student as a struggling learner in math; then Tier 2 data could suggest that the student does not correctly complete multidigit subtraction problems; and assessment conducted in Tier 3 could identify regrouping as the target skill, and additional analysis could suggest that the student has yet to sufficiently learn the skill and requires additional instruction in it. In addition to these formative data, designed to indicate for what skill an intervention is needed, the effectiveness of the interventions should be monitored with increasing frequency through the tiers.

Tier 1

Because the primary purpose of assessment in Tier 1 of an RTI model is to evaluate how much learning has occurred, data used within this tier should be global in nature. Moreover, multiskill measures correlate better with a global measure of math performance than do single-skill probes (VanDerHeyden & Burns, 2008). Thus CBM with multiskill probes should be administered three times each year as a universal screening tool.

TABLE 6.1. Description of a Comprehensive Assessment System for Multitiered Interventions

Tier	Who is assessed	Who conducts the assessment	How often assessed	Type of probe
Tier 1	All students in a group format	Teacher	3 times per year	• Multiskill general outcome measure (GOM)
Tier 2	Approximately 15–20% of students in a small-group format	Interventionist	At least every other week	• Single-skill specific subskill mastery measures (SSMM) to identify intervention targets • GOM and SSMM to monitor progress
Tier 3	Approximately 5% of students individually administered	Interventionist	At least once each week	• SSMM to identify intervention targets • Error analysis to identify procedural difficulties • Conceptual assessments to determine whether the underlying concept is understood • GOM and SSMM to monitor progress

There are three ways to interpret math CBM data within Tier 1; one that examines group scores and two that focus on individual student data. VanDerHeyden and Burns (2008) collected multiskill CBM data and compared those data with group-administered accountability math test scores to identify empirically derived proficiency criteria. The results suggested that 17 DCPM were necessary to demonstrate proficiency among second- and third-grade students and that 29 DCPM were needed for fourth- and fifth-grade students. Only approximately 7% of second and third graders and 13% of fourth and fifth graders scored above these math CBM criteria but did not score proficiently on the state test (VanDerHeyden & Burns, 2008). Thus the first approach to interpreting math CBM data in Tier 1 is to compare the class median with these criteria.

The DCPM score for each student in Tier 1 is recorded, and a class median, grade mean, and grade standard deviation are computed. Next, the data are used to rule out potential classwide or grade-level problems, which is best accomplished for math by comparing the class medians and grade means to the aforementioned proficiency criteria. A class median is used because the number of students in any one class is often small enough (e.g., less than 30 students) that the mean could be influenced by an extreme score. It is probably safe to use mean scores for grade levels because combining two or more classes often results in enough data (i.e., more than 30 students) to make the mean acceptably stable.

If a classwide problem exists, it may be more efficient to apply an intervention to the class than to pull students out individually for interventions at the selected level (Tier 2). For example, VanDerHeyden and Burns (2005) implemented a peer-assisted learning strategy to teach math facts in classrooms with a classwide problem. The classroom intervention led to immediate gains in skill so that the classwide problem was no longer evident after a few weeks, and student scores increased significantly within the school year and across cohorts (VanDerHeyden & Burns, 2005).

The first step in implementing the classwide intervention is to use single-skill probe assessment data to better identify specific instructional needs (i.e., what exactly to teach). SSMM probes are administered using the curriculum sequence of skills, starting with the current skill and working backward (e.g., double-digit addition, then single-digit subtraction, then single-digit addition) until the class median falls within the instructional level (14–31 DCPM for second and third graders and 24–49 DCPM for fourth- and fifth-grade students; Burns et al., 2006). Classroom instruction and classwide interventions would then focus on the skill (e.g., single-digit subtraction) at which the class median fell within the instructional-level range. Weekly SSMM probes are also administered to monitor progress within the skill. The instructional focus changes once the class median of the SSMM exceeds the relevant proficiency standard, at which time the next skill in the sequence would be taught and an SSMM of that skill would be conducted at least weekly. VanDerHeyden and colleagues (VanDerHeyden & Burns, 2005; VanDerHeyden, Witt, & Gilbertson, 2007; VanDerHeyden, Witt, & Naquin, 2003) have consistently demonstrated the effectiveness of identifying and remediating classwide problems in math while monitoring progress with SSMM.

After a classwide problem is remediated or ruled out, individual student scores can then be examined to identify students for Tier 2 using a normative approach. Students who score at or below a normative criterion (e.g., the 20th percentile, the 25th percentile, or more than 1 standard deviation below the mean) are identified as requiring more intensive intervention. Alternatively, schools could simply compare individual student scores with instructional-level criteria (Burns et al., 2006), described in the following subsection, and any student who scores below the appropriate criterion would be identified for a Tier 2 intervention.

Tier 2

Assessment within Tier 2 relies on GOM data to identify students who need intervention, but instructional decisions within Tiers 2 and 3 rely heavily on SSMM data (Burns & Coolong-Chaffin, 2006). Moreover, single-skill and multiskill probes both lead to data that are dependable for instructional decisions, but neither seems to generalize well to the other (Hintze et al., 2002). Thus a comprehensive assessment system for math at Tier 2 would include both SSMM (single-skill) and GOM (multiskill) data.

After a classwide problem is remediated, or if one does not exist to begin with, individual students are then identified as needing a Tier 2 intervention. Students within the lowest 15th–20th percentile on a grade-level GOM would receive a more targeted intervention, and SSMM probes would be administered to identify which skill in the instructional sequence would be the appropriate starting point. Thus SSMM probes are administered in a progressively easier sequence (e.g., double-digit subtraction without regrouping, then double-digit addition, then single-digit subtraction, then single-digit addition) until the score for a particular SSMM falls within an instructional level, and the intervention process starts with that skill.

Deno and Mirkin (1977) presented fluency criteria to determine an instructional level for math of 21–40 DCPM for students in first–third grades and 41–80 DCPM for fourth–twelfth graders. However, the Deno and Mirkin (1977) standards were not based on research. A recent study found empirically derived instructional-level criteria of 14–31 DCPM for second and third graders and 24–49 DCPM for fourth- and fifth-grade students (Burns et al., 2006). Scores below the lowest end of the instructional-level range fall within the frustration level and suggest that the skill is too difficult for the child, and those that exceed the highest score of the instructional-level range fall within the mastery (or independent) category. Practitioners should administer single-skill probes until the task that represents an instructional level is identified for students in Tier 2 using the criteria derived by Burns et al. (2006). After the instructional-level skill is identified, interventions for that skill could be implemented for a small group, and the appropriate single-skill probes should be administered frequently (e.g., once each week or every other week) until the students in the group demonstrate mastery of the skill; a new skill is then remediated.

Multiskill CBM probes are used to collect GOM data within Tier 2 to monitor the effectiveness of interventions. These data are interpreted by examining the level of the score and the slope of student progress across the duration of the intervention. The level of the score could be interpreted with the VanDerHeyden and Burns (2008) criteria for student proficiency (e.g., 17 DCPM for second and third graders and 29 DCPM for fourth and fifth graders) but also could be examined through a normative approach in which scores would be judged as representing adequate skill once they fell at or above a local or national norm (e.g., at or above the 25th percentile). Fuchs, Fuchs, Hamlett, Walz, and Germann (1993) present math growth rates for realistic and ambitious goals, which could be used to judge the slope with which the scores increased during the intervention.

Tier 3

As in Tiers 1 and 2, the monitoring of student progress is critically important, and multiskill math CBM data serve that purpose better than single-skill assessments (Fuchs et al., 2007). However, the level of problem analysis for children receiving Tier 3 interventions should match the severity of the need, and multiskill data may not provide enough information for instructional planning. Moreover, single-skill probes might be useful in targeting the skill deficit area but may not identify error patterns. Rivera and Bryant (1992) present an active and a passive means to assess the procedures students used to complete the task. A passive approach is one in which an error pattern is detected by examining completed multiskill probes to identify discrepancies between expected and actual performance for skill domains (Howell & Nolet, 2000). For example, a student may complete all of the problems on the sheet that involve multi-digit addition and single-digit multiplication but may not correctly complete 1-digit-by-2-digit multiplication despite its being part of the grade-level curriculum. However, this passive error analysis suggests discrepancies only for skill domains, and additional information may be needed (Kelley, 2008). Thus Rivera and Bryant (1992) suggest passively identifying error patterns that lead to the problem being incorrectly completed and reteaching that skill (e.g., regrouping).

A second approach to identifying error patterns involves a more active assessment in which the student is asked to complete one of two tasks. First, the student is asked to "think out loud" as he or she completes problems. This will allow the student to verbally articulate the errors being made (Rivera & Bryant, 1992). For example, consider the following problem:

$$\begin{array}{r} 32 \\ -15 \\ \hline 23 \end{array}$$

The student might say something like "5 minus 2; I can't subtract 5 from 2, so I'll take 2 from 5, which is 3." Then the procedure for regrouping could be explicitly taught. This particular example could probably be assessed with passive means and is a simple and common error, but it demonstrates the first approach to active assessment. If the child does not articulate the error, he or she is provided with a second example of the problem type and asked to be the teacher and teach the evaluator how to complete it. It is likely that one of these two approaches will identify the specific procedural error being made (Rivera & Bryant, 1992), which can then be directly and explicitly remediated.

Math CBM data in Tier 3 should also be used to determine a student's functioning within the learning hierarchy, which can be best accomplished with both fluency and accuracy scores. Although several scholars have emphasized using the learning hierarchy to drive academic interventions (Ardoin & Daly, 2007; Christ, 2008; Daly, Lentz, & Boyer, 1996), criteria with which to judge where to place student functioning within the hierarchy are not well established. Remediation efforts tend to focus on the acquisition and fluency phases of the hierarchy. Accuracy of the skill is the primary outcome of acquisition, and fast completion of the task is of primary importance in the fluency phase. Thus the data on accuracy with which items are completed are used to evaluate whether students are functioning in the acquisition phase. Meta-analytic research found large effects for drill tasks, such as math computation, as long as the task contained at least 50% known items, with the largest mean effect for tasks that contained 90% known items (Burns, 2004). Therefore, completion of a task with at least 90% correct (e.g., 18 items correct in 1 minute out of a possible 20) suggests that a student has successfully

acquired the skill, and less than 90% correct suggests the need for an acquisition intervention. Certainly, students who obtain a high percentage of incorrect responses require an intensive acquisition intervention, or perhaps they should receive remediation in the prerequisite skills (e.g., intervention in single-digit multiplication may be needed if they complete 10 out of 30 digits correct on a three-digit multiplication probe). Moreover, students who exhibit poor accuracy could also be administered a conceptual assessment to make sure they understand the underlying concepts and are not simply completing the procedures erroneously.

After a student correctly completes 90% of the responses, as measured with sensitive metrics such as digits correct as opposed to items correct, he or she is ready to become more proficient (i.e., fast) in the skill, and fluency data become critically important. The instructional-level criteria found by Burns and colleagues (2006) can again be useful guides. A student who scores within the instructional level is progressing through the proficiency stage, and one who scores above the highest end of instructional-level range (e.g., 24–49 DCPM for fourth- and fifth-grade students) on a single-skill probe is deemed proficient with this skill. When a student scores above the instructional-level range (e.g., 55 DCPM for a fourth grader) on three consecutive single-skill probes, the focus then shifts to maintenance and generalization, and monthly retention probes are used (Burns et al., 2006).

Conclusion

School psychology has always been committed to quality assessment practices, but perhaps the data from past practices resulted in a less direct relationship to student learning. RTI represents a significant change in paradigm in that now assessment's primary function is to identify an effective intervention rather than a disability diagnosis. In other words, the term *diagnosis* may no longer be used exclusively in reference to identifying a child with a disability but now may represent identifying areas of specific deficit and prescribing interventions to address them. Valid diagnostic paradigms are based on data that lead to treatments with known outcomes (Cromwell, Blashfield, & Strauss, 1975). Conducting benchmark procedural assessments, SSMM, and conceptual assessments for children in Tiers 2 and 3 and monitoring the effectiveness of interventions with GOM could result in a well-developed instructional plan with highly predictable outcomes.

Precision teaching research has consistently shown that identifying component tasks and providing explicit instruction with individualized practice opportunities has increased math skills (Chiesa & Robertson, 2000; Johnson & Layng, 1992, 1996; Miller & Heward, 1992). However, there is much more to learn about quality math assessment, instruction, and intervention. That research is currently under way. Through adequately targeting math interventions based on the principles of measurement and human learning, we can enhance student learning for all children, which is the ultimate goal for education, RTI, and school psychology.

References

AIMSweb. (2006). *Measures/norms*. Eden Prairie, MN: Edformation.

Ardoin, S. P., & Daly, E. J., III. (2007). Introduction to the special series: Close encounters of the instructional kind—how the instructional hierarchy is shaping instructional research 30 years later. *Journal of Behavioral Education, 16*, 1–6.

Badian, N. (1999). Persistent arithmetic, reading, or arithmetic and reading disability. *Annals of Dyslexia, 49*, 45–70.

Barnett, D. W., Daly, E. J., Jones, K. M., & Lentz, F. E. (2004). Response to intervention: Empirically based special service decisions from single-case designs of increasing and decreasing intensity. *Journal of Special Education, 38*, 66–79.

Beatty, R., & Moss, J. (2007). Teaching the meaning of the equal sign to children with learning disabilities: Moving from concrete to abstractions. In W. G. Martin, M. E. Strutchens, & P. C. Elliott (Eds.), *The learning of mathematics: Sixty-ninth yearbook* (p. 27–42). Reston, VA: National Council of Teachers of Mathematics.

Bisanz, J., & LeFevre, J. (1992). Understanding elementary mathematics. In J. I. D. Campbell (Ed.), *The nature and origins of mathematical skills* (pp. 113–136). Amsterdam: North-Holland Elsevier Science.

Boaler, J. (1998). Open and closed mathematics: Student experiences and understandings. *Journal for Research in Mathematics Education, 29*, 41–62.

Briars, D. J., & Siegler, R. S. (1984). A featural analysis of preschoolers' counting knowledge. *Developmental Psychology, 20*, 607–618.

Burns, M. K. (2004). Empirical analysis of drill ratio research: Refining the instructional level for drill tasks. *Remedial and Special Education, 25*, 167–175.

Burns, M. K. (in press). Formative evaluation in school psychology: Using data to design instruction. *School Psychology Forum*.

Burns, M. K., & Coolong-Chaffin, M. (2006). Response to intervention: Role of and effect on school psychology. *School Psychology Forum, 1*(1), 3–15.

Burns, M. K., & Gibbons, K. (2008). *Response to intervention implementation in elementary and secondary schools: Procedures to assure scientific-based practices*. New York: Routledge.

Burns, M. K., Tucker, J. A., Frame, J., Foley, S., & Hauser, A. (2000). Interscorer, alternate-form, internal consistency, and test–retest reliability of Gickling's model of curriculum-based assessment for reading. *Journal of Psychoeducational Assessment, 18*, 353–360.

Burns, M. K., VanDerHeyden, A. M., & Jiban, C. (2006). Assessing the instructional level for mathematics: A comparison of methods. *School Psychology Review, 35*, 401–418.

Canobi, K. H. (2004). Individual differences in children's addition and subtraction knowledge. *Cognitive Development, 19*, 81–93.

Canobi, K. H., Reeve, R. A., & Pattison, P. E. (1998). The role of conceptual understanding in children's addition problem solving. *Developmental Psychology, 34*, 882–891.

Canobi, K. H., Reeve, R. A., & Pattison, P. E. (2002). Young children's understanding of addition concepts. *Educational Psychology, 22*, 513–532.

Canobi, K. H., Reeve, R. A., & Pattison, P. E. (2003). Patterns of knowledge in children's addition. *Developmental Psychology, 39*, 521–534.

Chiesa, M., & Robertson, A. (2000). Precision teaching and fluency training: Making maths easier for pupils and teachers. *Educational Psychology in Practice, 16*, 297–310.

Christ, T. J. (2008). Best practices in problem analysis. In A. Thomas & J. Grimes (Eds.), *Best practices in school psychology* (5th ed., Vol. 2, pp. 159–176). Bethesda, MD: National Association of School Psychologists.

Christ, T. J., Johnson-Gros, K. N., & Hintze, J. M. (2005). An examination of alternate assessment durations when assessing multiple-skill computational fluency: The generalizability and dependability of curriculum-based outcomes within the context of educational decisions. *Psychology in the Schools, 42,* 615–622.

Christ, T. J., & Vining, O. (2006). Curriculum-based measurement procedures to develop multiple-skill mathematics computation probes: Evaluation of random and stratified stimulus-set arrangements. *School Psychology Review, 35,* 387–400.

Cowan, R., Dowker, A., Christakis, A., & Bailey, S. (1996). Even more precisely assessing children's understanding of the order-irrelevance principle. *Journal of Experimental Child Psychology, 62,* 84–101.

Cromwell, R., Blashfield, R., & Strauss, J. (1975). Criteria for classification systems. In N. Hobbs (Ed.), *Issues in the classification of children* (pp. 4–25). San Francisco: Jossey-Bass.

Daly, E. J., III, Lentz, F. E., & Boyer, J. (1996). The instructional hierarchy: A conceptual model for understanding the effective components of reading interventions. *School Psychology Quarterly, 11,* 369–386.

Daly, E. J., III, & McCurdy, M. (2002). Getting it right so they can get it right: An overview of the special series. *School Psychology Review, 31,* 453–458.

Deno, S. L. (1985). Curriculum-based measurement: The emerging alternative. *Exceptional Children, 52,* 219–232.

Deno, S. L., & Mirkin, P. K. (1977). *Data-based program modification: A manual.* Reston, VA: Council for Exceptional Children.

Edformation. (2005). *AIMSweb progress monitoring and improvement system.* Retrieved September 18, 2007, from *www.aimsweb.com/.*

Fuchs, L. S., & Deno, S. L. (1991). Paradigmatic distinctions between instructionally relevant measurement models. *Exceptional Children, 57,* 488–500.

Fuchs, L. S., & Fuchs, D. (1991). Curriculum-based measurements current applications and future directions. *Preventing School Failure, 35*(3), 6–11.

Fuchs, L. S., Fuchs, D., Compton, D., Bryant, J. D., Hamlett, C. L., & Seethaler, P. M. (2007). Mathematics screening and progress monitoring at first grade: Implications for responsiveness to intervention. *Exceptional Children, 73,* 311–330.

Fuchs, L. S., Fuchs, D., Hamlett, C. L., & Stecker, P. M. (1991). Effects of curriculum-based measurement and consultation on teacher planning and student achievement in mathematics operations. *American Educational Research Journal, 28,* 617–641.

Fuchs, L. S., Fuchs, D., Hamlett, C. L., Walz, L.,

& Germann, G. (1993). Formative evaluation of academic progress: How much growth can we expect? *School Psychology Review, 22,* 27–48.

Fuchs, L. S., Fuchs, D., Hamlett, C. L., & Whinnery, K. (1991). Effects of goal line feedback on level, slope, and stability of performance with curriculum-based measurement. *Learning Disabilities Research and Practice, 6,* 66–74.

Fuchs, L. S., Fuchs, D., & Karns, K. (2001). Enhancing kindergarteners' mathematical development: Effects of peer-assisted learning strategies. *Elementary School Journal, 101,* 495–510.

Fuchs, L. S., Fuchs, D., & Maxwell, L. (1988). The validity of informal reading comprehension measures. *Remedial and Special Education, 9*(2), 20–28.

Fuchs, L. S., Hamlett, C. L., & Fuchs, D. (1999). *Monitoring basic skills progress: Basic math concepts and applications* (2nd ed.). Austin, TX: Pro-Ed.

Gersten, R., & Chard, D. (1999). Number sense: Rethinking arithmetic instruction for students with mathematical disabilities. *Journal of Special Education, 33,* 18–28.

Gresham, F. M. (2002). Responsiveness to intervention: An alternative approach to the identification of learning disabilities. In R. Bradley & L. Danielson (Eds.), *Identification of learning disabilities: Research to practice* (pp. 467–519). Mahwah, NJ: Erlbaum.

Haring, N. G., & Eaton, M. D. (1978). Systematic instructional technology: An instructional hierarchy. In N. G. Haring, T. C. Lovitt, M. D. Eaton, & C. L. Hansen (Eds.), *The fourth R: Research in the classroom* (pp. 23–40). Columbus, OH: Merrill.

Helwig, R., Anderson, L., & Tindal, G. (2002). Using a concept-grounded curriculum-based measure in mathematics to predict statewide test scores for middle school students with LD. *Journal of Special Education, 36,* 102–112.

Hiebert, J., & Lefevre, P. (1986). Conceptual and procedural knowledge in mathematics: An introductory analysis. In J. Hiebert (Ed.), *Conceptual and procedural knowledge: The case of mathematics* (pp. 1–28). Hillsdale, NJ: Erlbaum.

Hintze, J. M., Christ, T. J., & Keller, L. A. (2002). The generalizability of CBM survey-level mathematics assessments: Just how many samples do we need? *School Psychology Review, 31,* 514–528.

Hofmeister, A. M. (2004). Education reform in mathematics: A history ignored? *Journal of Direct Instruction, 4*(1), 5–11.

Hosp, M. K., Hosp, J. L., & Howell, K. W. (2007). *The ABCs of CBM: A practical guide to curriculum-based measurement*. New York: Guilford Press.

Howell, K. W., Hosp, J. L., & Kurns, S. (2008). Best practices in curriculum-based evaluation. In A. Thomas & J. Grimes (Eds.), *Best practices in school psychology* (5th ed., pp. 349–362). Bethesda, MD: National Association of School Psychologists.

Howell, K. W., & Nolet, V. (2000). *Curriculum-based evaluation: Teaching and decision making*. Belmont, CA: Wadsworth.

Kelley, B. (2008). Best practices in curriculum-based evaluation and math. In A. Thomas & J. Grimes (Eds.) *Best practices in school psychology* (5th ed., pp. 417–438). Bethesda, MD: National Association of School Psychologists.

Kratochwill, T. R., & Bergan, J. R. (1990). *Behavioral consultation in applied settings: An individual guide*. New York: Plenum Press.

Johnson, K. R., & Layng, T. V. J. (1992). Breaking the structuralist barrier: Literacy and numeracy with fluency. *American Psychologist, 27*, 1475–1490.

Johnson, K. R., & Layng, T. V. J. (1996). On terms and procedures: Fluency. *Behavior Analyst, 19*, 281–288.

Lee, J., Grigg, W., & Dion, G. (2007). *The nation's report card: Mathematics 2007*. Washington, DC: U.S. Department of Education, National Center for Education Statistics, Institute of Education Sciences.

Linn, R. L., & Gronlund, N. E. (2000). *Measurement and assessment in teaching* (8th ed.). Upper Saddle River, NJ: Merrill/Prentice Hall.

Manzo, K. K., & Galley, M. (2003). Math climbs, reading flat on '03 NAEP. *Education Week, 23*(12), 1–18.

Miller, A. D., & Heward, W. L. (1992). Do your students really know their math facts? *Intervention in School and Clinic, 28*(2), 98–104.

Moss, J., & Case, R. (1999). Developing children's understanding of the rational numbers: A new model and an experimental curriculum. *Journal for Research in Mathematics Education, 30*, 122–147.

National Council of Teachers of Mathematics. (2000). *Principles and standards for school mathematics*. Reston, VA: Author.

Rittle-Johnson, B., & Siegler, R. S. (1998). The relation between conceptual and procedural knowledge in learning mathematics: A review. In C. Donlan (Ed.), *The development of mathematical skill* (pp. 75–110). Hove, UK: Psychology Press.

Rivera, D. M., & Bryant, B. R. (1992). Mathematics instruction for students with special needs. *Intervention in School and Clinic, 28*, 71–86.

Saffer, N. (1999). Core subjects and your career. *Occupational Outlook Quarterly, 43*(2), 26–40.

Shapiro, E. S. (2004). *Academic skills problems: Direct assessment and intervention* (3rd ed.). New York: Guilford Press.

Shapiro, E. S., Keller, M. A., Lutz, J. G., Santoro, L. E., & Hintze, J. M. (2006). Curriculum-based measures and performance on state assessment and standardized tests: Reading and math performance in Pennsylvania. *Journal of Psychoeducational Assessment, 24*, 19–35.

Shinn, M. R., & Shinn, M. M. (2004). *AIM-Sweb training workbook administration and scoring of mathematics curriculum-based measurement (M-CBM) for use in general outcome measurement*. Eden Prairie, MN: Edformation.

Tilly, W. D. III. (2002). Best practices in school psychology as a problem-solving enterprise. In A. Thomas & J. Grimes (Eds.), *Best practices in school psychology* (4th ed., Vol. 1, pp. 21–36). Bethesda, MD: National Association of School Psychologists.

Upah, K. R. F., & Tilly, W. D. III. (2002). Best practices in designing, implementing, and evaluating quality interventions. In A. Thomas & J. Grimes (Eds.), *Best practices in school psychology* (4th ed., pp. 483–502). Bethesda, MD: National Association of School Psychologists.

VanDerHeyden, A. M., & Burns, M. K. (2005). Using curriculum-based assessment and curriculum-based measurement to guide elementary mathematics instruction: Effect on individual and group accountability scores. *Assessment for Effective Intervention, 30*(3), 15–29.

VanDerHeyden, A. M., & Burns, M. K. (2008). Examination of the utility of various measures of mathematics proficiency. *Assessment for Effective Intervention, 33*, 215–224.

VanDerHeyden, A. M., Witt, J. C., & Gilbertson, D. (2007). A multi-year evaluation of the effects of a response to intervention model on identification of children for special education. *Journal of School Psychology, 45*, 225–256.

VanDerHeyden, A. M., Witt, J. C., & Naquin, G. (2003). Development and validation of a process for screening referrals to special education. *School Psychology Review, 32*, 204–227.

Ysseldyke, J., Burns, M., Dawson, P., Kelley, B., Morrison, D., Ortiz, S., et al. (2006). *School psychology: A blueprint for training and practice: III*. Bethesda, MD: National Association of School Psychologists.

Chapter 7

Assessment of Skills in Written Expression within a Problem-Solving Model

Kristin A. Gansle
George H. Noell

Literacy for *all* children is increasingly recognized as one of the critical outcomes of education by scholars, policy makers, and educators in the United States (No Child Left Behind, 2001; Snow, Burns, & Griffin, 1998). It is necessary to read *and* to write to be literate. Like trends of increasing expectations in mathematics and science, the expectations of what it means for students to be literate writers have steadily increased over time. Early writing instruction tended to focus on transcription of teachers' dictation, with emphasis on generative prose emerging subsequent to emphasis on simple textual forms (Bransford, Brown, & Cocking, 2000). In the 1930s, expectations continued to evolve, with written expression becoming more of an instructional focus within primary schools (Alcorta, 1994; Schneuwly, 1994). As the 20th and 21st centuries have unfolded, the expectations that students employ increasingly sophisticated prose, be conscious of audience, write for a variety of purposes, and generate original ideas have all become evident in curriculum, standardized assessment, and educational discourse.

As has become evident from a number of sources, such as the National Assessment of Educational Progress (NAEP), emphasis, expectations, curriculum, and assessments do not necessarily translate into results. For example, the 2002 NAEP data (the latest assessment for which data are available at this writing) showed that only 24–31% of the students at grades 4, 8, and 12 performed at the *Proficient* level on the writing assessment (National Center for Education Statistics [NCES], 2003). Clearly, many students are neither meeting grade level expectations nor becoming effective written communicators during their K–12 years (Greenwald, Persky, Ambell, & Mazzeo, 1999; Persky, Daane, & Jin, 2003). Poor written literacy outcomes are both far too common and likely to have far too dire effects on students' educational outcomes, vocational training opportunities, employment performance, and future income (Graham & Perin, 2007). The ability to write effectively is an increasingly necessary skill for socialization, citizenship, and work in the information age.

Recognizing that expressive literacy is critical to full participation in society and that many students do not achieve the necessary skills is an obvious call to action for school psychologists. However, successful assessment and intervention in written expression must address at least two challenges that are distinct from those that confront educators in reading and mathematics. First, written expression often appears to suffer from benign neglect in comparison with reading in terms of scholarship and policy (see National Institute of Child Health and Human Development, 2000, and the Reading First component of No Child Left Behind, 2001). Frequently, although educators, parents, and policy makers will agree that writing is important, they appear to perceive reading as the more important of the two tasks. Indeed, referrals for evaluation and intervention are dominated by concerns regarding reading rather than writing (Bramlett, Murphy, Johnson, Wallingsford, & Hall, 2002; Noell, Gansle, & Allison, 1999). At both the individual-student level and the systemic level, it can be difficult to convince parents and educators to devote a level of resources to writing similar to what they are willing to devote to reading.

A second major challenge to assessment and intervention in writing is that, unlike in reading, mathematics, science, and social sciences, a correct response cannot be easily defined. In response to most writing demands, students can produce a nearly infinite number of correct, weak, and incorrect responses. In written expression, no simple equivalent of $3 + 4 = 7$ exists. As is described in the following sections regarding assessment strategies for written expression, this ambiguity about what is good or good enough in written expression is a recurrent challenge confronting students, educators, and school psychologists. It has implications for the selection of dimensions of writing to quantify and for setting standards for acceptable performance. The difficulty inherent in designating which dimensions of writing to assess has also contributed to the absence of convergence on broadly accepted measures in written expression similar to words read correctly (WRC) in 1 minute in reading. There is considerable disagreement about which skills might represent capstone writing skills that indicate competent practice, and each may be measured in a variety of ways. Also, unlike reading or mathematics, there are no widely accepted standards for fluency in written expression for students in elementary school at different grade levels.

The assessment process described in this chapter attempts to layer the classic stages of problem-solving assessment over a writing process that has its own distinct iterative stages. The stages of the problem-solving process include problem identification, problem analysis, plan implementation, and progress evaluation/monitoring (Bergan & Kratochwill, 1990). Within those stages, the assessment process described attends to skills, motivational variables, and the context for writing. The general approach described in this chapter emphasizes the distinction between the author and secretarial roles in writing (Smith, 1982). The author role emphasizes developing and organizing the narrative, and the secretarial role emphasizes producing text that executes the plan.

Assessment of the writing process includes consideration of the multistage process of writing that incorporates at least planning, transcribing, reviewing, and revising (Isaacson, 1985). Planning, organizing, and developing the message according to the purpose of the composition usually comes first, followed by transcribing or putting ideas to paper through longhand writing, dictation, or typing. Transcribing depends on skills such as handwriting, spelling, capitalization, grammar, and punctuation. Reviewing involves the assessment of the match of the product with the purpose of the composition, as well as the composition's match to the conventions of writing. Revising will include making whatever revisions are necessary to improve what was judged inadequate in the reviewing stage. Although there is a sequential nature to the process, the stages are not mutually exclusive; indeed, competent writers tend to do all of these things at the same time (Howell & Nolet, 2000).

The balance of this chapter describes a problem-solving approach to the assessment of written expression based on the problem-solving model (Bergan & Kratochwill, 1990). The major questions addressed in this chapter are the common core questions that form the backbone of the problem-solving process (see Figure 7.1). The major sections of this chapter focus in turn on identifying when a problem in written expression is evident, specifying what the problem is, identifying what actions might improve performance, and assessing the efficacy of interventions. The challenges in selecting measures of written expression and setting standards for adequate performance become increasingly salient across stages of the problem-solving process.

Stage	Assessment foci	Data sources
Problem identification	*Screening* to proactively identify struggling students	**National**: published, norm-referenced achievement tests (e.g., ITBS) **Regional**: published, norm-referenced, state-specific achievement tests **Local**: teacher nomination, district norms on CBM-WE measures
	Problem assessment to identify what the concerns are in written expression	Teacher and student interviews Review permanent products Observations Task-analysis-driven skills assessment
Problem analysis	What changes in the environment might support improved student achievement?	Hypotheses suggested by integrating data from the problem assessment: data describing environment and academic performance Brief experimental analysis
Intervention implementation and progress monitoring	Is the intervention that is being provided effective?	Short-term outcomes derived from remediation activities Long-term outcomes from a long-term global outcome measure such as CBM

FIGURE 7.1. Stages of assessment for written expression.

Problem Identification

Educational programs vary widely in the degree to which they are proactive, or antecedent-based, versus reactive, or consequent-based, regarding student achievement (DuPaul & Weyandt, 2006). Reactive models in education might be described as a traditional wait-to-fail approach. In a reactive model, all students are provided core academic programming, and additional resources are focused on students once they fall sufficiently behind that their functioning is qualitatively distinct from that of peers and is a source of concern to teachers and/or parents. The emergence of problem solving, response to intervention (RTI), and preventive service delivery models in education occurred partially in response to the failings of a wait-to-fail approach (Elliott, Huai, & Roach, 2007). A wait-to-fail approach withholds resources when problems are emerging, are small in magnitude, and are responsive to intervention. In contrast, problem-solving or preventive approaches attempt to identify deficits in achievement at the point at which they begin to emerge and to intervene while the prognosis for improvement is still relatively positive.

It is not conceptually difficult to appreciate the logical appeal of intervening when problems are small and malleable in a preventive and problem-solving approach. The challenge is to create and maintain systems that provide early detection and intervention for problems when their intensity is low. In school psychology, the early detection process has historically been described as *screening*. Screening typically refers to the provision of brief, simple, repeatable assessments to many or all students. These brief assessments are designed to detect students whose performance on current academic tasks is lagging sufficiently behind such that additional assessment or intervention is warranted. It is important to note that in order for screening assessments to be practical (i.e., that they not consume most of the available resources for intervention), it is critical that they either capitalize on tasks that are already naturally occurring or that they be simple.

Screening: Who Might Be in Trouble with Writing?

Academic screening is traditionally used to identify children who may need additional assistance to succeed in the general curriculum. Students' skills are generally compared with those of their peers during screening. Accuracy, efficiency, and early use in students' academic careers are desirable characteristics of good screening instruments (Elliott et al., 2007). Despite the clear benefits of early, proactive identification of children at risk for failure (e.g., Campbell, Ramey, Pungello, Sparling, & Miller-Johnson, 2002), educators frequently wait for students to fail and/or use assessments that lack validity evidence (Donovan & Cross, 2002; Elliott et al., 2007). A variety of methods are available to screen children's writing skills that range from teacher nomination to standardized achievement data that schools routinely collect. Screening methods tend to use a global appraisal of student skills rather than specific skills-based assessment, as the data are quickly collectible from large numbers of students.

Teachers as Screeners

Screening may take the form of informal review of classroom work, in which the teacher functions as the test of whether the student is meeting expectations. The level of precision with which teachers are asked to provide judgments regarding students' skills may range from a simple request for teacher nomination of students experiencing difficulties with written expression to requesting structured ratings of specific writing skills that are germane to the students' current grade placement. For example, ratings at the end of first grade might ask about spelling, penmanship, capitalization, and punctuation in the context of writing simple sentences. In contrast, fifth-grade ratings might inquire about mechanics more globally, about grammar, outlining, narrative formation, proofreading, and clarity of prose for the audience. Teachers tend to be more accurate judges of student achievement when provided a structure for describing that achievement (Elliott et al., 2007). For example, correlations of structured teacher ratings of student skills with standardized achievement scores are over .6 (Demaray & Elliott, 1998; Hoge & Coladarci, 1989). The following suggestions may prove helpful for practitioners who wish to devise a brief teacher rating form to screen students in writing:

1. Review appropriate end-of-grade expectations for writing as published by state departments of education, school districts, and/or text publishers.

2. Identify capstone skills for the grade level of the students you wish to screen.
3. Break down capstone skills into four to six key component skills.
4. Create a simple form on which the writing skills of an entire class can be rated on a single page on the five or so dimensions of the capstone task that was identified by circling the rating that describes each student's writing skills in the component skill areas.

In addition, Figure 7.2 provides an example of a rating form for screening for one grade-level expectation in writing for third-grade students in Louisiana. Given the low cost of implementation and their easy availability, data based on structured teacher reports of writing skills should be a facet of school-wide screening for academics (Elliott et al., 2007).

Standardized Achievement Tests

To state the obvious, standardized achievement tests are poor screening instruments. They are too expensive and infrequent, and the lag between test completion and scoring is typically too long for them to be an ideal screening tool. As a result school psychologists would typically not recommend the *adoption* of standardized achievement tests as screening tools. However, standardized testing is now widespread in the United States, and it would be inefficient *not* to use data that are already available to provide an indicator of student needs in tested grades.

For screening purposes, group tests are likely to be used to provide general information regarding student skills. School districts often administer annual assessments for statewide accountability systems. In varying levels of detail, these tests tend to provide student scores for areas such as mechanics, usage, expression, and total language. For example, the Iowa Tests of Basic Skills (ITBS; Hoover, Dunbar, & Frisbie, 2005) is a nationally available, commonly used group test of academic skills that gives language scores in spelling, capitalization, punctuation, and usage/expression. Validity is generally accepted as strong, and internal consistency and equivalent-form reliability coefficients range between the mid .80s and the low .90s, with subtest reliability somewhat lower (Engelhard & Lane, 2004).

Third-Grade ELA Grade Level Expectation

Write compositions of two or more paragraphs that are organized with the following: a central idea; a logical, sequential order; supporting details that develop ideas; and transitional words within and between paragraphs.

Please rate each student as to how often he or she does what is described at the top of the column while writing.

1 = never   2 = occasionally   3 = often   4 = usually   5 = almost always

Student	Writes 2 or more paragraphs	Communicates a central idea	Communicates distinct sequential order	Provides details sufficient to develop ideas	Uses transitional words within and between paragraphs	Total
A						
B						
C						
D						
E						
F						
G						

FIGURE 7.2. Grade-level expectation with sample rating scale.

Scores for group achievement tests are traditionally norm-referenced or reported as standard scores, percentile ranks, and age or grade equivalents, and they can be used to screen and flag students whose performances are below those of a percentage of their peers or below some predetermined cut score. Although these scores provide information regarding how individual students' scores compare with those in their grades or age groups, they have limited treatment validity or utility in providing recommendations of target skills for remediation or goals for intervention (Cone, 1989; Hayes, Nelson, & Jarrett, 1987). However, they can serve to identify students whose poor performances should trigger follow-up assessment.

Curriculum-Based Measurement

Curriculum-based measurement (CBM) was designed to provide special educators with a way to measure progress on specific skills that was not possible with norm-referenced testing. It provides valid measurements of student performance that can be adminis-

tered repeatedly to evaluate the effects of instruction (Bradley & Ames, 1977; Christ & Silberglitt, 2007; Deno, 1985, 1986, 1989; Deno, Marston, & Tindal, 1985). However, CBM has also been used successfully to screen students in a variety of academic skill areas. As CBM became more commonly used during its formative period, efforts were made to determine how larger groups of students were functioning so that the performance of those experiencing difficulties in the general curriculum could be compared across classes, schools, and districts (Shinn, 1988). The data from these groups are considered "norms" in that they provide a standard sot that individual students' performances can be compared with the performances of students from their specific educational systems (Stewart & Kaminski, 2002). Norms are especially pertinent to screening for academic deficits in that they provide systems-level data that may help educators identify students functioning at the lower end of the distribution who may need additional instruction or practice with basic skills. Districts may set their own cut marks to determine the size of the group of students who may be referred for additional evaluation or assistance.

According to the standard procedures for CBM writing originally described by Shinn (1989), students are provided with a picture, a half-sentence story starter, or a sentence that serves as a prompt for them to write. They are first told to think about the topic for 1 minute without writing and then told to write for a specific period of time. Validity coefficients for CBM—Written Expression (CBM-WE) measures are strongest when 3-minute or 5-minute writing samples are gathered from students and are similar across the types of prompts used (McMaster & Espin, 2007). For example, concurrent validity coefficients with the Test of Written Language (TOWL; Hammill & Larsen, 1996) range from .69 to .88, and those with the Developmental Scoring System (DSS; Lee & Canter, 1971) range from .76 to .88 (McMaster & Espin, 2007).

Some of the most common and best validated CBM-WE measures include total words written (TWW), words spelled correctly (WSC), correct word sequences (CWS), and percentages of the totals, as described subsequently. For TWW, results are reported as the total number of words the student writes during the period, including those that are spelled incorrectly. Numbers do not count. WSC is a subset of TWW and includes only those words that are spelled correctly, even if the choice of word is not correct in the context of the sentence written. Results may be reported as the number of WSC in the course of the time period of the passage or as the proportion of TWW that are spelled correctly (number spelled correctly divided by the TWW × 100 = %WSC). CWS is intended to assess the grammatical correctness of the writing sample by decreasing the credit assigned for sheer volume when "word salad" (Shinn, 1989) has been generated: Any two neighboring words that are correctly spelled and grammatically and syntactically correct within the writing sample are counted as one correct writing sequence. Results are reported as a count of the number of CWS written during the 3- or 5-minute assessment. For example, in the following sentence,

^ Save ^ som ^ pie ^ for ^ him ^ and ^ I ^ ,

there are eight possible word sequences, each marked with a caret. The second and third are incorrect because *som* is an incorrectly spelled word, and the seventh and eighth are also incorrect because *I* should have been *me*. Percent CWS can be calculated by dividing the number of CWS by the total number of word sequences and multiplying by 100 (%CWS). The score for this example would be four CWS out of eight total word sequences, or an accuracy of 50%. Correct minus incorrect word sequences, which in the preceding example would be 4 minus 4, or 0, has been found to be moderately correlated with district writing tests for middle school students (Espin et al., 2000). Measures such as TWW, correct letter sequences, CWS, and WSC have been found to have significant correlations with criterion measures of writing such as the TOWL or the Stanford Achievement Test, as well as adequate reliability (Deno, Marston, & Mirkin, 1982; Deno, Mirkin, & Marston, 1980; Gansle, Noell, VanDer-Heyden, Naquin, & Slider, 2002; Marston & Deno, 1981; Videen, Deno, & Marston, 1982). In addition, a growing body of literature describes the measurement of a variety of common and alternate curriculum-based measures, including adequate reliability data and moderate validity coefficients with widely accepted standardized assessments of written expression (e.g., Espin, De La Paz, Scierka, & Roelofs, 2005; Espin, Scierka, Skare, & Halverson, 1999; Espin et al., 2000; Gansle et al., 2002; 2004; Marston, 1989). Although some of these alternative measures have shown promise as tools for measuring written expression, additional research is indicated before they could be adopted for common use by assessment teams in schools.

Parker, Tindal, and Hasbrouck (1991) evaluated several CBM-WE measures for the purpose of screening to identify students experiencing difficulty with writing. They measured several aspects of student writing samples that were collected in fall and spring: TWW, WSC, CWS, %WSC, and %CWS. Whereas most of the measures did not distinguish among low performers, Parker et al. (1991) found that in the second through fifth grades, %WSC was the best tool for screening purposes as the distribution of scores was relatively normally distributed, whereas for the other measures collected the distribution of scores was skewed positively or negatively depending on the grade level.

Problem Identification: What Is the Problem with Writing?

Once students have been identified who are having difficulty with written expression, additional and more detailed assessment will be needed to identify the specific areas of concern. The general approach to this stage of the assessment might be described as curriculum-based assessment (CBA). In contrast, CBM, described previously, is a series of global outcome measures that were developed to permit frequent monitoring of student progress on tasks that are psychometrically sound and closely linked to critical global educational outcomes such as literacy. CBA is a diverse collection of assessment procedures that employ CBM and other direct measures of academic performance to answer assessment questions, guide intervention design, and evaluate program success (Mercer & Mercer, 2005). CBA is an umbrella term under which a variety of possible activities, including interviews, permanent product review, fluency-based probes, accuracy-based probes, and curriculum-based measurement, reside (Shapiro, 2004). CBA also involves task analysis of the curriculum prior to frequent measurement of student performance on those curricular tasks (Salvia, Ysseldyke, & Bolt, 2007). CBA investigates academic behavior in relation to the specific events that precede and follow it, examining behavior in the context of the environment and events that continue from day to day (Sulzer-Azaroff & Mayer, 1991). For the purpose of assessment for problems with written language, teacher interviews, permanent product reviews, fluency and accuracy probes, direct observations in the classroom, and student interviews are recommended.

Initially, the CBA assessment will focus on identifying and defining the breakdowns in the writing process. One of the elements that the assessment will eventually turn to is the distinction between what have been described as the writing demands of the author and those of the secretary (Howell & Nolet, 2000; Smith, 1982). Writers' author role requires students to generate ideas, organize those ideas, and then communicate them in clear and interesting ways. In contrast, the secretary role requires the transcription of the ideas into conventionally acceptable prose that at a minimum does not distract from the authors' ideas and that ideally enhances them. Different students will struggle with different aspects of writing. Some students will report that they simply cannot think of anything to write about, others will have ideas that excite them but have difficulty organizing their ideas into coherent prose, and others will struggle with fundamental mechanics such as grammar, spelling, and punctuation.

To examine writing skills, it is helpful to have information regarding teacher demands, curriculum demands, student skills, and student work habits, as each may be related to poor performance in the classroom. In other words, evaluation of the problem should contain more than just assessment of academic skills in isolation, as the context of the instructional environment is likely to play a part in determination of success or failure for the student (Shapiro, 2004). It may be the case that skills are more evident under some demands than others, and this information can prove invaluable during problem analysis (described later in the chapter).

Interviews

Because of their simplicity, brevity, and efficiency, teacher interviews are often used as a first step in the assessment process (Shapiro, 2004). The interview phase should include questions about a variety of writing-relevant issues, which are included in Table 7.1 with some examples of possible questions. Information about what happens in the classroom at the times that the student exhibits problems with writing should be collected from the teacher, as this may contribute to the problem analysis. The interviewer should gather more specific information regarding areas of concern to help focus more direct assessment activities (Witt, Daly, & Noell, 2000). For example, an interviewer would typically inquire about work habits, timeliness of assignment completion, maturity of writing content, grammar, mechanics, and organizational skills. If the student generally works hard in class and produces timely

TABLE 7.1. Data Collection Using Teacher Interview Questions for Writing Concerns

Focus	Example questions
Curriculum	1. Are you using a published curriculum? If so, which one? 2. On what skills are students currently working?
Typical classroom performance	3. How would you describe the behavior of your class as a group? 4. How would you describe the academic work of your class as a group? 5. Is your class's work and behavior comparable to those of other classes you have had in past years?
Classroom management	6. Do you have a formal system for teaching students classroom expectations and routines? 7. What consequences do you use for student behavior? 8. What consequences do you use for student academic work?
Progress monitoring	9. How do you monitor your students' academic progress in language arts? 10. Are you doing anything differently to monitor the progress of the student whom you have referred?
Programmed academic consequences	11. Are there planned consequences for academic work in your classroom? What are they?
Target student: work habits	12. Please describe the target student's work habits in language arts. 13. Are these work habits consistent with those in other content areas (e.g., mathematics)? 14. Is homework a problem for this student?
Target student: academic work	15. Does the target student complete language arts assignments on time? 16. Does the target student follow directions? 17. What aspects of the target student's writing are problematic? 18. Are the problems specific to writing, or are they evident in other areas as well?

work but his or her writing samples are immature in content and organizational structure, this would suggest a very different pattern of follow-up assessment from that of a student who is generally off task and produces few if any products.

Although many students will not have substantial insight into their writing difficulties, it can prove very helpful to interview students briefly early in the assessment process. In some cases, students will be able to identify key factors that may influence intervention design. For example, students who report difficulty generating ideas or understanding directions and/or a general dislike of writing will have identified factors that need to be addressed during intervention design. Students should be asked to describe not only the steps that are used when writing but also areas that are problematic for them in writing. For example, if the student's writing samples contain many errors in capitalization and punctuation, the

student should be asked about how to correct the errors. If the student cannot correct the errors, instruction would be indicated, rather than a consequence-based procedure, such as reward for accurate error correction for a student who has the necessary skills and can fix the errors but does not do so on assignments.

Review of Writing Samples: Permanent Products

Writing samples will provide information about the student's current writing performance and skills and will help guide more detailed assessment. Review of permanent products should answer the following questions.

1. Does the student *complete assignments*? Is the problem the quality of the assignments written or poor assignment completion rate?
2. Has the student *followed directions*?

Failure is likely to follow noncompliance with directions, which may result from lack of understanding, lack of skills to comply, or lack of motivating consequences for compliance. It may be necessary to retrieve the directions from the teacher, as they will not always be obvious from review of assignments.

3. Does the student *write fluently*? Is there enough text to meet the requirements of the assignment?

4. Is *assignment difficulty appropriate* to common grade-level expectations? If difficulty is too high relative to student skills and prior instruction, the student may not produce work sufficient to earn passing scores.

5. Does the student *write legibly*? Clearly, if the teacher cannot read the text, the student cannot earn credit for completed work.

6. Does the student follow *conventions* of written language, including mechanics, grammar, spelling, and punctuation?

7. Does the student competently *generate content*, including constructing sentences, paragraphs, narrative, and expository text?

Review of permanent products should help identify what the problems are with the final writing product. For example, it may be obvious that the student does not communicate well through writing. It is important to look at the specific errors observed in the writing samples for information regarding such conventions as which mechanics, grammar, or spelling errors the student makes (Howell & Nolet, 2000). However, for issues such as content, organization, and style, initially it may not be clear where the breakdown in the writing process occurs. Additional assessment may be necessary to isolate this breakdown. It is important to acknowledge, when reviewing permanent products, that the conditions under which they were created may be largely unknown. Direct assessment under known conditions can be an invaluable tool for getting a more accurate picture of student skills in writing.

Setting standards for performance is an additional issue that emerges when assessing student writing samples and that is relevant to varying degrees for the following assessment activities. The issue of standard setting is particularly troublesome, as writing is a multiple-dimensional activity, the expectations for which change as the age and maturity of the students do. For school psychologists who have not spent a good deal of time reading first or final drafts of third-grade essays on "What I Did on My Summer Vacation," it may not be clear whether the sample in front of them is a strong or weak writing sample. Solving this dimension of the assessment problem may require reviewing the work of competent peers and published standards to develop reasonable assessment standards for the specific concerns that are evident (for a more detailed discussion, see, e.g., Kelley, Reitman, & Noell, 2003).

Direct Observation

Direct observation of the student and teacher in the classroom during writing instruction and independent writing time may help clarify what the students' work habits look like in context and may ultimately contribute to the problem analysis phase that follows. As a practical matter, the same observational occasions that contribute to the assessment of work habits can contribute to the descriptive assessment of the context, as well. As a result, both environmental and student-level variables are discussed in this section. These data may support or disconfirm concerns regarding student work habits, instruction, the classroom context, and how these variables interact (Kelley et al., 2003; Witt et al., 2000).

Information concerning environmental variables may be collected through direct observation of the student's work habits and may provide information relevant to the assessment of the student's skills problem. The school psychologist may find that variables unrelated to the presumed reasons for difficulties may contribute significantly to the observed deficits. For example, if the student is not attending to the task when asked to write or is placed in a location in the classroom that is not conducive to sustained work engagement, writing is likely to be negatively affected, regardless of whether or not a skill problem is present. Instructional variables may also be contributing to the problem. For example, instruction regarding tenses of irregular verbs is unlikely to be very effective for a student who cannot yet differentiate verbs from nouns.

Evidence regarding the teacher's delivery of prompts or instructions and student work habits during writing assignments would be the main foci of direct observation for writing problems. The direct observation should be used to collect information regarding *teacher behavior*, *student compliance* and *work habits*, and *peer behavior* during the period devoted to writing in the classroom. This observation would be conducted to get an objective picture of the antecedents that precede writing problems, the writing behavior itself, and the consequences that follow behavior—both appropriate behavior (e.g., student working diligently on writing assignments) and inappropriate behavior (e.g., student is wandering around the room during journal writing time). Rather than through strict adherence to interval recording procedures, writing behaviors will be better assessed by looking at the following variables in a more general manner:

1. *Teacher behavior.* What is the routine that the teacher uses to open lessons? Does the teacher clearly indicate what the student is supposed to do during the time devoted to writing? If the student does not understand what the desired behavior is, compliance will be attenuated as a result. Further, does the teacher provide corrective and positive feedback to the students in the classroom? Is there sufficient positive feedback to maintain desired student writing behavior?

2. *Student compliance and work habits.* Does the student comply with teacher instructions? If initial compliance occurs, does the student remain engaged throughout the period during which students write? Good initial compliance that decreases with the duration of the period devoted to writing may indicate that the assignment is not at the student's instructional level, that it is either too easy or too hard for the student to maintain attention.

3. *Peer behavior.* What are the other students in the classroom doing? What are the students close to the target student doing? It is possible that the target student is interested more in what the nearby students are doing than in the assignment or that the level of activity in the classroom is too high for any of the students to get much writing done. If the

nearby students are too active for the target student to maintain attention to the task, a solution to the problem might be something as simple as moving the student's desk to a quieter and more teacher-accessible location in the room.

Task Analysis and Detailed Skill Assessment

The final part of the problem identification phase for many students will be a more fine-grained and detailed assessment of specific skills. However, it would be inefficient to have a standardized task analysis and skill assessment that was applied indiscriminately to all students. For example, in one case, prior assessment data may suggest a wealth of writing volume produced with poor mechanics and nearly incomprehensible grammar. In this case the detailed assessment would likely focus on guided editing of prior work to determine whether the student lacks the requisite skills to proofread and correct his or her work. In another case, assessment data may indicate that writing mechanics, grammar, and spelling all meet or exceed grade-level expectations but that concerns are evident regarding the quality and organization of ideas. This section summarizes an approach to this detailed assessment organized around the concepts of author functions versus secretarial functions (Smith, 1982) and the four-stage writing process (Isaacson, 1985) that were introduced previously.

Paradoxically, the detailed assessment of writing typically will begin not with writing, but with talking. In order to write, one needs to have something to say. This corresponds to the author role and the planning stage of writing. Initial assessment typically will begin by presenting students with a grade-appropriate writing task and prompting them to talk through the planning stage. Typically, the school psychologist should act as the scribe at this point so that students can attend to ideas. The goal of the planning stage assessment is to have the students create a developmentally appropriate writing *plan* with as few *writing demands* as possible. For a first-grade student, that might simply be saying a sentence aloud that was intended to be written. For a second-grade student, it might be planning a well-thought-out paragraph, and for a fifth-grade student it might consist of outlining an essay. The key consideration at this stage is that until the student has a well-developed plan, consideration of writing mechanics may be premature.

The second stage of the writing process is dominated by the secretarial role: transcribing. For assessment purposes, the task is simply to ask students to write the composition they had planned during the development and planning stage. Depending on age, context, and expectations, this may be done in script, in print, or by typing (Howell & Nolet, 2000). The school psychologist's key foci at this stage of the assessment are to watch the student's work habits and to ensure a minimum of distractions so that the assessment of skills is not contaminated by competing behaviors and classroom distractions (Noell, Ardoin, & Gansle, 2009).

Once the initial draft is complete, the next stage is to observe the completion of the reviewing process. It is important to talk with students to prompt description of thoughts concerning the writing product and to get a sense of whether mechanical issues such as punctuation and content are being addressed. This stage of the assessment has two key goals. The first is to determine whether or not students can identify and correct their grammatical and mechanical errors. The second is to determine whether or not students can proofread their writing for content. In other words, do the students ask and answer the questions of whether the prose makes sense and whether it adequately expresses the thoughts or goals that were originally intended?

The final phase of assessment should consist of directing the students to review, assess, and revise the draft appropriately. The critical consideration at this stage is whether students can recognize and correct their own errors. Some students will recognize that words are misspelled and that paragraphs do not make sense but still struggle with how to correct these problems. A last target in observing and interacting with students through the writing process assessment is consideration of students' work habits. How long can they work before they become fatigued? Are they restless and inattentive? Are they able to organize their own work, or are they dependent on directions and cues?

Problem Analysis

Problem analysis is commonly described as assessment and analysis designed to identify the reason that a problematic behavior occurs, and it is a common feature of consultation, problem solving, RTI, and secondary prevention (Beavers, Kratochwill, & Braden, 2004; Bergan & Kratochwill, 1990). Problem analysis as it has been classically framed has been developed to identify reasons that students engage in problematic behaviors and has been nearly synonymous with functional assessment (Carr & Durand, 1985; Iwata, Dorsey, Silfer, Bauman, & Richman, 1982; O'Neill et al., 1997). For example, a student may engage in disruptive behavior to escape academic demands or to obtain attention. Problem analysis has examined what students obtain (i.e., positive reinforcement) or escape from (i.e., negative reinforcement) as a result of the target behavior. However, in the context of academic skill problems, the target of concern is typically not the occurrence of a behavior but the absence or the poor quality of the behavior. When behaviors are absent, it is not possible to analyze the environmental context to identify what is maintaining them. Furthermore, for many academic deficits, the origin of the problem will be in complex instructional histories that may not be readily accessible at the time of assessment (Daly, Witt, Martens, & Dool, 1997). In some cases, however, the classroom observations, interviews, and review of permanent products may *suggest* proximal issues that may be interfering with student performance. For example, ambiguous instructions, infrequent feedback, limited opportunities to practice, and a noisy, distracting classroom may all contribute to poor performance. Prior to implementing an individualized intervention, it would be prudent to target classroom factors that may explain the referral concern and that may have a negative impact on the performance of all students.

In many instances, no environmental factors will be implicated in the referred student's poor writing skills, and assessment will move to planning for an individualized intervention. Problem analysis for academic skill deficits commonly will focus on specification of the skill breakdowns, identifying effective instructional supports, and devising remediation strategies that maximize opportunities to practice skills with feedback that will ameliorate the identified deficits. For example, if a student's weakness is in proofing and correcting work, practice opportunities might be developed for proofing and correcting sentences in a cover–copy–compare (e.g., Skinner, McLaughlin, & Logan, 1997) or peer-tutoring format (e.g., Harris, Graham, & Mason, 2006; Saddler & Graham, 2005). In contrast, if the primary deficits are related to topic generation and planning, the primary initial intervention activity might consist of identifying essay topics and developing rich outlines of those topics using traditional outlines or a story map (e.g., Vallecorsa & deBettencourt, 1997). This work could then be reviewed, revised, and reinforced with an adult or peer tutor. The keys to the process are to isolate the critical skills that are in need of rapid development, to devise a practice strategy that provides effective prompts and feedback, and to develop a practice schedule that will permit the student to catch up to his or her peers. Description of the range of intervention elements that may be combined to meet students' needs is beyond the scope of this chapter. Readers are encouraged to read McCurdy, Schmitz, and Albertson, Chapter 18 in this volume, describing interventions for written expression.

Brief experimental analysis (BEA) is an additional tool for problem analysis that can aid in the examination of the influence of environmental conditions on student performance. BEA has increasingly been used as an assessment tool for poor academic performance (e.g., Duhon et al., 2004; Malloy, Gilbertson, & Maxfield, 2007). *Functional analysis* is a set of procedures designed to identify the variables that control the occurrence of behaviors (Hanley, Iwata, & McCord, 2003). A BEA is an abbreviated procedure in which only one session is typically conducted per phase or condition, whereas in a full functional analysis the number of sessions could easily reach 40–60 over an extended period of time (Northup et al., 1991), making it unlikely to be of use in a school setting. For example, Noell, Freeland, Witt, and Gansle (2001) applied a BEA to oral reading fluency. In this study students were exposed to a baseline condition, a reward condition, an instruction condition, and a combined instruction–reward condition. Each condi-

tion was presented for a single brief session, and then the entire sequence was repeated, constituting a minimal reversal condition. Subsequent extended analyses tested the efficacy of the conditions that were identified as most promising in the BEA, and, in 83% of cases, the extended analysis supported the result obtained in the BEA.

Duhon and colleagues (2004) provide an example of assessment-driven intervention design in which the target behaviors included written expression. The assessment did not include the reversal conditions that are needed to complete a BEA (e.g., Daly et al., 1997; Eckert, Dunn, & Ardoin, 2006) but, instead, implemented each condition for a single session and developed skill-versus-performance deficit hypotheses from this nonexperimental assessment. The goal of the assessment was to differentiate students whose poor academic performance could be described as a performance deficit, having skills but lacking motivation, rather than a skill deficit. Students whose performances improved when they were told that they would have access to rewards would be considered students with performance deficits. These students have the skills necessary to achieve, but the environmental contingencies do not support adequate performance. Subsequent extended experimental analyses built around this assessment-driven heuristic supported the hypotheses developed in this brief nonexperimental assessment.

BEA can be used to differentiate between different skill set difficulties that may be implicated in students' writing problems. For example, conditions could be developed that place heavier demands on the author role or on the secretarial role in writing. This type of BEA would begin with the provision of specific information regarding the composition to be written. In one condition, this could take the form of a list or outline of ideas, of verbal instructions regarding specific content, or even of a picture that the student would be asked to describe in writing. When given rich content and asked to write, is the student able to generate adequate text? Alternatively, another condition could take the form of a structured checklist. Students would be provided with a simple writing prompt with a detailed checklist of what the structure of desired text should include. For a paragraph, a checklist might include a topic sentence, three or four supporting details, and a concluding sentence. For a sentence, a checklist might include a subject, a predicate or verb, descriptors of both (if desired), capital letters for the first word and proper nouns, and ending punctuation. Checklists such as this would be adapted to the requisite parts of the writing assignments given. Data would be reviewed examining the content, quality, and volume of writing under each condition. If the student produced a strong product when given considerable support for the author role, intervention would likely focus on developing these skills. Alternatively, if the student produced a stronger product when provided procedural supports, then intervention would focus on grammar, syntax, and mechanics.

Progress Monitoring

The central reason to engage in the type of problem-solving process described herein is to develop and implement an intervention that improves student functioning. Successful intervention requires a sound plan, implementation of that plan, and monitoring of student performance to evaluate student progress and the adequacy of the intervention to improve it. This chapter focuses on assessment. Companion chapters in this volume provide more detailed consideration of intervention design for written assessment and supporting intervention implementation.

Progress monitoring is critical due to its demonstrated link to students' educational gains (Fuchs, Fuchs, Hamlett, & Stecker, 1991; Fuchs, Fuchs, Hamlett, Walz, & Germann, 1993; Jones & Krouse, 1988). However, recognizing and accepting its importance does not indicate *which* assessment should be utilized in progress monitoring. We recommend a blended strategy that includes both short-term and long-term elements. The short-term strategy should most profitably be embedded in the remedial strategy. For example, if students are proofreading and correcting sentences, what percentage of errors are they detecting and correcting? Alternatively, if the goal is to generate essay topics and supporting outlines, how many appropriate headings and detailed subheadings do students develop per working

session? The keys to this type of proximal short-term assessment are that it should be naturally integral to the remedial activity and highly informative regarding the immediate intervention target (e.g., generating essay topics and supporting outlines).

Optimally, progress monitoring will also include one or more long-term global outcome assessments such as a CBM. This long-term strategy should be implemented less often than the short-term remedial strategy, but it should be designed to be relatively constant across a somewhat long duration of intervention. The long-term assessment strategy might blend CBM writing probes with an assessment rubric that captures key developmentally appropriate dimensions of writing. Ideally, the long-term progress monitoring strategy would be implemented frequently, but depending on its complexity and duration, it may not be practical to implement it more than once per week. This is particularly true in a domain such as writing in the upper grades, in which completing and revising essays is a time-consuming task. A long-term progress monitoring strategy should occur frequently enough to help guide decision making, should be simple enough to be frequently repeatable, and should sample a sufficiently advanced skill that it can be maintained over a relatively long period of time.

Conclusion

The problem-solving process guides assessment in written language through a number of important steps. Screening determines whether there is a problem with students' writing in comparison with national, regional, and/or local data. Problem identification can be determined through the use of teacher interviews, reviews of writing samples, skill and accuracy assessments, student interviews, and direct observations in the classroom. A brief functional analysis may provide some important information regarding why the problem is happening in terms of the environmental supports for desired and undesirable behavior and their interaction with student skills. During assessment, it is important to be aware that the data collected must serve the purpose of the assessment. Ideally, the written language assessment will result in valid treatment (Cone, 1989; Hayes et al., 1987) by contributing directly to the selection of intervention components tailored specifically to the deficits observed during the assessment.

References

Alcorta, M. (1994). Text writing from a Vygotskyan perspective: A sign-mediated operation. *European Journal of Psychology of Education, 9,* 331–341.

Beavers, K. F., Kratochwill, T. R., & Braden, J. P. (2004). Treatment utility of functional versus empiric assessment within consultation for reading problems. *School Psychology Quarterly, 19,* 29–49.

Bergan, J. R., & Kratochwill, T. R. (1990). *Behavioral consultation and therapy.* New York: Plenum Press.

Bradley, M. M., & Ames, W. S. (1977). Readability parameters of basal readers. *Journal of Reading Behavior, 11,* 175–183.

Bramlett, R. K., Murphy, J. J., Johnson, J., Wallingsford, L., & Hall, J. D. (2002). Contemporary practices in school psychology: A national survey of roles and referral problems. *Psychology in the Schools, , 39,* 327–335.

Bransford, J. D., Brown, A. L., & Cocking, R. R. (2000). *How people learn: Brain, mind, experience, and school.* Washington, DC: National Academy Press.

Campbell, F. A., Ramey, C. T., Pungello, E., Sparling, J., & Miller-Johnson, S. (2002). Early childhood education: Young adult outcomes from the Abecedarian Project. *Applied Developmental Science, 6,* 42–57.

Carr, E. G., & Durand, V. M. (1985). Reducing behavior problems through functional communication training. *Journal of Applied Behavior Analysis, 18,* 111–126.

Christ, T. J., & Silberglitt, B. (2007). Estimates of the standard error of measurement for curriculum-based measures of oral reading fluency. *School Psychology Review, 36,* 130–146.

Cone, J. D. (1989). Is there utility for treatment utility? *American Psychologist, 44,* 1241–1242.

Daly, E. J., III, Witt, J. C., Martens, B. K., & Dool, E. J. (1997). A model for conducting a functional analysis of academic performance problems. *School Psychology Review, 26,* 554–574.

Demaray, M. K., & Elliott, S. N. (1998). Teachers' judgments of students' academic functioning: A comparison of actual and predicted performances. *School Psychology Quarterly, 13,* 8–24.

Deno, S. L. (1985). Curriculum-based measurement: The emerging alternative. *Exceptional Children, 52,* 219–232.

Deno, S. L. (1986). Formative evaluation of individual student programs: A new role for school psychologists. *School Psychology Review, 15,* 358–374.

Deno, S. L. (1989). Curriculum-based measurement and special education services: A fundamental and direct relationship. In M. R. Shinn (Ed.), *Curriculum-based measurement: Assessing special children* (pp. 1–17). New York: Guilford Press.

Deno, S. L., Marston, D., & Mirkin, P. K. (1982). Valid measurement procedures for continuous evaluation of written expression. *Exceptional Children, 48,* 368–371.

Deno, S. L., Marston, D., & Tindal, G. (1985). Direct and frequent curriculum-based measurement: An alternative for educational decision making. *Special Services in the Schools, 2,* 5–27.

Deno, S. L., Mirkin, P. K., & Marston, D. (1980). *Relationships among simple measures of written expression and performance on standardized achievement tests* (Research Report No. 22). Minneapolis: University of Minnesota Institute for Research on Learning Disabilities.

Donovan, M. S., & Cross, C. T. (Eds.). (2002). *Minority students in gifted and special education.* Washington, DC: National Academy Press.

Duhon, G. J., Noell, G. H., Witt, J. C., Freeland, J. T., Dufrene, B. A., & Gilbertson, D. N. (2004). Identifying academic skill and performance deficits: The experimental analysis of brief assessments of academic skills. *School Psychology Review, 33,* 429–443.

DuPaul, G. J., & Weyandt, L. L. (2006). School-based interventions for children and adolescents with attention-deficit/hyperactivity disorder: Enhancing academic and behavioral outcomes. *Education and Treatment of Children, 29,* 341–358.

Eckert, T. L., Dunn, E. K., & Ardoin, S. P. (2006). The effects of alternate forms of performance feedback on elementary-aged students' oral reading fluency. *Journal of Behavioral Education, 15,* 149–162.

Elliott, S. N., Huai, N., & Roach, A. T. (2007). Universal and early screening for educational difficulties: Current and future approaches. *Journal of School Psychology, 45,* 137–161.

Engelhard, G., Jr., & Lane, S. (2004). Iowa Tests of Basic Skills, Forms A & B. In H. D. Hoover et al. (Ed.), *Mental Measurements Yearbook.* Lincoln, NE: Buros Institute of Mental Measurements.

Espin, C. A., De La Paz, S., Scierka, B. J., & Roelofs, L. (2005). The relationship between curriculum-based measures in written expression and quality and completeness of expository writing for middle school students. *Journal of Special Education, 38*, 208–217.

Espin, C. A., Scierka, B. J., Skare, S., & Halverson, N. (1999). Criterion-related validity of curriculum-based measures in writing for secondary school students. *Reading and Writing Quarterly: Overcoming Learning Difficulties, 15*, 5–27.

Espin, C., Shin, J., Deno, S. L., Skare, S., Robinson, S., & Benner, B. (2000). Identifying indicators of written expression proficiency for middle school students. *Journal of Special Education, 34*, 140–153.

Fuchs, L. S., Fuchs, D., Hamlett, C. L., & Stecker, P. M. (1991). Effects of curriculum-based measurement and consultation on teacher planning and student achievement in mathematics operations. *American Educational Research Journal, 28*, 617–641.

Fuchs, L. S., Fuchs, D., Hamlett, C. L., Walz, L., & Germann, G. (1993). Formative evaluation of academic progress: How much growth can we expect? *School Psychology Review, 22*, 27–48.

Gansle, K. A., Noell, G. H., VanDerHeyden, A. M., Naquin, G. M., & Slider, N. J. (2002). Moving beyond total words written: The reliability, criterion validity, and time cost of alternate measures for curriculum-based measurement in writing. *School Psychology Review, 31*, 477–497.

Gansle, K. A., Noell, G. H., VanDerHeyden, A. M., Slider, N. J., Naquin, G. M., Hoffpauir, L. D., et al. (2004). An examination of the criterion validity and sensitivity of alternate curriculum-based measures of writing skill. *Psychology in the Schools, 41*, 291–300.

Graham, S., & Perin, D. (2007). A meta-analysis of writing instruction for adolescent students. *Journal of Educational Psychology, 99*, 445–476.

Greenwald, E., Persky, H., Ambell, J., & Mazzeo, J. (1999). *National assessment of educational progress: 1998 report card for the nation and states.* Washington, DC: U.S. Department of Education.

Hammill, D. D., & Larsen, S. C. (1996). *TOWL: Test of Written Language.* Upper Saddle River, NJ: Pearson.

Hanley, G. P., Iwata, B. A., & McCord, B. E. (2003). Functional analysis of problem behavior: A review. *Journal of Applied Behavior Analysis, 36*, 147–185.

Hansen, J. B., Bucy, J. E., & Swerdlik, M. E. (2004). Test of Written Language, Third Edition. In D. D. Hammill & S. C. Larsen (Eds.), *Mental Measurements Yearbook.* Lincoln, NE: Buros Institute of Mental Measurements.

Harris, K. R., Graham, S., & Mason, L. H. (2006). Improving the writing, knowledge, and motivation of struggling young writers: Effects of self-regulated strategy development with and without peer support. *American Educational Research Journal, 43*, 295–340.

Hayes, S. C., Nelson, R. O., & Jarrett, R. B. (1987). The treatment utility of assessment: A functional approach to evaluating assessment quality. *American Psychologist, 42*, 963–974.

Hoge, R. D., & Coladarci, T. (1989). Teacher-based judgments of academic achievement: A review of the literature. *Review of Educational Research, 76*, 777–781.

Hoover, H. D., Dunbar, S. B., & Frisbie, D. A. (2005). *Iowa tests of basic skills.* Itasca, IL: Riverside.

Howell, K. W., & Nolet, V. (2000). *Curriculum-based evaluation: Teaching and decision making* (3rd ed.). Atlanta, GA: Wadsworth.

Isaacson, S. (1985). Assessing written language. In C. S. Simon (Ed.), *Communication skills and classroom success: Assessment methodologies for language-learning disabled students* (pp. 403–424). San Diego, CA: College Hill.

Iwata, B. A., Dorsey, M., Silfer, K., Bauman, K., & Richman, G. (1982). Toward a functional analysis of self-injury. *Journal of Applied Behavior Analysis, 27*, 197–209.

Jones, E. D., & Krouse, J. P. (1988). The effectiveness of data-based instruction by student teachers in classrooms for pupils with mild handicaps. *Teacher Education and Special Education, 11*, 9–19.

Kelley, M. L., Reitman, D., & Noell, G. H. (2003). *Practitioner's guide to empirically based measures of school behavior.* New York: Kluwer Academic/Plenum.

Lee, L. L., & Canter, S. M. (1971). Developmental sentence scoring: A clinical procedure for estimating syntactic development in children's spontaneous speech. *Journal of Speech and Hearing Disorders, 36*, 315–340.

Malloy, K. J., Gilbertson, D., & Maxfield, J. (2007). Use of brief experimental analysis for selecting reading interventions for English language learners. *School Psychology Review, 36*, 291–310.

Marston, D., & Deno, S. L. (1981). *The reliability of simple, direct measures of written expression* (Research Report No. 50). Minneapolis: University of Minnesota Institute for Research on Learning Disabilities.

Marston, D. B. (1989). A curriculum-based measurement approach to assessing academic performance: What it is and why do it. In M. R. Shinn (Ed.), *Curriculum-based measurement: Assessing special children* (pp. 18–78). New York: Guilford Press.

McMaster, K., & Espin, C. (2007). Techinical

features of curriculum-bsed measurement in writing. *Journal of Special Education, 41,* 68–84.

Mercer, C. D., & Mercer, A. R. (2005). *Teaching students with learning problems* (7th ed.). Upper Saddle River, NJ: Pearson.

National Center for Education Statistics. (2003). *The nation's report card: Writing 2002.* Washington, DC: U.S. Department of Education, Institute of Education Sciences.

National Institute of Child Health and Human Development. (2000). *Report of the National Reading Panel. Teaching children to read: An evidence-based assessment of the scientific research literature on reading and its implications for reading instruction: Reports of the subgroups* (NIH Publication No. 00-4754). Washington, DC: U.S. Government Printing Office.

No Child Left Behind Act of 2001, Pub. L. No. 107-110, 20 U.S.C. § 6301 *et seq* (2002).

Noell, G. H., Ardoin, S. P., & Gansle, K. A. (2009). Academic assessment. In J. L. Matson & F. Adrasik (Eds.), *Assessing childhood psychopathology and developmental disabilities and treating childhood psychopathology and developmental disabilities* (pp. 311–340). New York: Springer.

Noell, G. H., Freeland, J. T., Witt, J. C., & Gansle, K. A. (2001). Using brief assessments to identify effective interventions for individual students. *Journal of School Psychology, 39,* 335–355.

Noell, G. H., Gansle, K. A., & Allison, R. (1999). Do you see what I see? Teachers' and school psychologists' evaluations of naturally occurring consultation cases. *Journal of Educational and Psychological Consultation, 10,* 107–128.

Northup, J., Wacker, D., Sasso, G., Steege, M., Cigrand, K., Cook, J., et al. (1991). A brief functional analysis of aggressive and alternative behavior in an outclinic setting. *Journal of Applied Behavior Analysis, 24,* 509–522.

O'Neill, R. E., Horner, R. H., Albin, R. W., Sprague, J. R., Storey, K., & Newton, J. S. (1997). *Functional assessment of problem behavior: A practical assessment guide* (2nd ed.). Pacific Grove, CA: Brooks/Cole.

Parker, R. I., Tindal, G., & Hasbrouck, J. (1991). Progress monitoring with objective measures of writing performance for students with mild disabilities. *Exceptional Children, 58,* 61–73.

Persky, H., Daane, M., & Jin, Y. (2003). *The nation's report card: Writing.* Washington, DC: U.S. Department of Education.

Saddler, B., & Graham, S. (2005). The effects of peer-assisted sentence-combining instruction on the writing performance of more and less skilled young writers. *Journal of Educational Psychology, 97,* 43–54.

Salvia, J., Ysseldyke, J. E., & Bolt, S. (2007). *Assessment in special and inclusive education* (10th ed.). Boston, MA: Houghton Mifflin.

Schneuwly, B. (1994). Tools to master writing: Historical glimpses. In J. V. Wertsch & J. D. Ramirez (Eds.), *Literacy and other forms of mediated action: Vol. 2. Explorations in socio-cultural studies* (pp. 37–44). Madrid, Spain: Fundación Infancia y Aprendizaje.

Shapiro, E. S. (2004). *Academic skills problems: Direct assessment and intervention* (3rd ed.). New York: Guilford Press.

Shinn, M. R. (1988). Development of curriculum-based local norms for use in special education decision making. *School Psychology Review, 17,* 61–80.

Shinn, M. R. (1989). *Curriculum-based measurement: Assessing special children.* New York: Guilford Press.

Skinner, C. H., McLaughlin, T. F., & Logan, P. (1997). Cover, copy, and compare: A self-managed academic intervention effective across skills, students, and settings. *Journal of Behavioral Education, 7,* 295–306.

Smith, F. (1982). *Writing and the writer.* New York: Holt, Rinehart, & Winston.

Snow, C. E., Burns, M. S., & Griffin, P. (1998). *Preventing reading difficulties in young children.* Washington, DC: National Academy Press.

Stewart, L. H., & Kaminski, R. (2002). Best practices in developing local norms for academic problem solving. In A. Thomas & J. Grimes (Eds.), *Best practices in school psychology* (4th ed., pp. 737–752). Bethesda, MD: National Association of School Psychologists.

Sulzer-Azaroff, B., & Mayer, G. R. (1991). *Behavior analysis for lasting change.* Fort Worth, TX: Holt, Rinehart & Winston.

Vallecorsa, A. L., & deBettencourt, L. U. (1997). Using a mapping procedure to teach reading and writing skills to middle grade students with learning disabilities. *Education and Treatment of Children, 20,* 173–188.

Videen, J., Deno, S., & Marston, D. (1982). *Correct word sequences: A valid indicator of proficiency in written expression* (Research Report No. 84). Minneapolis: University of Minnesota, Institute for Research in Learning Disabilities.

Witt, J. C., Daly, E., & Noell, G. H. (2000). *Functional assessments: A step-by-step guide to solving academic and behavior problems.* Longmont, CO: Sopris West.

Chapter 8

Selecting Academic Interventions for Individual Students

Edward J. Daly III
Kristi L. Hofstadter
Rebecca S. Martinez
Melissa Andersen

[A] wise man has something better to do than to boast
of his cures, namely to be always self-critical.
—PHILIPPE PINEL (1749–1826)

Although it might seem strange to start a chapter on selecting academic interventions with a rather dour quote reminding us to be always self-critical of our presumed "cures," anyone who has facilitated interventions in the schools knows that if school psychologists fail to carefully scrutinize their intervention recommendations, our clients, constituents, and the public will. In spite of the sobering quote, there is good reason to be enthusiastic about the tools for intervention that are available to school psychologists. Yet one must be cautious about becoming overly confident about one's ability to select effective interventions. Psychology has had a long love affair with the practice of predicting which interventions will work based on available psychological assessment information. The school psychologist often confidently shares intervention recommendations with teachers and parents based on a psychological profile derived from testing information. Unfortunately, outcomes often have not met expectations, even for ideas that have a great deal of intuitive appeal (Kavale & Forness, 1999).

The danger in being overly confident about an intervention (before showing that it actu-

ally works for a particular student) is that an ineffective intervention has potential to create disappointment in our clients and, worse yet, may actually cause harm by delaying or denying appropriate services. Given that an intervention (by definition) requires additional work on the part of a teacher or parent, he or she is not likely to tolerate a series of ineffective interventions for very long before turning to someone else for help. It behooves us as a profession, therefore, to approach the task of selecting and recommending interventions with a critical eye before giving in to the impulse to merely select the first intervention that catches our attention.

An understanding of the context in which interventions will be applied (classrooms and schools in this case) is critical to selecting effective interventions. Currently, the response-to-intervention (RTI) movement is leading schools to adopt multi-tier prevention and intervention models as the basis for addressing all students' instructional needs (Glover, DiPerna, & Vaughn, 2007; Jimerson, Burns, & VanDerHeyden, 2007). RTI service delivery models are characterized by (1) regular evaluation through universal screening and progress monitoring, (2) stra-

TABLE 8.1. Three Principles for Selecting High-Quality Academic Interventions

1. Know why and when academic intervention strategies work.
2. Select intervention components that match the student's instructional needs.
3. Prove that the intervention is valid for the student.

tegically selected interventions that increase in intensity across multiple intervention tiers, and (3) data-based decision rules for changing interventions and for determining eligibility for special education services. Other chapters in the book deal with the first and third elements of RTI models (i.e., regular evaluation and data-based decision rules). So, although these aspects of RTI relate to the topic of selecting interventions, the focus of this chapter is on explaining and demonstrating the use of three principles for structuring strategically selected interventions within a framework for RTI and systematic problem solving. School psychologists' effectiveness at selecting interventions within multitier intervention models will be greater if they adhere to the three principles of effective intervention that appear in Table 8.1. Each is dealt with in turn as we explain how to go about selecting academic interventions on an individual basis.

Knowing Why and When Academic Intervention Strategies Work

The Role of Active Treatment Ingredients

The notion of strategically selected interventions implies that interventions are selected based on students' instructional needs within an organizational and administrative structure for the use of existing resources (e.g., the use of Title I teachers to assist with supplemental interventions at a higher level tier in schools in which this is permissible). The most common way in which RTI is done in schools is through a standard intervention protocol that is delivered to all students who failed to meet criterion levels of performance ("benchmarks") in a schoolwide screening (Daly, Martens, Barnett, Witt, & Olson, 2007; Wanzek & Vaughn, 2007). The standard intervention protocol is a preplanned,

packaged intervention (meaning that it contains multiple instructional components) that is routinely administered to all students who fail to meet benchmark performance levels. (See Linan-Thompson & Vaughn, Chapter 16; Chard, Keterlin-Geller, Jungjohann, & Baker, Chapter 17; and McCurdy, Schmitz, & Albertson, Chapter 18, of this volume for content-specific recommendations about what standard intervention protocols should include in the areas of reading, math, and writing, respectively.)

What distinguishes the standard intervention protocol at higher tiers from the core curriculum is that it (1) supplements (not supplants) the curriculum and (2) also "intensifies" instruction in some way for the student who is not responding to regular classroom instruction in the core curriculum. Therefore, if Tier 1 is regular education instruction in the core curriculum, Tier 2 should represent more intense instruction than Tier 1 (in part because it is supplemental to regular education instruction). In the same manner, Tier 3 should be characterized by even more intense intervention than Tier 2. Intensifying instruction or intervention is essentially a matter of increasing *treatment strength*. Yeaton and Sechrest (1981) define treatment strength as "the a priori likelihood that a treatment could have its intended outcome. Strong treatments contain large amounts in pure form of those ingredients that lead to change" (p. 156). To design a sustainable intervention of appropriate treatment strength or adjust an ongoing intervention means correctly establishing the appropriate *duration* of intervention sessions, their *intensity* (in terms of dosage and frequency of intervention sessions), and their *complexity* for multicomponent interventions, as well as knowing what the "ingredients" are that make a treatment effective.

The active treatment ingredients are what cause behavior to change. An apparently intense treatment might not be a strong treatment at all. For example, having students engage in gross motor activities (e.g., practicing appropriate crawling on the floor) in an attempt to improve reading scores (an intervention) may be more intense (certainly physically) than what the teacher has done to date to address reading concerns, but it is certainly a weaker treatment than modeling correct responding and having the student practice reading error words correctly. Selecting appropriate treatment strength depends on one's ability to identify what will make the treatment effective and why it was effective or not. If this is not done *prior to* intervention, then even an apparently strong treatment (e.g., crawling on the floor) may be totally irrelevant, exposing the child and the teacher to an ineffective intervention.

Another element of treatment strength is treatment integrity, which refers to the extent to which an intervention is implemented as designed (Gresham, 1989). An intervention full of potent treatment ingredients is useless if implementation is poor (e.g., if some steps are regularly left out) or inconsistent (e.g., if the intervention is done only once or twice a week instead of four times a week as planned). Because this issue is addressed more thoroughly elsewhere (see Noell, Chapter 30, this volume), we limit ourselves to pointing out that consistent implementation may be partially affected by the degree to which stakeholders (e.g., teachers and parents) are confident that the intervention is a reasonable solution to the problem. When the school psychologist can explain why an intervention is more likely to work under a particular set of circumstances, teachers and parents are more likely to be convinced and may actually carry out the intervention as intended. Certainly, without a clear understanding of why it is important, it is likely that the teacher or parent may abandon the intervention as irrelevant or carry out only the easiest (but not most necessary) parts of the intervention. Furthermore, the intervention should be no more complex than it absolutely needs to be. Also, it should fit well into the current instructional routines while minimizing demands on the person carrying out the intervention.

Identifying Active Treatment Ingredients by Their Effect on the Academic Response (a Functional Approach)

Strong interventions start from a sound, empirically supported conceptual basis that allows one to identify the active treatment ingredients. For example, in the field of applied behavior analysis (ABA), the conceptual basis for analyzing the relationship between environmental events and behavior is the three-term contingency (antecedent–behavior–consequence; Cooper, Heron, & Heward, 2007). The central event in the three-term contingency is the occurrence of behavior, in this case an academic response of some type (e.g., writing the correct numbers in the correct columns for a computation problem). In this light, student achievement refers simply to the probability of a student getting the right answer under the appropriate conditions (e.g., in the classroom when the teacher gives an exercise to complete, when taking the SATs for college entrance, interpreting measurements correctly in a chemistry lab). By extension, an academic performance problem is nothing more than a behavioral deficit, which means that the response is not occurring as frequently as it should following relevant environmental events (e.g., the teacher instructs students to answer all the problems on a page). Indeed, the response may not be occurring at all.

The goal of all academic intervention is deceptively simple: Increase active student responding during instructional time (Greenwood, 1996; Heward, 1994). For any appropriate curricular exercise, anything that increases active responding (where there was previously a deficit in responding) is a functional intervention component. In ABA, intervention components are referred to as controlling variables that have stimulus functions. Stimuli that occasion, reinforce, or punish behavior are said to have a stimulus function because they reliably predict the occurrence or nonoccurrence of behavior (Daly, Martens, Skinner, & Noell, 2009). For academic performance problems, stimulus functions increase correct responses when they are desired. For example, in a case of poor writing skills (a behavior deficit), an analysis might be conducted by the school psychologist to determine whether the child can or cannot perform the skill under highly motivating conditions (Lentz, 1988). If the child *can* perform the skill under highly motivating conditions (e.g., when offered his or her favorite reward contingent on problem completion) but is simply choosing to do other things, then differential reinforcement might be used as the intervention. If the child *cannot* perform the desired writing skill even with the promise of the most tantalizing rewards contingent on problem completion, then modeling, prompting, and error correction might be added to a differential reinforcement plan. If the school psychologist carries out an assessment that accurately identifies the function of a problem behavior, he or she can work with teachers and parents to rearrange the environment to increase behavior over time in ways that directly relate to why the problem is occurring. For example, if the writing deficit is occurring as a function of poorly arranged consequences for behavior (a "won't-do" problem—the child can but "won't" do it), more effective rewards would be considered. On the other hand, if the writing deficit is occurring because of nonexistent skill repertoires when the teacher asks the student to write (a "can't do" problem because the child cannot do it even if he or she wants to), explicit instruction in how to write through modeling, explanations, error correction, and adjusting task difficulty level are called for rather than merely offering rewards to "do better."

Knowing why and when academic intervention strategies work is best achieved within a functional approach to selecting interventions for academic performance problems. The functional approach outlined in this chapter is based on the principles of functional assessment. Miltenberger (2008) defines functional assessment as "the process of gathering information about the antecedents and consequences that are functionally related to the occurrence of a problem behavior. It provides information that helps you determine why a problem is occurring" (p. 276). When the antecedents and consequences of academic performance problems are understood, an intervention that is appropriate to the child's instructional needs can be selected. Although this does not imply 1:1 instruction, it does imply that the intervention is individualized to address the problem for this student. Grouping might occur when students have similar instructional needs. Or classroom instruction might be supplemented for an individual student simply by having the student engage in additional practice relative to his or her peers, if the need for more practice is what is indicated by the functional assessment. In this case, the student could practice with a peer, parent, classroom tutor, or anyone available to help.

A functional approach implies that the child's academic performance is problematic because of an instructional mismatch: The problem is not with the child but with the arrangement of antecedents and consequences relative to the child's current instructional needs. It may be that (1) antecedents of appropriate behavior (e.g., directions for a writing exercise, explanation of available rewards for completing the writing exercise) are not clear enough; (2) antecedents of inappropriate behavior (e.g., an eager buddy in the next seat preparing to fling paper clips at peers) may be too clear and evoke the wrong behavior (e.g., joining the peer in the mischievous activity instead of completing class work); (3) consequences of appropriate behavior are not strong or frequent enough (e.g., getting a good grade or teacher praise); or (4) consequences of inappropriate behavior (e.g., seeing the surprised reaction of a peer smarting from a paper clip sting) are stronger than the consequences of appropriate behavior. Selecting the right intervention, therefore, depends on understanding *why* the current instructional arrangement is not functionally relevant to the student's current instructional and motivational needs.

Finally, note that a functional approach treats interventions as composed of various components that can be dissected as either antecedents or consequences. For example, modeling (i.e., demonstrating) the correct response, providing a partial answer to help a student, and allowing a student to choose which instructional task to do are antecedents, whereas providing computer time contingent on accurate problem completion, correcting errors, and having a student graph his or her performance are consequences that might increase the future probability of behavior. Any combination of these strategies might work for a particular child for whom there is an instructional mismatch. Therefore, a functional approach to intervention is one that seeks to add the right combination of antecedents and consequences to current instruction to increase academic performance. As such, intensity is increased (with no more complexity than is absolutely necessary); the intervention is differentiated based on student need (because it provides the combination of antecedents and consequences needed for this particular child); and the approach can be applied to academic interventions at any tier within a multitier intervention model.

Selecting Intervention Components that Match the Student's Instructional Needs

Multi-tiered intervention models contain differentiated interventions across all tiers to meet the diverse needs of all students in the school. Therefore, although there are instructional groupings and standard intervention protocols, the purpose is to meet the needs of *every* student. RTI forces schools to decide on the appropriateness of instruction for *all* students (based on universal screening and progress monitoring) and makes differentiation a part of the very organizational fabric of effective schoolwide instruction. Thus interventions are unavoidably individualized even if students are grouped (Daly et al., 2007). Differentiation, however, can and should occur within tiers as well. For example, a teacher might use a peer-tutoring intervention prior to reading group instruction in the core curriculum (Tier 1) to increase a student's practice with reading texts before trying a more complex and costly intervention (e.g., placement in a Tier 2 intervention). The point is that, regardless of tier, the individual and his or her response to instruction is *always* the basis for instructional and intervention decisions. Although individualized 1:1 intervention is likely to be rare in schools, school psychologists must know how to help teachers modify or differentiate interventions both within and across all tiers. There always will be a place for individual problem solving even as multitier intervention models become the predominant mode of delivering interventions in schools.

Students' instructional needs are defined functionally in terms of instructional and/or motivational factors over which teachers have control. To the degree that those needs are similar, students can be grouped effectively for instruction and intervention. However, it is critical to be sure that the intervention addresses why there is a problem in the first place. In reviewing the literature on academic interventions, Daly, Witt, Martens, and Dool (1997) identified five reasons why students do not get the right answer when they should (see Table 8.2). They refer to them as "reasonable hypotheses for academic deficits" that can be used as a point of departure for selecting intervention components. As an illustration of the first reasonable hypothesis (i.e., "They don't want

TABLE 8.2. Five Reasons Why Students Do Not Get the Right Answer

1. They don't want to do it.
2. They need more time doing it.
3. They need more help (because of a need for more prompting and feedback, an accuracy problem, a fluency problem, or a generalization problem).
4. They haven't had to do it that way before.
5. It's too hard.

to do it"), consider Chris, who demonstrates that he does not want to "do it" by failing to complete math worksheets in Mrs. Ramirez's class until Mrs. Ramirez offered him 10 minutes of computer time for putting completed worksheets in the assignment bin. In this case, Mrs. Ramirez improved the reinforcing consequences for appropriate behavior, which was sufficient to resolve the problem and meant that she did not need to try something more complex, such as giving him supervised practice. On the other hand, Sandy failed to complete math exercises on money that involved selecting appropriate combinations of coins as a multiple-choice task until Mrs. Ramirez had Sandy practice coin identification using a simulated shopping activity. As a result, Sandy's coin-identification and money-counting skills improved significantly. The naturalistic task (the simulated shopping activity) was much more motivating than the paper-and-pencil exercises.

Sometimes, students may simply need more time to do it (the second reasonable hypothesis). For example, Ronnie, a first-grade student, was referred for reading difficulties because the teacher was sure he had a learning disability. Classroom observations revealed that during the entire language arts block devoted to teaching reading, Ronnie read aloud only 4 minutes per day. Although Ronnie might have ultimately had a learning disability, a simpler solution would be to start by increasing the amount of time that he is reading aloud on a daily basis, assuming that a high-quality curriculum is used for reading instruction.

Some problems will require more complex solutions: The students need a specific form of help (the third reasonable hypothesis). Needing help can manifest itself in at least one of four ways: needing more prompting and feedback, having an accuracy problem, having a fluency problem, or having a generalization problem. For instance, Jim, who consistently earns Ds on his American history tests, was called on infrequently and mostly gave incorrect answers when he was called on, until his teacher used response cards with the entire class (requiring him to answer every teacher question) and the teacher began praising him explicitly for his correct answers. Increasing prompting of responding and feedback for responses was sufficient to improve Jim's performance. Jim is now more actively engaged (through answering frequent questions) and receives considerably more feedback about the correctness of his responses.

A student might need help because he or she has an accuracy problem. For example, Tanika was found to read phonetically regular words with consonant combinations with only 60% accuracy until the teacher explained the phonics rule, modeled correct reading of words, had her reading group practice a variety of words, and provided error correction for incorrect responses.

Sometimes, accuracy is not the problem. The student may not be fluent with the skill, as in the case of Jake, who took 20 minutes to complete five math computation problems. At that rate, Jake would never be prepared to take on more difficult math problems. In this case, Jake's teacher should probably have him practice more to become fluent. His teacher might accelerate Jake's fluency by giving him feedback on how accurately and quickly he completes problems and perhaps offering rewards for beating fluency (i.e., time-based) criteria (e.g., beating his last score within an established time frame).

A student might need help of a different type. For instance, although Matthew is quite adept at reading long-vowel words on flash cards, he has difficulty generalizing correct reading of those words to text. Therefore, he would probably benefit from instruction that explicitly had him practice reading those words in connected text, in addition to his flash card instruction.

The fourth reasonable hypothesis, "They haven't had to do it that way before," relates to whether the curricular exercise is actually teaching what the student needs to learn (Vargas, 1984). For example, if Emily's spelling instruction consists simply of circling the correct choice among three alternative spellings, she is less likely to spell the words correctly during writing assignments than if her instruction required her to actually practice by writing out spelling words. In Bill's case, he thinks he has outsmarted his teacher by figuring out that if he matches the number of blank spaces on his vocabulary exercise to the number of letters in his vocabulary word, he can get the correct answer without even having to know what the word means. This, too, is a case of the student getting the right answer for the wrong reason. Examples such as this should cause us to investigate the quality of instructional exercises to be sure they are actually teaching the student the right way of giving the correct response.

Finally, some students do not make progress because the instructional exercises are just too difficult—the fifth reasonable hypothesis. For instance, an oral reading fluency assessment reveals that Zach, a fourth grader, is reading only 19 words correctly per minute in typical fourth-grade reading material. In this case, Zach is not likely to progress until the difficulty level of the material is adjusted.

The descriptive examples of reasons for academic deficits and possible solutions just described are grounded in the behavior-analytic three-term contingency described earlier. The learning trial, a synonym for the three-term contingency, has been shown to be an important contributor to academic learning (Heward, 1994). When learning trials are increased, students learn more (Skinner, Fletcher, & Henington, 1996). The learning trial consists of an instructional antecedent (usually the teacher presenting a problem or an instructional exercise), a student response, and a consequence that either reinforces a correct response or corrects an incorrect response. Within a functional approach, learning trials are at the heart of all academic interventions. As noted earlier, when an academic performance deficit exists, it indicates that instructional antecedents and consequences for academic responding are not correctly aligned with the student's proficiency level. As such, functional relationships between the instructional exercise (the antecedent that should evoke a response) and student responding need to be properly established.

You can use the learning trial to diagnose the instructional mismatch. First, examine just how much active responding is occurring during the problematic instructional time. Chances are it is low (that's why the student was referred for a problem). If active responding is low, it means that practice and feedback (a nontechnical description of the learning trial construct) are low as well. Therefore, looking for ways to increase practice and feedback is a simple but functionally relevant way to start intervening.

But can it be that simple? It would seem that academic interventions, particularly for students with severe problems, are clearly more complex than that. Nonetheless, the learning trial is at the heart of all academic instruction, and all interventions are merely an elaboration on the learning trial. Here is the reason. The technical term in ABA for the learning trial (or the sequence of practice and feedback) is *differential reinforcement*. Differential reinforcement, which stands on about three-quarters of a century of research within humans and across species (Catania, 1998; Rilling, 1977), is the process by which behavior comes under the control of environmental stimuli. When a response (e.g., orally reading "Willie") is reinforced (e.g., teacher says "Correct!") in the presence of an antecedent stimulus (e.g., a flash card with the word "Willie" on it) and corrected when an incorrect response is given, this configuration of letters comes to have control over the response, such that the response is more likely in the presence of the antecedent stimulus in the future. Over time and with effective instruction, the response is correctly applied to the appearance of the word in other contexts and then becomes functional for achieving other tasks (e.g., recognizing the name "Willie" on a list of names). Differential reinforcement is the core behavioral process that governs learning. It is not, however, the only process that does so. This is why more complex interventions are often necessary.

Before we move on to demonstrating how to elaborate on differential reinforcement to strengthen academic interventions, we want to stress the importance of applying effective consequences to behavior. Consequences are what *cause* behavior change (Miltenberger, 2008). Consequences that reliably follow a response govern whether it will occur in the future or not. If the response is more likely as a function of a particular consequence, then the consequence is a reinforcer. For example, if extra computer time is available contingent on increased problem completion and if problem completion improves, then the extra time is a reinforcer. If the response is less likely as a function of a particular consequence, the consequence is a punisher. For example, having a student practice spelling words that she spelled incorrectly may actually cause her to be more careful in the future and make fewer spelling mistakes. The point is that the most sophisticated intervention will have no effect if it does not lead to functional consequences for the learner. For this reason, it is best to keep the simple model of the learning trial at the heart of intervention efforts and to understand the components of interventions according to their properties as relevant antecedents or consequences. Therefore, the most efficient way to start with academic interventions is by strengthening the positive consequences for desired behavior. If the consequences are effective, active student responding will increase.

A contrast was made in an earlier example between a writing deficit that occurred because the student could perform the skill but simply chose not to perform as expected and the case in which the student could not perform the skill regardless of how "juicy" the consequences might be. These examples illustrate a heuristic distinction made by Lentz (1988) between a performance deficit (i.e., "won't do") and a skill deficit (i.e., "can't do") that is extremely useful for guiding intervention selection. Differential reinforcement using more effective consequences is sufficient to resolve the performance deficit. An intervention of this type could be carried out in a variety of ways. The teacher could offer coveted classroom privileges (e.g., being the line leader, taking the attendance list to the principal, computer time) or could allow someone else to administer consequences (e.g., parents allowing privileges at home, visiting the school psychologist) when a student reaches a criterion level of performance on academic exercises. For skill deficits, the solution is more complex. Protocols for differentiating performance versus skill deficits can be found in Daly et al. (1997) and Duhon et al. (2004). Duhon et al.'s protocol is particularly useful because it can be applied to entire classrooms.

For the student who has a skill deficit, differential reinforcement will not be sufficient, because differential reinforcement assumes that the behavior is occurring with at least some regularity in the first place so that it can then be reinforced to be strengthened. The intervention needs to be tailored to increase the probability of a response so that it can then be reinforced. Therefore, response-prompting strategies are what is called for (Wolery, Bailey, & Sugai, 1988). A response prompt is a type of behavioral prosthetic in that it makes a response more likely to occur so that it can then be appropriately dealt with by the environment (e.g., reinforced for a desired behavior). For example, if a student is unable to read a word and if the teacher models correct reading of the word, then the model (an antecedent added to the instructional antecedent) increases the chances that the student will read the word correctly when the teacher re-presents the word. It is an adjunct to the stimulus that should evoke the correct response (i.e., the word on a page or on a flash card). Eventually, response prompts need to be faded so that the natural stimulus (e.g., the reading word, a math problem) evokes the correct response without any additional assistance. Antecedent prompting strategies should be used to simply jump-start active student responding so that it can be reinforced and come under the control of natural classroom contingencies.

In the academic intervention literature, the instructional hierarchy (IH; Ardoin & Daly, 2007; Daly, Lentz, & Boyer, 1996; Haring & Eaton, 1978) has emerged as a particularly useful heuristic for understanding how to add to learning trials through response prompts and sequentially structured contingencies. According to the IH, response strength for a behavior deficit progresses from nonexistent to accurate to fluent to widely generalizable with effective teaching. Conceptualized in terms of instructional goals for proficiency, the teacher first helps the student become accurate in responding. When responding is initially accurate, it is usually not very fast. The next level of proficiency is fluency. Instruction is configured to improve responding so that it is rapid. When responding is accurate and fluent, it is more likely to generalize across time and across tasks. Response prompting to improve initial accuracy may include modeling, partial prompts, and delayed prompts. At this point, every response should be given a consequence (either reinforcement or corrective feedback). All practice should be supervised to guard against the student's practicing errors.

When responding is largely accurate but slow, the teacher should turn to fluency-based instruction by increasing practice opportunities (which need not be supervised as carefully because responding is accurate) and making reinforcement available contingent on improved rate of responding (e.g., 30 correct problems completed in 5 minutes). Self-recording of performance on a graph may increase the potency of the reinforcement plan because it provides direct feedback to the student on fluency level and because visible performance improvements on a graph may become reinforcing. Response fluency is a prerequisite to the kind of broad generalization teachers would like to see of the skills they are teaching in the classroom. A more extensive discussion of generalization strategies can be found in Chapter 29, this volume, by Daly, Barnett, Kupzyk, Hofstadter, and Barkley (see also Daly et al., 2007, for generalization strategies and how they work). Table 8.3 contains a list of functionally relevant strategies that can be added to learning trials to make interventions match the reason for the problem more carefully. The reader is referred to Witt, Daly, and Noell (2000) for a more extensive treatment of the topic.

When treatment ingredients have been selected, they need to be turned into procedures. This process of "operationalizing" the intervention is best done by developing an intervention protocol that specifies exactly what the intervention agent should do. An example of a reading fluency intervention protocol frequently used by my (EJD) research team (e.g., Daly, Bonfiglio, Mattson, Persampieri, & Foreman-Yates, 2005) can be found in Figure 8.1. When working with students, we actually use this intervention protocol as a "mix and match" treatment plan. In other words, intervention components are selected based on the student's instructional need (usually determined through a brief experimental analysis, which is described later

TABLE 8.3. Intervention Components Matched to Five Reasons Why Students Do Not Get the Right Answer

Antecedents	Functional reasons	Consequences
• Give the student choices of tasks or how to do the task • Make the task more interesting/stimulating, and/or naturalistic	They don't want to do it	• Improve rewards (quality, frequency immediacy) for desired academic behavior relative to whatever is reinforcing undesired behavior • Give performance feedback on number correct per time unit (e.g., number of computation problems completed in 4 minutes)
• Increase time allocated for active responding	They need more time doing it	
• Increase clarity and precision of explanations for how to do the exercise, modeling, prompting of correct responses (e.g., offering partial answers and letting the student finish the response) • Teach the student to request more help • Supervise problem completion more carefully (e.g., by watching them perform five problems before having them practice independently)	They need more help	• Give performance feedback • Correct errors
• Revise curricular exercises to ensure student is practicing correctly • Align curricular exercises with naturalistic demands	They haven't had to do it that way before	
• Adjust difficulty level	It's too hard	

in the chapter). Although some students may need all components (i.e., reward, listening passage preview, repeated readings, phrase-drill error correction, and syllable segmentation error correction), most students need only a combination of components. The protocol, however, illustrates some of the intervention components (antecedents and consequences) discussed up to this point. For reinforcement, a reward contingency is explained prior to the instructional session, and the contingency is applied after the student reads the high-word-overlap generalization passage (explained in detail subsequently) at the end of the session.

Listening passage preview calls for the instructor to model accurate and fluent reading. The repeated readings technique is used in this protocol by having the student read the passage twice (with the phrase-drill error correction procedure inserted between readings). There are two forms of error correc-

tion in the protocol. With phrase-drill error correction, error words (based on a previous reading of the passage) are modeled by the instructor, who then has the student practice reading the phrases containing the error words three times (to assure more practice with connected text). For words that are read incorrectly a second time, the word is broken into syllables while the instructor models and prompts the student to practice the syllables and then the word. Suitable components can be chosen on a case-by-case basis and combined into a sequence of intervention steps that delivers the appropriate antecedents (i.e., explanations, prompting, modeling) and consequences (i.e., error correction, reward, performance feedback). For other types of academic performance problems (e.g., math, writing), the procedures will obviously look different, but the principles (antecedents and consequences) are the same.

Materials

☐ Examiner Copy of the Instructional Passage

☐ Student Copy of the Instructional Passage

☐ Examiner Copy of the Corresponding High-Word-Overlap Generalization Passage (with predetermined goal*)

☐ Student Copy of the Corresponding High-Word-Overlap Generalization Passage

☐ Stopwatch

☐ Pen or Pencil

☐ Highlighter

☐ Rewards

☐ Tape Recorder and Tape

*A bracket should be placed in the **Generalization Passage** after the third word following the number of correctly read words per min from screening. For example, if the student read 36 correct words per min during screening, place a bracket after the 39th word.

Record Beginning Time _____

Explanation of Reward Contingency

☐ 1. Place several rewards in front of the child and say: "YOU WILL HAVE THE CHANCE TO EARN ONE OF THESE REWARDS FOR READING THIS STORY" (*point to the generalization passage*).

☐ 2. Say "LET'S CHOOSE A REWARD. CHOOSE ONE OF THE THINGS BEFORE YOU TO WORK FOR."

☐ 3. Place the chosen reward so that it is visible to the student and, if possible, sitting on top of the generalization passage, but beyond his or her reach.

☐ 4. Say: "FIRST, WE WILL PRACTICE READING THIS STORY [*point to the instructional passage*]. PRACTICING THIS STORY [*point to the instructional passage*] WILL MAKE IT EASIER TO EARN THE REWARD IN THIS STORY [*point to the generalization passage*]. THEY HAVE A LOT OF THE SAME WORDS."

Listening Passage Preview (Instructional Passage)

☐ 5. Present the Student Copy of the **Instructional Passage** to the student, saying: "HERE IS A STORY THAT I WOULD LIKE FOR YOU TO READ. HOWEVER, I AM GOING TO READ THE STORY TO YOU FIRST. PLEASE FOLLOW ALONG WITH YOUR FINGER, READING THE WORDS TO YOURSELF AS I SAY THEM."

☐ 6. Using the Examiner Copy of the **Instructional Passage**, read the <u>entire passage</u> at a comfortable reading rate (approx. 130 words per minute), making sure that the student is following along with a finger. Prompt the student to follow along if he or she is not doing so.

Student Reading 1 (Instructional Passage)

☐ 7. Say: "NOW I WANT YOU TO READ THE STORY. YOU ARE GOING TO PRACTICE READING THIS STORY A COUPLE OF TIMES TO HELP YOU GET BETTER AT READING. EACH TIME I WILL TELL YOU HOW FAST YOU HAVE READ THE STORY AND HOW MANY WORDS YOU MISSED. READ THE STORY ALOUD. TRY TO READ EACH WORD. IF YOU COME TO A WORD YOU DON'T KNOW, I WILL TELL IT TO YOU. BE SURE TO DO YOUR BEST READING. DO YOU HAVE ANY QUESTIONS?"

☐ 8. Say, "BEGIN!" and start the stopwatch when the student says the first word.

☐ 9. While the student is reading the passage aloud, follow along on the Examiner Copy **highlighting** errors. If the student hesitates on a word for more than 3 seconds, say the word and **highlight** it.

☐ 10. Make a bracket and write the number "**1**" after the first minute of reading, *but* have the student read the whole passage aloud. [The number **1** indicates that this is where you stopped after the first reading.]

☐ 11. Say, "THAT TIME, YOU READ _____ WORDS PER MINUTE AND MADE _____ ERRORS."

(cont.)

FIGURE 8.1. Example of a multicomponent reading fluency intervention protocol.

Phrase Drill (Instructional Passage)

☐12. Say: "YOU MISSED [SEVERAL/A COUPLE OF/NO] WORDS. WE ARE GOING TO PRACTICE THE WORDS YOU MISSED." Show the student where each error word is highlighted in the passage.

☐13. Point to the first word read incorrectly and say: "THIS WORD IS _____." Have the student say the word. Point to the beginning of the sentence containing the error word and say, "PLEASE READ THIS SENTENCE THREE TIMES. GO ALL THE WAY TO HERE [point to closest punctuation; e.g., period, question mark]." Have the student read the sentence containing the error word **three times**. If more than one error occurs in the sentence, model and prompt correct reading of each word once in the sentence and have the student read the sentence only three times (regardless of the number of errors in the sentence). Do the same for each of the highlighted words.

Student Reading 2 (Instructional Passage)

☐14. Say, "NOW I WOULD LIKE FOR YOU TO READ THE STORY FROM THE BEGINNING AGAIN. ARE YOU READY? "

☐15. Say, "BEGIN!" and start the stopwatch when the student says the first word. While the student is reading the passage aloud, follow along on the Examiner Copy **underlining** errors. If the student hesitates on a word for more than 3 seconds, say the word and **underline** it.

☐16. Make a bracket and write the number **2** after the first minute of reading, but have the student read the whole passage aloud. [The number **2** indicates that this is where you stopped after the second reading.]

☐17. Say, "THAT TIME, YOU READ _____ WORDS PER MINUTE AND MADE _____ ERRORS." [Say the two2 appropriate statements regarding fluency and errors:]
☐"YOU READ THE STORY FASTER THIS TIME, AND ... " [or]
☐"YOU DID NOT READ THE STORY FASTER THIS TIME, AND ... "
☐"YOU MADE FEWER ERRORS THIS TIME." [or]
☐"YOU DID NOT MAKE FEWER ERRORS THIS TIME."

Syllable Segmenting and Blending Lesson (Instructional Passage)

☐18. Say: "WE ARE GOING TO PRACTICE SOME OF THE DIFFICULT WORDS." [You will work only with words missed during both student readings. These words will be both **underlined and highlighted**.]

☐19. Turn the Examiner Copy of the instructional passage towards the student. For each **underlined and highlighted** error word in the passage, cover all but the first **syllable** of the error word with an index card. Say, "THESE LETTERS SAY _____. NOW YOU SAY IT." Wait for a response and say, "GOOD!" [If the student makes an error or fails to respond, say, "THESE LETTERS SAY _____. SAY IT. GOOD!"] Repeat this step for all of the syllables in the word, successively exposing each syllable until the student practices all of the syllables in the word. Do this for every **underlined and highlighted** word.

☐20. Returning to the first error word, cover all but the first syllable of the error word with an index card and say, "NOW SAY THE SOUNDS AND THEN SAY THE WORD." Expose the first syllable and have the student say the sounds. [If the student makes an error or fails to respond, say, "NO. THESE LETTERS SAY _____. SAY IT. GOOD!"] Expose each successive syllable, following the same procedure. With all syllables exposed, say, "SAY THE WORD." [If the student makes an error, say, "NO. THE WORD IS _____. SAY IT. GOOD!"] Do this for every **underlined and highlighted** word.

Reward and Assessment (High-Word-Overlap Generalization Passage)

☐21. Remove the Instructional Passage and replace it with the Generalization passage.

☐22. Say: "NOW I WOULD LIKE FOR YOU TO READ THIS STORY. THIS TIME YOU CAN EARN THE REWARD FOR DOING WELL. IN ORDER TO EARN THE _____ [say the name of the chosen reward] YOU HAVE TO BEAT YOUR LAST SCORE [based on screening results], WHILE MAKING NO MORE THAN THREE ERRORS. WHEN I SAY 'BEGIN,' START READING ALOUD AT THE TOP OF THE PAGE [point to the top of the page] AND READ ACROSS THE PAGE [demonstrate by pointing]. TRY TO READ EACH WORD. IF YOU COME TO A WORD YOU DON'T KNOW, I WILL TELL IT TO YOU. DO NOT STOP READING UNTIL I SAY 'STOP'. BE SURE TO DO YOUR BEST READING."

(cont.)

FIGURE 8.1. *(cont.)*

☐23. Say, "BEGIN!" and start the stopwatch when the student says the first word. While the student is reading the passage aloud, follow along on the Examiner Copy **putting a slash through** errors. If the student hesitates on a word for more than 3 seconds, say the word and **put a slash through it**.

☐24. Make a bracket after **ONE MINUTE** and tell the student to stop reading.

☐25. When the student finishes the passage, count the number of error words.

    ☐ A.   If the student met the goal with no more than three errors, say, "THAT TIME, YOU READ __ WORDS PER MINUTE AND MADE _____ ERRORS. GREAT WORK! YOU MET THE GOAL AND EARNED THE REWARD!" Deliver the reward to the student.

    ☐ B.   If the student did not meet the goal and/or made more than 3 errors, say "THAT TIME, YOU READ _____ WORDS PER MINUTE AND MADE _____ ERRORS. NICE TRY. BUT YOU DID NOT MEET THE GOAL. NEXT TIME YOU READ FOR ME, YOU WILL HAVE A CHANCE TO EARN A REWARD."

Record Ending Time _____

FIGURE 8.1. *(cont.)*

Proving That the Intervention Is Valid for the Student

In line with legal and policy mandates for scientifically valid and research-based interventions in psychology and a number of other fields (Kratochwill et al., 2009), a critical component of RTI is the use of a scientifically valid curriculum and interventions (Batsche et al., 2005; Glover, DiPerna, & Vaughn, 2007). This means that school psychologists and other educators should be scouring the research literature, searching for the most effective interventions available, while applying the most stringent criteria for rigorous research to assure a sufficient research base. Unfortunately, although reviewing the research literature is necessary, it is not sufficient, as a well-supported intervention carries no guarantee that it will work for a particular student. Over 100,000 research studies have been conducted on reading since 1966 (National Reading Panel, 2000), yet generalizability of reading research to actual classroom conditions has been quite weak (Lyon & Moats, 1997), which is not surprising in light of the probable differences in methods used, participant characteristics, and circumstances between a research study and a particular child referred for an academic performance problem. In an influential document on RTI, Batsche et al. (2005) point out:

> Selection and implementation of scientifically based instruction/intervention markedly increases the probability of, but does not guarantee, positive individual response. Therefore, individual response is assessed in RtI and the modifications to instruction/intervention or goals are made depending on results with individual students. (p. 5)

Practitioners need more than a list of research-based interventions; they also need a *method* for investigating whether a particular intervention is effective for a particular child under a particular set of circumstances. Not until a research-based intervention has been proven to work for a particular student is it a valid intervention, a process we refer to as *local validation* (Daly, Kupzyk, Bossard, Street, & Dymacek, in press). Local validation is done only on a case-by-case basis through a strong evaluation design (see Daly et al., Chapter 29, this volume). With respect to selecting the intervention, it means that the right combination of active treatment ingredients is chosen to work for the child in question.

A self-critical approach to providing cures is not a negative aspect of the school psychologist's job but involves the application of standards of quality and measurement of our ability to uphold those standards. Directly subjecting one's idea for an effective intervention to the impartial and dispassionate jury of objective and standardized measurement through repeated measures over time (as is done within the problem-solving model) is quite humbling when one realizes that the "cure" might not work. But this is the price that is paid for adhering to the problem-solving model. Being an effective problem solver (also known as scientist–practitioner) means treating one's ideas, plans, preferred methods of doing things, and cures with circumspection until clear evidence has been gathered that it was, in fact, the right thing to do for a particular individual or group of students and setting about to gather objective evidence about the correctness of the "cure" (local validation).

Using Brief Experimental Analysis to Identify Potential Interventions

The ultimate test of an intervention's effectiveness is established by repeatedly measuring student performance over time (see Marcotte & Hintze, Chapter 5; Burns & Klingbeil, Chapter 6; and Gansle & Noell, Chapter 7 of this volume for descriptions of how to do this). However, through a recent innovation—brief experimental analysis (BEA)—that borrows single-case experimental design elements (Daly et al., Chapter 29, this volume), it is possible to test potential intervention strategies *before* they are recommended to a teacher. Although there is no guarantee that they will work when the teacher applies the intervention in the classroom, a BEA can at least rule out potentially ineffective interventions. Derived from the methodology of ABA, the primary focus of BEA is the antecedent and consequent variables (e.g., opportunities to respond, reinforcement contingencies) that maintain academic behavior rather than the academic behavior in question (e.g., reading difficulty), which alone provides very little information regarding appropriate action (Gresham, Watson, & Skinner, 2001). BEA, an abbreviated experimental analysis of academic performance using single-case design elements, involves directly manipulating relevant instructional antecedents and consequences while measuring the impact on the academic performance as a basis for selecting intervention components.

Previous research has demonstrated that BEA leads to significantly idiosyncratic response to intervention across students with similar academic concerns that can and should be taken into account in instructional planning (Daly, Martens, Dool, & Hintze, 1998; Daly, Martens, Hamler, Dool, & Eckert, 1999; Jones & Wickstrom, 2002). Additionally, extended analyses in which selected strategies are implemented and evaluated over multiple sessions have provided evidence that results of BEAs are generally consistent over extended periods of time (Daly, Murdoch, Lillenstein, Webber, & Lentz, 2002; Jones &

Wickstrom, 2002; Noell, Freeland, Witt, & Gansle, 2001; McCurdy, Daly, Gortmaker, Bonfiglio, & Persampieri, 2007; VanAuken, Chafouleas, Bradley, & Martens, 2002). Whereas experimental analysis has been applied to various academic areas, such as reading comprehension, math, and writing (Daly et al., 1998; Duhon et al., 2004; Hendrickson, Gable, Novak, & Peck, 1996; McComas et al., 1996; Noell et al., 1998; VanAuken et al., 2002), the primary focus of BEA research has been reading fluency, making curriculum-based measurement (CBM) probes of oral reading fluency (ORF) the most commonly used measure. Although variations of the BEA model have been developed, all approaches incorporate the same basic foundation. All variations of BEA target academic performance and incorporate repeated measurements within and across conditions, evidence-based interventions that are sequentially organized according to conceptual and/or logistical considerations, and single-case design elements (Hendrickson et al., 1996; Wilber & Cushman, 2006), each of which is discussed in turn.

Although intervention strategies vary to some degree in the BEA literature, a common set of evidence-based reading intervention components has been used for reading fluency interventions (Daly, Andersen, Gortmaker, & Turner, 2006); these components are listed in Table 8.4. Testable intervention components in BEAs have been conceptualized along the lines of differentiating performance deficits from skill deficits, with the IH guiding the selection of instructional components for skill deficits. After treatments are selected and sequenced in order of efficiency and functional relevance, the BEA proceeds with administration of baseline and treatment conditions in rapid succession. Each condition is administered once until an effective intervention is identified. In order to demonstrate effectiveness, the treatment must lead to a visible increase in responding (e.g., reading fluency). In some cases, criteria for improvements have been used. The criteria used in previous literature include a 20% increase over baseline performance (e.g., Jones & Wickstrom, 2002), a 30% increase over baseline (Daly, Persampieri, McCurdy, & Gortmaker, 2005) and literature-based criterion-referenced scores, reflecting mastery rates (e.g., Daly et al., 1999). The least intrusive intervention that helps the student

TABLE 8.4. Reading Intervention Components

Component	Description	Purpose
Incentive	The student is offered a reward, contingent on increased reading performance	Implemented to identify performance deficits (Daly et al., 2002)
Listening passage preview	Before reading the passage, the student follows along while the examiner reads the passage aloud	Provides modeling of fluent, accurate reading (Daly & Martens, 1994)
Repeated readings	The student reads the same passage repeatedly, two to four times	Increases opportunities to respond (Rashotte & Torgeson, 1985)
Phrase drill	Phrases containing student-produced errors are highlighted by the examiner, and the student is asked to read each phrase (up to 15 total phrases) three times each, with immediate error correction	Provides corrective feedback and practice responding accurately (O'Shea, Munson, & O'Shea, 1984)
Instructional difficulty level	The student is asked to read a passage one grade level below the current reading level	Tests instructional match by isolating the effects of lowering the difficulty level (Jones, Wickstrom, & Daly, 2008)
Syllable segmentation	Using an index card, the examiner covers each error word, revealing one syllable at a time while simultaneously modeling the correct pronunciation. The student then reads each syllable and pronounces the word independently	Provides corrective feedback and practice blending syllables to form words (Daly, Bonfiglio, Mattson, Persampieri, & Foreman-Yates, 2006)

reach the criterion is then chosen for application in the natural setting. Further analysis, including a minireversal (Daly et al., 1997) or extended analysis, can be used to increase confidence in BEA findings before continued implementation.

Variations of the BEA Model

Several versions of the BEA have been developed, including the component approach, the interaction approach, the dismantling approach, and the single-instructional-trial approach. The component approach, the initial conceptualization of the BEA model (Daly et al., 1997), consists of implementing each treatment component individually, in order of increasing intensity. The least intrusive yet effective component is then identified, and a minireversal, which includes a return to baseline and reintroduction of the selected component, is conducted to replicate the effects of the intervention, providing evidence of experimental control. On successful replication, the strategy can be confidently recommended as the primary component of an intervention package. The purpose of the

component approach is to identify the most effective combination of intervention components for a particular individual, such as motivation, practice, corrective feedback, or instructional match (Jones, Wickstrom, & Daly, 2008).

The most commonly implemented BEA model is the interaction approach, in which intervention components are added sequentially, using a stacking approach (Daly et al., 1998; Daly et al., 1999; VanAuken et al., 2002). The model is similar to the component approach; however, the most effective treatment package, rather than a single component, is identified and replicated. The purpose of the interaction approach is not to isolate the effects of components but to identify the intervention package that exerts the greatest control over academic responding (Jones et al., 2008). The interaction approach more closely resembles instruction within the natural classroom environment, because it incorporates multiple strategies (Daly, Bonfiglio, Mattson, Persampieri, & Foreman-Yates, 2006). The evaluation of combined strategies is particularly useful when treatments interact to produce greater gains than the effects of isolated components would suggest. However, due to the fact that all components are not independently evaluated, it is possible that an equally effective, less intrusive strategy is overlooked in some cases.

A relatively recent model, the dismantling approach, includes the initial introduction of a strong treatment package followed by removal of components in order of decreasing intensity until the most manageable yet effective intervention is identified (Daly et al., 2005; Daly, Bonfiglio, et al., 2006). The purpose of this approach is to produce immediate effects while simultaneously identifying a sustainable intervention package. The dismantling approach provides the unique opportunity to compare effects of a strong instructional package with effects produced by packages containing fewer components. Thus less intrusive strategies can be selected and confidently expected to produce results similar to more complex, multicomponent interventions.

A Single-Instructional-Trial Approach

Daly, Andersen, et al. (2006) provide guidelines for implementing a brief analysis that has been condensed to fit into a single instructional trial. Three conditions—treatment package, reward-only, and control—are evaluated. Daly, Andersen, et al. (2006) use one instructional passage in which the entire treatment package—including reward, listening passage preview, repeated reading, phrase drill, and syllable segmentation—is delivered. Next, three assessment passages are employed to obtain a measure of each condition. One high-word-overlap passage is used to assess the treatment package implemented during instruction, and two low-word-overlap passages are assigned to reward-only and control conditions. The high-word-overlap passage contains many of the same words as the original instructional passage (e.g., 80% of the same words), but it is written as a different story. This passage allows the examiner to test for generalization of fluent word reading to a different context (i.e., instructed words in a different passage). The low-word-overlap passages must be of the same difficulty level to allow for a fair test of how effective the instructional condition is relative to a reward-only condition (measured in one of the low-overlap passages) and a control condition (the other low-word-overlap passage).

Possible results include identifying the total package as the most effective condition, identifying the reward-only condition as similarly effective to the total package, and obtaining undifferentiated results, in which all three conditions produce similar effects. The purpose of this approach is to identify an effective treatment within one instructional trial using a skills-versus-performance deficit framework. In spite of the fact that the single-trial approach significantly reduces the amount of time needed to identify an effective intervention, the time saved is of little use if the intervention package is too cumbersome to be implemented. Optional dismantling of the total package is offered to account for this problem; however, the additional steps of dismantling remove the time-saving strength of this approach.

Although there is not one commonly espoused BEA model, there may be benefits to using one approach versus another, depending on various factors. For example, in a school setting in which treatment integrity is generally low, an approach that offers the most simple yet effective intervention, such as the component approach, would be most likely to produce results. Recommending a complex treatment package in such a setting may result in reduced treatment adherence or complete lack of implementation. Additional research is necessary to determine which approach is the best choice according to various factors, such as setting, student variables, and available resources.

Results from extended analyses and ongoing progress monitoring indicate that brief analyses result in selection of effective interventions (Daly et al., 2002; Jones & Wickstrom, 2002; Noell et al., 2001; McCurdy et al., 2007; VanAuken et al., 2002). However, it is unclear whether the use of BEA leads to the selection of interventions that improve achievement more than generally effective treatment packages. For instance, it may be that a feasible evidence-based treatment package and packages derived from BEA procedures typically produce similar long-term student growth. In this case, rather than implementing BEA as a first step in problem analysis, the use of BEA could be reserved for nonresponsive students, thus reducing the time lapse between problem identification and initial intervention implemen-

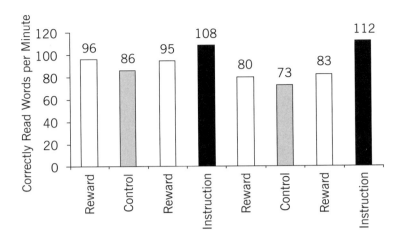

FIGURE 8.2. Example of a brief experimental analysis ("treatment testing").

tation. An example of BEA results appears in Figure 8.2. In this case, an instructional condition was administered twice, a reward-only condition was administered four times, and a control condition was administered twice. The results suggest that the student responded best to the instructional condition.

Conclusion

For a student experiencing academic difficulties, no intervention or the wrong intervention can have long-term consequences as the school curriculum becomes progressively harder. Those who take a critical approach to practice are more likely to be careful about the interventions they choose and recommend to others: Reasonable grounds for interventions should be sought in empirical, theoretical, rational, and logistical considerations for any intervention administered to any student. A problem-solving focus forces school psychologists to take a critical view of practice and strategically and continuously test for solutions. Until we get it right, the students under our care will not get it right. Fortunately, the task of helping students get it right is simplified conceptually when one uses active student responding as the key to both diagnosing and solving the problem. To date, the best we can do is to increase active student responding during

instructional time. This chapter examined a robust yet simple conceptual model—the learning trial—as the basis for intervention and described some ways in which the school psychologist can elaborate on it to select an intervention that is a better "fit" for the student than what he or she is currently receiving instructionally. Of course, the best way to determine fit is to try it on for size and hold it up to the objective mirror of the data. The BEA methodology may help psychologists do just that before they make any recommendations to the teacher about how instruction can be improved for a particular student.

References

Ardoin, S. P., & Daly, E. J., III. (2007). Introduction to the special series: Close encounters of the instructional kind—how the instructional hierarchy is shaping instructional research 30 years later. *Journal of Behavioral Education, 16*, 1–6.

Batsche, G., Elliott, J., Graden, J. L., Grimes, J., Kovaleski, J. F., Prasse, D., et al. (2005). *Response to intervention: Policy considerations and implementation.* Alexandria, VA: National Association of State Directors of Special Education.

Catania, A. C. (1998). *Learning* (4th ed.). Upper Saddle River, NJ: Prentice Hall.

Cooper, J. O., Heron, T. E., & Heward, W. L. (2007). *Applied behavior analysis* (2nd ed.). New York: Macmillan.

Daly, E. J., III, Andersen, M., Gortmaker, V., & Turner, A. (2006). Using experimental analysis to identify reading fluency interventions: Connecting the dots. *Behavior Analyst Today*, 7, 133–150.

Daly, E. J., III, Bonfiglio, C. M., Mattson, T., Persampieri, M., & Foreman-Yates, K. (2005). Refining the experimental analysis of academic skill deficits: Part I. An investigation of variables affecting generalized oral reading performance. *Journal of Applied Behavior Analysis*, 38, 485–498.

Daly, E. J., III, Bonfiglio, C. M., Mattson, T., Persampieri, M., & Foreman-Yates, K. (2006). Refining the experimental analysis of academic skill deficits, Part II: An investigation of the use of brief experimental analysis for identifying reading fluency interventions. *Journal of Applied Behavior Analysis*, 39, 323–331.

Daly, E. J., III, Kupzyk, S., Bossard, M., Street, J., & Dymacek, R. (in press). Taking RTI "to scale": Developing and implementing a quality RTI process. *Journal of Evidence-Based Practices for Schools*.

Daly, E. J., III, Lentz, F. E., & Boyer, J. (1996). The instructional hierarchy: A conceptual model for understanding the effective components of reading interventions. *School Psychology Quarterly*, 11, 369–386.

Daly, E. J., III, & Martens, B. K. (1994). A comparison of three interventions for increasing oral reading performance: Application of the instructional hierarchy. *Journal of Applied Behavior Analysis*, 27, 459–469.

Daly, E. J., III, Martens, B. K., Barnett, D., Witt, J. C., & Olson, S. C. (2007). Varying intervention delivery in response to intervention: Confronting and resolving challenges with measurement, instruction, and intensity. *School Psychology Review*, 36, 562–581.

Daly, E. J., III, Martens, B. K., Dool, E. J., & Hintze, J. M. (1998). Using brief functional analysis to select interventions for oral reading. *Journal of Behavioral Education*, 8, 203–218.

Daly, E. J., III, Martens, B. K., Hamler, K. R., Dool, E. J., & Eckert, T. L. (1999). A brief experimental analysis for identifying instructional components needed to improve oral reading fluency. *Journal of Applied Behavior Analysis*, 32, 83–94.

Daly, E. J., III, Martens, B. K., Skinner, C. H., & Noell, G. H. (2009). Contributions of applied behavior analysis. In T. B. Gutkin & C. R. Reynolds (Eds.), *The handbook of school psychology* (4th ed., pp. 84–106). New York: Wiley.

Daly, E. J., III, Murdoch, A., Lillenstein, L., Webber, L., & Lentz, F. E. (2002). An examination of methods for testing treatments: Conducting experimental analyses of the effects of instructional components on oral reading fluency. *Education and Treatment of Children*, 25, 288–316.

Daly, E. J., III, Persampieri, M., McCurdy, M., & Gortmaker, V. (2005). Generating reading interventions through experimental analysis of academic skills: Demonstration and empirical evaluation. *School Psychology Review*, 34, 395–414.

Daly, E. J., III, Witt, J. C., Martens, B. K., & Dool, E. J. (1997). A model for conducting a functional analysis of academic performance problems. *School Psychology Review*, 26, 554–574.

Duhon, G. J., Noell, G. H., Witt, J. C., Freeland, J. T., Dufrene, B. A., & Gilbertson, D. N. (2004). Identifying academic skills and performance deficits: The experimental analysis of brief assessments of academic skills. *School Psychology Review*, 33, 429–443.

Glover, T. A., DiPerna, J. C., & Vaughn, S. (2007). Introduction to the special series on service delivery systems for response to intervention: Considerations for research and practice. *School Psychology Review*, 36, 523–525.

Greenwood, C. R. (1996). The case for performance-based instructional models. *School Psychology Quarterly*, 11, 283–296.

Gresham, F. M. (1989). Assessment of treatment integrity in school consultation and prereferral intervention. *School Psychology Review*, 18 37–50.

Gresham, F. M., Watson, T. S., & Skinner, C. H. (2001). Functional behavioral assessment: Principles, procedures, and future directions. *School Psychology Review*, 30, 156–172.

Haring, N. G., & Eaton, M. D. (1978). Systematic instructional procedures: An instructional hierarchy. In N. G. Haring, T. C. Lovitt, M. D. Eaton, & C. L. Hansen (Eds.), *The fourth R: Research in the classroom* (pp. 23–40). Columbus, OH: Merrill.

Hendrickson, J. M., Gable, R. A., Novak, C., & Peck, S. (1996). Functional assessment as strategy assessment for teaching academics. *Education and Treatment of Children*, 19, 257–271.

Heward, W. L. (1994). Three "low-tech" strategies for increasing the frequency of active student response during group instruction. In R. Gardner, III, D. M. Sainato, J. O. Cooper, T. E. Heron, W. L. Heward, J. W. Eshleman, et al. (Eds.), *Behavior analysis in education: Focus on measurably superior instruction* (pp. 283–320). Pacific Grove, CA: Brooks/Cole.

Jimerson, S. R., Burns, M. K., & VanDerHeyden, A. M. (Eds.). (2007). *Handbook of response to intervention: The science and practice of assessment and intervention*. New York: Springer.

Jones, K. M., & Wickstrom, K. F. (2002). Done in sixty seconds: Further analysis of the brief assessment model for academic problems. *School Psychology Review, 31*, 554–568.

Jones, K. M., Wickstrom, K. F., & Daly, E. J., III. (2008). Best practices in the brief assessment of academic problems. In A. Thomas & J. Grimes (Eds.), *Best practices in school psychology* (6th ed., pp. 489–501). Washington, DC: National Association of School Psychologists.

Kavale, K. A., & Forness, S. R. (1999). Effectiveness of special education. In C. R. Reynolds & T. B. Gutkin (Eds.), *Handbook of school psychology* (3rd ed., pp. 984–1024). New York: Wiley.

Kratochwill, T. R., Eaton Hoagwood, K., Frank, J. L., Mass Levitt, J., Olin, S., Hunter Romanelli, L., et al. (2009). Evidence-based interventions and practices in school psychology: Challenges and opportunities for the profession. In T. B. Gutkin & C. R. Reynolds (Eds.), *Handbook of school psychology* (4th ed., pp. 497–521).

Lentz, F. E. (1988). Effective reading interventions in the regular classroom. In J. L. Graden, J. E. Zins, & M. J. Curtis (Eds.), *Alternative educational delivery systems: Enhancing instructional options for all students* (pp. 351–370). Washington, DC: National Association of School Psychologists.

Lyon, G. R., & Moats, L. C. (1997). Critical conceptual and methodological considerations in reading intervention research. *Journal of Learning Disabilities, 30*, 578–588.

McComas, J. J., Wacker, D. P., Cooper, L. J., Asmus, J. M., Richman, D., & Stoner, B. (1996). Brief experimental analysis of stimulus prompts for accurate responding on academic tasks in an outpatient clinic. *Journal of Applied Behavior Analysis, 29*, 397–401.

McCurdy, M., Daly, E., Gortmaker, V., Bonfiglio, C., & Persampieri, M. (2007). Use of brief instructional trials to identify small group reading strategies: A two experiment study. *Journal of Behavioral Education, 16*, 7–26.

Miltenberger, R. G. (2008). *Behavior modification: Principles and procedures* (4th ed.). Belmont, CA: Wadsworth/Thomson Learning.

National Reading Panel. (2000). *Teaching children to read: An evidence-based assessment of the scientific research literature on reading and its implications for reading instruction*. Retrieved *www.nationalreadingpanel.org/*.

Noell, G. H., Freeland, J. T., Witt, J. C., & Gansle, K. A. (2001). Using brief assessments to identify effective interventions for individual students. *Journal of School Psychology, 39*, 335–355.

Noell, G. H., Gansle, K. A., Witt, J. D., Whitmarsh, E. L., Freeland, J. T., LaFleur, L. H., et al. (1998). Effects of contingent reward and instruction on oral reading performance at differing levels of passage difficulty. *Journal of Applied Behavior Analysis, 31*, 659–664.

O'Shea, L. J., Munson, S. M., & O'Shea, D. J. (1984). Error correction in oral reading: Evaluating the effectiveness of three procedures. *Education and Treatment of Children, 7*, 203–214.

Rashotte, C. A., & Torgeson, J. K. (1985). Repeated reading and reading fluency in learning disabled children. *Reading Research Quarterly, 20*, 180–188.

Rilling, M. (1977). Stimulus control and inhibitory processes. In W. K. Honig & J. E. R. Staddon (Eds.), *Handbook of operant behavior* (pp. 432–480). Englewood Cliffs, NJ: Prentice-Hall.

Skinner, C. H., Fletcher, P. A., & Henington, C. (1996). Increasing learning rates by increasing student response rates: A summary of research. *School Psychology Quarterly, 11*, 313–325.

VanAuken, T. L., Chafouleas, S. M., Bradley, T. A., & Martens, B. K. (2002). Using brief experimental analysis to select oral reading interventions: An investigation of treatment utility. *Journal of Behavioral Education, 11*, 163–179.

Vargas, J. S. (1984). What are your exercises teaching? An analysis of stimulus control in instructional materials. In W. L. Heward, T. E. Heron, D. S. Hill, & J. Trap-Porter (Eds.), *Focus on behavior analysis in education* (pp. 126–141). Columbus, OH: Merrill.

Wanzek, J., & Vaughn, S. (2007). Research-based implications from extensive early reading interventions. *School Psychology Review, 36*, 541–561.

Wilber, A., & Cushman, T. P. (2006). Selecting effective academic interventions: An example using brief experimental analysis for oral reading. *Psychology in the Schools, 43*, 79–84.

Witt, J. C., Daly, E. J., III, & Noell, G. H. (2000). *Functional assessments: A step-by-step guide to solving academic and behavior problems*. Longmont, CO: Sopris West.

Wolery, M., Bailey, D. B., Jr., & Sugai, G. M. (1988). *Effective teaching: Principles and procedures of applied behavior analysis with exceptional children*. Boston: Allyn & Bacon.

Yeaton, W. H., & Sechrest, L. (1981). Critical dimensions in the choice and maintenance of successful treatments: Strength, integrity, and effectiveness. *Journal of Consulting and Clinical Psychology, 49*, 156–167.

PART III

ASSESSMENT AND ANALYSIS

Focus on Social–Emotional and Behavioral Outcomes

Chapter 9

Schoolwide Analysis of Data for Social Behavior Problems

Assessing Outcomes, Selecting Targets for Intervention, and Identifying Need for Support

Kent McIntosh
Wendy M. Reinke
Keith C. Herman

The domain of student social behavior is not new to school psychologists, who have long been viewed as school district experts in issues regarding severe problem behavior and mental health. The primary underlying assumption of this expert model is that students with these challenges are categorically different from other students and can be understood and treated only by someone with substantial mental health training. The resulting implication is that working with students with significant behavior difficulties is beyond the expertise level of teachers and other school personnel and that the best method of providing support to these students is to refer them for psychoeducational evaluation. Yet decades of research have shown that classroom teachers can support student behavior (from mild to severe) through the use of evidence-based educational practices (Alberto & Troutman, 2003; Shinn, Walker, & Stoner, 2002; Sugai, Horner, et al., 2000; H. M. Walker, 2004; H. M. Walker, Ramsey, & Gresham, 2005). In many school districts today, school psychologists are now seen not as psychological experts in diagnosing and treating behavior disorders but as educational leaders in preventing and addressing problem behavior while promoting social competence for all students (McNamara, 2002; Sugai, Horner, & Gresham, 2002).

The traditional model of school psychology is a passive one. It used to be that universal behavior screening meant checking one's mailbox at the district office for new referrals. Our hope is that this traditional model is seen as ineffective for supporting student behavior and a poor use of school psychologists' skills. A more contemporary vision of the field places school psychologists in new roles focusing on prevention and early intervention in the area of social behavior (National Association of School Psychologists, 2006). The multi-tiered response to intervention (RTI) model provides a particularly salient picture in understand the changing role of school psychologists in this area (see Ervin, Gimpel Peacock, & Merrell, Chapter 1, and Hawkins, Barnett, Morrison, & Musti-Rao, Chapter 2, this volume). The traditional role of school psychologist as gatekeeper of special education is akin to the role of a nightclub bouncer—standing guard between Tiers 2 and 3, turning away students who do not meet criteria for emotional disturbance and letting in students who do. Contemporary school psychologists can take action across the tiers of behavior support by evaluating the effectiveness of universal behavior support and identifying at-risk students early. Activities include: (1) identifying and clarifying the core behavioral curriculum provided to all students, (2) assessing outcomes of schoolwide efforts to reduce problem behavior and promote prosocial behavior, (3) ensuring that services provided at all tiers are exemplary, and (4) screening students to determine which students need more (or less) support than they are currently receiving.

A critical but often overlooked role in all of the activities just described is the coordination of data collection, analysis, and action planning to improve student outcomes (Horner, Sugai, & Todd, 2001). Though school psychologists may be most familiar with data collected for individual decision making, collection and analysis of data at the schoolwide level is optimal for several reasons. First, the use of schoolwide data allows limited resources to be allocated effectively by focusing efforts beyond the individual student, allowing for greater impact. If the analysis takes place at the classroom level, teachers may need to identify their own resources to help a small number of students in their classrooms with specific concerns. If the analysis is schoolwide, the school's resources can be used to assist all students, including grouping by need, if indicated (e.g., a group to support students with anxiety or depression). Second, the use of data at the school level provides school personnel with the ability to efficiently and effectively locate entire settings of the school for intervention (e.g., hallways, assemblies, or school bus) to support entire groups of students. And third, collecting schoolwide data may provide some foundational data (e.g., screening, baseline data, contextual information, what has been tried) for assessment of individuals who do not respond to schoolwide intervention.

This chapter describes the selection, collection, and use of schoolwide data for decision making in the domain of student social behavior. Emphasis is placed on designing and adapting systems of data that are valid, reliable, and useful in making important decisions about the effectiveness of schoolwide behavior support; on how to improve the behavior support provided to students; and on identifying student needs for support.

Particular emphasis is placed on identifying existing data on problem behavior incidents (such as office discipline referrals and suspension data) that may be used to answer multiple questions, as well as selecting additional measures to answer questions not addressed by existing datasets. Finally, we provide a case study using behavior data to assess outcomes, to identify areas for intervention, and to screen for students needing more support.

Schoolwide Data Decision Making: Three Basic Questions

Despite the utility and many benefits of data, data collection in today's schools often lacks purpose: Data are collected at great expense but not used for decision making (Horner et al., 2001). Effective use of data depends on a careful planning process that starts with asking important questions, then selecting the right tools for answering these questions, and finally using those data to make informed decisions. With an eye to predicting and preventing ineffective use of data, we explore a few important questions to ask when collecting and using data. These questions should drive the selection of measures, creation of systems, and regular analysis of data to make informed decisions. Three basic questions for data collection and decision making are listed in Table 9.1 (along with specific questions teams may ask) and are described in the following paragraphs. Though the uses and examples come from the domain of social behavior, these questions represent a data decision-making process that could be used in a broad range of school team decision-making processes, such as academic instruction or special education eligibility determination.

Question 1: Is the Current Plan Achieving Intended Outcomes?

The first purpose of this question is to assess the outcomes of current efforts. This is a critical step: It identifies how well the current plan is working to support student behavior (a related question, Is the plan being implemented as intended? is covered by Noell, Chapter 30, this volume). Even if there is no formal behavior support pro-

TABLE 9.1. Questions for Data Collection and Decision Making (Schoolwide Social Behavior)

Basic question	Sample questions
Question 1: Is the current plan achieving intended outcomes?	• Is the plan working as well as or better than it did last year?
	• Is a change in the plan needed?
	• Are the behavior needs of all students being adequately met?
	• Do the students have the skills to do what is expected?
	• Are at least 80% of students effectively supported by our schoolwide behavior curriculum?
	• Do the students in the Tier 2 anxiety group use coping skills effectively?
Question 2: What areas need improvement?	• Which grade levels need additional social skills training?
	• What physical areas of the school are perceived as less safe?
	• Which classroom routines do students need to be retaught?
	• Why are parent management training sessions poorly attended?
	• Why do students behave well in assemblies and poorly at lunch?
Question 3: Which students need additional support?	• Which students have received two or more ODRs in the first month of school?
	• Which students are not adequately responding to the Tier 2 check-in–check-out intervention?
	• Which students are consistently showing signs of anxiety or depression?

gram, all schools have informal, hidden behavior curricula that are taught when individual school personnel address instances of prosocial and problem behavior. Question 1 is aligned with the problem identification phase of the problem-solving (PS) model (Bergan & Kratochwill, 1990; Tilly, 2008; see also Gimpel Peacock et al., Chapter 1, this volume).

It may seem peculiar to start by determining outcomes, but starting with important, valued outcomes is a critical feature of effective data systems (Sugai & Horner, 2005). When teams start with a favored data system before considering what they want to measure, they risk a mismatch between what is being measured and what they want to know. Generally, people do not buy a watch and then discover what they want to do with it; they want to tell time, so they buy a watch. Yet, in this age of data-based accountability, it is more likely that educators will make this mistake. Data systems and educational reforms that are implemented without a clear, agreed-on goal in mind are not likely to be sustained (McIntosh, Horner, & Sugai, 2009). But by starting with an outcome in mind, teams can design the most appropriate system to measure that outcome. It is only when outcomes and an adequate data system are identified that teams can see whether current efforts are adequate or whether changes in their plans are needed.

So what are common desired outcomes for school teams? Certainly academic excellence, independent functioning, and social competence are cited as broad outcomes. In the social behavior domain, some common desired outcomes are as follows: (1) predictable, orderly, and safe schools, which allow instruction to occur and which are free from violence, harassment, and drug abuse; (2) social competence for all students, including the ability to form and maintain positive relationships with peers, to work effectively with adults and supervisors in higher education and the workplace, and to be responsible, caring citizens in the community; and (3) social–emotional resilience, including the skills to function independently, to use appropriate self-care skills, and to maintain physical and emotional health. Schools vary to the degree to which they value some of these outcomes over others.

Teams may also identify secondary outcomes, or beneficial side effects of their plans. If primary outcomes are achieved (e.g., a safe school environment, students focusing on learning, and teachers spending more time on instruction than behavioral correction), some secondary outcomes may be expected, such as improvements in student literacy (Ervin, Schaughency, Goodman, McGlinchey, & Matthews, 2006; Goodman, 2005; McIntosh, Chard, Boland, & Horner, 2006) and in the quality of the school workplace (Bradshaw, Koth, Bevans, Ialongo, & Leaf, 2008), and reduced referrals for out-of-school placement (Lewis, 2007). Assessing these outcomes may be as simple as linking to existing data systems for other school initiatives, and it can pay off greatly in terms of relating the importance of an ongoing initiative to newer, higher priority initiatives in areas other than social behavior (McIntosh, Horner, & Sugai, 2009).

Outcomes assessment can be completed at the district, school, class, program, or individual level. The answer may be that the current efforts are producing acceptable results and that outcomes are being met, or the data may indicate that there is a need to formalize or improve the quality of schoolwide, classwide, or Tier 2 or 3 behavior support. If the outcomes are deemed insufficient, the team may collect and analyze data to address question 2.

Question 2: What Areas Need Improvement?

Once a school team determines that changes are needed (based on its response to question 1), the focus of the analysis may logically move toward identifying the reasons that outcomes were not realized and what areas are of concern. The initial analysis may provide some detail but may not be sufficient to determine *why* goals were not met. Utilizing schoolwide data systems allows analysis at the systemic level with an eye toward identifying areas for improvement. The dual purposes of this question are to identify specific areas in which the current plan is not working and then to explore potential causes of the problem. This question is aligned with the problem-analysis phase of the PS model.

Though we describe a logical progression from assessing outcomes to analysis of areas for improvement, our experience is that teams are tempted to bypass this question

and move directly to proposing solutions. This strategy, though appealing due to perceived efficiency, often results in haphazard adoption of new programs that do not address the school's actual needs. In this case, school teams may abandon a practice that was previously effective for another practice that is chosen spuriously for reasons as random as a recently attended workshop. For example, a middle school with significant needs may stop teaching schoolwide expectations and adopt a popular, non-evidence-based drug abuse prevention curriculum, with potentially disastrous consequences (Severson & James, 2002). A team analysis of schoolwide data to identify specific needs should precede selection of interventions or strategies, as these decisions should be based on the nature of the problem. It is only once specific areas are targeted and understood that effective changes can be made.

School teams can understand the nature of the problems through a careful analysis of specific areas in which problem behavior is common or prosocial behavior is not occurring. These areas could be physical settings of the school (e.g., school entry area, cafeteria), but they may also be specific student behaviors that indicate gaps in the schoolwide curriculum (e.g., lack of empathy, vandalism), interventions that have been ineffective (e.g., attendance programs), or missing components of a comprehensive program (e.g., parent outreach and education). Once problem areas are identified, the team can then ask why these areas are problematic. The problem may be apparent based on the existing data, or it may be necessary to collect more information to determine why the problems exist. The analysis of this question leads directly to what should be done (i.e., assessment data leads to intervention selection), and after implementation, question 1 is asked again. As an additional note, it is also helpful to assess what is working well in other areas to gain insight into successes and to build on strengths.

Question 3: Which Students Need Additional Support?

The final question asked is one of individual response to intervention. As it is clear that not all students will respond to the schoolwide intervention (Vaughn, Linan-Thompson, & Hickman, 2003; Walker et al., 1996), a critical use of data is to identify individuals who require additional support (Tier 2 or 3) to be successful. A proactive approach to student support involves active screening for inadequate RTI. This process improves the odds that students are identified and assisted early, before behavior becomes entrenched in maladaptive patterns and is more difficult to remediate (Walker & Sprague, 1999). Without a regular and structured screening process, school personnel may fail to identify students until problems have reached a point of crisis. This may be due to overlooking signs that are difficult to observe, to habituation to the behavior, or to a desire to help the student succeed with typical support (Sprague et al., 2001).

Depending on the data used in the system, screening may simply involve generating a list of students who need additional assessment and support beyond the schoolwide level of intervention. A more useful system allows school team members to identify the specific needs of students. For example, a screening system may indicate which students need additional social skills training, reteaching and supervision at specific times of the day, or referral to treatment for anxious behavior. In addition, the system may indicate the level of additional support that is needed for the student to be successful. For some students, an efficient Tier 2 level of support is all that is needed (e.g., reteaching of routines and/or expectations, a targeted social skills group, or daily report card intervention). For others, the data may indicate an immediate need for an individualized Tier 3 intervention. Yet even with a system that indicates the type and level of support needed, further assessment is sometimes needed to match a student's needs to available interventions (Carter & Horner, 2007; March & Horner, 2002; McIntosh, Campbell, Carter, & Dickey, 2009). This question may span both the problem identification and problem analysis phases of the PS model if the system both identifies students and indicates a specific type of support that is needed.

Additionally, it is sometimes (and happily) necessary to consider the extent to which a student is receiving more support than is necessary and to move students down the tiers of support (Campbell, 2008; McIntosh & Av-Gay, 2007). This is helpful to the school system because it frees up resources for other students in need, but it is also helpful to the individual student because it increases independent functioning and may reduce stigma.

Considerations

Some considerations are necessary to keep in mind when asking the three questions identified here. First, these questions are not mutually exclusive—preferably data should answer more than one question. For example, teams might answer question 1 by counting the number of students who did not respond to the universal intervention and comparing that number with an outcome goal (e.g., 80% of students with less than two office discipline referrals). The team would use the same data to answer question 3 by identifying the students with two or more office discipline referrals as those who need additional help. In addition, the team could use the same data to answer question 2 by identifying patterns of behavior that indicate problem areas or groups who need additional instruction (e.g., students having trouble getting on the buses to get home or requesting teacher assistance correctly). Measures that may be used to answer multiple questions are more valuable because of the expense of data collection. In the same vein, measures that can be used to answer only one question should be added only after considering more efficient alternatives.

Similar to the contemporary approach to student behavior, data should be used to provide additional support to school personnel, not to punish them for their behavior. For instance, analysis of data at the schoolwide level may pinpoint a particular classroom in which elevated levels of problem behavior exist. Though ineffective teaching may be the cause of these problems, there are a variety of alternative explanations for this pattern of data, including a poor match between teacher and students, a large number of students with histories of challenging behavior, and other environmental influences (e.g., a large increase in class size). Instead of identifying personnel deficiencies, school teams could use the data to provide additional support within that classroom (e.g., coaching or mentoring for the classroom teacher, development of a targeted intervention within the classroom), and continued analysis of data will show whether the plan is effective. When school personnel feel that the data are being used to support them rather than to identify their weaknesses, they are more likely to use the measures as intended. However, if data systems are used to draw attention to their deficiencies, school personnel may choose not to report data accurately, and the system becomes invalid. This is a particular danger if administrators (school, district, or state) emphasize reductions in behavior incidents over accurate data collection.

Another consideration of data collection is the school psychologist's time. Often, when considering adding new systems, it is natural to question the value of adding another responsibility to an already burdensome workload. So, does taking a leadership role in developing and using data systems mean more work for the school psychologist? Perhaps at the onset, but when data decision-making and prevention practices are implemented effectively, the investment leads to fewer expensive and time-consuming individual assessments. The goal is to intervene before intensive assessment and support are needed. Though this may represent a significant change for some, this transformation of roles and the resulting early identification and treatment are likely to mean fewer difficult cases down the road, which benefits students *and* protects school psychologists' time.

Designing an Effective Data System

The term *data system* is used here to describe an overall structure that includes the measures used, the collection method, any tools used to organize and synthesize the raw data, and a process by which the data are used to make decisions. In a simple physiological analogy, the heart of the data system includes the actual measures and tools selected to collect data. The veins that transmit these data are the various steps taken to collect and organize it. Finally, the brain of the system is the process by which the data are accessed to make important decisions. As such, each part plays a vital role in the overall functioning of the system.

Suitability Criteria for Useful Measures in Data Systems

When designing a data system, it is critical to identify what information will be collected, and a primary concern is determining what would constitute good data. A system and a plan are worthless and potentially even harmful without good measurement. Therefore, it is vital to consider the elements of measures that would make them useful when selecting them. Following is a list of the four key aspects of measures that determine their worth to an effective data system. Later in the chapter, commonly used schoolwide behavior assessment measures are discussed in the context of these criteria. Though it is beyond the scope of this chapter to provide a detailed discussion of all of these aspects, some points are worth noting. Useful measures should:

1. Answer important questions.
2. Be technically adequate (valid and reliable).
3. Be efficient.
4. Demonstrate treatment utility (adapted from Horner et al., 2001).

Answering Important Questions

Measures should be selected based on the extent to which they help answer the three questions presented earlier, preferably multiple questions. Data that will not actively be used for decision making should not be part of a data system.

Being Technically Adequate

To be used effectively, data must be accurate and trustworthy; measures without acceptable levels of validity and reliability do not meet these criteria. In some areas, valid and/or reliable systems-level measures may not exist. In these situations, data should be collected from multiple sources, compared with other results, and treated with caution.

Being Efficient

It is critical to create a system that stresses efficient rather than all-encompassing use of data because of the intensive workload of today's teachers, the vast majority of whose time is best spent teaching. In addition, data systems should be easy to convert into graphs that are readily interpretable. In this digital era, an electronic data system is almost a necessity, given the relative ease with which numbers can be summed, averaged, and graphed almost instantly (Cordori, 1987; May et al., 2006). Even entering handwritten data into a computer program may be more efficient because it is so easy to graph with basic spreadsheet programs.

Demonstrating Treatment Utility

Another key consideration in the quality of measures is their treatment utility, the extent to which a measure provides information that informs the selection of effective interventions (Hayes, Nelson, & Jarrett, 1987). As noted earlier, a superior assessment tool provides information not only on what outcomes are being met and whether changes are needed but also on *what* specific changes are needed. Reliable indications for steps to take, areas for focus, or interventions to utilize will improve a measure's value to school teams and the efficiency and effectiveness of the data system.

How to Transform Measures into a Coherent, Efficient Data System

Now that we have described what questions to ask and how to evaluate measures for their utility, it is time to explore a process for selecting measures to form a coherent data system. There are two main methods used to design data systems. The first method is to use the information presented earlier to select an array of measures (e.g., observation, rating scales, and multiple-gating screening measures) that are chosen specifically to answer the questions completely and to meet the criteria described previously. This method involves the most time and effort, but it is most likely to produce accurate, useful data for decision making. The second method is to identify only measures currently used in schools, often as a district or state requirement (e.g., current discipline data, attendance data, achievement data, or grades). This method, though the more efficient choice, may not lead to accurate and valid answers to important questions.

A more realistic approach is to integrate the two methods, maximizing both effectiveness and efficiency. The first step is to identify the measures that are already collected on a regular basis (monthly or more frequently) and that are available for decision making. Each of the measures can be evaluated based on the extent to which it can be used to answer the basic questions and on its suitability as an effective, efficient measure. Once this initial assessment is completed, the team can assess what other measures, if any, will need to be added to answer all of the questions with some accuracy. When selecting new measures, a key point is to implement only what is most efficient to get results, especially considering the resources used not only in collecting but also in entering, summarizing, and graphing results (Horner et al., 2001). As such, when weighing the suitability of existing data versus adding new measures, it is preferable to utilize existing data whenever possible but to recognize their limitations as well.

One example outside of the educational realm that may be instructive is the data system the park wardens use to count grizzly bears in Nahanni National Park in Canada's Northwest Territories. Though park wardens often sight grizzly bears as part of their regular duties, the resources needed to directly observe all bears in the area would not only be cost-prohibitive but would also cause harm to the bears and the environment. Instead, the wardens put in place a system to estimate bear counts by identifying trees that bears use as scratching posts and testing the DNA of the hairs left behind, a permanent product of bear activity. These data are combined with existing direct observations of bear activity to provide an estimated count of bears in the area. Though this system may not provide the exact number of bears, the resulting data represent an efficient method of adding a measure to bolster data already collected.

The final and often overlooked step in data system design is to create the framework for using the data system, a data-decision-making cycle. To be useful to school teams, data need not only answer important questions and meet criteria but also to be used in regular cycles of decision making (e.g., during monthly team meetings). This process includes bringing graphs of data to meetings and discussing the data as an early agenda item at every meeting. When used consistently in this fashion, the data systems often drive the agenda for the entire meeting. Effective data systems specify: (1) who will collect the data, (2) who will enter and graph the data, (3) when the data will be analyzed and discussed, (4) who will bring the data to meetings, and (5) who will create and carry out action plans based on the data.

Measures Commonly Used for Schoolwide Behavior Decision Making

The following are descriptions of measures that are often used by school teams in their data systems for schoolwide social behavior support. For each general group of data, measures are described briefly, along with an evaluation of their suitability for decision making, including (1) decision-making utility, (2) technical adequacy, (3) efficiency, and (4) treatment utility. This is not an exhaustive list by any means but rather a list from which to start making decisions about primary behavior outcomes.

Office Discipline Referrals

Office discipline referrals (ODRs) are a class of forms used to document events of significant problem behavior in schools. Most schools already collect ODRs in some way or another; they may be called incident forms, discipline tracking forms, or behavior log entries (Tobin, Sugai, & Colvin, 2000). If the ODR forms specify useful information about the incident and are used systematically and consistently, they represent existing data that are uniquely valuable for efficient and effective schoolwide decision making (Horner et al., 2001; Sugai, Sprague, Horner, & Walker, 2000; Wright & Dusek, 1998). To a certain extent, suspension data may also be used for decision making, though the use of these data alone is less preferable than in conjunction with ODRs—the extreme behavior has already occurred, and lower level behaviors, which might be used to predict and prevent problems, are not assessed.

ODRs provide an indication of the level of problem behavior for individuals, areas of the school, or the school as a whole. School personnel complete ODRs when they observe student behavior and determine that the behavior warrants a referral (Sugai, Sprague et al., 2000). Useful information in an ODR form includes: student name(s), name of referring staff member, the problem behavior, date, time of day, location, possible antecedent of problem behavior, possible function of problem behavior (i.e., hypothesized reasons why the behavior is occurring), others involved, and administrative decision (May et al., 2006; Tobin et al., 2000). Figure 9.1 provides a sample ODR form that includes these features.

Once completed, ODRs are typically entered into a computer program for tallying, summarizing, and graphing to answer questions about behavior (Cordori, 1987). A variety of computer programs are available for this use, from Web-based applications designed specifically for entering and analyzing ODRs, such as the School-Wide Information System (SWIS; May et al., 2006), to spreadsheets using common computer applications. When graphs are produced and used, decision making is greatly facilitated. Specific data that are helpful for school teams are graphs of the average numbers of referrals per day (standardized for number of students), types of problem behavior, locations of referrals, time of day, and students with multiple referrals (Horner et al., 2001; Todd, Sampson, & Horner, 2005). Programs that can also combine these questions (e.g., types of behavior by location) are valuable for "drilling down" to explore further data analysis questions (Tobin et al., 2000).

Decision-Making Utility

ODRs are particularly well suited to decision making and answering all three basic questions of schoolwide data. To answer question 1 (*Is the current plan achieving intended outcomes?*), teams may use a number of different criteria. First, schools may calculate the total number of ODRs for the year and compare the result with past years (Wright & Dusek, 1998). This procedure can give an index of improvement and can identify whether current efforts are making a difference. Second, schools may compare their number of referrals per day with a standardized general criterion, such as ODRs per day per 100 students. For schools in the SWIS

Name: _____

Date: _____ **Time:** _____

Teacher: _____

Grade: K 1 2 3 4 5 6 7 8

Referring Staff: _____

Location

☐ Playground   ☐ Library

☐ Cafeteria   ☐ Bathroom

☐ Hallway   ☐ Arrival/Dismissal

☐ Classroom   ☐ Other _____

Minor Problem Behavior	Major Problem Behavior	Possible Motivation
☐ Inappropriate language ☐ Physical contact ☐ Defiance ☐ Disruption ☐ Dress code ☐ Property misuse ☐ Tardy ☐ Electronic violation ☐ Other _____	☐ Abusive language ☐ Fighting/physical aggression ☐ Overt defiance ☐ Harassment/bullying ☐ Dress code ☐ Tardy ☐ Inappropriate display aff. ☐ Electronic violation ☐ Lying/cheating ☐ Skipping class ☐ Other _____	☐ Obtain peer attention ☐ Obtain adult attention ☐ Obtain items/activities ☐ Avoid peer(s) ☐ Avoid adult ☐ Avoid task or activity ☐ Don't know ☐ Other _____

Administrative Decision	
☐ Loss of privilege ☐ Time in office ☐ Conference with student ☐ Parent contact	☐ Individualized instruction ☐ In-school suspension (____ hours/ days) ☐ Out-of-school suspension (____ days) ☐ Other _____

Others involved in incident: ☐ None ☐ Peers ☐ Staff ☐ Teacher ☐ Substitute ☐ Unknown

☐ Other _____

Other comments:

FIGURE 9.1. Office disciplinary referral (ODR) form with features that enhance data decision making and treatment utility. From Todd and Horner (2006). Copyright 2006 by the University of Oregon. Reprinted by permission.

database in the 2007–2008 school year, the average ODRs per day per 100 students was as follows: elementary schools, 0.34; middle schools, 0.92; high schools, 1.05 (current statistics can be found at the SWIS website, *www.swis.org*). For example, a middle school with 1,000 students may set a goal of no more than 10 ODRs per day (and examine results monthly). If ODRs are above these averages, schools may conclude that their schoolwide efforts could be improved. Alternatively, schools may look at the number of students with multiple referrals to determine what percentage of students is supported by the current schoolwide behavior support plan. School teams may identify criteria for effectiveness based on general patterns reported in the literature (Horner,

Sugai, Todd, & Lewis-Palmer, 2005). For example, if the number of students without two or more ODRs is below a certain criterion (e.g., 85% of students in elementary school, 80% in middle school/junior high school, and 75% in high school), the team may determine that their schoolwide plan needs improvement.

To answer question 2 (*What areas need improvement?*), schools may analyze graphs of ODRs to determine problem locations, times of day, or prevalence of particular problem behaviors (Tobin et al., 2000). These graphs may indicate that the areas of the school to target for intervention could include a specific location, a particular offense, or, if computer programs allow fine-tuned analysis, even a particular grade level's lunchtime. Once areas for improvement are identified, potential interventions could include reteaching the expectations in these areas or with these students or adding additional supervision and/or a reinforcement system targeting expected behaviors specific to the nature of the problems. A more detailed example of this process is included in a case study at the end of this chapter.

ODRs may also be used to answer question 3 (*Which students need additional support?*). School teams may set criteria to identify students who are not responding to the schoolwide intervention and who require more support to be successful in the social–emotional realm (Tobin et al., 2000; Wright & Dusek, 1998). The most common criterion is receiving two or more ODRs in 1 year (Horner et al., 2005). This threshold has been validated in research showing that students with two or more ODRs have significantly higher ratings of problem behavior on behavior scales such as the Behavior Assessment Scale for Children—2 (Reynolds & Kamphaus, 2004) and Social Skills Rating Scale (Gresham & Elliott, 1990) than students with zero or one ODR (McIntosh, Campbell, Carter, & Zumbo, in press; B. Walker, Cheney, Stage, & Blum, 2005). Some school teams also add a more proactive criterion for referring students: If students receive three or more minor referrals (for low-level problem behaviors that do not warrant an ODR) within 1 week, they are identified for further assessment and support.

Technical Adequacy

The validity of ODRs has been studied extensively. In two studies, Irvin and colleagues (Irvin et al., 2006; Irvin, Tobin, Sprague, Sugai, & Vincent, 2004) concluded that there is evidence of acceptable construct validity for using ODRs in schoolwide and individual decision making. As described in the previous paragraph, there is sufficient evidence for concurrent validity with standardized individual behavior rating scales (McIntosh et al., in press; Walker, Cheney, et al., 2005). In addition, there is considerable evidence for the predictive validity of ODRs: ODRs are associated with future negative outcomes, including suspension, expulsion, delinquency, dropout, and academic fail-

ure (McIntosh, Horner, Chard, Boland, & Good, 2006; Morrison, Anthony, Storino, & Dillon, 2001; Tobin & Sugai, 1999). However, it is important to note that ODRs are most closely associated with externalizing behaviors (e.g., aggression or disruption) and do not always capture internalizing behaviors (e.g., anxiety, depression, or somatization), especially mild behaviors (McIntosh et al., in press).

Because they are used widely by a variety of school personnel, ODRs are subject to a number of threats to reliability (Kern & Manz, 2004; Martens, 1993). Therefore, it is necessary for schools to improve reliability through analysis of data and training for accurate use. Schools using ODRs are advised to complete regular reliability trainings, including defining what specific behaviors should result in ODRs, as opposed to warnings or simple reteaching (Sugai, Lewis-Palmer, Todd, & Horner, 2001). In addition, school and district administrators must take care not to promote a goal of reducing ODRs over using them accurately. If reliability is a concern for schools, teams may complete direct observation of problem behavior in specific settings to confirm or disconfirm ODR data (Cushing, Horner, & Barrier, 2003).

Another threat to the reliability of ODRs is biased use. Considering the ethnic disproportionality in punishment and representation in special education (Skiba, Michael, Nardo, & Peterson, 2002; Skiba et al., 2008), it is important to consider whether students receive different rates of ODRs based on bias, not on actual behaviors. Some data systems allow easy analysis of ODR data by ethnicity. For example, the SWIS ethnicity report can be used to determine whether some groups are referred or suspended more often than their proportion of the student body would predict (May et al., 2006).

Efficiency

Schools may already be required to collect some kind of behavior referral data, and using existing information is an efficient method of data collection. ODRs are generally viewed as easier to collect when a checklist (as opposed to a narrative) format is used. When school personnel can complete a form by marking boxes rather than writing an account of the behavior, instruction is less likely to be affected by documentation, and ODRs are more likely to be used when needed. With appropriate and readily available technology, ODRs can be entered with minimal resources, and using a computer program with easy graph generation will make ODRs easy to use in decision making (Cordori, 1987).

Treatment Utility

ODR forms with adequate information fields can be used to select appropriate systems-level and individual interventions. As shown in the discussion of question 2 earlier, patterns of ODRs can be used to target physical locations of the school, levels of intervention, times of day, or groups of students for specialized support (Tobin et al., 2000). In addition to identifying students who require additional support, ODRs may also be used to indicate particular interventions based on indicated function of problem behavior. Recent studies have demonstrated how patterns of ODRs can be used to generate preliminary behavioral hypothesis statements (including behavior, antecedents, and consequences) to be confirmed by interviews and/ or direct observation (March & Horner, 2002; McIntosh, Horner, Chard, Dickey, & Braun, 2008).

Multiple-Gating Screening Measures

In contrast to common individual behavior rating scales (poorly suited to schoolwide analysis due to time intensiveness of administration and summary), multiple-gating screening measures have been proposed as rating scale systems with increased utility for schoolwide decision making (Patterson, Reid, & Dishion, 1992; Severson, Walker, Hope-Doolittle, Kratochill, & Gresham, 2007). Multiple-gating measures are systems of progressively intensive measures to identify students at risk for negative outcomes (Lochman, 1995; Patterson et al., 1992; Sprague et al., 2001). Multiple-gating measures include a series of stages. The first stage (or gate) of a multiple-gating system involves a relatively inexpensive screening that is conducted schoolwide. Only the students identified by this stage progress to the next stage,

which includes more intensive screening. At each stage, the assessment becomes increasingly more expensive and time-consuming, but fewer students are assessed (Sprague & Walker, 2005).

One commonly used multiple-gating screening measure in school settings is the Systematic Screening for Behavior Disorders (SSBD; Walker & Severson, 1992). The SSBD is used to identify elementary school students with elevated risk for either externalizing or internalizing behavior disorders, and a version for use in preschools is also available (Feil, Severson, & Walker, 1998). The SSBD has been studied extensively, and results have demonstrated its effectiveness in identifying students in need of additional support with accuracy, cost-effectiveness, and consumer acceptance (Walker & Severson, 1994; Walker et al., 1988, 1990). The SSBD's multiple-gating procedure consists of three stages: (1) teacher ranking, (2) teacher rating, and (3) systematic direct observation. In stage 1, general education teachers rank-order students in their classrooms according to level of concern in two categories: externalizing behaviors and internalizing behaviors. In stage 2, teachers rate their top three ranked students in each category (identified in stage 1) on checklists of adaptive and maladaptive behaviors. Students who exceed the normative cutoff points on these checklists move on to stage 3. In stage 3, a trained observer (e.g., school psychologist) records the target students' academic engaged time and peer social behavior in both classroom and playground settings. Normatively derived cutoff points are then used to determine which students warrant referral for individual evaluation. Students moving through two stages are candidates for Tier 2 interventions, and those moving through all three stages are candidates for Tier 3 interventions.

Currently, the SSBD is out of print, and its norms are outdated. As a result, some schools have devised their own measures based on the logic of the SSBD gating system, but with updated measures at each stage (II. Muscott, personal communication, March 28, 2008). For stage 1, teams may use the same rank ordering as the SSBD (selecting the top three students in externalizing and internalizing categories). For the six students in each class who pass on to stage 2, teachers would complete a brief screener, such as the Behavioral and Emotional Screening System (Kamphaus & Reynolds, 2008). Students scoring in the elevated range of this measure would pass on to stage 3. At stage 3, students would be monitored frequently by the classroom teacher using a daily behavior report card system, such as those used in a check-in–check-out program (Crone, Horner, & Hawken, 2003). After 2 weeks of monitoring, each student's need for support can be assessed through the daily ratings of appropriate and problem behavior (Cheney, Flower, & Templeton, 2008). Though this method incorporates portions of the SSBD with updated measures of behavior, caution is advised in relying on such a system before research is undertaken to evaluate the overall system.

Decision-Making Utility

Multiple-gating measures are particularly well suited to answer question 3 (*Which students need additional support?*). Measures such as the SSBD are designed to identify students with externalizing, as well as internalizing, problems who may go undetected by a screening system based only on ODRs. In addition, these systems may be more proactive than ODR systems for early identification of students who need additional support, as teams may identify students exhibiting early symptoms of distress rather than waiting for ODRs to be issued. However, multiple-gating systems may not be useful for answering questions 1 and 2. If the measure always yields the same number of student nominations at stage 1, these data are not informative about overall school climate or student needs. A close analysis of results could identify patterns of behavioral needs of students, but analysis of the data in this way is likely to be prohibitive due to the time involved.

Technical Adequacy

Each system will need to be assessed individually to determine its psychometric properties. In general, there is evidence that teachers are accurate in nominating students who need additional support, though additional training may be needed to identify students with internalizing problem behavior with

accuracy (Davis, 2005). The SSBD in particular has strong research evidence supporting its reliability and validity as a screening tool (Walker & Severson, 1994; Walker et al., 1988; Walker et al., 1990).

Efficiency

Implementing a multiple-gating screening measure is clearly less efficient than utilizing existing data, but using these screeners can be more efficient and cost-effective than utilizing individual rating scale systems (Walker & Severson, 1994). When considering the features of some measures (e.g., assessment of externalizing *and* internalizing behavior, utility for early identification), the multiple-gating measures may be valuable tools for school teams to consider, particularly if teams use them to replace existing screening systems.

Treatment Utility

Though these measures are designed primarily to *identify* students who are at risk, some information may be generated that could guide intervention design. For example, a school team may use the information from rating scales administered in each of the stages to identify specific problems or prosocial skill deficits for targeting. In addition, the team may use more direct data from the final stage to determine areas of concern and to identify baseline levels of behavior for progress monitoring. However, most multiple-gating measures are unlikely to yield information about antecedents or about maintaining consequences of problem behavior for function-based support.

Measures Assessing Levels of Prosocial Behavior

Most existing schoolwide measures, including those described earlier, measure problem behavior exclusively. Though documenting levels of problem behavior is important, successful schoolwide interventions focus not only on the reduction of problem behavior but also on the promotion of prosocial behavior. Optimally, effective schoolwide data systems would measure both desired and undesired behavior. Currently, there are few valid and efficient options in schools, and more research is needed to produce measures that are worthy of wide use. The following sections briefly describe some measures that show potential utility for measuring prosocial behavior for schoolwide decision making.

Rating Scales That Focus on Positive Behaviors

One limitation of traditional rating scales, including the SSBD, is that they tend to overemphasize problem behaviors and often fail to tap prosocial behaviors. Recently, Hosp, Howell, and Hosp (2003) reviewed the usefulness of commonly used rating scales as tools for planning and monitoring behavior support. Two scales, the Behavioral and Emotional Rating Scale (Epstein & Sharma, 1998) and the Walker–McConnell Scale of Social Competence and School Adjustment (H. M. Walker & McConnell, 1995) included a broad range of items assessing prosocial behavior. Yet in terms of schoolwide decision making, use of these rating scales still suffers from the same drawbacks (e.g., time intensity, difficulty of summarizing schoolwide rating scale data) mentioned in the previous section.

Positive Behavior Referrals

Some school teams choose to document positive behavior referrals as a complement to their systems for tracking ODRs. These often come in the form of tickets and cards that are issued for displays of desirable behavior. For instance, students might receive positive referrals for helping their peers, for following directions the first time, for managing a conflict appropriately, or for walking quietly in the halls. Such systems help schools track the ratio of positive to negative interactions between adults and students, the location and time that positive behaviors are more and less likely to be noted, and students whose positive behaviors are or are not being noticed. These may be used to identify areas of strength, skills to target for further instruction, and effectiveness of schoolwide interventions. However, positive referrals are rarely used in this way, and no studies to date have examined their psychometric properties for assessing schoolwide behavior. And as with ODRs, use may not be consistent across teachers without explicit training.

Direct Observation Procedures

Though schoolwide observations of behavior may be cost-prohibitive, brief direct observation measures can be used to assess levels of desired behavior in specific settings. If the data system identifies locations of concern for intervention (question 2), the team may use direct observation to collect information on prosocial behavior. The School-Wide Observation System (Smith, 2007) assesses levels of student prosocial and problem behavior, as well as adult–student interactions in common areas in the school. The measure allows school teams to calculate probabilities of student prosocial and problem behaviors based on levels of adult supervision and staff–student interactions. If teaching practices are a concern, the team could assess desired teaching behavior, such as delivery of praise and provision of opportunities for academic responding, through the Brief Classroom Interaction Observation (Reinke & Lewis-Palmer, 2007). Brief direct observation methods hold promise for tracking positive behavior in students, though the benefits of using these measures (e.g., low inference measurement, specific information for assessing and improving a particular location) must be weighed against their associated costs (e.g., resource intensity, narrow focus; Wright & Dusek, 1998).

Social Skills/Social–Emotional Skills Inventories

School teams can also use brief skills inventories or rubrics to rate groups of students on their use of prosocial skills and to assess the effects of their schoolwide behavior curriculum. Some states and provinces have adopted standards for social–emotional competencies that all students are expected to acquire by given grade levels, similar to the academic content standards that are established for student learning. For instance, the Missouri School Counselor Association (2007) has specified grade-level expectations in prosocial behavior, such as respect for self and others, healthy and safe choices, and coping skills. Within these criteria, the competency standard for kindergarten students in the transition concept is to "identify how school expectations are different from home, day-care, or pre-school." The British Columbia Ministry of Education (2001) has developed a rubric for four areas of social responsibility and specific behaviors that indicate competence through four rating levels (from "not yet within expectations" to "exceeds expectations"). When these criteria are skill-based and specify actual student behaviors, teachers can use these standards to assess prosocial behavior in a consistent, coherent manner.

Teachers can use observation and decision rules to determine whether they need to reteach behavior expectations to all students or to just a few. For instance, if fewer than 80% of students demonstrate the behavior fluently and independently, then the behavior should be retaught to all students. However, if over 80% are fluent, teachers should teach only the students who need additional instruction or practice (Haring, Lovitt, Eaton, & Hansen, 1978). In this way, competency standards for social behavior development are highly compatible with RTI approaches. But, as with the other methods focused on measuring prosocial behavior, efforts to establish social–emotional standards have much room for growth and improvement. In particular, further work is needed to clearly define behavior expectations for each grade level, how these expectations might vary based on geographic and cultural differences, and how to measure schoolwide competencies in a reliable and valid manner.

Case Study: Kennedy Middle School

This section describes an applied example of using data to make decisions about the state of social behavior support. The school and data are fictitious, but the information presented here mirrors a number of trends we have observed in actual schools. The school, Kennedy Middle School, is a public middle school with 1,000 students in grades 6–8. The school is in its third year of implementing a schoolwide positive behavior support program (Horner et al., 2005).

The school has implemented a data system that monitors ODRs, suspensions, and attendance data through SWIS (May et al., 2006). The school secretary enters the ODRs daily, and the school vice principal prints relevant graphs and brings them to monthly meetings at which the team reviews the data and creates action plans. All figures

represent typical output graphs from SWIS. To maximize the reliability of the data, the school administration holds a training at the start of each school year, with the following goals: (1) describing how the data are used, (2) emphasizing accuracy over reductions in incidents, and (3) providing a flowchart that indicates when to write ODRs and when to handle incidents without ODRs. In addition to the data described earlier, the team collects data documenting fidelity of implementation and perceptions of impact (from staff, students, and families).

At the monthly schoolwide behavior team meeting in November, the team reviewed data from the first 2 months of the school year and all of the previous year. The goals of the meeting were to answer the basic questions of schoolwide decision making and make the necessary changes to improve behavior support. The team would then report a summary of this information and selected graphs at the next faculty meeting.

The first goal of the team is to answer question 1 (*Is the current plan achieving intended outcomes?*). To address this question, the team has set three goals: an absolute goal of fewer 10 ODRs per day per month for each month (reviewed monthly), improvement compared with the previous year's data (reviewed monthly), and 80% of students with 0–1 ODRs (reviewed yearly). As seen in Figure 9.2, the rate of ODRs in September was below both the absolute goal and the previous year's level, but the rate in October both exceeded the absolute goal and equaled the previous year's rate. From the previous ODR year-end report, the team noted that only 60% of students had 0–1 ODRs the previous year. Given these data, the team determined that the current plan was not working as well as desired and that changes in the schoolwide plan could be made to support students more effectively.

The team then set out to determine what specific areas could be targeted to improve the school's current efforts (question 2: *What areas need improvement?*). The goal in answering this question was to analyze the nature of the problem and pinpoint what changes needed to be made. Figures 9.3 and 9.4 are graphs that show distributions of ODRs by type of problem behavior and location to date for the current school year. From these data, the team determined that

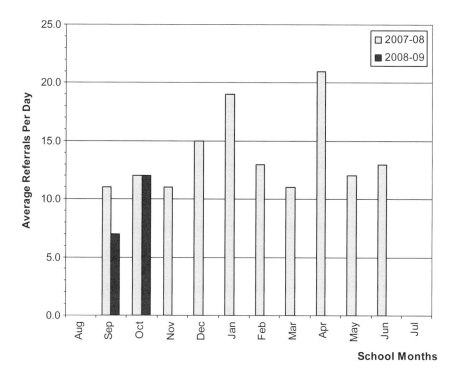

FIGURE 9.2. Average ODRs per day per month multiyear graph.

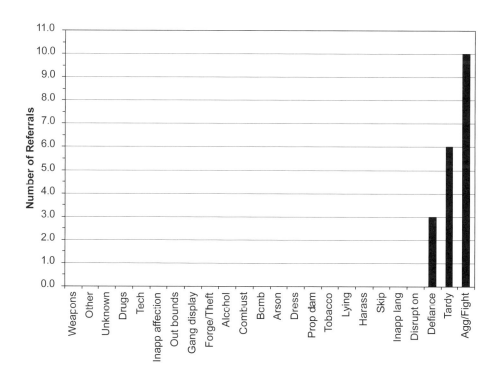

FIGURE 9.3. ODRs by type of problem behavior graph.

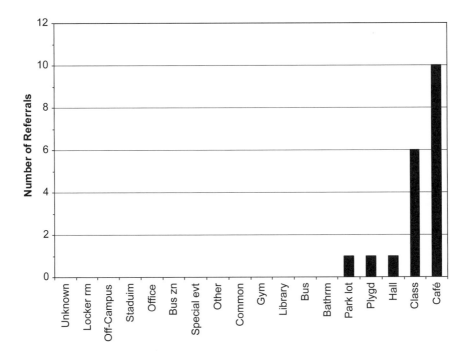

FIGURE 9.4. ODRs by location graph.

student fighting and tardies were problem behaviors that needed immediate intervention and that the cafeteria was of particular concern.

Though these data provide some indication of areas to target, the data system can provide more specific information to the team. Rather than addressing these problems with a broad plan, the team decided to drill down to explore further the potential causes of the school's challenges. During a 5-minute break, the vice principal produced the graphs in Figures 9.5–9.7 based on the existing data. Because the data indicated fighting as the highest frequency problem behavior, the vice principal produced a graph of locations where ODRs for fighting were issued, shown in Figure 9.5. As shown, the location with the highest frequency of fighting was the cafeteria. This graph allowed the team to target fighting in the cafeteria as a significant challenge for the school. The vice principal also generated a graph of ODRs by grade level in the cafeteria, shown in Figure 9.6, because the ODRs by time of day graph indicated that the grade 8 lunch period may be a cause of specific concern. This graph

confirmed that levels of ODRs for grades 6 and 7 were acceptable and that the grade 8 lunch period was a setting that clearly needed to be addressed. Figure 9.7, displaying tardies by time of day, caused some concern among the team about the start of the school day, but the majority of tardies came after the grade 8 lunch period. The team hypothesized that these tardies may have been due to the disruption caused by the fighting during lunch.

The team then used this specific information to create an action plan to address the specific problems identified. During the discussions, the team also noted the low level of ODRs in the hallways, in contrast to the previous year's graphs that showed hallways as the location with the most ODRs. This location had been targeted for improvement the preceding year, and team members noted the success of the intervention implemented (teachers reteaching expectations and supervising the halls from their doorways during passing period; Colvin, Sugai, Good, & Lee, 1997; Kartub, Taylor-Greene, March, & Horner, 2000). The team decided to build on this strength by implementing a similar

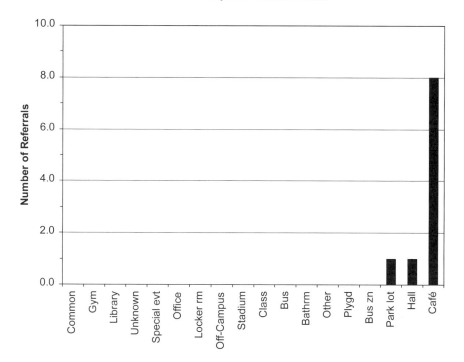

FIGURE 9.5. Custom graph: ODRs by location—fighting only.

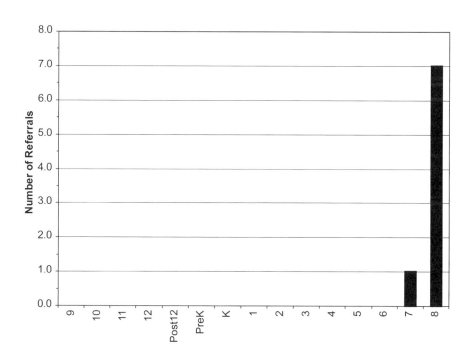

FIGURE 9.6. Custom graph: ODRs by grade level—cafeteria only.

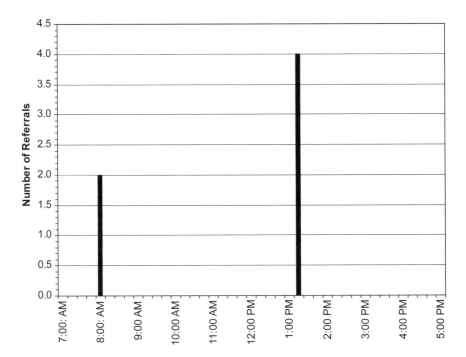

FIGURE 9.7. Custom graph: ODRs by time of day—tardies only.

plan for the cafeteria. Because only one grade level's lunch period was identified, the team could create a plan that was more efficient than targeting all grade levels. The team decided to (1) reteach the cafeteria expectations to the grade 8 students, (2) have the school counselor teach the grade 8 students conflict resolution skills (using typical cafeteria disputes as examples), (3) increase the level of active adult supervision during the grade 8 lunch period by reassigning aides, and (4) consider implementing a lunchtime recognition system to reinforce prosocial behavior if the cafeteria location still had the most ODRs in November. The team also decided that in place of intervention, they would monitor tardiness in November; they reasoned that tardies were likely to decrease if lunchtime fighting was reduced.

To identify students needing additional assessment and support (question 3), the team relied on both ODRs and teacher nominations for screening purposes. The team identified 41 students with moderate behavior needs (two to three ODRs or teacher referral) who might benefit from their current targeted intervention, a check-in–check-out daily feedback and mentoring intervention (Crone

et al., 2003). Five students already had five or more ODRs; the team referred these students to the school-based behavior support team for individual behavior support and used the existing ODR information to begin creating initial hypotheses about what was contributing to problem behaviors.

The data system created by the school team at Kennedy Middle School serves as the critical means by which the school assesses how well their schoolwide system is working, what support is needed, and who would benefit from additional support. Rather than relying solely on staff perceptions to determine effectiveness of support and what should be done, the team uses the data objectively to determine what changes are likely to produce the biggest improvements in student behavior at the school.

Conclusion: The Big Ideas

As seen in this chapter, school-based data decision making in the area of social behavior can greatly benefit from an examination of data through a structured problem-solving process. Though it may be tempting to adopt resource-intensive measurement systems or to implement programs without analyzing data, a careful approach that utilizes existing and suitable data to identify areas to target is the most likely avenue to effective and efficient behavior support. Even after measures are identified, a data system is not complete without a decision-making process that uses visual representations of data to drive decisions about schoolwide behavior support. Using data to provide proactive and preventive behavior support is a uniquely powerful way to create a safe teaching and learning environment, to foster the development of respect and compassion, and to encourage lifelong social and emotional competence.

Acknowledgment

We wish to extend our gratitude to Leslie MacKay for creating the figures in this chapter.

References

Alberto, P. A., & Troutman, A. C. (2003). *Applied behavior analysis for teachers* (6th ed.). Upper Saddle River, NJ: Merrill Prentice Hall.

Bergan, J. R., & Kratochwill, T. R. (1990). *Behavioral consultation and therapy*. New York: Springer.

Bradshaw, C. P., Koth, K., Bevans, K. B., Ialongo, N., & Leaf, P. J. (2008). The impact of school-wide positive behavioral interventions and supports on the organizational health of elementary schools. *School Psychology Quarterly, 23*, 462–473.

British Columbia Ministry of Education. (2001). *BC performance standards. Social responsibility: A framework*. Victoria, British Columbia, Canada: Author. Retrieved October 10, 2007 from *www.bced.gov.bc.ca/perf_stands/social_resp.htm*.

Campbell, A. L. (2008). *Stimulus fading within check-in check-out*. Unpublished doctoral dissertation, University of Oregon.

Carter, D. R., & Horner, R. H. (2007). Adding functional behavioral assessment to First Step to Success: A case study. *Journal of Positive Behavior Interventions, 9*, 229–238.

Cheney, D., Flower, A., & Templeton, T. (2008). Applying response to intervention metrics in the social domain for students at risk of developing emotional or behavioral disorders. *Journal of Special Education, 42*, 108–126.

Colvin, G., Sugai, G., Good, R. H., & Lee, Y.

(1997). Effect of active supervision and precorrection on transition behaviors of elementary students. *School Psychology Quarterly, 12*, 344–363.

Cordori, M. (1987). A computer-based recording system for analyzing disciplinary referrals. *NASSP Bulletin, 71*, 42–43.

Crone, D. A., Horner, R. H., & Hawken, L. S. (2003). *Responding to problem behavior in schools: The Behavior Education Program*. New York: Guilford Press.

Cushing, L. S., Horner, R. H., & Barrier, H. (2003). Validation and congruent validity of a direct observation tool to assess student social climate. *Journal of Positive Behavior Interventions, 5*, 225–237.

Davis, C. A. (2005). *Effects of in-service training on teachers' knowledge and practices regarding identifying and making a focus of concern students exhibiting internalizing problems*. Unpublished doctoral dissertation, University of Oregon.

Epstein, M. H., & Sharma, J. (1998). *Behavioral and Emotional Rating Scale: A strength-based approach to assessment*. Austin, TX: Pro-Ed.

Ervin, R. A., Schaughency, E., Goodman, S. D., McGlinchey, M. T., & Matthews, A. (2006). Merging research and practice agendas to address reading and behavior schoolwide. *School Psychology Review, 35*, 198–223.

Feil, E. G., Severson, H., & Walker, H. M. (1998). Screening for emotional and behavioral delays: The early screening project. *Journal of Early Intervention, 21*, 252–266.

Goodman, S. (2005, October). *Implementation of reading and behavior support at the state level*. Paper presented at the Positive Behavioral Interventions and Supports Forum, Chicago, IL.

Gresham, F. M., & Elliott, S. N. (1990). *Social skills rating system*. Circle Pines, MN: American Guidance Service.

Haring, N. G., Lovitt, T. C., Eaton, M. D., & Hansen, C. L. (1978). *The fourth R: Research in the classroom*. Columbus, OH: Merrill.

Hayes, S. C., Nelson, R. O., & Jarrett, R. B. (1987). The treatment utility of assessment: A functional approach to evaluating assessment quality. *American Psychologist, 42*(11), 963–974.

Horner, R. H., Sugai, G., & Todd, A. W. (2001). "Data" need not be a four-letter word: Using data to improve schoolwide discipline. *Beyond Behavior, 11*(1), 20–26.

Horner, R. H., Sugai, G., Todd, A. W., & Lewis-Palmer, T. (2005). Schoolwide positive behavior support. In L. Bambara & L. Kern (Eds.), *Individualized supports for students with problem behaviors: Designing positive behavior plans* (pp. 359–390). New York: Guilford Press.

Hosp, J. L., Howell, K. W., & Hosp, M. K. (2003). Characteristics of behavior rating scales: Implications for practice in assessment and behavioral support. *Journal of Positive Behavior Interventions, 5,* 201–208.

Irvin, L. K., Horner, R. H., Ingram, K., Todd, A. W., Sugai, G., Sampson, N. K., et al. (2006). Using office discipline referral data for decision making about student behavior in elementary and middle schools: An empirical evaluation of validity. *Journal of Positive Behavior Interventions, 8,* 10–23.

Irvin, L. K., Tobin, T. J., Sprague, J. R., Sugai, G., & Vincent, C. G. (2004). Validity of office discipline referral measures as indices of school-wide behavioral status and effects of school-wide behavioral interventions. *Journal of Positive Behavior Interventions, 6,* 131–147.

Kamphaus, R. W., & Reynolds, C. R. (2008). *Behavioral and Emotional Screening System.* Bloomington, MN: Pearson.

Kartub, D. T., Taylor-Greene, S., March, R. E., & Horner, R. H. (2000). Reducing hallway noise: A systems approach. *Journal of Positive Behavior Interventions, 2,* 179–182.

Kern, L., & Manz, P. (2004). A look at current validity issues of school-wide behavior support. *Behavioral Disorders, 30,* 47–59.

Lewis, T. J. (2007, July). *Functional assessment and positive behavior support plans.* Paper presented at the Office of Special Education Programs Forum, Washington, DC.

Lochman, J. (1995). Screening of child behavior problems for prevention programs at school entry. *Journal of Consulting and Clinical Psychology, 63,* 549–559.

March, R. E., & Horner, R. H. (2002). Feasibility and contributions of functional behavioral assessment in schools. *Journal of Emotional and Behavioral Disorders, 10,* 158–170.

Martens, B. K. (1993). Social labeling, precision of measurement, and problem solving: Key issues in the assessment of children's emotional problems. *School Psychology Review, 22,* 308–312.

May, S., Ard, W. I., Todd, A. W., Horner, R. H., Glasgow, A., Sugai, G., et al. (2006). *School-Wide Information System.* Eugene, OR: University of Oregon, Educational and Community Supports.

McIntosh, K., & Av-Gay, H. (2007). Implications of current research on the use of functional behavior assessment and behavior support planning in school systems. *International Journal of Behavior Consultation and Therapy, 3,* 38–52.

McIntosh, K., Campbell, A. L., Carter, D. R., & Dickey, C. R. (2009). Differential effects of a direct behavior rating intervention based on function of problem behavior. *Journal of Positive Behavior Interventions, 11,* 82–93.

McIntosh, K., Campbell, A. L., Carter, D. R., & Zumbo, B. D. (in press). Concurrent validity of office discipline referrals and cut points used in school-wide positive behavior support. *Behavioral Disorders.*

McIntosh, K., Chard, D. J., Boland, J. B., & Horner, R. H. (2006). Demonstration of combined efforts in school-wide academic and behavioral systems and incidence of reading and behavior challenges in early elementary grades. *Journal of Positive Behavior Interventions, 8,* 146–154.

McIntosh, K., Horner, R. H., Chard, D. J., Boland, J. B., & Good, R. H. (2006). The use of reading and behavior screening measures to predict non-response to school-wide positive behavior support: A longitudinal analysis. *School Psychology Review, 35,* 275–291.

McIntosh, K., Horner, R. H., Chard, D. J., Dickey, C. R., & Braun, D. H. (2008). Reading skills and function of problem behavior in typical school settings. *Journal of Special Education, 42,* 131–147.

McIntosh, K., Horner, R. H., & Sugai, G. (2009). Sustainability of systems-level evidence-based practices in schools: Current knowledge and future directions. In W. Sailor, G. Dunlap, G. Sugai, & R. H. Horner (Eds.), *Handbook of positive behavior support* (pp. 327–352). New York: Springer.

McNamara, K. (2002). Best practices in the promotion of social competence in the schools. In A. Thomas & J. P. Grimes (Eds.), *Best practices in school psychology* (4th ed., pp. 911–927). Bethesda, MD: National Association of School Psychologists.

Missouri School Counselor Association. (2007). *Standards for social–emotional competencies.* Warrensburg, MO: Missouri Center for Career Education. Retrieved October 14, 2007, from *missouricareereducation.org/curr/cmd/guidanceplacementG/GLE.html.*

Morrison, G. M., Anthony, S., Storino, M., & Dillon, C. (2001). An examination of the disciplinary histories and the individual and educational characteristics of students who participate in an in-school suspension program. *Education and Treatment of Children, 24,* 276–293.

National Association of School Psychologists. (2006). *School psychology: A blueprint for training and practice: III.* Bethesda, MD: Author.

Patterson, G. R., Reid, J. B., & Dishion, T. J. (1992). *Antisocial boys.* Eugene, OR: Castalia Press.

Reinke, W. M., & Lewis-Palmer, T. L. (2007). Improving classroom management. *Principal*

Magazine [Web-exclusive content], *86*(4). Retrieved August 8, 2008, from *www.naesp.org/principal.*

Reynolds, C. R., & Kamphaus, R. W. (2004). *Behavior Assessment Scale for Children* (2nd ed.). Circle Pines, MN: AGS.

Severson, H. H., & James, L. (2002). Prevention and early interventions for addictive behaviors: Health promotion in the schools. In M. R. Shinn, H. M. Walker, & G. Stoner (Eds.), *Interventions for academic and behavior problems: II. Preventive and remedial approaches* (pp. 681–701). Bethesda, MD: National Association of School Psychologists.

Severson, H. H., Walker, H. M., Hope-Doolittle, J., Kratochwill, T. R., & Gresham, F. M. (2007). Proactive, early screening to detect behaviorally at-risk students: Issues, approaches, emerging innovations, and professional practices. *Journal of School Psychology, 45,* 193–223.

Shinn, M. R., Walker, H. M., & Stoner, G. (Eds.). (2002). *Interventions for academic and behavior problems: II. Preventive and remedial approaches* (2nd ed.). Bethesda, MD: National Association of School Psychologists.

Skiba, R. J., Michael, R. S., Nardo, A. C., & Peterson, R. L. (2002). The color of discipline: Sources of racial and gender disproportionality in school punishment. *Urban Review, 34,* 317–342.

Skiba, R. J., Simmons, A. B., Ritter, S., Gibb, A. C., Rausch, M. K., Cuadrado, J., et al. (2008). Achieving equity in special education: History, status, and current challenges. *Exceptional Children, 74,* 264–288.

Smith, B. W. (2007, May). *School-Wide Observation (SW-OBS) System: A direct observation assessment of changes in student–teacher interaction patterns.* Paper presented at the International Association for Positive Behavior Support Conference, Boston, MA.

Sprague, J. R., & Walker, H. M. (2005). *Safe and healthy schools: Practical prevention strategies.* New York: Guilford Press.

Sprague, J. R., Walker, H. M., Stieber, S., Simonsen, B., Nishioka, V., & Wagner, L. (2001). Exploring the relationship between school discipline referrals and delinquency. *Psychology in the Schools, 38,* 197–206.

Sugai, G., & Horner, R. H. (2005). School-wide positive behavior supports: Achieving and sustaining effective learning environments for all students. In W. H. Heward (Ed.), *Focus on behavior analysis in education: Achievements, challenges, and opportunities* (pp. 90–102). Upper Saddle River, NJ: Pearson Prentice-Hall.

Sugai, G., Horner, R. H., Dunlap, G., Hieneman, M., Lewis, T. J., Nelson, C. M., et al. (2000). Applying positive behavior support and functional behavioral assessment in schools. *Journal of Positive Behavior Interventions, 2,* 131–143.

Sugai, G., Horner, R. H., & Gresham, F. M. (2002). Behaviorally effective school environments. In M. R. Shinn, H. M. Walker, & G. Stoner (Eds.), *Interventions for academic and behavior problems: Preventive and remedial approaches* (2nd ed., pp. 315–350). Bethesda, MD: National Association of School Psychologists.

Sugai, G., Lewis-Palmer, T. L., Todd, A. W., & Horner, R. H. (2001). *School-wide Evaluation Tool (SET).* Eugene, OR: University of Oregon, Educational and Community Supports. Retrieved August 8, 2008, from *www.pbis.org.*

Sugai, G., Sprague, J. R., Horner, R. H., & Walker, H. M. (2000). Preventing school violence: The use of office discipline referrals to assess and monitor school-wide discipline interventions. *Journal of Emotional and Behavioral Disorders, 8,* 94–101.

Tilly, W. D. (2008). The evolution of school psychology to science-based practice: Problem-solving and the three-tiered model. In A. Thomas & J. P. Grimes (Eds.), *Best practices in school psychology* (5th ed., pp. 17–36). Bethesda, MD: National Association of School Psychologists.

Tobin, T. J., Sugai, G., & Colvin, G. (2000). Using disciplinary referrals to make decisions. *NASSP Bulletin, 84,* 106–117.

Tobin, T. J., & Sugai, G. M. (1999). Using sixth-grade school records to predict school violence, chronic discipline problems, and high school outcomes. *Journal of Emotional and Behavioral Disorders, 7,* 40–53.

Todd, A. W., & Horner, R. H. (2006). *SWIS documentation project: Referral form examples.* Eugene, OR: University of Oregon, Educational and Community Supports.

Todd, A. W., Sampson, N. K., & Horner, R. H. (2005). Data-based decision making using office discipline referral data from the School-Wide Information System (SWIS). *Association for Positive Behavior Support Newsletter, 2*(2), 3.

Vaughn, S., Linan-Thompson, S., & Hickman, P. (2003). Response to instruction as a means of identifying students with reading/learning disabilities. *Exceptional Children, 69,* 391–409.

Walker, B., Cheney, D., Stage, S. A., & Blum, C. (2005). Schoolwide screening and positive behavior supports: Identifying and supporting students at risk for school failure. *Journal of Positive Behavior Interventions, 7,* 194–204.

Walker, H. M. (2004). Commentary: Use of evidence-based intervention in schools: Where we've been, where we are, and where we need to go. *School Psychology Review, 33,* 398–407.

Walker, H. M., Horner, R. H., Sugai, G., Bullis, M., Sprague, J. R., Bricker, D., et al. (1996). Integrated approaches to preventing antisocial behavior patterns among school-age children and youth. *Journal of Emotional and Behavioral Disorders, 4,* 194–209.

Walker, H. M., & McConnell, S. R. (1995). *The Walker–McConnell Scale of Social Competence and School Adjustment.* San Diego, CA: Singular.

Walker, H. M., Ramsey, E., & Gresham, F. M. (2005). *Antisocial behavior in school: Strategies and best practices* (2nd ed.). Pacific Grove, CA: Brooks/Cole.

Walker, H. M., & Severson, H. (1992). *Systematic screening for behavior disorders* (2nd ed.). Longmont, CO: Sopris West.

Walker, H. M., & Severson, H. (1994). Replication of the systematic screening for behavior disorders (SSBD) procedure for the identification of at-risk children. *Journal of Emotional and Behavioral Disorders, 2,* 66–78.

Walker, H. M., Severson, H., Stiller, B., Williams, N., Shinn, M., & Todis, B. (1988). Systematic screening of pupils in the elementary age range at risk for behavioral disorders: Development and trial testing of a multiple gating model. *Remedial and Special Education, 9*(3), 8–14.

Walker, H. M., Severson, H., Todis, B., Block-Pedego, A., Williams, G., Haring, N., et al. (1990). Systematic screening for behavior disorders (SSBD): Further validation, replication, and normative data. *Remedial and Special Education, 11,* 32–46.

Walker, H. M., & Sprague, J. R. (1999). The path to school failure, delinquency and violence: Causal factors and some potential solutions. *Intervention in School and Clinic, 35,* 67–73.

Wright, J. A., & Dusek, J. B. (1998). Compiling school base-rates for disruptive behavior from student disciplinary referral data. *School Psychology Review, 27,* 138–147.

Chapter 10

Assessing Disruptive Behavior within a Problem-Solving Model

Brian K. Martens
Scott P. Ardoin

As discussed by Ervin, Gimpel Peacock, and Merrell in Chapter 1, this volume, a major paradigm shift is occurring with respect to the delivery of psychological services in the schools (e.g., Reschly, 2004). Historically, these services were dominated by the refer–test–place (RTP) model in which children were identified as needing additional services by their regular education teacher (*refer*), evaluated for eligibility by a multidisciplinary team of support personnel (*test*), and provided services by a special education teacher (*place*). Each person was responsible for a different aspect of the child's case, and this allowed school professionals to go about their business of assessment and treatment independently of each other and of the context in which problem behavior initially occurred (Christenson & Ysseldyke, 1989; Erchul & Martens, 2002). Because individuals conducting the assessments were rarely involved in treatment and because treatment rarely occurred in the regular education setting, this model also encouraged a child-centered assessment focus. That is, school psychologists and other assessment personnel spent the majority of their time describing children's traits and dispositions as important correlates of classroom behavior independent of the classroom ecology itself.

This focus, in turn, did little to inform special education programming (i.e., the treatment phase of the RTP model), which proceeded largely in isolation and without the benefit of systematic outcome evaluation.

The problem-solving model of behavioral consultation has emerged as a viable alternative to the RTP sequence, shifting a good deal of the responsibility for school-based intervention from special to regular education. This shift has necessitated a much closer coordination of activities among school professionals, who must now work together to design, implement, and evaluate treatment programs in regular classroom settings. Regardless of the treatment context (e.g., prereferral intervention, response to intervention, or positive behavioral support models), many of these programs are implemented by regular classroom teachers and involve significant changes in their instructional, managerial, and evaluation activities (Martens & DiGennaro, 2008). In order to inform these changes and to evaluate treatment effectiveness, the problem-solving model involves assessment goals and strategies that are very different from those used in the traditional RTP model.

Within the RTP model, tests are administered primarily for the purpose of assessing the amount of a psychological attribute, trait, or construct a student possesses relative to a normative sample (nomothetic assessment). Tests used for this purpose are typically composed of items measuring a broad array of behavioral indicators. Because these tests measure global indicators of student performance and because the obtained scores are compared with national samples, assessment results generally fail to identify specific behaviors that should be targeted through intervention. That is, although standardized measures can suggest general areas for remediation, they provide little information regarding *why* a student is choosing to engage in specific behaviors and/or *what* skills a student does and does not possess. Another limitation of measures that are core to the RTP model is that they are generally insensitive to short-term changes in student behavior, as they are intended to measure stable internal dispositions (Fletcher et al., 1998; Hayes, Nelson, & Jarrett, 1986; Marston, Mirkin, & Deno, 1984).

Within a problem-solving model, decisions are based on data that are compared with a student's past behavior, as well as the behavior of his or her peers. Comparing students' behavior with that of their peers, as opposed to a national standardization sample, can provide information about the extent to which the local environment supports appropriate behavior for all children (e.g., Ardoin, Witt, Connell, & Koenig, 2005). Measures used within a problem-solving model focus on specific behaviors or skills that are targeted for change as a function of intervention. In response to intervention (RTI) applications, data regarding the level and rate of behavior change also become the primary source of information used to determine a student's eligibility for special education (Ardoin & Christ, 2008; Speece, Case, & Molloy, 2003; Vaughn & Fuchs, 2003).

A basic premise of this chapter is that research in the areas of behavioral assessment and applied behavior analysis provides a strong foundation for application of the problem-solving model to students' inappropriate classroom behavior. Research in these areas has long recognized the necessity of evaluating the context in which behavior occurs when determining students' intervention needs. Furthermore, behavioral assessment

methods have been developed for assessing both nomothetic (i.e., relative to others) and idiographic (i.e., relative to oneself over time) changes in children's behavior, two features that are essential for measures being used to evaluate intervention effectiveness.

In order to evaluate a student's problem behavior and to develop an effective intervention plan, quality assessment measures must be employed. The quality of behavioral assessment measures, however, cannot be adequately judged by traditional indices of reliability and validity because these measures are based on a different set of assumptions than are psychological measures (Hayes et al., 1986). We begin the chapter by discussing the assumptions that underlie the development, use, and interpretation of behavioral assessment measures. Based on this set of assumptions, we identify common reasons why children engage in disruptive classroom behaviors that can be viewed as targets of the behavioral assessment process. We then describe three criteria by which the quality of behavioral assessment data should be evaluated, namely, their accuracy, sensitivity, and treatment utility (Hayes et al., 1986). Measurement strategies and approaches to data interpretation that meet these criteria in the assessment of disruptive behavior are discussed in each section.

Assumptions of Behavioral Assessment

Presented in Table 10.1 is a list of the four major assumptions of behavioral assessment. These assumptions are discussed in the following section and contrasted with

TABLE 10.1. Assumptions of Behavioral Assessment

1. Behavior is situation specific and will vary depending on the conditions surrounding its occurrence.

2. Behavior is an important focus of assessment in its own right, not just as an indicator of some underlying disorder.

3. Situational determinants of behavior can be understood only by collecting repeated measures of the same individual over time.

4. Conditions surrounding behavior as antecedents and consequences can be altered to produce desired changes in behavior.

the corresponding position taken by traditional approaches to assessing psychological aptitudes and traits (hereafter referred to as psychological assessment).

Situational Specificity and the Sign–Sample Distinction

All assessment strategies are limited by the inability to measure every possible behavior from the population of behaviors under consideration. Rather, measures are designed to sample a subset of behaviors that are believed to be important indicators or to be representative of a particular domain (e.g., impulsivity, depression, aggression). How these samples of behavior are obtained and interpreted, however, represents an important difference between psychological assessment and behavioral assessment. As described by Goldfried and Kent (1972), psychological assessment is concerned primarily with measuring children's underlying personality characteristics or traits as a means of predicting behavior. As such, psychological measures tend to be removed in time and place from the behavior of actual concern (e.g., self-report inventories) and to focus on characteristics believed to be internal to the child, and they are designed to detect differences between children rather than within children over time or across situations (Goldfried & Kent, 1972; Gresham & Carey, 1988). For example, a child's score on a self-report inventory of anxiety is expected to be similar regardless of who administers the test, on what day, or in what setting. Test scores should also be similar regardless of which particular items are administered, as long as the item sets are theoretically related to the personality trait of interest. In fact, this expectation underlies all parallel-forms approaches to estimating test reliability. From the perspective of psychological assessment, responses to test items are viewed as "signs" of the child's aptitude or trait, the latter of which is viewed as more important, more stable, and more predictive than the sample of behaviors on which it was based (Goldfried & Kent, 1972). Moreover, these "signs" can be collected at any point in time or in any setting to reveal the child's true score.

In contrast, the first major assumption of behavioral assessment is that children's be-havior is situation specific and therefore likely to vary as a function of who is present, the setting or activity in which behavior is measured, and even the method of measurement itself (Campbell & Fiske, 1959; Chafouleas, Christ, Riley-Tillman, Briesch, & Chanese, 2007; Epkins & Meyers, 1994; Kazdin, 1979). Given the expectation that behavior will be variable across situations, responses to test items are viewed as "samples" of behavior that must be obtained under different conditions (Goldfried & Kent, 1972). Unlike psychological assessment, measuring behavior at a single point in time or in one setting (i.e., collecting only one sample) is viewed as unlikely to yield a representative score. Rather, in behavioral assessment, samples of behavior are collected in all situations of primary concern to caregivers (e.g., classroom, lunchroom, playground). Once collected, these divergent samples can be averaged to produce a global indicator of the child's functioning, or true score (Gresham & Carey, 1988). A more common strategy in behavioral assessment, however, is to examine the extent to which behavior differs across settings and over time (Cone, 1977). Examining these differences can lead to hypotheses about what situational variables might be contributing to problem behavior, thereby suggesting potential intervention alternatives.

Direct Measurement and Intrasubject Variability

As the name suggests, behavioral assessment strategies are concerned with measuring children's actual behavior. That is, a second major assumption of behavioral assessment is that problem behaviors such as noncompliance, aggression, or self-injury are an important focus of assessment in their own right, not just indicators of some underlying disorder (Nelson & Hayes, 1979). Being concerned with measuring the occurrence of behavior, behavioral assessment strategies tend to be more direct than their psychological counterparts. Cone (1977) suggested that psychological measures can be ordered along a continuum of directness to the extent that they measure the actual behavior of clinical or educational relevance at the actual time and place of its occurrence. Systematic observation and self-monitoring of behavior in the natural environment anchor the direct end of the continuum. Self- or informant reports of behavior represent more indirect methods, as they are removed in both time and place from the behavior's original occurrence. In contrast, interviews, reviews of records, standardized measures, and projective tests fall at the indirect end of the continuum. It is not surprising, then, that direct, systematic observation is the *sine qua non* of behavioral assessment (Hintze, 2005; Martens, DiGennaro, Reed, Szczech, & Rosenthal, 2008).

As measures fall closer to the indirect end of the continuum, it becomes less meaningful to administer them repeatedly in order to obtain multiple samples of behavior (i.e., different scores). In fact, many standardized measures are designed to yield similar scores across repeated administrations, thereby demonstrating high levels of test–retest reliability (Crocker & Algina, 1986). More direct behavioral assessment measures, however, were designed to be administered repeatedly. For example, observational coding systems can be used to measure a child's engaged time and off-task behavior on consecutive days, in different content areas (e.g., math and reading), or with different teachers. Similarly, reading fluency can be assessed using curriculum-based measurement methods several times a week or following different instructional interventions to evaluate reading progress (Ardoin et al., 2004). Repeated measurement of the same child over time is related to the third major assumption of behavioral assessment, namely, that situational determinants of behavior can be understood only by comparing children with themselves rather than with each other (Hayes et al., 1986).

With most psychological measures, data are collected on a child at one point in time, and this score is compared with the standardization sample (i.e., a focus on *inter*subject variability). Although these data allow the child to be scaled high or low relative to others of the same age or grade level, they reveal nothing about potential changes in that child's behavior over time or across settings. Only by collecting repeated measures on the same child can one evaluate absolute changes in behavior in terms of level, trend, and variability over time (Johnston & Pennypacker, 1980). Perhaps more important,

variability in a child's behavior over time (i.e., *intra*subject variability) can be correlated with events surrounding its occurrence to suggest potential variables that may be controlling the occurrence or nonoccurrence of problem behavior.

Emphasis on Functional versus Structural Relations

As noted, psychological measures are used to scale children as high or low with respect to an aptitude or trait in relation to their same-age or grade-level peers. When a battery of tests is administered, a child may be scaled in a variety of domains, revealing a complex picture of that child's relative strengths and weaknesses. In so doing, psychological assessment attempts to understand why children engage in problem behavior by focusing on other, related dimensions of their psychological profiles or structures of characteristics (i.e., structural relations). Thus a child who engages in severe aggressive behavior may score significantly higher than his or her peers on measures of depression and anxiety, suggesting that these characteristics may be potentially causing his or her problem behavior when, in fact, they are merely describing the problem in global terms.

Rather than viewing problem behavior as the result of other child characteristics, a fourth major assumption of behavioral assessment is that problem behavior is related to events surrounding its occurrence (Nelson & Hayes, 1979). In our experience as researchers and clinicians, children's problem behavior does not occur constantly and is rarely unpredictable. Rather, changes in behavior are often correlated with one or more events surrounding their occurrence, thereby evidencing a pattern. Broadly speaking, events surrounding the occurrence of problem behavior can be categorized as antecedents or consequences. Antecedents refer to general conditions that exist prior to the occurrence of behavior, such as time of day, difficulty of assigned work, or instructional arrangement, as well as specific events that immediately precede behavior, such as the issuing of commands, withdrawal of teacher attention, or comments from a peer. Consequences refer to events that follow behavior either in the form of responses from teachers or peers (e.g., reprimands, laughter) or as a direct result of engaging in the behavior (e.g., stimulation, reduced anxiety).

Relating variability in behavior to events surrounding its occurrence can reveal an equally complex picture of behavior–environment relations. Thus one goal of behavioral assessment in a problem-solving model is to understand why children engage in problem behavior by focusing on its immediate antecedents and consequences. Mapping these antecedent–behavior–consequence (ABC) relations is termed a *functional behavior assessment* (FBA; Witt, Daly, & Noell, 2000). (The reader is referred to Jones and Wickstrom, Chapter 12, this volume, for a detailed discussion of FBA procedures and how the resulting data can be used to inform the design of school-based interventions.) FBA requires a different set of strategies from those used in psychological assessment because the latter focuses exclusively on the child. Moreover, because the conditions surrounding each child's behavior are unique, assessment strategies useful in conducting an FBA must be flexible enough to capture these differences but structured enough to produce reliable data. For these reasons, a comprehensive FBA is a multistage process that includes interviews with direct-care providers, structured informant reports, systematic observation of problem behavior under different antecedent conditions, and sequential recording of behavior and its consequences in the natural environment (Drasgow & Yell, 2001; Martens & DiGennaro, 2008; Martens et al., 2008; Sterling-Turner, Robinson, & Wilczynski, 2001).

If done correctly, an FBA can reveal patterns in antecedents or consequences that are associated with the occurrence or nonoccurrence of problem behavior. For example, an FBA may reveal that a child's aggressive behavior occurs at high rates during reading instruction in general and following the assignment of cooperative seat work in particular but at low rates during lunch. When aggressive behavior does occur during reading, the child is immediately sent out of the room to the office, allowing escape from work and negatively reinforcing inappropriate behavior.

A second goal of behavioral assessment is concerned with how to interpret patterns in ABC data such as these. Specifically, which of the observed antecedents and consequences are "functionally related" to problem behavior and how? The term *functionally related* has a specific meaning in this context and refers to events in the environment that, when changed or manipulated, will produce changes in children's behavior (i.e., behavior is a function of these events). Functional relations refer to important, controllable, and causal influences on student learning in the sense that manipulating these variables is sufficient to change behavior (Christenson & Ysseldyke, 1989; Erchul & Martens, 2002; Johnston & Pennypacker, 1980). Developing hypotheses about potential functional variables requires a theoretical framework for translating observed patterns in ABC data. Because it is concerned with the stimulus functions of behavioral antecedents and consequences, applied behavior analysis is the model most commonly used to interpret FBA data (e.g., Daly, Martens, Skinner, & Noell, 2009; Martens & Eckert, 2000).

Common Reasons for Classroom Behavior Problems

Children engage in aberrant or inappropriate behavior for a variety of reasons, including organic disorders, physical illnesses, skill deficits, poor academic instruction, and even the unwitting reinforcement of problem behavior by direct-care providers (Christenson & Ysseldyke, 1989; Sturmey, 1995; Witt, VanDerHeyden, & Gilbertson, 2004). The latter two categories are particularly relevant to the assessment and treatment of disruptive classroom behavior because they represent functional variables over which teachers and consulting school psychologists have control (Daly, Witt, Martens, & Dool, 1997). As such, these categories also represent important assessment targets for designing effective school-based interventions in a problem-solving model.

Inadequate Classroom Instruction

A considerable amount of research has shown that many classroom behavior problems are related to inadequate instructional and managerial practices by teachers (Witt et al., 2004). Key among these practices are (1) poorly matched curriculum materials, (2) failure to alter instruction to suit students' proficiency levels, and (3) an absence of classroom rules and routines. Instructional match refers to a correspondence between the difficulty level of assigned material and students' ability (e.g., Martens & Witt, 2004). Research has shown that students engage in higher levels of problem behavior and lower levels of on-task behavior when they are assigned difficult or frustrational-level tasks (Gickling & Armstrong, 1978; Weeks & Gaylord-Ross, 1981). At the same time, students also show lower levels of engagement when tasks are too easy or at their independent level. One reason for these findings is that overly difficult or easy tasks (i.e., those with a poor instructional match) contain aversive properties that children attempt to escape by engaging in problem behavior (Weeks & Gaylord-Ross, 1981). When teachers allow escape by terminating the task, sending the child out of the class-room, or switching to an easier task, the problem behavior is negatively reinforced. In contrast, when difficult tasks are introduced gradually, when students are given enough assistance to complete difficult tasks with few or no errors, or when easy items are interspersed with difficult items, engagement increases (e.g., Gickling & Armstrong, 1978; McCurdy, Skinner, Grantham, Watson, & Hindman, 2001).

Effective teaching is also a dynamic process that requires teachers to closely monitor student performance and then to tailor their instructional practices to the student's changing proficiency level (Fuchs & Fuchs, 1986; Martens & Eckert, 2007). Similar to the consequences of poor instructional match, failing to adjust instruction to meet a student's changing needs can also make learning aversive. According to the instructional hierarchy (IH; Ardoin & Daly, 2007; Daly et al., 1997; Haring, Lovitt, Eaton, & Hansen, 1978), children progress through a series of stages when learning academic skills, with each stage corresponding to a different proficiency level. During acquisition, children are learning to perform a new skill accurately with few or no errors, and therefore they require assistance in the form of modeling, prompting, and error correction. When children can perform a skill accurately

over repeated occasions, the focus of learning shifts to fluency building. Fluency refers to a combination of accuracy and speed that characterizes competent performance in the natural environment (Binder, 1996). Building fluency requires practice of the skill beyond an accuracy criterion, or what has been termed *overlearning* (Driskell, Willis, & Copper, 1992). With continued practice, skill performance becomes increasingly efficient and enters the maintenance stage. During maintenance, continued progress toward mastery requires practice under more demanding conditions. Once maintenance is achieved, children must learn to perform the skill fluently under conditions that differ from those of training, or what is termed *generalization*. Generalization rarely occurs spontaneously but must be programmed by arranging practice opportunities under varying conditions and with diverse materials (Ardoin, McCall, & Klubnik, 2007). Finally, in order to truly master a skill, the learner must be able to modify the skill to solve complex problems.

From the perspective of the IH, continuing to model and prompt the performance of a skill that a child can already perform fluently may slow progress and lead to disruptive or off-task behavior. Conversely, assigning complex application problems (a generalization-level activity) when a child is still at the acquisition stage may lead to frustration and escape-motivated problem behavior.

Finally, research on effective teaching has shown that well-run and -managed classrooms can serve a proactive function by preventing many behavior problems before they occur (Gettinger, 1988). Teachers in well-run classrooms have an explicit set of rules for desired student behavior, communicate these rules to students via public posting and class discussions, and provide consistent consequences for compliance with these rules (Witt et al., 2004). Similarly, behavior problems often occur when students are unclear about what is expected of them and/or are not held accountable for their academic performance. Effective teachers have clearly defined procedures for housekeeping routines such as procuring needed materials or transitioning from one activity to another, and they require students to practice these procedures at the beginning of the year (e.g., Emmer, Evertson, & Anderson, 1980).

Reinforcement of Problem Behavior by Direct-Care Providers

Although problem behavior may initially result from a variety of causes, as noted earlier, it may persist or even be strengthened by social reinforcement from direct-care providers (e.g., Carr, Newsom, & Binkoff, 1976). Put another way, children learn what to say and do based on the consequences of their actions, and many problem behaviors are learned (i.e., instrumental) in the settings in which they occur (Martens & Witt, 2004).

Although the specific reinforcer that maintains problem behavior is often unique for each child (e.g., a "talking to" by the teacher, being sent to the office), they can be classified into the three broad categories of social positive reinforcement, social negative reinforcement, and automatic reinforcement (Iwata, Vollmer, & Zarcone, 1990). Social positive reinforcement includes any consequences given by another person in the child's environment (i.e., socially mediated) that provide the child with desired attention, tangible items, or activities contingent on problem behavior. Social negative reinforcement includes any consequences delivered by another person that allow the child to escape or avoid undesired situations, such as difficult or boring tasks, contingent on problem behavior. The key to negatively reinforcing consequences is that they allow the child to escape something aversive, thereby increasing occurrences of the problem behavior that led to such escape. Finally, automatic reinforcement refers to consequences that are not socially mediated but that occur as a direct result of engaging in the behavior. Examples of automatic reinforcement include the self-stimulatory consequences of repetitive body motions or the relieving consequences of self-directed actions such as scratching when one has a rash.

How prevalent are these various categories of reinforcement in maintaining problem behavior in children? Hanley, Iwata, and McCord (2003) identified 277 published articles reporting functional analyses of behavior through the year 2000. A functional analysis is an assessment procedure that involves the experimental manipulation of reinforcers for problem behavior. Specifically, a child is exposed to a series of brief (e.g., 5- or 10-minute) test and control conditions

designed to mimic reinforcement for problem behavior in the natural environment. In each test condition, a different category of reinforcement is delivered contingent on occurrences of problem behavior. Problem behavior is expected to increase under the test condition that contains the type of reinforcement the child has come to expect and/or prefers in the natural environment (Iwata, Dorsey, Slifer, Bauman, & Richman, 1982/1994).

Of the functional analysis articles reviewed by Hanley et al. (2003), 70% involved children and approximately one-third were conducted in school settings. Of the 536 different individual datasets reported across the studies, over 95% found differentiated results or a clear increase in problem behavior during one of the test conditions evaluated. In terms of the prevalence of reinforcer categories, 35.4% of behaviors were maintained by social positive reinforcement in the form of attention or delivery of tangible items, 34.2% of problem behaviors were maintained by social negative reinforcement in the form of escape from task demands, and 15.8% were maintained by automatic reinforcement. These results suggest that in approximately 70% of the cases, significant adults or peers in the individual's environment were reinforcing the occurrence of problem behavior. In such instances, the quality of behavioral assessment is judged by the extent to which the data collected help to identify what modifications must be made so reinforcement for problem behavior is eliminated, reversed, or weakened (Martens, Witt, Daly, & Vollmer, 1999).

Assessment Strategies for Problem Behavior

Accuracy

Key to the development of an effective intervention is addressing the question of what behaviors should be targeted through intervention. The answer to this question may seem obvious, as one might expect that the target and goal of intervention should be to eliminate the undesirable behavior for which a referral was made. However, designing an intervention that simply targets the elimination of an undesirable behavior can lead to a greater reliance on punishment and the potential worsening of student behavior

(Vollmer & Northup, 1996). Effective interventions ensure that a student has the necessary skills to engage in appropriate behavior and that more reinforcement is available for appropriate than for inappropriate behavior, thereby increasing the likelihood of its occurrence (Billington & DiTommaso, 2003).

To increase the probability of accurately identifying intervention targets, assessments must be conducted to identify events in the classroom environment that are promoting and maintaining inappropriate student behavior and the reasons that appropriate behavior is not occurring at higher rates. The behavior of individual students varies over time and across settings, as do the antecedents and consequences of student behavior. This variability requires the collection of data from multiple settings and sources, thus increasing the complexity and time demands of conducting quality behavioral assessments. However, identifying variability in student behavior and its relationship to systematic variability in the antecedents and consequences of such behavior increases the probability of intervention success (Cone, 1977). To identify these systematic relationships, quality behavioral assessments involve the collection of both indirect and direct assessment data through teacher interviews, behavioral rating scales, evaluation of student records, and direct observations of the behavior of teachers, peers, and, of course, the target student (Martens et al., 1999).

A first step in accurately identifying the target of intervention is to conduct a problem identification interview with the referring teacher(s). The goals of this interview are to (1) gain a clear understanding of the teacher's concerns and prioritize these concerns; (2) operationally define a target problem behavior; (3) obtain estimates of the frequency, intensity, and duration of the problem behavior; (4) develop tentative goals for change; and (5) identify potential antecedents, sequences, and consequences of the problem behavior (Erchul & Martens, 2002). Table 10.2 provides a list of questions that might be beneficial in addressing the aforementioned interviewing objectives. The information collected through this interview is important in hypothesis and intervention development regardless of its accuracy, as it provides the teacher's perception of his or her own behavior, the behavior of the referred student, and the behavior of the student's peers. Understanding the teacher's perception is also important when considering the level of resources that will need to be provided to the teacher in implementing an intervention.

Unfortunately, humans' perceptions and attributions are not always accurate, and thus the data collected through teacher interviews, although not intentionally misleading, may not be an accurate representation of the severity of the behavior or its antecedents and consequences (Macmann & Barnett, 1999; Meehl, 1986; Nisbett & Ross, 1980). It is therefore necessary that additional sources of data be collected. Teachers should be asked to assist in this data collection, as they are the individuals most likely to be interacting with the child when problem behavior occurs. It is, however, essential that procedures be developed that allow the teacher to collect objective data using the operational definitions specified during the problem identification interview. Having teachers collect data is especially important when problem behavior does not occur at a high rate (i.e., less than five incidents per hour). With low-frequency behaviors, it is unlikely that direct classroom observations conducted by a school psychologist will yield a sufficient number of samples to allow for the development of hypotheses regarding the function of behavior and thus the accurate selection of intervention targets.

Another valuable indirect method of collecting data is to administer behavior rating scales such as the Behavior Assessment System for Children—Second Edition (Reynolds & Kamphaus, 2004) or the Child Behavior Checklist (Achenbach & Rescorla, 2001) to individuals who interact with the child across various settings. Such scales generally require raters to estimate the frequency and intensity of behaviors across a specified period of time (e.g., 1 week; 3 months). Each of the questions posed is intended to provide an estimation of the degree to which the student rated engages in one of a constellation of undesirable (e.g., anxiety, attention problems, conduct problems, learning problems) or desirable (social skills, leadership) behaviors measured by the scale. This information can be useful for making clinical diagnoses, as well as providing indirect information that can lead to the accurate identification of be-

TABLE 10.2. Useful Questions to Pose as Part of a Problem Identification Interview

Goal A: Gain a clear understanding of the teacher's concerns and prioritize these concerns.

1. What behaviors is the student engaging in that cause you concern?
2. Can you rank-order these behaviors as those that interfere most to least with the child's learning and/ or the learning of the child's peers? Are there any behaviors that you believe might result in the child hurting himself or others?
3. Are any of these behaviors related, so that addressing one behavioral concern might eliminate one of the other behavioral concerns?

Goal B: Operationally define behaviors.

1. Can you describe the top two or three behaviors in such a way that a substitute teacher would be able to tell you whether or not the behavior occurred?
2. Do you have any classroom rules that might interfere with the substitutes' understanding of whether the student is engaging in this behavior? For instance, if we record out-of-seat behavior, do you let students stand next to their desks while working, or must they stay in their seats?
3. Do you think that it would be easiest to record the behavior in terms of the number of times that the behavior occurs within an hour or a day, the amount of time that it occurs within an hour or a day, or the level of intensity at which the behavior occurs?
4. If we use this measure of recording, will we lose any information? For instance, if the number of times the child is out of his or her seat is recorded, we might record only that he or she leaves the seat, even if he or she is out of the seat for 10 minutes.

Goal C: Obtain estimates of the frequency, intensity, and duration of problem behavior.

1. If we were to estimate how often each behavior occurs, would it be best to talk about their frequency within the period of an hour, a day, or a week?
2. During the last hour, day, or week, how many times did the student engage in the behavior? How long did each behavior last? To what level of intensity did the student engage in the behavior?
3. Is this frequency, duration, or intensity representative of the child's typical behavior? If not, can you give estimates of the child's typical behavior?

Goal D: Develop tentative goals for change.

1. How often do you believe other students engage in these behaviors? What levels of frequency, duration, and intensity do you think would be acceptable in your classroom?
2. Realizing that it is unlikely that we can completely eliminate these behaviors, what might a good short-term goal be?
3. Instead of focusing entirely on these inappropriate behaviors, it would be great if we could pay greater attention to what the child might do instead in order to access what he or she is trying to get. What might some of these behaviors be? How often are they currently occurring?

Goal E: Identify potential antecedents, sequences, and consequences of problem behavior.

1. Is there any time of the day when you believe the behavior is more likely to occur?
2. Is there any specific event (e.g., assignment, directions, removal of toy, being reprimanded) that typically precedes the occurrence of each behavior?
3. Are there certain events that you feel certain would result in the child's engaging in the behavior?
4. Are there any behaviors that the student engages in that provides you with a sign that other problematic behaviors might occur if nothing is done to prevent them from occurring?
5. When the child engages in each behavior, how do the children around the child respond?
6. When the child engages in each behavior, how do you respond?
7. When the child engages in each behavior, how do the adults around the child respond?
8. Are you currently doing anything systematically to try to reduce the occurrence of the behavior?
9. Have you in the past tried any interventions that you found to be effective or ineffective? For how long did you use this intervention, and why did you decide not to use it anymore?

Note. Adapted from Erchul and Martens (2002). Adapted with permission from William P. Erchul.

haviors to be targeted through intervention. For instance, similarity of findings across raters and settings suggests that problem behavior is pervasive and is potentially a deficit of the child that will require skill training (e.g., social skills, self-monitoring). On the other hand, differences in scores across raters and settings suggest that either (1) the raters differ in their perceptions of the child's behavior or (2) the child's behavior differs across settings potentially as a function of differences in the antecedents and consequences for appropriate and inappropriate behavior between settings. Differences in ratings necessitates that direct observations be conducted across settings in an attempt to identify the source(s) of the differences. The accurate identification of behaviors to target through intervention is largely dependent on the accurate identification of these source(s) of variability.

Another means by which valuable indirect assessment data can be collected is through a review of the student's school records (e.g., grades, office referrals, details of previous attempted interventions). Analysis of these records might highlight a pattern in the events that precede problem behavior and/or might assist in identifying a specific life event that resulted in the appearance of problem behavior (Irvin et al., 2006; Radford & Ervin, 2002).

Shared patterns among indirect assessment methods can assist in streamlining subsequent direct observations. For instance, if the pattern across indirect assessment data indicates that behavior is worse in one setting than in others, direct assessments should be conducted with a focus on how the identified setting differs from other settings. Inconsistency in the patterns across indirect assessment methods may suggest sources of inaccurate data, requiring a more comprehensive direct assessment.

Similar to collection of indirect assessment data, direct assessment data should be collected across multiple settings using multiple methods. The probability of identifying the appropriate target of intervention is increased by conducting direct assessments of the environment (e.g., quality of instruction) in which the target student is engaged, as well as directly evaluating the antecedents and consequences specific to the student's behavior. Information regarding

the quality of instruction can help in determining whether a student's lack of skills is a problem specific to the target student or a common problem among peers and thus potentially a function of the general classroom instruction. Observations of the learning environment should include an assessment of whether teachers are providing students with modeling of skills being taught, as well as opportunities for students to practice the skills, paired with performance feedback for accurate and inaccurate responding. The impact of teacher instruction should also be assessed by sampling the performances of other students within the class and comparing peer performances with the target student's performance. Evidence that most students are having academic difficulties suggests that students are being provided with ineffective instruction and/or poor instructional match (Martens & Witt, 2004). Failure to obtain information regarding the general quality of instruction being provided to students might result in misattributing a skill deficit to a characteristic of the student (e.g., memory problems) when instead the problem is a function of poor classroom instruction (e.g., no corrective feedback; Witt et al., 2004). For instance, failure by the teacher to gain student attention prior to providing instructions, to provide clearly stated and goal-directed instructions, and/or to frequently reinforce compliance with instructions might result in student noncompliance and an attribution that the student is unable to follow multiple-step directions.

Even in the presence of quality instruction, behavior is likely to be problematic in the absence of a quality behavior management plan. Quality behavior management plans both ensure that students have the needed skills to engage in appropriate behavior and support the occurrence of appropriate over inappropriate behavior. Assessment of the behavior management plan is also important because behavioral interventions developed for individual students are more likely to be successful when implemented in conjunction with a schoolwide or classwide plan. Interventions that supplement an existing plan are more likely to be implemented as designed, thus increasing the probability of intervention success (Detrich, 1999). In order to assess the quality of a behavior management plan, teachers should be asked to list their classroom rules, procedures for teaching rules, and the means by which the appropriate behavior is reinforced. The accuracy of this information should then be evaluated by assessing students' knowledge of the behavior management plan (Nelson, Martella, & Galand, 1998; Rosenberg, 1986) and whether the probability of appropriate behavior is greater than that of inappropriate behavior. Even in the presence of reinforcement for appropriate behavior, aberrant behavior may occur more frequently if it requires less effort to engage in, if it has a greater probability of being reinforced, and/or if the quality of reinforcement for aberrant behavior is greater (Martens & Ardoin, 2002). Assessment procedures might include determining (1) the proportion of occurrences of reinforcement for appropriate versus inappropriate behavior; (2) whether teachers are more frequently engaging in preventative and reinforcement-based procedures as opposed to reactive punitive procedures; and (3) the allocation of time to transitions, classroom instruction, and unstructured time during which students are without clear instructional objectives.

A final component of direct behavioral assessment procedures is to conduct systematic observations of the target student as a means of identifying the antecedents and/or consequences that potentially maintain problem behavior. ABC observations, which involve either transcribing or coding the events that surround student behavior, can be useful in identifying commonly occurring antecedents and consequences of student behavior (Witt et al., 2000). Although computer-based programs are available to assist in these observations, within school settings pencil-and-paper ABC recording procedures are typically used. As first described by Bijou, Peterson, and Ault (1968), narrative ABC recording procedures involve dividing a sheet of paper into three columns, with the left column labeled A (antecedents), the middle column labeled B (behaviors of target student), and the right column labeled C (consequences). During observations, behaviors engaged in by the students are written in the middle column, and the behaviors of others that precede (antecedents) and follow (consequences) each of the target student's behaviors are recorded in the appropriate columns (Witt et al., 2000).

More structured ABC observations can be conducted by recording both positive and negative student behaviors that have been operationally defined prior to data collection (e.g., Martens et al., 2008). Important antecedents and consequences to attend to during these observations include (1) format of instruction (small or large group, seat work, subject matter, structured or unstructured); (2) proximity of teachers, adults, or peers to target student; (3) removal or presentation of attention; (4) types of teacher commands or directives; (5) transitions between subject areas; (6) positive or negative verbal and nonverbal communications directed toward target student and peers; and (7) positive or negative verbal and nonverbal communication between target student and peers. Natural variability in the antecedents and consequences of behavior mandates that multiple observations be conducted before one can have confidence that observed trends and behavioral sequences accurately represent the antecedents and consequences that are potentially maintaining a problem behavior (e.g., Hintze & Matthews, 2004).

Treatment Utility

Once all forms of indirect and direct assessment data have been collected, it is time again to meet with the teacher in order to conduct a problem analysis interview. Purposes of this interview include developing (1) reasonable intervention goals based on baseline levels of behavior, (2) a hypothesis about the function of problem behavior, and (3) an intervention based on the hypothesized function of problem behavior (Erchul & Martens, 2002). See Table 10.3 for questions that might be useful in structuring this interview. The decisions made during this meeting are based largely or exclusively on the data collected through the indirect and direct assessment procedures described previously. The treatment utility of collected data is determined by the extent to which these data allow an accurate determination of why inappropriate behavior is occurring and why appropriate behavior is not occurring at desired levels.

When interpreting indirect and direct assessment data, it is important to remember several factors key to the development of an effective intervention. First, it must be re-

TABLE 10.3. Useful Questions to Pose as Part of a Problem Analysis Interview

Goal A: Develop reasonable goals based on baseline levels of behavior.

1. Based on the data that were collected, it seems that the child is engaging in problem behavior approximately X times per hour. What type of goal can we establish that will result in a decrease in the behavior that the student will likely be able to achieve?
2. Based on the data that we collected, it seems that the child engaged in a more appropriate behavior X times within the given period. What type of goal can we establish that will result in an increase in the behavior that the student will likely be able to achieve?

Goal B: Develop a hypothesis of the function of problem behavior.

1. Looking at the data that were collected, is there any event that typically preceded the problem behavior?
2. Looking at the data collected, what one or two things seem to be consistently happening after the student engages in each problem behavior?
3. What might the student be getting out of these consequences?
   a. Escape: Are these consequences allowing the student to (1) somehow get out of work, (2) get help with his or her work, (3) reduce the amount of work, (4) get away from certain people, or (5) get out of the classroom?
   b. Escape: Do we have evidence that the student can do what he or she is being asked to do when the behavior occurs?
   c. Attention: Are these consequences allowing the student to get positive or negative attention from peers, teachers, parents, or administrators that he or she might otherwise not be getting?
   d. Attention: If the student had not engaged in these problem behaviors, what is the likelihood that the student would have been successful in what he or she was doing? How likely would it have been that the student would have received something positive as a result of doing the correct thing?
   e. Tangible item: Are these consequences allowing the student to get some sort of food or tangible reward that he or she would have otherwise not received or would have received after desired behavior?

Goal C: Develop an intervention based on the hypothesized function of problem behavior.

1. Do we have evidence that the child knows how to engage in appropriate behavior?
2. Do we have evidence that the child can be successful doing the work that he or she is being assigned?
3. Given that our information suggests that the reason the student is behaving inappropriately is for (attention/escape/tangible reward), what would be an appropriate behavior that the child could engage in that would get him or her access to this same thing?
4. What might be done to make it easier for the student to get (attention/escape/tangible reward) for appropriate behavior than for inappropriate behavior?
   a. Do we know that the student can do this behavior?
   b. Have you seen the child do this behavior before?
   c. Does the amount of effort required for the student to do the appropriate behavior exceed that for the inappropriate behavior? How could we reduce the amount of effort required by the student to engage in the appropriate behavior?
5. What could be done so that the student is less likely to want to gain (attention/escape/tangible reward)?
6. What can be done to decrease the likelihood that when the student engages in inappropriate behavior he or she gets access to (attention/escape/tangible reward)?
7. How much effort is going to be required of you to implement this intervention? What do you need to be successful in implementing this intervention? Are you willing to implement this intervention?

Note. Adapted from Erchul and Martens (2002). Adapted with permission from William P. Erchul.

membered that if a behavior is occurring with any frequency, it means that that behavior is likely being reinforced. At every moment of a school day, students are choosing what behavior to engage in. Their decisions are based on several factors, including the probability of reinforcement for engaging in each behavioral choice. Martens and colleagues (2008) describe a potentially useful technique re-

ferred to as contingency space analysis to determine how reinforcement is distributed for children's appropriate and inappropriate behavior. The procedure involves first conducting a series of sequential observations in which occurrences of potentially reinforcing consequences from others are recorded following both the presence and absence of problem behavior during brief intervals (e.g.,

15 second). For example, sequential recordings may reveal that in 8 out of 10 intervals in which a child engaged in aggressive behavior toward a peer, the classroom teacher issued a reprimand (i.e., a .80 probability of attention following aggression). Conversely, the teacher provided attention in only 1 of the 10 intervals in which the child was not aggressing but was working quietly instead (i.e., a .10 probability of attention following the absence of aggression). We might assume further that the teacher rarely allowed the child to escape task demands for either aggression (.10) or its absence (.10) and that the child was generally left alone when behaving appropriately (i.e., .80 probability of no consequence). When considered separately, these conditional probabilities indicate the schedule on which each category of behavior is potentially reinforced. In this example, it would appear that teacher attention is delivered on a nearly continuous schedule for aggressive behavior but on a lean schedule for other, more appropriate behavior (e.g., on task). Considered together, these probabilities can be plotted in coordinate space to indicate the degree to which each consequence is delivered *contingently* on aggressive behavior (plotted along the *y*-axis) or its absence (plotted along the *x*-axis; Martens et al., 2008). Figure 10.1 depicts a sample contingency space analysis of the

consequences for aggression just described. As shown in the figure, attention (circle) is provided contingent on aggression, escape (triangle) is rarely allowed for either aggression or its absence, and appropriate behavior is ignored far more than aggression (i.e., no consequence, depicted by the square).

Although a contingency space analysis can help in determining how reinforcement is distributed across behaviors, it fails to account for other factors that determine which behavior a child may choose to engage in at any given moment (Billington & DiTommaso, 2003). A second factor that must be considered when developing an intervention is whether appropriate behavior is in the student's repertoire and whether the effort required by a student to engage in appropriate behavior exceeds that of aberrant behavior. Students will not engage in behaviors that they lack and, all else being equal (e.g., quality of reinforcement), they are less likely to engage in appropriate behaviors that require more effort than aberrant behavior (Billington & DiTommaso, 2003).

A final factor that must be considered when developing interventions is that the function of student behavior is not necessarily consistent across settings. This variation can be due to numerous factors, including changes in antecedents, sources of reinforcement, and effort required to engage in ap-

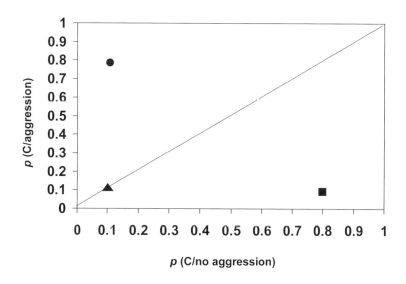

FIGURE 10.1. A sample contingency space analysis of attention (circle), escape (triangle), and no consequence (square) for aggressive behavior and its absence.

propriate or inappropriate behaviors, as well as changes in the value of reinforcers due to satiation or deprivation (e.g., Fisher, Piazza, & Chiang, 1996; Ringdahl & Sellers, 2000). For instance, time-out might function as a reinforcer in one setting in which it results in escape from effortful task demands but as a punisher in a second setting in which task demands require little effort and the time in the environment is abundant with reinforcement.

The treatment utility of assessment data is based on its usefulness in developing interventions specific to the child and the environment that is supporting the child's inappropriate behavior. Treatment utility is therefore determined by the extent to which data help in determining (1) the proportion of reinforcement provided for appropriate and inappropriate behavior, (2) the quality of reinforcement provided for appropriate and inappropriate behavior, (3) the effort required by the child to engage in appropriate versus inappropriate behavior, (4) how these factors interact to promote high rates of aberrant behavior, and (5) which factor(s) might be targeted through intervention to increase the probability that the student chooses to engage in appropriate behavior.

Sensitivity

Despite collecting multiple sources of assessment data, one cannot be certain of its accuracy in identifying potential maintaining variables without experimentally manipulating the antecedents and consequences of behavior. It is therefore essential that procedures be employed to evaluate intervention effects. Failure to evaluate an intervention might result in the continued implementation of an ineffective intervention or, worse yet, an intervention that increases aberrant behavior. It is therefore important to consider the methods by which the intervention will be evaluated prior to implementing the intervention. In considering how to evaluate intervention effectiveness, it is important to remember that, although a teacher's perceptions of changes in student behavior must be considered, these perceptions are fallible given the teacher's involvement in intervention implementation. Teacher bias can be reduced if the behaviors recorded are discrete, easily observable (e.g., raising a hand to an-

swer questions), and operationally defined. Another unbiased source of data that can be collected by teachers is permanent products, including data collected on a student's percentage of accuracy, percentage of work completed, and time to complete assignments and homework (Witt et al., 2000).

Unfortunately, many behaviors targeted through intervention (e.g., time on task) do not fall within categories that can easily be collected by a teacher and thus require more sophisticated data recording procedures. Although it is unreasonable to expect a teacher to conduct behavioral observations daily, a reasonable alternative is a teacher behavioral report card (Chafouleas et al., 2007). Teacher behavioral report cards differ from behavior rating scales in that (1) student behavior is rated over a shorter period of time, such as an hour per day as opposed to a week per month; (2) teachers provide their estimates of the rate or level at which the student engaged in the behaviors of interest as opposed to behaviors believed to be signs of an underlying disorder; and (3) they are meant to be sensitive to changes in behavior over time. Although research suggests that teacher behavior report cards are sensitive to changes in behavior, generalizability across raters is poor (Chafouleas et al., 2007). Thus ratings provided by one teacher will not necessarily match those of a second teacher observing the same behavior. The individual who completes the ratings must therefore be kept constant across the monitoring period. In order to increase the accuracy and sensitivity of teacher ratings, it is important to provide operational definitions of targeted behaviors, specific directions regarding what constitutes the various scores on the associated Likert-type scale, and performance feedback. Accuracy and sensitivity are also likely to be greater with shorter (1 hour) as opposed to longer (1 academic day) rating periods. Behavioral report cards can be created and easily reproduced for specific behaviors of concern by using the Behavior Reporter behavior report card generator at *www.interventioncentral.com.*

Data collected by a teacher should be supplemented by behavioral observations conducted by a trained observer, using observational procedures known to be accurate and sensitive to changes in student behavior. Possible data collection procedures include measures of latency or duration, as well as interval recording procedures. Observations that are compared with each other as a means of evaluating intervention effects should ideally be conducted at the same time of day and setting; otherwise, differences in observed behavior may be a function of time or setting as opposed to true intervention effects. Although it is essential to use measures that are sensitive to changes in behavior, it is critical to remember that sensitive measures will also be sensitive to changes in behavior as a function of variables other than those manipulated as part of the intervention.

Monitoring intervention effects is important for several reasons. First, inaccurate identification of the variable(s) that were maintaining inappropriate behavior might actually increase rates of inappropriate behavior. Second, although the intervention might produce behavior change in the desired direction, objective data allows the determination of whether behavior has reached normative levels. Finally, by monitoring intervention effects, one can make an educated decision regarding when it is appropriate to begin fading components of the intervention, ultimately allowing for the natural environment to maintain appropriate behavior.

Conclusions

According to Hayes et al. (1986), the strategies used to assess disruptive behavior within a problem-solving model are designed to accomplish three goals: "selecting a target behavior, selecting a treatment, or evaluating treatment outcome" (p. 476). As discussed in this chapter, accomplishing these goals requires a multimethod, multisource approach to collecting information about the child, the child's instructional environment, and the immediate antecedents and consequences of the child's behavior. During the first phase of assessment, variability in children's behavior is correlated with events surrounding its occurrence to suggest potential maintaining variables. This phase is completed when it is clear what needs to be manipulated and why in order to increase desired behavior and decrease problem behavior. During the second phase of assessment, potential maintaining variables are manipulated as part of treat-

ment while desired changes in behavior are closely monitored. This phase is completed when it is clear that treatment produced the intended effects.

Conducting a comprehensive behavioral assessment poses unique challenges to school psychologists and other support personnel who are used to conducting psychological assessments. We recognize that the domain sampling and functional relation goals of behavioral assessment can be strategically demanding. We also realize that evaluating changes in children's behavior over time (i.e., intrasubject variability) and translating ABC patterns into potential maintaining variables can be conceptually demanding. As noted by Wolery, Bailey, and Sugai (1984), however, the effectiveness of any behavior-change strategy relies in large part on the use of assessment tools to identify students' needs and to evaluate student progress. Because behavioral assessment is ultimately about "understanding and … altering behavior" (Nelson & Hayes, 1979, p. 13), we believe that its focus on events in a child's environment that can be manipulated to produce desired changes in behavior make it uniquely suited for use in a problem-solving model.

References

Achenbach, T. M., & Rescorla, L. A. (2001). *Manual for the ASEBA School-Age Forms and Profiles.* Burlington: University of Vermont, Department of Psychiatry

Ardoin, S. P., & Christ, T. J. (2008). Evaluating curriculum-based measurement slope estimates using data from tri-annual universal screenings. *School Psychology Review, 37,* 109–125.

Ardoin, S. P., & Daly, E. J., III. (2007). Introduction to the Special Series: Close encounters of the instructional kind—How the instructional hierarchy is shaping instructional research 30 years later. *Journal of Behavioral Education, 16*(1), 1–6.

Ardoin, S. P., McCall, M., & Klubnik, C. (2007). Promoting generalization of oral reading fluency: Providing drill versus practice opportunities. *Journal of Behavioral Education, 16*(1), 55–70.

Ardoin, S. P., Witt, J. C., Connell, J. E., & Koenig, J. (2005). Application of a three-tiered response to intervention model for instructional planning, decision making, and the identification of children in need of services.

Journal of Psychoeducational Assessment, 23(4), 362–380.

Ardoin, S. P., Witt, J. C., Suldo, S. M., Connell, J. E., Koenig, J. L., Resetar, J. L., et al., (2004). Examining the incremental benefits of administering a maze and three versus one curriculum-based measurement reading probes when conducting universal screening. *School Psychology Review,* 33, 218–233.

Bijou, S. W., Peterson, R. F., & Ault, M. H. (1968). A method to integrate descriptive and experimental field studies at the level of data and empirical concepts. *Journal of Applied Behavior Analysis,* 1, 175–191.

Billington, E. J., & DiTommaso, N. M. (2003). Demonstration and applications of the matching law in education. *Journal of Behavioral Education,* 12(2), 91–104.

Binder, C. (1996). Behavioral fluency: Evolution of a new paradigm. *Behavior Analyst,* 19, 163–197.

Campbell, D. T., & Fiske, D. W. (1959). Convergent and discriminant validation by the multitrait–multimethod matrix. *Psychological Bulletin,* 56, 81–105.

Carr, E. G., Newsom, C. D., & Binkoff, J. A. (1976). Stimulus control of self-destructive behavior in a psychotic child. *Journal of Abnormal Child Psychology,* 4, 139–153.

Chafouleas, S. M., Christ, T. J., Riley-Tilman, T. C., Briesch, A. M., & Chanese, J. A. M. (2007). Generalizability and dependability of direct behavior ratings to assess social behavior of preschoolers. *School Psychology Review,* 36, 63–79.

Christenson, S. L., & Ysseldyke, J. E. (1989). Assessing student performance: An important change is needed. *Journal of School Psychology,* 27, 409–425.

Cone, J. D. (1977). The relevance of reliability and validity for behavioral assessment. *Behavior Therapy,* 8, 411–426.

Crocker, L., & Algina, J. (1986). *Introduction to classical and modern test theory.* New York: Holt, Rinehart & Winston.

Daly, E. J., III, Martens, B. K., Skinner, C. H., & Noell, G. H. (2009). Contributions of behavioral psychology. In T. B. Gutkin & C. R. Reynolds (Eds.), *The handbook of school psychology* (4th ed., pp. 84–106). New York: Wiley.

Daly, E. J., III, Witt, J. C., Martens, B. K., & Dool, E. J. (1997). A model for conducting a functional analysis of academic performance problems. *School Psychology Review,* 26, 554–574.

Detrich, R. (1999). Increasing treatment fidelity by matching interventions to contextual variables within the educational setting. *School Psychology Review,* 28, 608–620.

Drasgow, E., & Yell, M. L. (2001). Functional behavioral assessments: Legal requirements and challenges. *School Psychology Review,* 30, 239–251.

Driskell, J. E., Willis, R. P., & Copper, C. (1992). Effect of overlearning on retention. *Journal of Applied Psychology,* 77, 615–622.

Emmer, E. T., Evertson, C. M., & Anderson, L. M. (1980). Effective classroom management at the beginning of the school year. *Elementary School Journal,* 80, 219–231.

Epkins, C. C., & Meyers, A. W. (1994). Assessment of childhood depression, anxiety, and aggression: Convergent and discriminant validity of self-, parent-, teacher-, and peer-report measures. *Journal of Personality Assessment,* 62, 364–381.

Erchul, W. P., & Martens, B. K. (2002). *School consultation: Conceptual and empirical bases of practice* (2nd ed.). New York: Kluwer Academic/Plenum.

Fisher, W. W., Piazza, C. C., & Chiang, C. L. (1996). Effects of equal and unequal reinforcer duration during functional analysis. *Journal of Applied Behavior Analysis,* 29, 117–120.

Fletcher, J. M., Francis, D. J., Shaywitz, S. E., Lyon, G. R., Foorman, B. R., Stuebing, K. K., et al. (1998). Intelligent testing and the discrepancy model for children with learning disabilities. *Learning Disabilities Research and Practice,* 13(4), 186–203.

Fuchs, L. S., & Fuchs, D. (1986). Effects of systematic formative evaluation: A meta-analysis. *Exceptional Children,* 53, 199–208.

Gettinger, M. (1988). Methods of proactive classroom management. *School Psychology Review,* 17, 227–242.

Gickling, E. E., & Armstrong, D. L. (1978). Levels of instructional difficulty as related to on-task behavior, task completion, and comprehension. *Journal of Learning Disabilities,* 11, 32–39.

Goldfried, M. R., & Kent, R. N. (1972). Traditional versus behavioral personality assessment: A comparison of methodological and theoretical assumptions. *Psychological Bulletin,* 77, 409–420.

Gresham, F. M., & Carey, M. P. (1988). Research methodology and measurement. In J. C. Witt, S. N. Elliott, & F. M. Gresham (Eds.), *Handbook of behavior therapy in education* (pp. 37–65). New York: Plenum.

Hanley, G. P., Iwata, B. A., & McCord, B. E. (2003). Functional analysis of problem behavior: A review. *Journal of Applied Behavior Analysis,* 36, 147–185.

Haring, N. G., Lovitt, T. C., Eaton, M. D., & Hansen, C. L. (1978). *The fourth R: Research in the classroom.* Columbus, OH: Merrill.

Hayes, S. C., Nelson, R. O., & Jarrett, R. B. (1986). Evaluating the quality of behavioral assessment. In R. O. Nelson & S. C. Hayes (Eds.), *Conceptual foundations of behavioral assessment* (pp. 463–503). New York: Guilford Press.

Hintze, J. M. (2005). Psychometrics of direct observation. *School Psychology Review, 34,* 507–519.

Hintze, J. M., & Matthews, W. J. (2004). The generalizability of systematic direct observations across time and setting: A preliminary investigation of the psychometrics of behavioral observation. *School Psychology Review, 33*(2), 258–270.

Irvin, L. K., Horner, R. H., Ingram, K., Todd, A. W., Sugai, G., Sampson, N. K., et al. (2006). Using office discipline referral data for decision making about student behavior in elementary and middle schools: An empirical evaluation of validity. *Journal of Positive Behavior Interventions, 8*(1), 10–23.

Iwata, B. A., Dorsey, M. F., Slifer, K. J., Bauman, K. E., & Richman, G. S. (1982/1994). Toward a functional analysis of self-injury. *Journal of Applied Behavior Analysis, 27,* 215–240 (reprinted from *Analysis and Intervention in Developmental Disabilities, 2,* 1–20).

Iwata, B. A., Vollmer, T. R., & Zarcone, J. R. (1990). The experimental (functional) analysis of behavior disorders: Methodology, applications, and limitations. In A. C. Repp & N. N. Singh (Eds.), *Perspectives on the use of nonaversive and aversive interventions for persons with developmental disabilities* (pp. 301–330). Sycamore, IL: Sycamore.

Johnston, J. M., & Pennypacker, H. S. (1980). *Strategies and tactics of human behavioral research.* Hillsdale, NJ: Erlbaum.

Kazdin, A. E. (1979). Situational specificity: The two-edged sword of behavioral assessment. *Behavioral Assessment, 1,* 57–75.

Macmann, G. M., & Barnett, D. W. (1999). Diagnostic decision making in school psychology: Understanding and coping with uncertainty. In C. R. Reynolds & T. B. Gutkins (Eds.), *The handbook of school psychology* (3rd ed., pp. 519–548). New York: Wiley.

Marston, D., Mirkin, P. K., & Deno, S. L. (1984). Curriculum-based measurement: An alternative to traditional screening, referral, and identification. *Journal of Special Education, 18,* 109–117.

Martens, B. K., & Ardoin, S. P. (2002). Training school psychologists in behavior support consultation. *Child and Family Behavior Therapy, 24,* 147–163.

Martens, B. K., & DiGennaro, F. D. (2008). Behavioral consultation. In W. P. Erchul & S. M. Sheridan (Eds.), *Handbook of research in school consultation* (pp. 147–170). New York: Erlbaum.

Martens, B. K., DiGennaro, F. D., Reed, D. D., Szczech, F. M., & Rosenthal, B. D. (2008). Contingency space analysis: An alternative method for identifying contingent relations from observational data. *Journal of Applied Behavior Analysis, 41,* 69–81.

Martens, B. K., & Eckert, T. L. (2000). The essential role of data in psychological theory. *Journal of School Psychology, 38,* 369–376.

Martens, B. K., & Eckert, T. L. (2007). The instructional hierarchy as a model of stimulus control over student *and* teacher behavior: We're close but are we close enough? *Journal of Behavioral Education, 16,* 83–91.

Martens, B. K., & Witt, J. C. (2004). Competence, persistence, and success: The positive psychology of behavioral skill instruction. *Psychology in the Schools, 41,* 19–30.

Martens, B. K., Witt, J. C., Daly, E. J., III, & Vollmer, T. R. (1999). Behavior analysis: Theory and practice in educational settings. In C. R. Reynolds & T. B. Gutkins (Eds.), *Handbook of school psychology* (3rd ed., pp. 638–663). New York: Wiley.

McCurdy, M., Skinner, C. H., Grantham, K., Watson, T. S., & Hindman, P. M. (2001). Increasing on-task behavior in an elementary student during mathematics seatwork by interspersing additional brief problems. *School Psychology Review, 30,* 23–32.

Meehl, P. E. (1986). Causes and effects of my disturbing little book. *Journal of Personality Assessment, 50,* 370–375.

Nelson, J. R., Martella, R., & Galand, B. (1998). The effects of teaching school expectations and establishing consistent consequences on formal office disciplinary actions. *Journal of Emotional and Behavioral Disorders, 6,* 153–161.

Nelson, R. O., & Hayes, S. C. (1979). Some current dimensions of behavioral assessment. *Behavioral Assessment, 1,* 1–16.

Nisbett, R., & Ross, L. (1980). *Human inferences: Strategies and shortcomings of judgments.* Englewood Cliffs, NJ: Prentice Hall.

Radford, P. M., & Ervin, R. A. (2002). Employing descriptive functional assessment methods to assess low-rate, high-intensity behaviors: A case example. *Journal of Positive Behavior Interventions, 4*(3), 146–155.

Reschly, D. (2004). Paradigm shift, outcomes, criteria, and behavioral interventions: Foundations for the future of school psychology. *School Psychology Review, 33,* 408–416.

Reynolds, C. R., & Kamphaus, R. W. (2004). *Behavior Assessment System for Children,* 2nd edition (BASC-2). Bloomington, MN: Pearson Assessments.

Ringdahl, J. E., & Sellers, J. A. (2000). The effects of different adults as therapists during functional analyses. *Journal of Applied Behavior Analysis, 33,* 247–250.

Rosenberg, M. (1986). Maximizing the effectiveness of structured classroom management programs: Implementing rule-review procedures with disruptive and distractible students. *Behavioral Disorders, 11,* 239–248.

Speece, D. L., Case, L. P., & Molloy, D. E. (2003). Responsiveness to general education instruction as the first gate to learning disabilities identification. *Learning Disabilities Research and Practice, 18,* 147–156.

Sterling-Turner, H. E., Robinson, S. L., & Wilczynski, S. M. (2001). Functional assessment of distracting and disruptive behaviors in the school setting. *School Psychology Review, 30,* 211–226.

Sturmey, P. (1995). Diagnostic-based pharmacological treatment of behavior disorders in persons with developmental disabilities: A review and a decision-making typology. *Research in Developmental Disabilities, 16,* 235–252.

Vaughn, S., & Fuchs, L. S. (2003). Redefining learning disabilities as inadequate response to instruction: The promise and potential problems. *Learning Disabilities Research and Practice, 18,* 137–146.

Vollmer, T. R., & Northup, J. (1996). Some implications of functional analysis for school psychology. *School Psychology Quarterly, 11,* 76–92.

Weeks, M., & Gaylord-Ross, R. (1981). Task difficulty and aberrant behavior in severely handicapped students. *Journal of Applied Behavior Analysis, 14,* 449–463.

Witt, J. C., Daly, E. J., & Noell, G. H. (2000). *Functional assessment: A step-by-step guide to solving academic and behavioral problems.* Longmont, CO: Sopris West.

Witt, J. C., VanDerHeyden, A. M., & Gilbertson, D. (2004). Troubleshooting behavioral interventions: A systematic process for finding and eliminating problems. *School Psychology Review, 33,* 363–383.

Wolery, M., Bailey, D. B., & Sugai, G. M. (1984). *Effective teaching: Principles and procedures of applied behavior analysis with exceptional students.* Needham, MA: Allyn & Bacon.

Chapter 11

Assessing Internalizing Problems and Well-Being

David N. Miller

Child and adolescent internalizing problems are often misunderstood and frequently overlooked by school personnel. The term *internalizing* indicates that these problems are developed, maintained, experienced, and exhibited largely within the individual (Miller & Nickerson, 2007a). In contrast to externalizing problems (e.g., conduct disorder, attention-deficit/hyperactivity disorder), which are overt, undercontrolled behaviors that are disruptive to others, internalizing problems (e.g., depressive disorders, anxiety disorders) are covert, overcontrolled behaviors that involve a high degree of subjective distress for the individual experiencing them (Merrell, 2008a). Internalizing problems are frequently underreported in schools, largely because they are often difficult to observe, and as a result they have been described as a *secret illness* (Reynolds, 1992).

Internalizing problems represent one end of the spectrum of human emotion, or affect. Traditional assessment and intervention services for children and youths in schools have emphasized the measurement and remediation of behavior and learning problems (Huebner & Gilman, 2004), including internalizing problems. For example, a goal for a middle school student identified as clinically depressed might be to have the

student report feeling nondepressed following treatment. An intervention that results in a student no longer feeling depressed, however, does not necessarily indicate that the student is experiencing a high level of happiness and well-being. Greenspoon and Saklofske (2001) and Suldo and Shaffer (2008) identified a subgroup of schoolchildren who reported low psychological distress but also low subjective well-being, findings that suggest that the absence of psychopathological symptoms is not necessarily concordant with optimal mental health (Huebner, Suldo, & Gilman, 2006). Similarly, not all children and youths with clinically significant levels of psychopathology experience poor quality of life (Bastiaansen, Koot, & Ferdinand, 2005).

In an effort to develop a more comprehensive perspective on human emotion and behavior, psychologists associated with the "positive psychology" movement (Seligman & Csikszentmihalyi, 2000) have recently advocated giving increased attention to positive indicators of well-being to complement psychology's traditional focus on negative indicators of disorder and disability (Huebner & Gilman, 2004). Although earlier work within positive psychology was directed toward adults, there has recently been greater

175

attention given to positive youth development (Larson, 2001), including an increased focus on strength-based assessment (Jimerson, Sharkey, Nyborg, & Furlong, 2004; Nickerson, 2007) and the assessment of well-being, life satisfaction, and quality of life in children and youths (Gilman & Huebner, 2003; Gilman, Huebner, & Furlong, 2009; Huebner & Gilman, 2004).

The purpose of this chapter is to provide a broad overview of the school-based assessment of internalizing problems and well-being in children and adolescents. Although the interest in assessing children's well-being is clearly increasing, this area remains an emerging and relatively new development in school psychology. As such, there is less information currently available on this topic, and therefore the coverage of it in this chapter is correspondingly less than the coverage given to assessing internalizing problems. To begin, an overview of internalizing problems in children and youths is provided.

A Brief Overview of Internalizing Problems in Children and Adolescents

Terminology: Symptoms, Syndromes, and Disorders

To properly understand internalizing problems and their assessment, it is first necessary to become familiar with several key terms, including *symptom*, *syndrome*, and *disorder*. These terms are sometimes mistakenly used interchangeably, but there are important distinctions between them. A *symptom* is a specific behavioral or emotional characteristic associated with particular types of disorders or problems. For example, one symptom of depression is depressed mood. In contrast, a *syndrome* is a collection of symptoms. For example, the combination of depressed mood, fatigue, sleep problems, and feelings of low self-esteem would indicate the syndrome of depression. A *disorder* exists when a collection of symptoms or a syndrome meets specific diagnostic criteria based on standard classification systems (Merrell, 2008a), such as the *Diagnostic and Statistical Manual of Mental Disorders* (DSM-IV-TR; American Psychiatric Association, 2000).

A disorder always includes both a syndrome and symptoms, and a syndrome always includes symptoms. Symptoms, however, do not always constitute a syndrome or a disorder, and a syndrome is not always formally diagnosable as a disorder (Merrell, 2008b). For the purposes of this chapter, the general term *problem* is typically used instead of symptom, syndrome, or disorder. An *internalizing problem* should therefore be interpreted as meaning any internalizing symptom, syndrome, or disorder that affects an individual to the point of causing clinically significant and sustained levels of subjective distress. It should be noted, however, that although it is not usually necessary to differentiate among the terms *symptom*, *syndrome*, and *disorder*, such differentiation may be very important when conducting assessments of internalizing problems and communicating information to other professionals (Merrell, 2008a).

Types of Internalizing Problems

Although the symptoms of internalizing disorders are numerous and complex, researchers have found that there are four main types of specific problem clusters within this general category. These problems include *depression*, *anxiety*, *somatic problems* (i.e., physical problems with no known organic basis), and *social withdrawal* (Merrell, 2008b). Common depressive disorders include major depression, dysthymia, and bipolar disorder. Examples of anxiety disorders in children and youths include generalized anxiety disorder, school phobia/refusal, obsessive–compulsive disorder, posttraumatic stress disorder, panic disorder, and separation anxiety. Somatic problems can include headaches, stomachaches, pain with no known medical cause, and otther physical complaints. Other problems often considered to have an internalizing component include selective mutism and the eating disorders of anorexia nervosa and bulimia. Finally, although they are not characterized as specific disorders, suicidal behavior (i.e., suicidal thoughts, suicide attempts, suicide completion) and self-injury (i.e., the self-destruction of body tissue without deliberate suicidal intent) are internalizing problems affecting a significant number of children and youths (Miller & McConaughy, 2005). These and other internalizing problems may appear as distinct symptoms, but they frequently tend to exist together in a co-occurring or *comorbid* relationship. As such, it often is useful to study the assessment of these problems within a common framework (Merrell, 2008b).

For a more detailed discussion of child and adolescent internalizing problems, including information on their prevalence, gender issues, comorbidity rates, and how these disorders are developed and maintained, the reader is referred to Evans et al. (2005), Mash and Barkley (2003, 2007), and Merrell (2008a, 2008b).

The Purposes of Assessment

As indicated by Ervin, Gimpel Peacock, and Merrell in Chapter 1 (this volume), assessment is integral to the problem-solving process—both at the initial stages of identifying what the problem is and why it is occurring and at the later stage of determining whether an intervention is successful. Thus the school-based assessment of internalizing problems should provide a solid foundation for understanding the problems that have been identified, as well as data for monitoring and evaluating evidence-based interventions. A thorough assessment should provide much of the information needed to help solve problems by suggesting the development of effective, socially valid interventions targeted at the areas of primary concern (Tilly, 2008).

Assessing internalizing problems presents a number of challenges to the school psychologist. One of the most significant of these is that many of the characteristics associated with internalizing problems may not be readily observable by others in the student's environment. As such, obtaining a child's or adolescent's perceptions via self-report or individual interview typically is of much greater importance in the assessment of internalizing problems than of externalizing problems, which are generally much easier to assess through direct observation and teacher–parent informant reports (McMahon & Frick, 2007). An additional challenge is that students with suspected internalizing problems are often not referred by school personnel as often as students with externalizing problems, and as a result these students frequently are underidentified and underserved (Miller & Nickerson, 2007a).

A third challenge is that many school-based professionals may not be adequately trained to conduct comprehensive assessments of internalizing problems. For example, in their national survey of school psychologists, Miller and Jome (2008) found that a large majority of the sample perceived that they needed at least some and often significant additional training in the assessment of a variety of internalizing problems. Finally, although a variety of reliable and valid measures are available for identifying internalizing problems, there is currently less research available on how to accurately identify the various functions of internalizing problems and how these may be more directly linked to intervention within a problem-solving framework.

A Model for Assessing Internalizing Problems

Merrell (2008a, 2008b) has described a comprehensive problem-solving model that can be used by the school psychologist to assess internalizing problems. Referred to as the *multimethod, multisource, multisetting assessment* model, its essential feature is a broad-based approach to assessment so that an aggregated, comprehensive picture of functioning is obtained. In this assessment model, multiple methods of assessment (e.g., rating scales, self-report scales, interviews, direct observations) are used across multiple informants (e.g., students, teachers, parents–caregivers) and settings (e.g., school, home, community). A brief overview of issues to be considered in terms of assessment sources and settings is provided next, followed by a more extensive discussion of recommended assessment methods and practices.

Assessment Methods

Because each particular method, instrument, or source used in the collection of assessment data is subject to error variance, a comprehensive and aggregated approach can be useful for overcoming the limitations of any particular assessment component, thereby reducing the amount of error in assessment interpretation and analysis (Merrell, 2008b). Methods in the assessment of child and adolescent internalizing problems may potentially include *direct observations, record reviews, sociometric techniques, behavior rating scales, interviews, self-report measures*, and *projective–expressive techniques* (Merrell, 2008b).

Assessment Sources

The many potential sources of assessment information include the particular *student* who is being evaluated, his or her *parents or caregivers*, other *family members*, *teachers* and other *school personnel*, the student's *peer group*, and possibly *community-based informants* such as youth group leaders or other service providers (Merrell, 2008a). Some of these sources will typically be more valuable than others. In particular, for the school-based assessment of internalizing problems, the most important individuals to assess typically are the student, his or her parents or caregivers, and his or her teachers. Because internalizing problems involve internal perceptions and states, obtaining the student's self-report (through both interviews and self-report scales) is widely considered to be the most critical and usually the most essential method. Possible exceptions to this general rule are the assessment of very young children, children who are unwilling to provide information about themselves, or students with limited cognitive and verbal skills. In these situations, parents or caregivers and teachers may provide the most useful information (Merrell, 2008a).

Assessment Settings

The phrase *assessment settings* refers to the particular places in which assessment information is based rather than the actual setting in which data are collected or where meetings occur. For example, although parents or caregivers may meet with the school psychologist in her or his office to provide information about a child's emotional problems, the setting on which the assessment is based is the child's home. Possible settings for obtaining information include school, home, various clinics or agencies, or other community settings. Typically, the school and home settings will be the primary focus for conducting assessments of internalizing problems (Merrell, 2008a).

Recommended Assessment Methods and Practices

Practitioners interested in assessing internalizing problems in children and youths are presented with a variety of options, including the use of record reviews, sociometric techniques, and projective–expressive techniques (Merrell, 2008b). In comparison with other assessment techniques, however, these three methods typically do not provide as much clinically useful information, often lack empirical support for their utility, and are not as clearly linked to problem solving. In particular, the use of projective–expressive techniques (e.g., the Rorschach and thematic apperception tests or human figure drawings) with children and youths is highly controversial and has been frequently criticized, primarily because of their questionable or poor psychometric properties (Knoff, 2003; Lilienfeld, Wood, & Garb, 2000; Merrel, 2008b; Salvia & Ysseldyke, 2001) and their limited incremental and treatment validity (Gresham, 1993; Miller & Nickerson, 2006, 2007a). Practitioners are therefore encouraged to make use of reliable and valid (i.e., evidence-based) methods in the assessment of internalizing problems in children and youths and to engage in assessment practices designed to assist in problem identification, treatment selection, and plan evaluation within a problem-solving framework.

Evidence-based methods in the assessment of child and adolescent internalizing problems include self-report instruments, interviewing techniques, behavior rating scales, direct behavioral observations, functional behavioral assessment procedures, and other methods (e.g., progress monitoring, template matching, keystone behavior strategy) for linking assessment to intervention. Each of these methods can make valuable contributions to the problem-solving process and are described in greater detail next.

Self-Report Instruments

Self-report measures designed for use with children and adolescents have become increasingly popular, and in recent decades there have been substantial improvements in their technical characteristics (Eckert, Dunn, Guiney, & Codding, 2000). These instruments are not only a recommended method for assessing internalizing problems in children and youths, but are also widely considered an essential and perhaps the single most preferred method (Merrell, 2008b). Because many of the symptoms associated with depression, anxiety, and other internalizing problems are difficult if not impossible to detect through external methods of assessment (such as through direct observations and parent or teacher rating scales), and because a well-designed self-report measure provides a structured and norm-referenced method to evaluate these problems, these instruments are uniquely suited to and particularly useful for assessing internalizing problems (Rudolph & Lambert, 2007).

Several excellent self-report instruments are available for use with students in schools. These include personality inventories or general-purpose problem inventories that include internalizing symptom items and subscales (i.e., broadband measures), as well as self-report measures designed to measure particular internalizing problems, such as depression and anxiety (i.e., narrowband measures). Broadband self-report forms may include internalizing syndromes as part of a broad, comprehensive evaluation covering a variety of disorders. Perhaps the most well-known of this type of instrument is the Minnesota Multiphasic Personality Inventory—Adolescent (MMPI-A; Butcher et al., 1992), which contains 10 basic clinical scales, four of which (Depression, Conversion Hysteria, Social Introversion, Hypochondriasis) appear to specifically target internalizing problems. Additionally, 5 of the 15 adolescent "content" scales of the MMPI-A (Anxiety, Depression, Obsessiveness, Low Self-Esteem, Social Discomfort) are significantly related to internalizing problems. Other general-purpose, broadband self-report assessment instruments include the Personality Inventory for Youth (PIY; Lachar & Gruber, 1995), the Youth Self-Report (YSR; Achenbach, 2001a), the Adolescent Psychopathology Scale (APS; Reynolds, 1998), and the Behavior Assessment System for Children—Second Edition (BASC-2; Reynolds & Kamphaus, 2004). Each of these broadband measures has demonstrated adequate to strong levels of reliability and validity and can provide use-

ful information to school personnel. These broadband measures have the advantage of providing a comprehensive assessment of students' overall emotional and behavioral functioning. In particular, they can serve a valuable "screening" function by determining the presence of a wide variety of possible emotional and behavioral problems, which can then be more thoroughly assessed via various narrowband measures. Broadband measures have the disadvantage, however, of being time-consuming, and they may not be needed in situations in which assessment is focused specifically on internalizing problems. Moreover, the age range is more restricted for some (e.g., MMPI-A) than for others (e.g., BASC-2), and none of these broadband measures is particularly useful as an ongoing measure of plan evaluation within a problem-solving model.

Narrowband measures for internalizing problems are typically less broad in scope and are designed to evaluate particular internalizing problems and concerns. Examples of narrowband self-report instruments for the assessment of child and adolescent depression include the Children's Depression Inventory (CDI; Kovacs, 1991), the Reynolds Children's Depression Scale (RCDS; Reynolds, 1989), and the Reynolds Adolescent Depression Scale—Second Edition (RADS-2; Reynolds, 2002). Useful narrowband instruments for the assessment of anxiety include the Revised Children's Manifest Anxiety Scale (RCMAS; Reynolds & Richmond, 1985), the Multidimensional Anxiety Scale for Children (MASC; March, 1997), and the State–Trait Anxiety Inventory for Children (STAIC; Spielberger, Edwards, Montuori, & Lushene, 1973). The Internalizing Symptoms Scale for Children—Revised Edition (ISSC-R; Merrell & Walters, in press) is a self-report measure designed to assess a wide spectrum of internalizing problems, as well as positive and negative affect in children.

Each of these instruments possesses adequate to excellent psychometric properties, and several have an impressive degree of evidence to support their use in the assessment of internalizing problems (Rudolph & Lambert, 2007; Southam-Gerow & Chorpita, 2007). Moreover, the use of such measures typically is neither time- nor labor-intensive, and they do not require a significant amount of clinical skill or experience to use effectively. Perhaps most important, they can be useful tools in the problem-solving process. For example, the use of a narrowband measure for depression could be used not only to identify students who may be depressed but also to routinely monitor and evaluate treatment effectiveness. Additionally, student responses on particular items of self-report scales may have direct implications for intervention. For example, a student's response to a self-report scale of depression that indicates that he or she is thinking about suicide should lead the school psychologist to immediately conduct a suicide risk assessment and, if necessary, implement appropriate suicide prevention and intervention procedures.

Despite the clear advantages of self-report measures, school psychologists need to be cognizant of several issues when using them with children and youths. One such concern involves the cognitive maturity that is required for a child to adequately understand the various demands of self-report measures and to effectively differentiate between response options. In most cases, it is very difficult for children under 8 years of age to comprehend self-report questions and complete these instruments, and even children older than 8 may have difficulties if they have learning problems and/or cognitive deficits (Eckert et al., 2000). Another concern about self-report measures is the various types of response bias that may occur, including the possibility of students giving dishonest responses or endorsing items in a socially desirable manner (Merrell, 2008a). Despite these concerns, the use of self-report instruments should be considered an essential component in the assessment of child and adolescent internalizing problems. For a more detailed discussion of self-report measures with children and youths, the reader is referred to Mash and Barkley (2007), Merrell (2008a, 2008b), and Shapiro and Kratochwill (2000a, 2000b).

Interviews

Like self-report measures, interviews should be considered an essential technique for assessing internalizing problems in children and youths (Merrell, 2008a). In fact, some consider the individual student interview to be perhaps the most important element in this process (Hughes & Baker, 1991). Probably the oldest form of assessment, interviews vary in length, structure, and the degree to which they are formal or informal (Merrell, 2008a). In contrast to the more structured nature of self-report measures, in which individuals respond to specific, standardized questions, interviewing often is more flexible and open-ended and allows a greater variety of responses.

More than perhaps any other assessment technique, conducting effective interviews requires a high level of clinical skill, including interpersonal skills, observational skills, and a thorough knowledge of normal and abnormal development (Merrell, 2008a). In particular, the age and developmental level of the student being assessed are important aspects to consider when conducting student interviews (McConaughy, 2005). For example, when interviewing students in middle childhood (ages 6–11) the interviewer should utilize familiar settings and activities, provide contextual cues (e.g., pictures, examples), request language interaction, and avoid abstract questions and constant eye contact (Merrell, 2008b).

School psychologists should be cognizant of developmental factors when conducting interviews, including the child's verbal skill and degree of "emotional vocabulary" (Merrell, 2008a). This last phrase refers to the child's skill level at communicating nuanced and sometimes complex emotions and reactions. For example, the characteristics and symptoms that might be identified by a mature adolescent or adult as "tension" might be described as "feeling angry" by a younger or less sophisticated student. Or what might be described as "disappointment" in an older child might be referred to as "feeling sad" by a younger one (Merrell, 2008a).

Moreover, when interviewing children suspected of having internalizing problems, it is important to assess their developmental thought processes and self-talk (Hughes & Baker, 1991).

Cognitive models of internalizing problems stress the role that thinking plays in the development and maintenance of emotional distress, with particular attention given to the individual's belief systems, irrational thoughts, and attributions regarding events and behaviors (Beck, 1976). For example, interview responses that suggest a student may be engaging in cognitive distortions (e.g., "My girlfriend dumped me *and I will never meet anyone like her ever again*"; "No one likes me *and no one ever will*") indicates that the use of cognitive restructuring (Friedberg & McClure, 2002) might be considered as a major component of intervention. Conducting interviews with children and youths is perhaps the best method for assessing cognitive variables and the degree to which they may be contributing to the development or maintenance of internalizing problems.

As noted, interviews can range from being very structured, in which each question is sequential and standardized (e.g., Diagnostic Interview for Children and Adolescents— Fourth Edition; Reich, Welner, & Herjanic, 1997), to being highly unstructured and open-ended. For assessing internalizing problems, Merrell (2008a) recommends the use of semistructured or behavioral interviewing techniques, and preferably some combination of the two. The advantage of a combined approach is that these two interviewing methods potentially are more reliable and less time-intensive than unstructured, open-ended interviews, as well as more flexible and adaptable than structured interviews. In essence, they (1) provide information that addresses the specific concerns of the child (and family and teacher), (2) can be easily modified for particular circumstances, and (3) may be useful for making both special education classification and intervention decisions.

A semistructured interview is one in which the school psychologist does not have a list of standardized questions yet still has a specific focus or aim (McConaughy, 2005). For example, if there is a concern that a student may be experiencing anxiety, the interviewer might ask the student specific questions related to the extent to which the student has experienced particular symptoms. In this manner, the interviewer would be maintaining some structure in the interview, in contrast to a more unstructured, open-ended approach.

Merrell (2008b) recommends that semistructured interviews with children and youths include five domains of questioning, including interpersonal functioning, family relationships, peer relationships, school adjustment, and community involvement. For example, in assessing student perceptions regarding peer relationships, general areas of questioning should include number of close friends, preferred activities with friends, perceived peer conflicts, social skills for initiating friendships, and reports of peer rejection and/or loneliness (Merrell, 2008b). Although questions should be tailored to the specific needs and concerns of a particular student, these five domains can provide some useful structure when interviewing students suspected of experiencing internalizing problems.

Behavioral interviewing is a particular type of semistructured interview. The objective of behavioral interviewing is to obtain descriptive information about the problem(s), as well as the conditions under which the problems are evoked and maintained. The conceptual foundation of behavioral interviewing is in behavioral psychology generally and applied behavior analysis in particular. As such, although it can be used by school-based practitioners who identify with theoretical orientations other than behaviorism, the use of behavioral interviewing requires a basic background in behavioral theory for maximum effectiveness (Merrell, 2008a). Behavioral interviewing is a process that may be used to inform the interviewer about possible *functions* that internalizing problems may serve, as well as to analyze various *antecedents* and *consequences* of problem behaviors that might be involved in their elicitation and maintenance. It is often necessary to follow up behavioral interviews with direct, naturalistic observations of students in environments in which problem behaviors occur and to use this information to further develop and refine hypotheses about problem behaviors and how these might be modified through interventions (Merrell, 2008a). Although many internalizing problems are often difficult to identify using external methods of assessment, behavioral interviewing is recommended because of its flexibility and potential usefulness in intervention development. Moreover, behavioral interviewing is an important component of a thorough functional behavioral assessment, a procedure discussed in greater detail later in this chapter. Table 11.1 provides some suggested procedures for conducting behavioral interviews.

Finally, although the primary focus when interviewing should be on the student suspected of having internalizing problems, it is often desirable and necessary to interview the student's parents or caregivers, as well (Merrell, 2008a). Parents or caregivers can provide invaluable information in the interview process because they know the student best and are usually the only ones who can provide a complete developmental history and who know the idiosyncratic manner in which the student manifests his or her strengths and problems and how the student behaves across multiple environments. Merrell (2008b) recommends that school psychologists ask parents about possible internalizing problems in very concrete, specific ways and that they avoid using professional jargon or classification terminology. For example, rather than asking, "Has your child seemed depressed lately?" it is much better to ask parents or caregivers about their observations of specific symptoms or characteristics of depression, such as excessive sadness, poor self-esteem, possible changes in eating and sleeping patterns, irritability, and loss of interest in previously enjoyable activities. Asking parents questions in this manner helps to operationalize the internalizing problems of concern, leading more readily to the formulation of specific and measurable treatment goals.

Becoming a skillful and effective interviewer requires extensive training and supervised experience. For more detailed information on developmental and other aspects of clinical and behavioral interviewing, the reader is referred to Hughes and Baker (1991), McConaughy (2005), Merrell (2008a, 2008b), and Watson and Steege (2003).

Behavior Rating Scales

Like self-report measures, behavior rating scales have become very popular in recent years for assessing a variety of emotional and behavioral disorders in children and youths, including internalizing problems. Behavior rating scales are sometimes referred to as "third party" evaluation tools because they are completed by other persons ("third parties") who know the student and have the opportunity to observe him or her under various conditions (Merrell, 2008a). Rating scales provide a standard format for measuring the frequency and intensity of particular emotional or behavioral problems and concerns. Ratings are conducted by individuals who have been able to observe the child for a long period of time, most typically parents or caregivers and teachers. They are typically norm-referenced, which means that the school psychologist can compare ratings of a target child with those of a nationwide sample of other children across a variety of variables such as age, grade, and gender. Some examples of general-purpose behavior rating scales that include items and subscales for internalizing problems include the BASC-2 (Reynolds & Kamphaus, 2004), the Clinical Assessment of Behavior (CAB; Bracken & Keith, 2004), and the Achenbach

---

TABLE 11.1. Suggested Steps in Conducting Behavioral Interviews

Set the stage for the interview.

- Build rapport with the person to be interviewed.
- Describe the purpose of the interview
- Provide instructions on how to respond to questions (e.g., "be specific").

Identify the problem behaviors.

- Specify the problem or problems.
- Get an objective description of the problems.
- Identify conditions in the environment that surround the problem.
- Estimate how often, how intense, and how long the problem behaviors occur.

Prepare to analyze the problem behaviors.

- Identify appropriate strategies for follow-up observation of the problem behaviors.
- Begin to form hypotheses about the functions the problem behaviors may be serving.
- Begin to form hypotheses about the antecedents that may be eliciting the problem behaviors.
- Begin to form hypotheses about the consequences that may be maintaining the problem behaviors.
- Determine time and places to collect additional data and to use these data to develop intervention strategies.

System of Empirically Based Assessment (ASEBA) Child Behavior Checklist (CBCL) and Teacher's Report Form (TRF) for ages 6–18 (Achenbach, 2001b).

Child and adolescent behavior rating scales have a number of advantages for use in the assessment of internalizing problems. Some of these advantages include their low cost, high efficiency, utility in providing valuable input from informants in the student's environment, and generally higher levels of reliability and validity in comparison with many other assessment instruments. In addition, behavior rating scales completed by adults can provide valuable information that can contribute to effective problem solving. For example, adults in the student's environment may observe certain behavioral characteristics exhibited by the student of which he or she is unaware or which he or she perceives inaccurately. Adults are also more accurate observers of students' externalizing behavior problems, and the extent to which students with internalizing problems exhibit comorbid externalizing problems has important implications for treatment. Finally, although student self-reports and adult ratings of students' internalizing problems are often discrepant, they provide useful information regarding the degree to which problems are recognized across various environments and multiple informants.

Despite their many advantages, however, behavior rating scales also have some disadvantages. First, behavior rating scales do not measure behavior per se but rather *perceptions* of behavior. They are therefore prone to potential response bias (Merrell, 2008b). Second, because many internalizing problems are not easily observable by others external to the child, extra caution should be employed when rating scales are used for assessing internalizing problems. In general, reports coming directly from the student, either though self-report or interview, often are more useful than other informant reports for assessing internal experiences, such as feelings of sadness and low self-esteem (Rudolph & Lambert, 2007). Nevertheless, given the many strengths of behavior rating scales, they are a recommended and often essential method in the assessment of child and adolescent internalizing problems. For more information on the use of behavior rat-

ing scales, see Merrell (2008b), Rudolph and Lambert (2007), Shapiro and Kratochwill (2000a, 2000b), and Southam-Gerow and Chorpita (2007).

Direct Behavioral Observations

Although the assessment of internalizing problems through methods other than self-report and interviewing presents a variety of problems, some internalizing problems can be observed directly. In contrast to the self-report methods, which assess an individual's own perceptions of internalizing symptoms, and rating scales, which assess third-party perceptions of internalizing symptoms retrospectively, the purpose of direct behavioral observations is to assess internalizing symptoms as they occur (Merrell, 2008b). Examples of symptoms of depression that could be measured directly through behavioral observations include diminished motor and social activity, reduced eye contact with others, and slowed speech (Kazdin, 1988). Examples of symptoms of anxiety that could be assessed through direct observation include avoidance of feared or anxiety-provoking stimuli, facial expressions, crying, physical proximity to others, and trembling lip or voice (Barrios & Hartmann, 1997). These behaviors, as well as others, could also be assessed via self-monitoring (Cole & Bambara, 2000), although this procedure has not received substantial attention from researchers as an assessment method for internalizing problems.

Several observational techniques can be used to assess various internalizing problems. One example is the Behavioral Avoidance Test (BAT) for anxiety, which involves some variation of bringing an individual into proximity to or contact with the feared or anxiety-arousing stimuli and observing his or her subsequent behavior (Hintze, Stoner, & Bull, 2000). Overall, however, direct observational procedures will likely not be as useful as other methods (e.g., self-reports, interviews) for assessing many internalizing problems. They may be most useful when assessing internalizing problems that are more likely to be directly observable, such as school phobia/refusal or self-injury. Direct observation procedures may also be useful in linking assessment to intervention through the use of functional behavioral assessment, which is discussed next.

Functional Behavioral Assessment

A central concern of school psychology in the 21st century is linking assessment to intervention (Merrell, Ervin, & Gimpel Peacock, 2006). This linkage can perhaps best be seen in the process of functional behavioral assessment, which may be defined as "a collection of methods for gathering information about antecedents, behaviors, and consequences in order to determine the reason (function) of behavior" (Gresham, Watson, & Skinner, 2001, p. 158). (See Jones & Wickstrom, Chapter 12, this volume, for a discussion of this method.) To date, functional assessment approaches have demonstrated greater utility in assessing disruptive, externalizing behavior problems than in assessing internalizing problems. However, some research suggests that a functional approach can be useful in linking assessment to intervention for some internalizing problems, such as self-injury (Nock & Prinstein, 2004).

The utility of taking a functional approach to the assessment of internalizing problems can be clearly illustrated in the assessment of school phobia, which in many cases may not be a "phobia" per se but rather a form of school refusal (Kearney, Eisen, & Silverman, 1995) or some other problem, such as separation anxiety (Kearney, 2001). The assessment of students who are frequently absent from school should include observations and behavioral interviews designed to identify the antecedents and consequences of their absenteeism to determine its function. This form of assessment, in conjunction with rating scales, self-report forms of depression and anxiety, and other recommended practices as described earlier, is important not simply for identification purposes but also for effective problem solving.

For example, possible reasons for school absence include anxiety related to social aspects of schooling (e.g., public speaking), anxiety about separating from one's parents or caregivers, oppositional and noncompliant behavior, and negative parent or school influences (Kearney, 2003). Although one student could refuse to attend school because of performance anxiety related to public speaking and another could refuse to attend school because of fears about being bullied, in both cases the function of the behavior would be escape or avoidance. Further, although the function in both cases would be identical, the recommended interventions for each would be different based on the unique environmental contingencies and other variables operating to cause and maintain the avoidance behaviors. In the first case, directly working with the student and providing interventions in relaxation training, skills training in public speaking, and cognitive restructuring might be used. In the second case, interventions may include cognitive-behavioral strategies for the student, as well as better monitoring by school staff in areas in which the student is likely to be bullied.

In contrast, another student may engage in school refusal behavior not because of any anxiety experienced as a result of parental separation or because of any particular variables at school but, rather, because the student is allowed to stay home and watch television when he or she claims to be sick. In this situation, which is more accurately described as a form of school refusal rather than school phobia, the behavior is maintained as a result of positive reinforcement (i.e., watching television) rather than escape/avoidance. The emerging field of clinical behavior analysis (Dougher, 2000) is increasingly engaged in the assessment of internalizing problems, and school psychologists are encouraged to be cognizant of these developments.

Other Assessment Methods

In addition to functional assessment procedures, other recommended methods for assessing internalizing problems include progress monitoring, template matching, and the keystone behavior strategy, each of which is described briefly next.

Progress monitoring emerged largely as a result of curriculum-based measurement (CBM), a procedure originally developed in the 1980s for measuring, monitoring, and evaluating individual student achievement (Shinn, 1997). Research on progress monitoring of academic skills has found that it may lead to modifications in instructional procedures, as well as to improvements in student academic performance (Fuchs & Fuchs, 1986). Although to date most of the evidence for the utility of progress monitoring comes from the academic rather than social–emotional–behavioral domains of student performance, this procedure may also be potentially useful in the context of assessing internalizing problems. For example, a school psychologist providing cognitive-behavioral therapy for a group of high school students experiencing depression could teach these students to conduct brief, daily self-assessments of their depressive symptoms, as well as administering weekly self-report scales to these students during group therapy sessions (Merrell, 2008a).

Template matching is a procedure in which assessment data are first gathered on students who have been identified as exhibiting problem behaviors and are therefore targeted for intervention. These assessment data are then compared with the assessment profiles of higher functioning students who do not exhibit these same problems. Behavioral profiles of these higher functioning students then serve as "templates" for students exhibiting problem behavior. That is, the discrepancies between the behaviors of the higher and lower functioning students serve as the basis for developing appropriate interventions (Hoier & Cone, 1987). For example, a school psychologist attempting to provide social skills training for a student with particular social skills deficits might have the behaviors of a socially skilled peer serve as a template for desired behavior in the less socially skilled student. Although template matching has traditionally been used primarily in the context of academic and behavioral problems, there is no reason it could not be used to address social and emotional concerns associated with internalizing problems (Merrell, 2008a).

The keystone behavior strategy (Nelson & Hayes, 1986) is based on the notion that a set of responses or characteristics is often linked to a particular disorder and that altering one specific response or "keystone behavior" may produce positive changes in an entire set of responses. Merrell (2008a) provides an example of using the keystone behavior strategy in a case involving the treatment of a 14-year-old girl experiencing significant emotional distress and social problems. In this case, the assessment revealed that the girl was socially withdrawn and experienced significant anxiety when engaging in social situations. Although her social skills appeared adequate, she often failed to engage in social situations because of debilitating anxiety. This anxiety appeared to be caused primarily by her negative and unrealistic thoughts, which then led to increased social anxiety and further social withdrawal. Given this information, the school psychologist might decide to focus on the negative and unrealistic self-statements as the target for intervention rather than on social skills training or other behavioral methods for reducing anxiety, because the negative and unrealistic self-statements may be the "keystone" within the larger set of responses.

Finally, although assessing internalizing problems necessitates a focus on the assessment of negative emotions and subjective distress, an exclusive focus on this domain presents a one-sided and distorted view of students' overall emotional and behavioral functioning. As such, it will be important for school psychologists in the 21st century to become increasingly familiar with the assessment of positive as well as negative emotions, particularly given that the absence of disorder (e.g., depression) does not necessarily suggest the presence of well-being (e.g., happiness). The assessment of well-being and the variables associated with it is discussed in the next section.

The Assessment of Well-Being

In recent years there has been a growing movement within psychology toward placing a greater emphasis on the positive aspects of human nature (Linley, Joseph, Harrington, & Wood, 2006). This movement, known as *positive psychology*, has been defined as "the scientific study of ordinary human strengths and virtues" (Sheldon & King, 2001, p. 216) and is concerned with examining variables such as positive emotions, characteristics, and institutions (Seligman & Csikszentmihalyi, 2000). Positive psychology was developed in reaction to the "disease" model so prevalent in contemporary psychology, in which the assessment and treatment of psychological disorders is given primary emphasis rather than the assessment and promotion of mental health and wellness (Miller, Gilman, & Martens, 2008).

Since the definition and scope of positive psychology was introduced in a special issue of the *American Psychologist* (Seligman & Cskiszentmihalyi, 2000), it has received significant attention from a variety of applied psychological disciplines, including school psychology (e.g., Chafouleas & Bray, 2004; Gilman et al., 2009; Huebner & Gilman, 2003; Miller & Nickerson, 2007b). For example, increased attention has been given to the assessment of such positive constructs as hope (Snyder, Lopez, Shorey, Rand, & Feldman, 2003), positive self-concept (Bracken & Lamprecht, 2003), emotional competence (Buckley, Storino, & Saarni, 2003), and gratitude (Froh, Miller, & Snyder, 2007) in children and youths. These developments are consistent with a strength-based (rather than deficit-based) approach to assessment, which, like positive psychology, is receiving greater attention from school psychologists (Jimerson et al., 2004; Nickerson, 2007). Further, there are strong indications that the assessment of positive emotions and psychological well-being will be an important component of the practice of school psychology in the 21st century (Gilman et al., 2009). Two areas that are particularly important to assess include subjective well-being and overall life satisfaction, which are discussed next.

Assessing Subjective Well-Being and Life Satisfaction

A topic that has attracted substantial interest within positive psychology is how and why individuals experience their lives in positive ways (Gilman & Huebner, 2003). Researchers have traditionally distinguished between objective and subjective indicators associated with quality of life and well-being, with much of the research examining objective conditions (e.g., income level, age, gender, geographic location) and their association with well-being consistently resulting in small correlations (Diener, 2000; Lyubomirsky, 2007; Myers, 2000). These findings suggest that well-being is largely regulated by internal mechanisms rather than objective circumstances (Gilman & Huebner, 2003). As such, the assessment of well-being must in large part involve the assessment of subjective experience. Although *subjective well-being* (SWB) is not sufficient

for mental health, it appears to be necessary (Diener, 2000; Gilman & Huebner, 2003). Moreover, research in the area of SWB provides a valuable complement to psychology's traditional focus on disorder and has stimulated calls to formulate effective intervention strategies designed to promote positive SWB as part of comprehensive school programs (Gilman & Huebner, 2003).

SWB theoretically includes three components: positive affect, negative affect, and life satisfaction (Diener, Suh, Lucas, & Smith, 1999). The distinction between positive and negative affect is an important one, as research suggests that they are not simply opposite poles on a continuum (Huebner & Gilman, 2004). For example, studies of elementary students in grades 3–6 (Greenspoon & Saklofske, 2001) and middle school students in grades 6–8 (Suldo & Shaffer, 2008) identified four different groups of students based on their levels of psychopathology (PTH) and SWB. The four groups identified included students classified as being (1) high PTH–high SWB (symptomatic but content); (2) high PTH–low SWB (troubled); (3) low PTH–high SWB (complete mental health); and (4) low PTH–low SWB (vulnerable). This fourth group challenges one-dimensional models of mental health. Using only pathology-based measures, the low PTH–low SWB students would appear "healthy" even though their level of SWB is poor. The use of positively focused SWB measures would therefore appear to offer school psychologists the opportunity to develop more comprehensive assessments of children and youths and their adaptations to their life circumstances (Huebner & Gilman, 2004).

The experience of positive emotions can be a primary contributor to SWB (Seligman & Csikszentmihalyi, 2000). Increasing evidence suggests that positive emotions "broaden people's momentary thought–action repertoires, which in turn serves to build their enduring personal resources, ranging from physical and intellectual resources to social and psychological resources" (Fredrickson, 2001, p. 218). Because the affect domain represents an individual's rapidly changing experience of positive and negative emotions, however, *life satisfaction* is considered to be the more stable component of SWB, as well as the indicator most amenable for inclusion when examining youths' perceptions of their life circumstances (Huebner et al., 2006).

Life satisfaction may be defined as "a cognitive appraisal of life based on self-selected standards" (Huebner et al., 2006, p. 358). Although this appraisal is cognitive, it is largely based on the positive experiences and emotions that collectively contribute to life satisfaction and well-being. Research suggests that although most children and adolescents are generally satisfied with their lives, a minority appear very dissatisfied (Huebner, Suldo, Smith, & McKnight, 2004). Low life satisfaction is associated with several adverse outcomes, including those related to internalizing problems (e.g., depression, anxiety) and school adjustment. In contrast, high life satisfaction functions as a genuine psychological strength and actively fosters resilience and well-being (Huebner et al., 2006). For example, in a study examining the characteristics of adolescents who reported high levels of global life satisfaction, Gilman and Huebner (2006) found that high life satisfaction was associated with mental health benefits that were not found among youths reporting comparatively lower life satisfaction levels. Moreover, school experiences can strongly influence life satisfaction. For example, behavioral contexts (e.g., grades received, in-school conduct), social contexts (e.g., school climate), and cognitive contexts (e.g., academic personal beliefs, attachment to school) associated with school are all linked to students' global life satisfaction (Suldo, Shaffer, & Riley, 2008).

Over the past decade, several psychometrically sound life satisfaction scales for children and adolescents have been developed on the basis of unidimensional or multidimensional models (see Gilman & Huebner, 2000, for a psychometric review of many of these instruments). To date, most measures have been self-reports and have been primarily used to illustrate similarities and differences between life satisfaction and related psychological constructs, such as self-concept (Huebner et al., 2006). Given that life satisfaction is a meaningful indicator and determinant of well-being in children and youths (Huebner et al., 2006), school psychologists can and should become well versed in its assessment.

School psychologists may also find the assessment of well-being to be useful in the problem-solving process. For example, both students who are depressed and those who are not depressed but have low levels of life satisfaction may benefit from interventions designed to increase subjective well-being. One intervention that may be useful in promoting greater well-being, as well as other positive behaviors, is the experience and expression of gratitude (Froh et al., 2007). Research suggests that keeping a "gratitude journal," in which individuals self-monitor and record events, people, or things for which they are grateful, can lead to greater subjective well-being and increased prosocial behavior in adults (Emmons & McCullough, 2003), as well as students (Froh, Sefick, & Emmons, 2008). Similarly, children and youths who are assessed as being unrealistically pessimistic about the future could potentially benefit from various cognitive-behavioral strategies designed to promote greater levels of hope (Snyder et al., 2003) and optimism (Seligman, 2007). Various self-report measures of positive emotions and/or life satisfaction could then be used to monitor progress and treatment effectiveness.

The assessment of well-being in children and youths is a new and emerging development within school psychology, and more research in this area is clearly needed. It is clear, however, that assessing well-being provides a broader, more comprehensive perspective on emotions and behavior and that assessing problems in the absence of strengths provides an incomplete and distorted picture of children and youths. For more information on assessing well-being and life satisfaction, the reader is referred to several works by Huebner and his colleagues (Gilman & Huebner, 2000, 2003; Gilman et al., 2009; Huebner & Gilman, 2004; Huebner, Gilman, & Suldo, 2007; Huebner et al., 2004).

Conclusion

The assessment of internalizing problems has been and will continue to be an important role and function of school psychologists, and practitioners are encouraged to be cognizant of evidence-based assessment practices (Klein, Dougherty, & Olino, 2005;

Mash & Barkley, 2007; Mash & Hunsley, 2005; Silverman & Ollendick, 2005) for use in a problem-solving model so that these problems can be accurately identified and effectively treated. The assessment of positive emotions such as subjective well-being and life satisfaction is only beginning to be recognized as a meaningful and useful activity in school psychology, and it appears that this strength-based approach will be an important component of 21st-century practice (Gilman et al., 2009). Given that a central mission of schools is to promote the healthy development of *all* students (Huebner et al., 2006), school psychologists should possess the knowledge and skills to conduct assessments of both negative and positive emotions in children and youths, including the assessment of internalizing problems and well-being.

References

Achenbach, T. M. (2001a). *Youth self-report for ages 11–18*. Burlington, VT: Research Center for Children, Youth, and Families.

Achenbach, T. M. (2001b). *Teachers Report Form for ages 6–18*. Burlington, VT: Research Center for Children, Youth, and Families.

American Psychiatric Association. (2000). *Diagnostic and statistical manual of mental disorders* (4th ed., text rev.). Washington, DC: Author.

Barrios, B. A., & Hartmann, D. P. (1997). Fears and anxieties. In E. J. Mash & L. G. Terdal (Eds.), *Behavioral assessment of childhood disorders: Selected core problems* (2nd ed., pp. 196–262). New York: Guilford Press.

Bastiaansen, D., Koot, H. M., & Ferdinand, R. F. (2005). Psychopathology in children: Improvement of quality of life without psychiatric symptom reduction? *European Child and Adolescent Psychiatry, 14,* 354–370.

Beck, A. T. (1976). *Cognitive therapy and the emotional disorders*. New York: New American Library.

Bracken, B. A., & Keith, L. K. (2004). *Clinical assessment of behavior*. Lutz, FL: Psychological Assessment Resources.

Bracken, B. A., & Lamprecht, M. S. (2003). Positive self-concept: An equal opportunity construct. *School Psychology Quarterly, 18,* 103–121.

Buckley, M., Storino, M., & Saarni, C. (2003). Promoting emotional competence in children and adolescents: Implications for school psychologists. *Psychology in the Schools, 18,* 177–191.

Butcher, J. N., Williams, C. L., Graham, J. R., Archer, R. P., Tellegen, A., Ben-Porath, Y. S., et al. (1992). *Minnesota Multiphasic Personality Inventory—Adolescent: Manual for administration and scoring*. Minneapolis: University of Minnesota Press.

Chafouleas, S. M., & Bray, M. A. (2004). Introducing positive psychology: Finding a place within school psychology. *Psychology in the Schools, 41,* 1–5.

Cole, C. L., & Bambara, L. M. (2000). Self-monitoring: Theory and practice. In E. S. Shapiro & T. R. Kratochwill (Eds.), *Behavioral assessment in schools: Theory, research, and clinical foundations* (2nd ed., pp. 202–232). New York: Guilford Press.

Diener, E. (2000). Subjective well-being: The science of happiness and a proposal for a national index. *American Psychologist, 55,* 34–43.

Diener, E., Suh, E. M., Lucas, R. E., & Smith, H. L. (1999). Subjective well-being: Three decades of progress. *Psychological Bulletin, 125,* 276–302.

Dougher, M. J. (2000). (Ed.). *Clinical behavior analysis*. Reno, NV: Context Press.

Eckert, T. L., Dunn, E. K., Guiney, K. M., & Codding, R. S. (2000). Self-reports: Theory and research in using rating scale measures. In E. S. Shapiro & T. R. Kratochwill (Eds.), *Behavioral assessment in schools: Theory, research, and clinical foundations* (2nd ed., pp. 288–322). New York: Guilford Press.

Emmons, R. A., & McCullough, M. E. (2003). Counting blessings versus burdens: An experimental investigation of gratitude and subjective well-being in daily life. *Journal of Personality and Social Psychology, 84,* 377–389.

Evans, D. L., Foa, E. B., Gur, R. E., Hendin, H., O'Brien, C. P., Seligman, M. E. P., et al. (Eds.). (2005). *Treating and preventing adolescent mental health disorders*. New York: Oxford University Press.

Fredrickson, B. L. (2001). The role of positive emotions in positive psychology: The broaden-and-build theory of positive emotions. *American Psychologist, 56,* 218–226.

Friedberg, R. D., & McClure, J. M. (2002). *Clinical practice of cognitive therapy with children and adolescents: The nuts and bolts*. New York: Guilford Press.

Froh, J. J., Miller, D. N., & Snyder, S. F. (2007). Gratitude in children and adolescents: Development, assessment, and school-based intervention. *School Psychology Forum, 1*(3), 1–14.

Froh, J. J., Sefick, W. J., & Emmons, R. A. (2008). Counting blessings in early adolescents: An experimental study of gratitude and subjective well-being. *Journal of School Psychology, 46,* 213–233.

Fuchs, L. S., & Fuchs, D. (1986). Effects of systematic formative evaluations: A meta-analysis. *Exceptional Children, 53,* 199–208.

Gilman, R., & Huebner, E. S. (2000). Review of life satisfaction measures for adolescents. *Behaviour Change, 3,* 178–195.

Gilman, R., & Huebner, E. S. (2003). A review of life satisfaction research with children and adolescents. *School Psychology Quarterly, 18,* 192–205.

Gilman, R., & Huebner, E. S. (2006). Characteristics of adolescents who report very high life satisfaction. *Journal of Youth and Adolescence, 35,* 311–319.

Gilman, R., Huebner, E. S., & Furlong, M. J. (2009). *Handbook of positive psychology in schools.* New York: Routledge.

Greenspoon, P. J., & Saklofske, D. H. (2001). Toward an integration of subjective well-being and psychopathology. *Social Indicators Research, 54,* 81–108.

Gresham, F. M. (1993). "What's wrong with this picture?": Response to Motta et al.'s review of human figure drawings. *School Psychology Quarterly, 8,* 182–186.

Gresham, F. M., Watson, T. S., & Skinner, C. H. (2001). Functional behavioral assessment: Principles, procedures, and future directions. *School Psychology Review, 30,* 156–172.

Hintze, J. M., Stoner, G., & Bull, M. H. (2000). Analogue assessment: Research and practice in evaluating emotional and behavioral problems. In E. S. Shapiro & T. R. Kratochwill (Eds.), *Behavioral assessment in schools: Theory, research, and clinical foundations* (2nd ed., pp. 104–138). New York: Guilford Press.

Hoier, T. S., & Cone, J. D. (1987). Target selection of social skills for children: The template-matching procedure. *Behavior Modification, 11,* 137–164.

Huebner, E. S., & Gilman, R. (2003). Toward a focus on positive psychology in school psychology. *School Psychology Quarterly, 18,* 99–102.

Huebner, E. S., & Gilman, R. (2004). Perceived quality of life: A neglected component of assessments and intervention plans for students in school settings. *California School Psychologist, 9,* 127–134.

Huebner, E. S., Gilman, R., & Suldo, S. M. (2007). Assessing perceived quality of life in children and youth. In S. R. Smith & L. Handler (Eds.), *Clinical assessment of children and adolescents: A practitioner's guide* (pp. 347–363). Mahwah, NJ: Erlbaum.

Huebner, E. S., Suldo, S. M., & Gilman, R.

(2006). Life satisfaction. In G. C. Bear & K. M. Minke (Eds.), *Children's needs: III. Development, prevention, and intervention* (pp. 357–368). Bethesda, MD: National Association of School Psychologists.

Huebner, E. S., Suldo, S. M., Smith, L. C., & McKnight, C. G. (2004). Life satisfaction in children and youth: Empirical foundations and implications for school psychologists. *Psychology in the Schools, 41,* 81–93.

Hughes, J. N., & Baker, D. B. (1991). *The clinical child interview.* New York: Guilford Press.

Jimerson, S. R., Sharkey, J. D., Nyborg, V., & Furlong, M. J. (2004). Strength-based assessment and school psychology: A summary and synthesis. *California School Psychologist, 9,* 9–19.

Kazdin, A. E. (1988). Childhood depression. In E. G. Mash & L. G. Terdal (Eds.), *Behavioral assessment of childhood disorders* (2nd ed., pp. 157–195). New York: Guilford Press.

Kearney, C. A. (2001). *School refusal behavior in youth: A functional approach to assessment and treatment.* Washington, DC: American Psychological Association.

Kearney, C. A. (2003). Bridging the gap among professionals who address youths with school absenteeism: Overview and suggestions for consensus. *Professional Psychology: Research and Practice, 34,* 57–65.

Kearney, C. A., Eisen, A. R., & Silverman, W. K. (1995). The legend and myth of school phobia. *School Psychology Quarterly, 10,* 65–85.

Klein, D. K., Dougherty, L. R., & Olino, T. M. (2005). Toward guidelines for evidence-based assessment of depression in children and adolescents. *Journal of Clinical Child and Adolescent Psychology, 34,* 412–432.

Knoff, H. M. (2003). Evaluation of projective drawings. In C. R. Reynolds & R. W. Kamphaus (Eds.), *Handbook of psychological and educational assessment of children: Personality, behavior, and context* (pp. 91–158). New York: Guilford Press.

Kovacs, M. (1991). *The Children's Depression Inventory.* North Tonawanda, NY: Multi-Health Systems.

Lachar, D., & Gruber, C. P. (1995). *Multidimensional description of child personality: A manual for the Personality Inventory for Youth.* Los Angeles, CA: Western Psychological Services.

Larson, R. W. (2001). Toward a psychology of positive youth development. *American Psychologist, 55,* 170–183.

Lilienfeld, S. O., Wood, J. M., & Garb, H. N. (2000). The scientific status of projective techniques. *Psychological Science in the Public Interest, 1,* 27–65.

Linley, A. P., Joseph, S., Harrington, S., & Wood,

A. M. (2006). Positive psychology: Past, present, and (possible) future. *Journal of Positive Psychology, 1*, 3–16.

Lyubomirsky, S. (2007). *The how of happiness: A scientific approach to getting the life you want.* New York: Penguin.

March, J. S. (1997). *Multidimensional anxiety scale for children: Technical manual.* New York: Multi-Health Systems.

Mash, E. J., & Barkley, R. A. (Eds.). (2003). *Child psychopathology* (2nd ed.). New York: Guilford Press.

Mash, E. J., & Barkley, R. A. (Eds.). (2007). *Assessment of childhood disorders* (4th ed.). New York: Guilford Press.

Mash, E. J., & Hunsley, J. (2005). Evidence-based assessment of child and adolescent disorders: Issues and challenges. *Journal of Clinical Child and Adolescent Psychology, 34*, 362–379.

McConaughy, S. H. (2005). *Clinical interviews for children and adolescents: Assessment to intervention.* New York: Guilford Press.

McMahon, R. J., & Frick, P. J. (2007). Conduct and oppositional disorders. In E. J. Mash & R. A. Barkley (Eds.), *Assessment of childhood disorders* (4th ed., pp. 132–183). New York: Guilford Press.

Merrell, K. W. (2008a). *Helping students overcome depression and anxiety: A practical guide to internalizing problems* (2nd ed.). New York: Guilford Press.

Merrell, K. W. (2008b). *Behavioral, social, and emotional assessment of children and adolescents* (3rd ed.). Mahwah, NJ: Erlbaum.

Merrell, K. W., Ervin, R. A., & Gimpel Peacock, G. A. (2006). *School psychology for the 21st century: Foundations and practices.* New York: Guilford Press.

Merrell, K. W., & Walters, A. S. (in press). *Internalizing Symptoms Scale for Children—Revised Edition.* Austin, TX: PRO-ED.

Miller, D. N., Gilman, R., & Martens, M. P. (2008). Wellness promotion in the schools: Enhancing students' mental and physical health. *Psychology in the Schools, 45*, 5–15.

Miller, D. N., & Jome, L. M. (2008). School psychologists and the assessment of childhood internalizing disorders: Perceived knowledge, role preferences, and training needs. *School Psychology International, 29*, 500–510.

Miller, D. N., & McConaughy, S. H. (2005). Assessing risk for suicide. In S. H. McConaughy, *Clinical interviews for children and adolescents: Assessment to intervention* (pp. 184–199). New York: Guilford Press.

Miller, D. N., & Nickerson, A. B. (2006). Projective assessment and school psychology: Contemporary validity issues and implications for practice. *California School Psychologist, 11*, 73–84.

Miller, D. N., & Nickerson, A. B. (2007a). Projective techniques and the school-based assessment of childhood internalizing disorders: A critical analysis. *Journal of Projective Psychology and Mental Health, 14*, 48–58.

Miller, D. N., & Nickerson, A. B. (2007b). Changing the past, present, and future: Potential applications of positive psychology in school-based psychotherapy with children and youth. *Journal of Applied School Psychology, 24*, 147–162.

Myers, D. G. (2000). The funds, friends, and faith of happy people. *American Psychologist, 55*, 56–67.

Nelson, R. O., & Hayes, S. C. (Eds.). (1986). *Conceptual foundations of behavioral assessment.* New York: Guilford Press.

Nickerson, A. B. (2007). The use and importance of strength-based assessment. *School Psychology Forum, 2*(1), 15–25.

Nock, M. K., & Prinstein, M. J. (2004). A functional approach to the assessment of self-mutilative behavior. *Journal of Consulting and Clinical Psychology, 72*, 885–890.

Reich, W., Welner, Z., & Herjanic, B. (1997). *Diagnostic Interview for Children and Adolescents—IV computer program.* North Tonawanda, NY: Multi-Health Systems.

Reynolds, C. R., & Kamphaus, R. W. (2004). *Behavior Assessment System for Children—Second Edition.* Circle Pines, MN: AGS.

Reynolds, C. R., & Richmond, B. O. (1985). *Revised Children's Manifest Anxiety Scale.* Los Angeles, CA: Western Psychological Services.

Reynolds, W. M. (1989). *Reynolds Child Depression Scale.* Odessa, FL: Psychological Assessment Resources.

Reynolds, W. M. (Ed.). (1992). *Internalizing disorders in children and adolescents.* New York: Wiley.

Reynolds, W. M. (1998). *Adolescent Psychopathology Scale.* Odessa, FL: Psychological Assessment Resources.

Reynolds, W. M. (2002). *Reynolds Adolescent Depression Scale—Second Edition.* Odessa, FL: Psychological Assessment Resources.

Rudolph, K. D., & Lambert, S. F. (2007). Child and adolescent depression. In E. J. Mash & R. A. Barkley (Eds.), *Assessment of childhood disorders* (4th ed., pp. 213–252). New York: Guilford Press.

Salvia, J., & Ysseldyke, J. E. (2001). *Assessment in special and remedial education* (8th ed.). Boston, MA: Houghton Mifflin.

Seligman, M. E. P. (2007). *The optimistic child.* New York: Houghton Mifflin.

Seligman, M. E. P., & Csikszentmihalyi, M. (2000). Positive psychology: An introduction. *American Psychologist, 55,* 5–14.

Shapiro, E. S., & Kratochwill, T. R. (Eds.). (2000a). *Behavioral assessment in schools: Theory, research, and clinical foundations* (2nd ed.). New York: Guilford Press.

Shapiro, E. S., & Kratochwill, T. R. (Eds.). (2000b). *Conducting school-based assessments of child and adolescent behavior.* New York: Guilford Press.

Sheldon, K. M., & King, L. (2001). Why positive psychology is necessary. *American Psychologist, 56,* 216–217.

Shinn, M. R. (Ed.). (1997). *Advanced applications of curriculum-based measurement.* New York: Guilford Press.

Silverman, W. K., & Ollendick, T. H. (2005). Evidence-based assessment of anxiety and its disorders in children and adolescents. *Journal of Clinical Child and Adolescent Psychology, 34,* 380–411.

Snyder, C. R., Lopez, S. J., Shorey, H. S., Rand, K. L., & Feldman, D. B. (2003). Hope theory, measurement, and applications to school psychology. *School Psychology Quarterly, 18,* 122–139.

Southam-Gerow, M. A., & Chorpita, B. F. (2007). Anxiety in children and adolescents. In E. J. Mash & R. A. Barkley (Eds.), *Assessment of childhood disorders* (4th ed., pp. 347–397). New York: Guilford Press.

Spielberger, C. D., Edwards, C. D., Montuori, J., & Lushene, R. (1973). *State–Trait Anxiety Inventory for Children.* Redwood City, CA: Mind Garden.

Suldo, S. M., & Shaffer, E. J. (2008). Looking beyond psychopathology: The dual-factor model of mental health in youth. *School Psychology Review, 37,* 52–68.

Suldo, S. M., Shaffer, E. J., & Riley, K. N. (2008). A social-cognitive-behavioral model of academic predictors of adolescents' life satisfaction. *School Psychology Quarterly, 23,* 56–69.

Tilly, W. D. (2008). The evolution of school psychology to science-based practice: Problem solving and the three-tiered model. In A. Thomas & J. Grimes (Eds.), *Best practices in school psychology* (5th ed., pp. 17–36). Bethesda, MD: National Association of School Psychologists.

Watson, T. S., & Steege, M. W. (2003). *Conducting school-based functional behavioral assessments: A practitioner's guide.* New York: Guilford Press.

Chapter 12

Using Functional Assessment to Select Behavioral Interventions

Kevin M. Jones
Katherine F. Wickstrom

There are seven deadly sins, seven sacraments, and seven habits of highly effective people. It has been said that there are only seven jokes, and they have all been told. There are only seven letters of the musical alphabet, from which every note of every composition in Western music is derived. Despite the title of the song, Paul Simon (1976) lists only seven ways to leave your lover. There are also only seven tools in a mechanic's kit: hammer, screwdriver, ruler, wrench, WD-40, duct tape, and a knife. This may seem at odds with the facts, as there are 250- and 500-piece tool kits in many garages. But these additional tools perform the same functions associated with each of these seven basic tools, which are, respectively, to drive, pry, measure, fasten, lubricate, adhere, and cut. One hundred more tools would be nice, and might make certain jobs easier or faster, but just one fewer would leave a handyman with no solution to at least one common type of problem.

This chapter argues, using similar logic, that there are only seven interventions and that they have all been tried. With the emergence of evidence-based practices, every "new" intervention that appears in psychological or educational research is actually a derivative, unique package or a novel ap-plication of a handful of well-established behavior-change processes. By clarifying the number and types of basic intervention processes, the task of linking assessment to treatment becomes more explicit, and multidisciplinary team problem solving may become more fluent. In this chapter, the elements of one approach to linking assessment to treatment, called functional behavioral assessment (FBA), is introduced. The foundations for FBA are briefly described, followed by a thorough introduction of each necessary step in an FBA.

What Is FBA?

FBA is a systematic process for identifying variables that reliably predict and control problem behavior. The purpose of FBA is to improve the effectiveness, relevance, and efficiency of behavior intervention plans by matching treatment to the individual characteristics of the child and his or her environment (Sugai et al., 2000). A primary assumption is that the same behavior exhibited by two children can actually serve a different function, thus warranting different interventions. Conversely, different behaviors exhibited by two children can serve the same function. By identifying antecedents and consequences that are most closely associated with a target behavior *for that individual*, treatments based on FBA may enhance the effectiveness of behavior intervention plans in the following ways (Iwata, Vollmer, & Zarcone, 1990):

1. The antecedents and consequences that maintain adaptive responses can be strengthened.
2. The antecedents and consequences that maintain maladaptive behavior can be weakened, avoided, or "reversed" so that they are associated only with alternative, appropriate responses.
3. It is possible to avoid the unnecessary use of extrinsic rewards and punishments, which may temporarily work but, in the long run, fail to compete with existing antecedents and consequences currently maintaining problem behavior.
4. It is possible to avoid countertherapeutic interventions that inadvertently strengthen maladaptive behavior.
5. By clarifying assessment and those conditions that lead to behavior change, it is possible to increase fluency in linking assessment to intervention.

Foundations for FBA

The conceptual framework for FBA began with Skinner's (1953) radical behaviorism, which introduced the principles of reinforcement, punishment, extinction, and stimulus control. The earliest applications of these principles to clinical problems appeared in the emerging field of applied behavior analysis in the late 1960s, primarily targeting troublesome classroom behavior and tantrums. Extending these principles to perhaps *the* most extreme and chronic expressions of psychopathology, Carr (1977) proposed that self-injurious behavior may be maintained by discrete environmental or sensory events. Within a few years, Iwata, Dorsey, Slifer, Bauman, and Richman (1982) introduced a methodology for isolating and testing these motivating factors, and for the first time a technology of conducting a pretreatment *functional analysis* emerged. Over the next two decades, massive accumulations of functional analysis studies appeared, but

they were largely limited to highly controlled experimental settings and the most severe disabilities.

These early studies provided conceptual and empirical foundations for FBA, but the emergence of functional analysis into mainstream education and psychology was grounded in a philosophical shift among educators and clinicians toward *functional contextualism* (Biglan, 2004; Hayes & Wilson, 1995), which assumes that the ultimate goal of applied science is *effective action*. Given this assumption, traditional assessment paradigms that focus on classification and prediction are less prominent than those that contribute directly to behavior *change* and improved child outcomes. Within the past 20 years, several innovations aligned with this goal appeared in schools, including the emergence of behavioral consultation (Kratochwill & Bergan, 1990), a relatively complete shift toward behavioral methods for personality assessment in the schools (Shapiro & Heick, 2004), and outcomes-based reform in special education (Reschly, Tilly, & Grimes, 1999).

Amid these reforms, a "problem-solving" approach to service delivery emerged as a core foundation of evidence-based practices and schoolwide service delivery systems based on response to intervention (RTI). The problem-solving approach includes four thematic questions that provide a framework for assessment and intervention decisions (Tilly, 2008; see also Ervin, Gimpel Peacock, & Merrell, Chapter 1, this volume):

1. Is there a problem and what is it?
2. Why is the problem happening?
3. What can be done about the problem?
4. Did the intervention work?

This framework assumes that there are unique child, teacher, and setting factors that should be considered before deciding what should be done about a problem. In other words, what works for one case may be ineffective or even countertherapeutic for another. Functional analysis is, in fact, one of the few research-proven methods for establishing an interaction between problem characteristics and intervention effects.

Functional analysis became "law" with the reauthorization of Public Law 94-142 into Public Law 105-17 (Individuals with

Disabilities Education Act [IDEA]) in 1997. Amendments to this law recommended positive behavior supports to address behavior that impedes learning and introduced the term *functional behavioral assessment* as mandated practice before individualized education program (IEP) teams consider disciplinary action against children with disabilities. Most recently, the emergence of schoolwide positive behavior supports guided by FBA represents perhaps the most sophisticated stage in the evolution of any applied science (Sugai et al., 2000).

What Is an FBA?

Have you ever done something you didn't want to do? Have you ever *not* done something you wanted to do? If so, you may understand the distinction between FBA and other approaches to analyzing a problem. People often explain behavior in terms of thoughts, feelings, intentions, and traits: A child acts out or isolates himself because he *wants* attention, he *feels* insecure, or he *has* attention-deficit/hyperactivity disorder (ADHD). Thoughts, feelings, and other "private events" do indeed reliably predict behavior, but only *under some conditions*. For example, a boy may feel angry every time he hits a peer, but he does not hit a peer every time he gets angry. A teenage girl may be anxious before every failed test, but she does not fail a test every time she is anxious. Identifying the conditions under which these private events predict the occurrence or nonoccurrence of important behaviors is the goal of FBA and a critical path to problem solving.

There is no universally accepted model for conducting an FBA, and practical applications in schools vary considerably (Weber, Killu, Derby, & Barretto, 2005). It appears, however, that existing frameworks include most of the following components:

1. Clarify the purpose of assessment.
2. Define the problem.
3. Develop a progress monitoring system.
4. Identify variables that are functionally related to targeted responses.
5. Design interventions.
6. Evaluate interventions.

Step 1: Clarify the Purpose of Assessment

The first step is for school-based multidisciplinary teams to clarify the purpose of FBA, which may be quite different from more traditional assessment strategies. The explicit purpose of an FBA is to *better understand the conditions that increase or decrease the frequency, duration, or intensity of behavior*. Thus more time may be spent assessing the environment than the child. The purpose is not to identify all potential thoughts, feelings, or actions or to cluster these behaviors into personality structures. In fact, any scrutiny of form or topography (e.g., aggression, ADHD, mood) is likely to be irrelevant to the design of appropriate intervention because variability between children, even with the same diagnosis, is so common. For example, the aggressive behaviors of two children with ADHD may "look" the same, but one child engages in aggression to access adult attention, whereas the other engages in aggression to escape demands. Furthermore, the *same child with ADHD* may exhibit markedly different rates of disruptive behavior when the type of attention or difficulty level of the work is altered.

Step 2: Define the Problem

A problem can be defined in terms of skill deficits, performance deficits, and performance excesses. The second step in an FBA is to identify missing skills, performance deficits, and inappropriate responses that may interfere with skill development or performance.

Skill Deficits

The term *skill* refers to the form or topography of a behavior, such as smiling, driving a car, or talking back to a teacher. Skills are often acquired through teaching or modeling, and fluency is achieved through repetition, feedback, and positive contingencies (Witt, Daly, & Noell, 2000). Thus one type of problem arises when a child has not mastered an appropriate, desirable skill, such as accepting feedback from teachers, cooperating with others, or ignoring distractions.

Witt et al. (2000) referred to this situation as a "can't do" problem, and the logical intervention for skills problems is to provide elements of instruction.

Performance Deficit

Performance refers to the occurrence of mastered skills in relation to contextual expectations or demands. A performance *deficit* arises when a child has mastered a skill but does not perform the skill at an appropriate frequency, duration, or intensity. For example, a student may comprehend a civics chapter and display proficient writing skills, but he or she does not complete an essay assignment on time. Thus the skills are within the student's behavioral repertoire, but the expected performance is not demonstrated. Witt et al. (2000) referred to this situation as a "won't do" problem, and the logical intervention is to strengthen motivation.

Performance Excess

Performance excesses are the most frequently targeted problem in literature examples of FBA. A performance excess arises when a child has mastered an undesirable skill and performance exceeds contextual expectations or demands. Although the term *performance excesses* may seem awkward, it is more comprehensive than *behavioral excesses*, because it includes instances in which (1) a single episode is intolerable, (2) only high rates are intolerable, or (3) it depends on the context. The *occurrence* of a behavior such as crying, fighting, or self-injury is rarely a concern. *All* children engage in these behaviors. Rather, these behaviors are problematic when they occur too much or in too many contexts. Crying, for example, is a developmentally appropriate response when teased, when a loved one is ill, or when an exam is failed. Daily episodes for an entire month may evoke concern, however, as would inconsolable sobbing during work or leisure activities. Thus it is excess *performance* (i.e., frequency, duration, intensity) that typically results in referrals. This situation might best be framed as a "won't stop" problem, and the logical intervention is to weaken motivation.

Step 3: Develop a Progress Monitoring System

The third step in an FBA is to develop a measurement system that can be used to monitor the child's progress and response-to-intervention (RTI) in the target or natural setting. This task is more challenging for interventions that target performance rather than skills. Skills can be assessed easily through *analogue* assessments that feature carefully controlled tasks, demands, and feedback, such as curriculum-based measurement for academic skills or role play for social skills. Performance of these skills, however, is highly sensitive to changes in the environmental context, so progress monitoring must also be conducted in the natural classroom or social setting.

Direct Observation

By far the most popular choice for progress monitoring is directly observing behavior as it occurs. Direct-observation strategies might include frequency counts, teacher checklists, analysis of permanent products, or office disciplinary referrals. One common approach is interval recording, which involves dividing an observation period into equal intervals (e.g., 1 minute), and coding the occurrence or nonoccurrence of target behavior(s) during each interval. Interval length is roughly proportional to observation duration, which is determined by the frequency of the target behavior. For example, a 30-minute observation divided into 15-second intervals should be sufficient for talking out in class, whereas an observation over the entire school day, divided into seven 1-hour intervals, might be sufficient for monitoring the frequency of peer aggression. Figure 12.1 displays an example of an interval recording system. Each cell represents a 10-second interval, and within each interval four child codes and six environmental codes are recorded. The four child codes are *on task*, *off task*, *target 1*, and *target 2*. Off task is defined as passive staring away from the instructional focus for at least 3 consecutive seconds. The latter two codes are individualized for each child, which allows the same form to be used regardless of target concerns. One strategy that could apply to a wide range of referrals is to define target 1 as "active engaged time"

Name of student: _____   Date: _____   Observer: _____

Target Behavior(s)   t1 = _____   t2 = _____

Setting: _____

		Peer			Peer			Peer
1 on off t1 t2 T T- T+ P C- C+	2 on off t1 t2 T T- T+ P C- C+	3 on off t1 t2 T T- T+ P C- C+	4 on off t1 t2 T T- T+ P C- C+	5 on off t1 t2 T T- T+ P C- C+	6 on off t1 t2 T T- T+ P C- C+	7 on off t1 t2 T T- T+ P C- C+	8 on off t1 t2 T T- T+ P C- C+	9 on off t1 t2 T T- T+ P C- C+
10 on off t1 t2 T T- T+ P C- C+	11 on off t1 t2 T T- T+ P C- C+	12 on off t1 t2 T T- T+ P C- C+	13 on off t1 t2 T T- T+ P C- C+	14 on off t1 t2 T T- T+ P C- C+	15 on off t1 t2 T T- T+ P C- C+	16 on off t1 t2 T T- T+ P C- C+	17 on off t1 t2 T T- T+ P C- C+	18 on off t1 t2 T T- T+ P C- C+
19 on off t1 t2 T T- T+ P C- C+	20 on off t1 t2 T T- T+ P C- C+	21 on off t1 t2 T T- T+ P C- C+	22 on off t1 t2 T T- T+ P C- C+	23 on off t1 t2 T T- T+ P C- C+	24 on off t1 t2 T T- T+ P C- C+	25 on off t1 t2 T T- T+ P C- C+	26 on off t1 t2 T T- T+ P C- C+	27 on off t1 t2 T T- T+ P C- C+
28 on off t1 t2 T T- T+ P C- C+	29 on off t1 t2 T T- T+ P C- C+	30 on off t1 t2 T T- T+ P C- C+	31 on off t1 t2 T T- T+ P C- C+	32 on off t1 t2 T T- T+ P C- C+	33 on off t1 t2 T T- T+ P C- C+	34 on off t1 t2 T T- T+ P C- C+	35 on off t1 t2 T T- T+ P C- C+	36 on off t1 t2 T T- T+ P C- C+
37 on off t1 t2 T T- T+ P C- C+	38 on off t1 t2 T T- T+ P C- C+	39 on off t1 t2 T T- T+ P C- C+	40 on off t1 t2 T T- T+ P C- C+	41 on off t1 t2 T T- T+ P C- C+	42 on off t1 t2 T T- T+ P C- C+	43 on off t1 t2 T T- T+ P C- C+	44 on off t1 t2 T T- T+ P C- C+	45 on off t1 t2 T T- T+ P C- C+
46 on off t1 t2 T T- T+ P C- C+	47 on off t1 t2 T T- T+ P C- C+	48 on off t1 t2 T T- T+ P C- C+	49 on off t1 t2 T T- T+ P C- C+	50 on off t1 t2 T T- T+ P C- C+	51 on off t1 t2 T T- T+ P C- C+	52 on off t1 t2 T T- T+ P C- C+	53 on off t1 t2 T T- T+ P C- C+	54 on off t1 t2 T T- T+ P C- C+
55 on off t1 t2 T T- T+ P C- C+	56 on off t1 t2 T T- T+ P C- C+	57 on off t1 t2 T T- T+ P C- C+	58 on off t1 t2 T T- T+ P C- C+	59 on off t1 t2 T T- T+ P C- C+	60 on off t1 t2 T T- T+ P C- C+	61 on off t1 t2 T T- T+ P C- C+	62 on off t1 t2 T T- T+ P C- C+	63 on off t1 t2 T T- T+ P C- C+
64 on off t1 t2 T T- T+ P C- C+	65 on off t1 t2 T T- T+ P C- C+	66 on off t1 t2 T T- T+ P C- C+	67 on off t1 t2 T T- T+ P C- C+	68 on off t1 t2 T T- T+ P C- C+	69 on off t1 t2 T T- T+ P C- C+	70 on off t1 t2 T T- T+ P C- C+	71 on off t1 t2 T T- T+ P C- C+	72 on off t1 t2 T T- T+ P C- C+
73 on off t1 t2 T T- T+ P C- C+	74 on off t1 t2 T T- T+ P C- C+	75 on off t1 t2 T T- T+ P C- C+	76 on off t1 t2 T T- T+ P C- C+	77 on off t1 t2 T T- T+ P C- C+	78 on off t1 t2 T T- T+ P C- C+	79 on off t1 t2 T T- T+ P C- C+	80 on off t1 t2 T T- T+ P C- C+	81 on off t1 t2 T T- T+ P C- C+

VALIDITY CHECK:
Review these estimates of child and general classroom on-task rates with the teacher. Ask the following questions:
Is this estimate of the target child's behavior close to his/her average? YES NO
Is this estimate of the classroom (peer) behavior close to their average? YES NO

FIGURE 12.1. Sample interval recording sheet for functional behavioral assessment.

and target 2 as "disruptive behavior." Environment codes pertain to neutral, negative, or positive teacher attention, peer attention, and "programmed" negative or positive classroom consequences, such as posting an "A" paper or receiving a discipline referral, respectively. Partial-interval recording is used for all codes except on task, meaning that the code is circled if the event occurs during *any part* of the 10-second interval. On task, on the other hand, is circled only if no off-task or disruptive responses occur during any part of the interval. Defined in this manner, at least one code will be circled during each interval, which prevents the observer from losing his or her place when using a bug-in-ear or other device that signals the end of each 10-second interval.

The percentage of intervals marked on task is typically used for progress monitoring, and intervention goals may be established by oberving three randomly selected peers every third column (marked "peer") of intervals.

Direct Behavior Ratings

Another approach to monitoring behavior interventions is to incidentally observe behavior during an interval and then rate performance according to subjective "anchors." Direct behavior ratings (DBR; Chafouleas, McDougal, Riley-Tillman, Panahon, & Hilt, 2005) represent a hybrid measurement system that combines direct observation and ordinal ratings. Although formats vary, a common element of all DBRs is that the observed frequency, duration, or intensity of behavior during a specified interval is summarized using ordinal ratings, such as a Likert-type rating between 0 (*none of the time*) and 4 (*all of the time*). Because completing the brief ratings takes less time than coding behaviors continuously, DBRs can often be completed by teachers or other individuals already in the natural setting. When used to summarize both academics and behavior across an entire school day, this system may function as a *daily report card*.

Step 4: Identify Variables That Are Functionally Related to Target Responses

The relationship between behavior and environmental events can be described using three terms. The functions of behavior include *positive reinforcement* and *negative reinforcement*, and *antecedents* are events or conditions that precede behavior.

The Functions of Behavior

Positive Reinforcement

Positive reinforcement occurs when an event is presented contingent on the occurrence of behavior and strengthens performance (frequency, duration, intensity) of that behavior. Praise, feedback, and privileges are common examples of positive reinforcement *if these consequences increase performance*. It is im-

portant to note that positive reinforcement describes the actual, rather than intended, impact of instructional or environmental events on behavior, and thus it applies to those situations in which positive reinforcement is unintended as well. A teacher's reprimands may actually intensify a child's throwing of tantrums, and peer reactions may increase disruptive classroom antics—although the effects are undesirable, both would still be considered instances of positive reinforcement. Children with academic deficits are particularly at risk for inadvertent strengthening of maladaptive behavior through positive reinforcement because they have fewer achievement-oriented skills in their repertoire.

Negative Reinforcement

Negative reinforcement occurs when an event is removed or avoided contingent on the occurrence of behavior and strengthens performance of that behavior. This process usually begins with the presence of some aversive condition, such as a challenging task or physical threat, which establishes the motivation to escape the condition or reduce discomfort. The removal of threats, avoidance of deadlines, and withdrawal of physical proximity are common examples of negative reinforcement *if these consequences increase performance*. It is important to note that *both* positive and negative reinforcement increase performance, although the consequences are different: "Positive" refers to adding a desired event, whereas "negative" refers to removing or avoiding an undesired event.

Negative reinforcement may describe unintentional effects as well. A teacher who allows a child having a tantrum to "take a break" may actually increase the future probability of tantrums. In a similar manner, suspensions, office referrals, and other punitive consequences that allow temporary escape from schoolwork or performance demands may inadvertently strengthen problem behavior. Children with performance excesses are particularly at risk for inadvertent strengthening of maladaptive behavior through negative reinforcement because their behavior is so distracting to teachers and peers.

Nonsocially Mediated Reinforcement

Some behaviors seem to persist even in the absence of environmentally based positive or negative reinforcement. *Nonsocially mediated reinforcement* refers to positive or negative reinforcement that is a direct product of the behavior, rather than "extrinsic" sources. Thumb sucking or daydreaming may provide sensory stimulation, whereas increased activity levels or fidgeting may provide escape from unpleasant private experiences such as anxious thoughts or drowsiness. With the exception of some cases of self-injury, stereotypy, and habit disorders, empirical demonstrations of "automatic" reinforcement are rare and do not obviate the need for an FBA.

Nonsocially mediated reinforcement is not synonymous with *intrinsic motivation*, a term that has also been used to describe behavior that persists in the absence of any observed external or extrinsic consequences (Deci, 1975). It is true that some children read for pleasure, solve challenging math or social problems for fun, and eat chocolate because it makes them happy. But pleasure, fun, and happiness can also describe perceptions associated with all types of reinforcement, whether it is socially or nonsocially mediated. Thus the terms *intrinsic motivation* and *reinforcement* are redundant: *All sources of reinforcement, whether activities, objects, or social attention, are effective because they have intrinsic value due either to genetic endowment or acquired experience.*

Table 12.1 summarizes five categories of reinforcers that should be considered during an FBA. Although it is impossible to categorize reinforcers based solely on topography (e.g., Is a toy a tangible or an activity reinforcer?), this table provides a clear distinction based on the specified mode of action. For example, an object is a tangible reinforcer if its delivery results in possession of that object. If a consequence of behavior results in engagement in an activity (but not possession of an object), it is an activity reinforcer. Within each category, the table provides common examples of positive as well as negative reinforcers. For example, if a teacher praises a child for self-editing a journal entry and self-editing increases, then that form of teacher attention is a source of positive reinforcement. If corrective feedback is avoided, reduced, or attenuated (e.g., worded less harshly) and self-editing increases, then that form of teacher attention is a source of negative reinforcement.

The Role of Antecedents

An FBA is primarily concerned with the consequences of behavior, but there is also potential value in assessing the *antecedents*. Antecedents refer to preceding events that reliably predict the occurrence of behavior. Classification of antecedents is a confusing affair, but it appears that there are two types, and each is defined in terms of its prediction versus control of performance.

Discriminative Stimuli

Discriminative stimuli are events that predict consequences but do not necessarily

TABLE 12.1. Categories of Reinforcers

Category	Mode of action	Examples
Attention	Accessibility	• Praise, positive feedback, public posting, proximity • Reprimands, corrective feedback, stares, demerits
Tangible	Possession	• Badges, stickers, toys, awards, jewelry, certificates • Citations, disciplinary referral slips
Edible	Consumption	• Candy, dessert, spices, sweeteners • Vegetables, smaller portions
Activity	Engagement	• Games, duties, physical exertion, relocation • Assignments, sharing, chores, detention
Sensory	Stimulation	• Sounds, smells, sexual arousal, altered biochemical states • Extreme temperatures, pain, itch, confinement

influence their effectiveness. Discriminative stimuli are "cues," so to speak, that evoke certain behaviors because they have been associated with greater availability of reinforcement. For example, a traffic light is a discriminative stimulus for braking, in the case of red light, or accelerating in the case of a green light. Behavior, in each instance, seems to be controlled by the stimulus—although, in actuality, the antecedent simply predicts differential reinforcement: It is likely that braking at a red light has, in the past, prevented accidents or punitive social consequences such as the glare of fellow motorists, reprimands from passengers, or fines from police officers. The behavior remains quite sensitive to its consequences and may change abruptly if its consequences or their value are altered. For example, the red light may not predict braking if it occurs on a deserted street, if there are no police officers in sight, or if the passenger is 9 months pregnant and 6 centimeters dilated.

Discriminative stimuli include salient environmental events, such as time of day, type of classroom instruction, exposure to models, and reminders, but they may also include *other behaviors* observable only to the individual, such as making a grocery list or texting a friend. Because these events precede other behaviors, such as going to the supermarket or meeting others after class, it is common to attribute behavior to thoughts, feelings, and intentions. Once again, however, these antecedents may be discriminative or predictive, but they do not control responding.

Establishing Operations

Establishing operations are antecedent conditions that actually control responding by momentarily altering the value of a reinforcer. These are typically setting events rather than discrete, episodic antecedents, but the most important distinction is that they actually alter the effectiveness of the reinforcers. The most common example of an establishing operation is deprivation: If adult attention is maintaining a response, then it is more effective if the child has not received this form of attention for a long period of time, just as a hamburger will gain effectiveness if the child has not eaten in a while. Rhode, Jenson, and Reavis (1992) provide

several other examples of establishing operations to make any reinforcer more effective, including *immediacy* (i.e., it quickly follows the behavior), *magnitude* (e.g., size), and *schedule* (e.g., intermittent). Each of these manipulations change how much the person wants the reinforcer; discriminative stimuli, on the other hand, change a person's chances of getting the reinforcer (Michael, 1982).

Conroy and Stichter (2003) reviewed the existing literature to compose a list of antecedents in natural settings that have contributed to FBA. The authors identified five general categories of antecedents that may be discriminative stimuli or establishing operations. These categories include *change agents* (e.g., parent, peer), *instructional factors* (e.g., individual versus group work, passive versus active, length), *environmental* (e.g., noise level, transitions, seating), *social* (e.g., peer prompts, praise, gender), and *physiological* (e.g., lack of sleep, illness). All of these factors should be considered when conducting an FBA.

The most important and salient antecedent in schools is the presence of academic demands, which in some cases may momentarily alter the value of negative reinforcement and increase the probability of escape or avoidance (a reinforcement function). Completing long division problems, conjugating verbs, and chronicling historical events are aversive for many children, and a number of teaching practices may make these tasks more aversive or less aversive. Thus, the "default" motivation for high-frequency behavior observed during class work may become escape or avoidance as a result of a negative reinforcement contingency, and critical instructional factors such as difficulty level or response requirements act as establishing operations. This may be true even at the most molecular, individual-item level (Billington, Skinner, & Cruchon, 2004).

Methods for Conducting an FBA

There are three methods for conducting an FBA. The most common approaches in schools today appear to be indirect and descriptive approaches (Weber et al., 2005), whereas the most rigorous and informative is an actual experimental analysis. These are not mutually exclusive strategies, how-

ever, and thus are presented as a logical sequence.

All methods of FBA attempt to narrow
down specific, testable hypotheses regarding
those antecedents and consequences that affect skill deficits, performance deficits, and
performance excesses. Table 12.2 lists some
common variables to assess for each of the
three types of problems. If skill acquisition
and fluency are targeted, then assessment
should focus on instructional elements such
as modeling, practice, and corrective feedback. If mastered skills occur at low rates
in desired settings or contexts, then variables such as expectations, understanding
of consequences, and incentives should be
examined. An FBA targeting performance
excesses should thoroughly evaluate those
events that precede and follow maladaptive
responses. The various methods of FBA are
distinguished by whether they are used to
generate, observe, or test hypotheses.

Indirect Assessment

Indirect assessment is used to generate hypotheses. Strategies include structured interviews that provide a detailed account of situ-

ations in which the target behavior occurs,
including the most common antecedents
and consequences. This information may be
provided by teachers, parents, or the child,
and some variations feature the actual rating of hypotheses using Likert-type scales.
The primary characteristic of this method is
that information is provided retrospectively
by the child, parent, or teacher, rather than
directly observed.

There are many published interviews and
checklists that may be used, yet it is rare to
find a single instrument that addresses the
conditions that influence skill acquisition
and fluency, performance deficits, *and* performance excesses. Various formats can be
obtained from Larson and Maag (1998),
Witt et al. (2000), and Watson and Steege
(2003).

Descriptive Analysis

In the second method, performance is observed as changes occur in the target classroom or social setting, such as when the
class moves from one type of instruction to
another. The goal of descriptive analysis is to
verify hypotheses through systematic direct

TABLE 12.2. Critical Variables to Assess in FBA

Type of problem	Description
Skill deficit (can't do)	• There is no evidence of skill mastery. • Excessive prompts or assistance are given. • The steps in the desired skill are unclear. • Opportunities or prompts to demonstrate the skill are rare. • Opportunities to observe others demonstrate the skill are rare. • Opportunities to rehearse or practice the skill are rare.
Performance deficit (won't do)	• Behavioral expectations are unclear. • The consequences for expected performance are unclear. • Expectations and consequences are not posted. • Prompts for comprehending instructions are rare. • Incentives and positive consequences for expected performance are rare. • The rationale for expected performance is not communicated clearly.
Performance excess (won't stop)	• Teacher attention often follows performance. • Peer attention often follows performance. • Access to preferred objects or activities often follows performance. • Performance produces sensory stimulation. • Performance results in isolation from others. • Performance leads to assistance with the task. • Performance results in temporary escape from work. • Performance results in withdrawn or reduced demands. • Performance is more likely when demand is difficult or repetitive. • Performance is more likely when request or choice is denied. • Performance is more likely when there is a threat of punishment.

observation and empirical quantification. The probability of performance (frequency, duration, intensity) given a particular antecedent event or the probability of a consequence given performance may be quantified as it occurs under natural conditions.

One descriptive analysis approach is to simply examine behavior changes across clearly defined settings. Touchette, MacDonald, and Langer (1985) describe a "scatterplot" observation that is functionally identical to interval recording, but the intervals correspond to changes in instruction (e.g., large group vs. small group, written work vs. computer time) or environments (e.g., one per class period). If behavior rates are consistently associated with certain intervals, the team may be able to isolate a specific hypothesis by examining those factors present or absent in those intervals. For example, if disruptive behavior occurs at lower rates in the morning versus the afternoon, the team would further investigate instructional variables that occur more frequently during the morning, such as independent work or group instruction. If disruptive behavior occurs more frequently during independent work than group instruction, the team may examine consequences that are more likely during independent work, such as peer attention. In this manner, a range of hypotheses can be systematically observed.

Another potentially useful approach to descriptive analysis described by Lerman and Iwata (1993) is to calculate the conditional probabilities associated with certain consequences. In this approach, short-duration interval recording (refer again to Figure 12.1), is used during the instructional or social setting in which problem behavior occurs most frequently. Following the observation, conditional probabilities are calculated. For example, to determine the probability of teacher attention given an episode of on-task behavior, the following formula is used:

$$\frac{\text{\# intervals marked "on" followed by teacher attention}}{\text{\#intervals marked "on"}}$$

"Followed by" is defined as occurring in the same or next interval. If the child was on-task during 40 intervals and 6 of these were followed by teacher attention, the probability of teacher attention, given for on-task behavior, is .15. By substituting each behavior code (off, t1, t2) and each consequence (teacher, peer, programmed), the probability of each consequence, given the occurrence of target behaviors, can be compared. This method provides *relative* differences in the probabilities of consequences and may assist the team in evaluating the most likely consequences for both appropriate and inappropriate responding.

A strength of the descriptive analysis approach is that quantitative rather than anecdotal data are collected. A second strength is that the method is unobtrusive—the "natural" relationship between behavior, performance, and environmental events is observed. A weakness of this method, however, is that these relationships are correlational, and thus a descriptive analysis reveals prediction rather than control. It is conceivable, for example, that an event may reliably follow a behavior but have no impact on performance. For example, it is not likely that sneezing is maintained by peer attention, even if there is a .95 probability that sneezing will be followed by "Gesundheit," "God bless you," or "Cover your nose!" It is also unlikely that highly intermittent yet causal relationships will be identified. To use another example, teachers often respond to misbehavior with reminders, but more rarely with reprimands or even threats. If the misbehavior persists, however, the teacher may occasionally withdraw the original demand ("Fine with me, don't finish the work and get a bad grade"). A descriptive analysis in this case would reveal a high probability of teacher attention when, in fact, the misbehavior may be maintained by less frequent and intermittent escape from work.

Experimental Analysis

The most rigorous FBA is an experimental or "functional" analysis, during which specific hypotheses are directly tested through the direct manipulation of instructional and/or motivational variables. This method involves applying and removing antecedents or consequences of behavior, such as difficult tasks, teacher attention, or presence of peers, while observing the impact of these changes on problem behavior. Given its complexity and intrusiveness, this step is usually conducted only if other methods have failed to provide clarity regarding the most likely causal variables. The experimental rigor is a primary strength of this method, and procedures for conducting an experimental analysis of severe disruptive behavior, disruptive classroom behavior, and academic skills have been broadly applied and replicated.

A serious challenge to conducting an experimental analysis in school settings is that environmental events must be controlled so that the effects of one variable at a time are assessed. Also, when targeting performance excesses, it is often necessary to produce rapid escalation of aggression, disruption, or self-injury, which would be intolerable in a classroom setting. Due to the level of rigor and, in some cases, the potential danger to target children and others, most FBA models incorporating an experimental analysis have been conducted in analogue environments and by research investigators (Ervin et al., 2001).

One of the most influential technological advances in FBA was Iwata et al.'s (1982) experimental analysis of self-injury. In this study, nine children were exposed to a series of carefully arranged analogue conditions that isolated the effects of staff attention, access to toys or activities, instructional demands, and an impoverished environment. The findings indicated that the same form of behavior (i.e., self-injury) was maintained by markedly different socially and nonsocially mediated consequences across individuals. The multielement design presented by Iwata et al. (1982), which involved a series of rapidly changing, brief, and replicated conditions, has since been extended to a host of other problem behaviors such as habit disorders, aggression, disruptive classroom behavior, and social skills (Ervin et al., 2001).

Northup and Gulley (2001) provided a description of analogue assessment conditions that have been used to isolate the function of disruptive classroom behaviors such as being out of seat, vocalizations, or fidgeting. An *alone* condition, in which the child is isolated in a barren office with no work or toys, may be used to test for possible sources of nonsocially mediated or "automatic" reinforcement in the form of sensory stimulation. A second condition, in which disruptions are followed by a neutral reprimand or reminder, may be used to test the effects of positive reinforcement in the form of *teacher attention*. A third condition, in which disruptions are followed by disapproving comments from other children, may be used to test the effects of positive reinforcement in the form of *peer attention*. A final condition, in which difficult work is presented and disruptions are followed by temporary "time-out," may isolate the effects of negative reinforcement in the form of *escape* from task demands. It is important to note that isolation, reprimands, peer pressure, and time-out are used often in classrooms *to stop misbehavior*, yet research in this area has clearly indicated that these events may also escalate the problem.

Beyond a few examples involving children with ADHD or habit disorders, functional analyses of social skills, performance deficits, and performance excesses for typically developing children are rare. Interestingly, no published study has demonstrated how the "gold standard" of FBA methodology might be used for severe conduct problems (e.g., substance abuse, bullying, truancy) that are most likely scrutinized in disciplinary actions. Thus it is unclear how FBA is being used by IEP teams, as mandated by IDEA, when considering disciplinary action against children with disabilities. There is sufficient support at this time, however, for teams to utilize a broad range of FBA strategies to inform data-based decisions and improve the design of individual interventions and supports for *all* children (Sugai et al., 2000).

Step 5: Design Interventions

There are only seven interventions, and they have all been tried. This may seem at odds with the facts, as 141 chapters are needed to compile "best practices" in school psychology (Thomas & Grimes, 2008). There are few examples, however, of FBA for children without disabilities or high-frequency disabilities (Ervin et al., 2001), so interventions targeting the most common school-based concerns are typically evaluated without regard to behavioral function. This is unfortunate, because one of the advantages of FBA is to increase fluency in linking assessment to intervention, and without a broad empirical base any attempt to link an overwhelming collection of best practices to a handful of basic behavior change processes is speculative. But an attempt is made here nonetheless because a conceptual system is necessary for advancing research and practice (Baer, Wolf, & Risley, 1968). The seven intervention processes detailed in Table 12.3 are grounded in Iwata et al.'s (1990) model for linking nonaversive approaches to reducing problem behavior. We extended this framework to include skill and performance deficits, as well as punishment procedures. In this section, each type of problem and its relevant treatment focus is presented, along with a few examples of published strategies that appear to demonstrate these basic intervention processes.

Skill Acquisition through Teaching Interactions

If a desired response does not occur in any setting, the skill may not be acquired. For this type of problem, it is important that intervention involve teaching interactions that may include one or more of the following: modeling, instructions, and feedback. There are many research-based demonstrations of teaching appropriate skills, such as self-management, social initiations, and cognitive problem solving. Kearney and Silverman (1990) introduced an indirect FBA method for classifying cases of school refusal according to its socially mediated consequences. For five children who experienced excessive fear or avoidant behavior, relaxation training or appropriate self-talk was successfully increased through modeling, role play, and feedback. Colton and Sheridan (1998) utilized a 15-day behavioral social skills training program in teaching cooperative play

behaviors to three children with ADHD. Although variable, the data indicated a gradual improvement over the 15 days, which would be expected if the children were acquiring skills in a successive fashion.

Improving Fluency through Increased Opportunities to Respond

Problems may occur if a desired skill is acquired but fluent responding is not achieved. When fluency is poor, the skill is less likely to be maintained over periods of abstinence, or it may not generalize to new conditions. For example, hitting a golf ball takes practice, and if there are long breaks between opportunities to play, the proper technique may be learned, but mastery may be delayed or never achieved. Mastery of important social or adaptive skills requires frequent practice, and one method for increasing fluency is to provide frequent opportunities to respond. Although rate of responding is commonly targeted in the academic literature, there are few examples of fluency-based interventions in behavioral research. An important exception, however, is the Girls and Boys Town teaching model (Dowd & Tierney, 2005). This teaching model, which is arguably one of the most socially valid psychosocial intervention "packages" in existence, features a corrective teaching strategy that includes rehearsal and practice of a new, alternative skill. Among its many other components, this strategy increases opportunities to respond by using each episode of misbehavior as an opportunity to practice and gain fluency in an appropriate replacement skill.

Gortmaker, Warnes, and Sheridan (2004) provided another example of use of this strat-

TABLE 12.3. Linking Functional Assessment to Behavioral Interventions

Type of problem	Description	Focus of treatment
Skill deficit	Skill is not acquired Poor fluency	• Teaching interactions • Increase opportunities to respond
Performance deficit	Lack of motivation for appropriate behavior	• Alter establishing operations • Differential reinforcement
Performance excess	Too much motivation for inappropriate, competing behavior	• Alter establishing operations • Differential reinforcement • Extinction • Positive punishment • Negative punishment

egy to increase the rate of verbalizations for a child with selective mutism. Zero rates were observed in the classroom during baseline, yet the child spoke outside of the classroom and thus demonstrated the requisite conversational skills. Treatment involved programming common stimuli, which increased opportunities to engage in verbal interactions by introducing the child to more and more situations that paired discriminative stimuli (e.g., being outside) with new stimuli (e.g., the classroom teacher). The treatment process, along with the gradual increases in verbalizations observed across a lengthy intervention phase, suggests that the intervention increased fluency of an existing skill.

Altering Establishing Operations to Address Performance Deficits

If the child possesses a requisite desirable skill yet performance is below expectations, one choice of intervention is to alter motivation by maximizing variables that enhance the effectiveness of existing reinforcement. This strategy requires no changes in the consequences for performance but, rather, changes in those antecedents that control responding by altering the value of a reinforcer. A useful example of this strategy for a performance deficit is "behavioral momentum," which involves preceding difficult requests with a series of easy requests. Ducharme and DiAdamo (2005) increased rates of compliance for two girls with Down syndrome from less than 20% during baseline to at least 70% during treatment by issuing *only* demands that the child "almost always" completed (e.g., "hold this") for a period of time, then *only* demands the child "usually" completed, followed by demands the child "occasionally" completed. Finally, a return to baseline conditions, in which the child was given only low-probability demands, was reinstituted. Increases in compliance were not due to contingent teacher praise, which was provided throughout all phases, but were instead due to enhancing the strength of the demand–compliance–praise contingency through "errorless" prior experience. Other examples of enhancing establishing operations are increasing *intermittency* of positive reinforcement using the mystery motivator (Moore, Waguespack, Wickstrom, Witt, & Gaydos, 1994) and

increasing *immediacy* of positive reinforcement (Rhode et al., 1992).

Differential Reinforcement to Address Performance Deficits

Perhaps the most familiar and widely used intervention for increasing performance is differential reinforcement. Using differential reinforcement to establish stimulus control over desired performance is arguably the central element in positive behavioral interventions. Its variations include differential reinforcement of alternative response (DRA), zero rates (DRO), and lower rates (DRL). When derived from an FBA, each variation "reverses" the contingencies so that the source of reinforcement maintaining problem behavior no longer follows misbehavior and is accessed only when desired performance occurs. Differential positive reinforcement involves providing positive reinforcers contingent on desired performance. For example, Ervin, Miller, and Friman (1996) increased the positive social interactions of a 13-year-old girl by arranging for peers to provide public praise statements directed to the child's prosocial behavior. Swiezy, Matson, and Box (1992) produced immediate and dramatic increases in the compliance rates of four preschoolers using the "Good Behavior Game," which involved points toward prizes and teacher praise contingent on cooperative responses.

Increases in performance can also be achieved through differential negative reinforcement, which refers to the contingent removal of an aversive event when—and only when—an appropriate response or performance occurs. One example of this strategy is using "eye contact" when issuing commands (Hamlet, Axelrod, & Kuerschner, 1984). The procedure involves demanding eye contact with the child as an instruction is delivered; the child is not allowed to escape eye contact until compliance is initiated. Another example is provided by Doyle, Jenson, Clark, and Gates (1999), who issued "dot stickers" contingent on work production that students could use to cover up and thus "escape" some of the problems on math worksheets. It is conceivable that any strategy that intersperses escape, easy problems, and correct answers may increase productivity rates through differential negative reinforcement.

Altering Establishing Operations to Reduce Performance Excesses

For a child with a performance excess, one intervention choice involves minimizing those variables that establish the effectiveness of reinforcement. This strategy requires neither changes in consequences nor the introduction of new contingencies, and thus it may be viewed by teachers as more favorable and less intrusive than other interventions. Some examples of this intervention strategy are providing choice, curricular revision, and noncontingent reinforcement. Powell and Nelson (1997) allowed a 7-year-old boy with ADHD a choice among three assignments that were identical in length and difficulty. Compared with conditions in which he was not allowed a choice, the percentage of disruptive behavior was much lower and less variable, despite the same levels of teacher interaction across both conditions. Roberts, Marshall, Nelson, and Albers (2001) achieved similar effects for three male students who displayed severe off-task behavior in the classroom. For each child, curricular revision included providing the child with class work at his appropriate instructional level. Providing choice or reducing the level of difficult work may have reduced, for children in these two studies, the aversiveness of demands and thus motivation for escape-related behavior.

Altering establishing operations can be used to reduce maladaptive behavior maintained by positive reinforcement as well, and one strategy with unlimited treatment implications is *noncontingent reinforcement* (NCR). Introduced by Iwata and colleagues (Iwata et al., 1990), NCR refers to the fixed-time delivery of reinforcers—regardless of whether they follow appropriate or inappropriate responses. Although its effects are probably idiosyncratic, most evidence suggests that this strategy reduces problem behavior through satiation: When access to reinforcement is provided frequently enough, there is less motivation to engage in problem behaviors that previously served this function. For example, Jones, Drew, and Weber (2000) conducted an experimental analysis that revealed that the disruptive behavior of an 8-year-old boy with ADHD was maintained by access to peer attention. A treatment that involved access to play time on a fixed schedule with peers reduced disruptive behavior from 100% to 11%. NCR has been applied to a wide range of problem behaviors, including those maintained by socially mediated negative reinforcement and sensory stimulation, but thus far most of these demonstrations are limited to individuals with severe cognitive disabilities.

Differential Reinforcement to Decrease Performance Excesses

If the performance of inappropriate responses exceeds expectations, one intervention option is to reduce performance by reversing the contingencies. This intervention is topographically identical to differential reinforcement strategies to increase performance deficits, but its focus is to reduce problem behavior. Boyajian, DuPaul, Handler, Eckert, and McGoey (2001), for example, reduced levels of aggression maintained by positive reinforcement in the form of access to toys for one child from 98 per hour to zero by providing the same reinforcer only when the child engaged in appropriate requests. Broussard and Northup (1997) demonstrated that access to peer attention for the absence of misbehavior (i.e., DRO) is effective in reducing problem behavior maintained by peer comments and disapproval.

Sometimes it is useful to create a new contingency that successfully "competes" with existing contingencies. For example, token economies or other classroom-based reward systems do not specifically address behavioral function but may promote a more appropriate alternative response, while indirectly limiting access to those antecedents and consequences that maintain problem behavior. Stern, Fowler, and Kohler (1988) provided evidence that teaching a new skill may effectively reduce problem behavior. Two children with high levels of off-task and disruptive behavior were assigned the role of peer monitor. Their duties were to evaluate the behavior and work of a peer and to award points according to criteria. Immediate and dramatic decreases in problem behavior were observed and were equal to conditions in which these same children earned points themselves. Either condition is an example of differential positive reinforcement. As point earner, appropriate behavior was reinforced with feedback and points. As peer monitor, a completely *new* skill emerged that was *incompatible* with the problem behavior: It is not possible to carefully evaluate another's work while also engaging in disruptive behavior.

Extinction

It is also possible to reduce performance excesses by withholding the source of reinforcement. This strategy is rarely used in isolation, due to the possibility that problem behavior may escalate, at least initially, to intolerable levels or intensities. Umbreit (1995) used extinction of peer attention to reduce levels of disruptive behavior exhibited in a classroom setting by an 8-year-old boy with ADHD. A brief functional analysis indicated that the child's problem behaviors were maintained by peer attention, which was removed by changing seating arrangements so that the child was working alone or with peers who ignored his misbehavior. Reductions in disruptive behavior across several settings were immediate and dramatic.

Extinction of negative reinforcement is also possible. Taylor and Miller (1997) evaluated a time-out procedure targeting the disruptive behavior of four children with developmental disabilities but found that the strategy actually increased problem behavior for two of the children. An experimental analysis indicated that the problem behavior of these two children was maintained by escape from tasks, so that time-out actually *increased* disruptive behavior through negative reinforcement. Thus the teaching staff provided escape extinction, which involved manually prompting the child to engage in work so that disruptive behavior no longer resulted in escape from task demands. Results indicated that the strategy was effective in reducing problem behavior to zero rates.

Positive Punishment

To this point, all interventions have been linked to the suspected variables that maintain skills and performance. It is possible, however, to reduce problem behavior by using interventions that are irrelevant to the function of behavior, such as punishment. There are certainly risks involved in aversive control procedures (Iwata et al., 1990): Punishment may produce emotional responses such as withdrawal or aggression and does not directly teach or strengthen alternative responses. Punishment is, however, an intervention that has successfully been used and must be presented in any discussion of behavior change. Positive punishment occurs when an aversive event is presented contingent on the occurrence of behavior and weakens future performance (frequency, duration, intensity) of that behavior. Redirection, writing lines, and spanking are common examples of positive punishment *if these consequences reduce performance.* Punishment is defined by its actual, rather than intended, impact, and it is possible that many consequences such as reprimands or scoldings may inadvertently increase problem behavior maintained by teacher attention.

An example of positive punishment is provided by Sandler, Arnold, Gable, and Strain (1987). A peer confrontation procedure was initiated for three children with high rates of disruptive behavior. Peers were taught to respond to problem behavior by telling the target student the problem, why it is a problem, and what to do to solve the problem. For all three children, rates of disruptive behavior were reduced in response to peer confrontations. Using a milder strategy, Lobitz (1974) provided a demonstration that a visual prompt or cue may function as positive punishment. In this study, a red light was illuminated whenever two target children violated specified classroom rules. Observations indicated that the problem behavior of both children was reduced dramatically by the strategy. Despite no programmed consequences associated with the red light, the author hypothesized that the public display probably acquired aversive properties because it signified, to the child and to the entire class, that misbehavior had occurred.

Negative Punishment

Negative punishment occurs when an event is withdrawn contingent on the occurrence of behavior and weakens performance (frequency, duration, intensity) of that behavior. Time-out, fines, and removing privileges are common examples of negative punishment *if these consequences reduce performance.* The term *negative* may seem redundant when used to describe punishment, just as *positive* punishment may be viewed as a contradiction. As was the case with reinforcement, both terms refer to the same effect. In this case, however, the effect is a reduction in performance that is occasioned by either the removal of a desired event (negative punishment) or the application of an undesirable event (positive punishment). Once again, the importance of an FBA deserves mention, as it is possible that many consequences commonly used in schools, such as taking away recess or placing a child in time-out, may inadvertently increase problem behavior maintained by escape from work (Taylor & Miller, 1997).

One of the most common examples of negative punishment is a response-cost procedure. Response cost involves providing a child with tokens (or points) that can be exchanged at a later time for positive rewards. Contingent on problem behavior, the child loses one of these tokens. Reynolds and Kelley (1997) used a response-cost system with two preschool children that involved removing one smiley face from a chart each time aggressive behavior occurred; all remaining smiley faces were exchanged for rewards. The program effectively reduced the target behaviors, and both teachers and children rated the strategy as highly acceptable.

Step 6: Evaluate Interventions

The final step in FBA is to evaluate interventions designed to address the function of target behaviors. The ultimate purpose of conducting an FBA is to improve student outcomes, and this is accomplished by implementing a positive behavior support plan that features one or more interventions that address skill deficits, performance deficits, and performance excesses. The impact of behavior plans in nonresearch settings is typically evaluated through A–B "accountability" designs, with the first phase representing baseline and the next phase representing the sustained implementation of a treatment plan. The impact of interventions is typically evaluated through visual inspection of changes in level, variability, and trend between baseline and treatment phases. Visual inspection not only allows teams to evaluate treatment effects but may also be used as final confirmation of an FBA.

The relationship between indirect assessment, descriptive analysis, and experimental analyses is unknown and probably will stay that way. Although studies comparing the different methods have produced mixed results, their relationship in actual practice is complementary rather than competitive. As mentioned earlier, each method is used to systematically converge on a handful of hypotheses for a particular individual and setting. Thus each method is validated by the next and, ultimately, by the patterns of responding observed during treatment evaluation. Figure 12.2 displays the patterns of responding typically associated with skill deficits, performance deficits, and performance excesses when treatments are matched to the type of problem. If observations across varied settings and times during baseline reveal relatively low and stable patterns, the problem is likely to be a skill deficit (top panel). In response to a skills-based treatment, a gradually increasing slope will occur as steps in the skill are mastered and fluency is increased. In the case of a performance deficit (middle panel), responding will be highly variable during baseline, indicating that performance is associated with motivating variables that occur in some environments but not others. A treatment matched to this problem, such as differential reinforcement of the desired performance, will result in abrupt and relatively stable increases in responding. A performance excess (bottom panel) is also likely to be variable during baseline, because performance is a function of antecedents and consequences common to some, but not all, natural conditions. A treatment matched to the behavioral function, such as altering establishing operations, will result in abrupt and relatively stable decreases in responding.

Conclusions

Since FBA became law, its application to mainstream educational policy and practice has been a major topic of research, reviews, and textbooks. Although most research has focused on performance excesses, this chapter extends functional assessment to behavioral skill and performance deficits as well, thus highlighting its broader contribution to school-based positive behavior supports

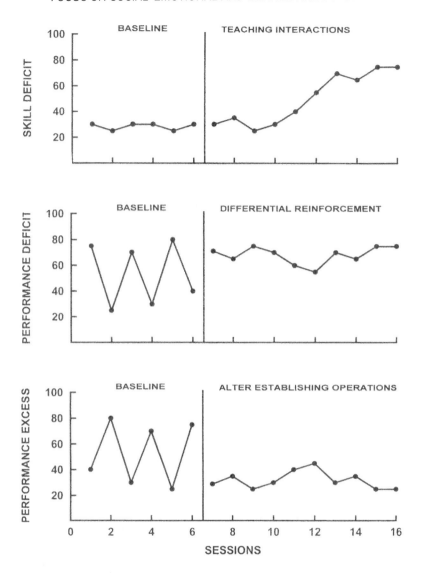

FIGURE 12.2. Patterns of response to intervention for skill deficits, performance deficits, and performance excesses.

(PBS) systems. In this chapter, a model is presented for matching the type of problem and its function to one of seven interventions. This simple model is intended to clarify the conceptual link between behavioral function and behavioral solutions. By "mapping out" data-based decision making, it may make the goal of team fluency in problem solving and confidence in intervention services more achievable (Barnett, VanDerHeyden, & Witt, 2007).

The seven interventions account for the most basic behavior change processes, and

thus this model is limited in scope to an analysis of behavior, rather than an analysis of interventions. In actual school settings, there are other, equally important dimensions of professional services that include, for example, methods to establish the most socially valid response requirements, designs for evaluating multiple treatment components, and strategies for promoting generalized outcomes. In retrospect, an analysis of behavior change is only one of seven tools needed to conduct an applied behavior analysis (Baer et al., 1968). One hundred more would be nice, and might make certain jobs easier or faster, but just one fewer would leave a school psychologist with no solution to at least one common type of service delivery problem.

References

Baer, D. M., Wolf, M. M., & Risley T. R. (1968). Some current dimensions of applied behavior analysis. *Journal of Applied Behavior Analysis, 1*, 91–97.

Barnett, D. W., VanDerHeyden, A. M., & Witt, J. C. (2007). Achieving science-based practice through response to intervention: What it might look like in preschools. *Journal of Educational and Psychological Consultation, 17*, 31–54.

Biglan, A. (2004). Contextualism and the development of effective prevention practices. *Prevention Science, 5*, 15–21.

Billington, E. J., Skinner, C. H., & Cruchon, N. M. (2004). Improving sixth-grade students' perceptions of high-effort assignments by assigning more work: Interaction of additive interspersal and assignment effort on assignment choice. *Journal of School Psychology, 14*, 89–103.

Boyajian, A. E., DuPaul, G. J., Handler, M. W., Eckert, T. L., & McGoey, K. E. (2001). The use of classroom-based brief functional analysis with preschoolers at-risk for attention-deficit/hyperactivity disorder. *School Psychology Review, 30*, 278–293.

Broussard, C., & Northup, J. (1997). The use of functional analysis to develop peer interventions for disruptive classroom behavior. *School Psychology Quarterly, 12*, 65–76.

Carr, E. G. (1977). The motivation of self-injurious behavior: A review of some hypotheses. *Psychological Bulletin, 84*, 800–816.

Chafouleas, S. M., McDougal, J. L., Riley-Tillman, T. C., Panahon, C. J., & Hilt, A. M. (2005). What do daily behavior report cards (DBRCs) measure? An initial comparison of DBRCs with direct observation for off-task behavior. *Psychology in the Schools, 42*(6) 669–676.

Colton, D. L., & Sheridan, S. M. (1998). Conjoint behavioral consultation and social skills training: Enhancing play behaviors of boys with attention-deficit/hyperactivity disorder. *Journal of Educational and Psychological Consultation, 9*, 3–28.

Conroy, M. A., & Stichter, J. P. (2003). The application of antecedents in the functional assessment process: Existing research, issues, and recommendations. *Journal of Special Education, 37*, 15–25.

Deci, E. L. (1975). *Intrinsic motivation.* New York: Plenum Press.

Dowd, T., & Tierney, J. (2005). *Teaching social skills to youth* (2nd ed.). Boys Town, NE: Boys Town Press.

Doyle, P. D., Jenson, W. R., Clark, E., & Gates, G. (1999). Free time and dots as negative reinforcement to improve academic completion and accuracy for mildly disabled students. *Proven Practice, 2*, 10–15.

Ducharme, J. M., & DiAdamo, C. (2005). An errorless approach to management of child noncompliance in a special education setting. *School Psychology Review, 34*, 107–115.

Ervin, R. A., Miller, P. M., & Friman, P. C. (1996). Feed the hungry bee: Using positive peer reports to improve the social interactions and acceptance of a socially rejected girl in residential care. *Journal of Applied Behavior Analysis, 29*, 251–253.

Ervin, R. A., Radford, P. M., Bertsch, K., Piper, A. L., Ehrhardt, K. E., & Poling, A. (2001). A descriptive analysis and critique of the empirical literature on school-based functional assessment. *School Psychology Review, 30*, 193–210.

Gortmaker, V. J., Warnes, E. D., & Sheridan, S. M. (2004). Conjoint behavioral consultation: Involving parents and teachers in the treatment of a child with selective mutism. *Proven Practice, 5*, 66–72.

Hamlet, C. C., Axelrod, S., & Kuerschner, S. (1984). Eye contact as an antecedent to compliant behavior. *Journal of Behavior Analysis, 17*, 553–557.

Hayes, S. C., & Wilson, K. G. (1995). The role of cognition in complex human behavior: A contextualistic perspective. *Journal of Behavior Therapy and Experimental Psychiatry, 26*, 241–248.

Iwata, B., Dorsey, M., Slifer, K., Bauman, K., & Richman, B. (1982). Toward a functional analysis of self-injury. *Analysis and Intervention of Developmental Disabilities, 2*, 3–20.

Iwata, B. A., Vollmer, T. R., & Zarcone, J. R. (1990). The experimental (functional) analysis of behavior disorders: Methodology, applications, and limitations. In A. C. Repp & N. N. Singh (Eds.), *Perspectives in nonaversive and aversive interventions with developmentally disabled persons* (pp. 301–330). Sycamore, IL: Sycamore.

Jones, K. M., Drew, H. A., & Weber, N. L. (2000). Noncontingent peer attention as treatment for disruptive classroom behavior. *Journal of Applied Behavior Analysis, 33*, 343–346.

Kearney, C. A., & Silverman, W. K. (1990). A preliminary analysis of a functional model of assessment and treatment for school refusal behavior. *Behavior Modification, 14*, 340–366.

Kratochwill, T. R., & Bergan, J. R. (1990). *Behavioral consultation in applied settings: An individual guide*. New York: Plenum.

Larson, P. J., & Maag, J. W. (1998). Applying functional assessment in general education classrooms: Issues and recommendations. *Remedial and Special Education, 19,* 338–349.

Lerman, D. C., & Iwata, B. A. (1993). Descriptive and experimental analysis of variables maintaining self-injurious behavior. *Journal of Applied Behavior Analysis, 26,* 293–319.

Lobitz, W. C. (1974). A simple stimulus cue for controlling disruptive classroom behavior. *Journal of Abnormal Child Psychology, 2,* 143–152.

Michael, J. (1982). Distinguishing between the discriminative and motivational functions of stimuli. *Journal of the Experimental Analysis of Behavior, 37,* 149–155.

Moore, L. A., Waguespack, A. M., Wickstrom, K. F., Witt, J. C., & Gaydos, G. R. (1994). Mystery motivator: An effective and time-efficient intervention. *School Psychology Review, 23,* 106–118.

Northup, J., & Gulley, V. (2001). Some contributions of functional analysis to the assessment of behaviors associated with attention-deficit/hyperactivity disorder and the effects of stimulant medication. *School Psychology Review, 30,* 227–238.

Powell, S., & Nelson, B. (1997). Effects of choosing academic assignments on a student with attention-deficit/hyperactivity disorder. *Journal of Applied Behavior Analysis, 30,* 181–183.

Reschly, D. J., Tilly, W. D. III, & Grimes, J. P. (Eds.). (1999). *Special education in transition: Functional assessment and noncategorical programming*. Longmont, CO: Sopris West.

Reynolds, L. K., & Kelley, M. L. (1997). The efficacy of a response cost-based treatment package for managing aggressive behaviors in preschoolers. *Behavior Modification, 21,* 216–230.

Rhode, G. R., Jenson, W. J., & Reavis, H. K. (1992). *The tough kid book*. Longmont, CO: Sopris West.

Roberts, M. L., Marshall, J., Nelson, J. R., & Albers, C. A. (2001). Curriculum-based assessment procedures embedded within functional behavioral assessments: Identifying escape-motivated behaviors in a general education classroom. *School Psychology Review, 30,* 264–277.

Sandler, A. G., Arnold, L. B., Gable, R. A., & Strain, P. S. (1987). Effects of peer pressure on disruptive behavior of behaviorally disordered classmates. *Behavioral Disorders, 12,* 104–110.

Shapiro, E. S., & Heick, P. F. (2004). School psychologist assessment practices in the evaluation of students referred for social/behavioral/emotional problems. *Psychology in the Schools, 41,* 551–561.

Simon, P. (1976). "*50 ways to leave your lover.*" On *Still Crazy After All These Years* [CD]. Warner Bros.

Skinner, B. F. (1953). *Science and human behavior*. New York: Macmillan.

Stern, G. W., Fowler, S. A., & Kohler, F. W. (1988). A comparison of two intervention roles: Peer monitor and point earner. *Journal of Applied Behavior Analysis, 21,* 103–109.

Sugai, G., Horner, R. H., Dunlap, G., Heineman, M., Lewis, T. J., Nelson, et al. (2000). Applying positive behavior support and functional behavioral assessment in schools. *Journal of Positive Behavior Interventions, 2,* 131–143.

Swiezy, N. B., Matson, J. L., & Box, P. (1992). The good behavior game: A token reinforcement system for preschoolers. *Child and Family Behavior Therapy, 14,* 21–32.

Taylor, J., & Miller, M. (1997). When timeout works some of the time: The importance of treatment integrity and functional assessment. *School Psychology Quarterly, 12,* 4–22.

Thomas, A., & Grimes, J. (Eds.). (2008). *Best practices in school psychology* (5th ed.). Bethesda, MD: National Association of School Psychologists.

Tilly, W. D. III. (2008). The evolution of school psychology to science-based practice: Problem solving and the three-tiered model. In A. Thomas & J. Grimes (Eds.), *Best practices in school psychology* (4th ed., pp. 17–36). Bethesda, MD: National Association of School Psychologists.

Touchette, P. E., MacDonald, R. F., & Langer, S. N. (1985). A scatter plot for identifying stimulus control of problem behavior. *Journal of Applied Behavior Analysis, 18,* 343–351.

Umbreit, J. (1995). Functional assessment and intervention in a regular classroom setting for the disruptive behavior of a student with attention-deficit/hyperactivity disorder. *Behavioral Disorders, 20,* 267–278.

Watson, T. S., & Steege, M. W. (2003). *Conducting school-based functional behavioral assessment: A practitioner's guide*. New York: Guilford Press.

Weber, K. P., Killu, K., Derby, K. M., & Barreto, A. (2005). The status of functional behavioral assessment (FBA): Adherence to standard practice in FBA methodology. *Psychology in the Schools, 42,* 737–744.

Witt, J. C., Daly, E. M., & Noell, G. (2000). *Functional assessments: A step-by-step guide to solving academic and behavioral problems*. Longmont, CO: Sopris West.

PART IV

IMPLEMENTING PREVENTION AND INTERVENTION STRATEGIES

Chapter 13

Guidelines for Evidence-Based Practice in Selecting Interventions

Karen Callan Stoiber
Jennifer L. DeSmet

Perhaps one of the most critical functions that school psychologists and other mental health practitioners perform is the selection of effective interventions. School psychologists typically are involved in selecting interventions as part of their key service delivery practices, including assessment, consultation, prevention, and therapeutic practices. Interventions refer to programs, products, practices, or policies intended to increase the skills, competencies, or outcomes in targeted areas (What Works Clearinghouse, 2007). The need for school-based interventions is demonstrated, at least in part, by prevalence data on children's mental health and learning difficulties. Approximately 15–20% of all school-age youths (or 15 million children) exhibit developmental, emotional, or problem behaviors requiring psychosocial intervention, with many more at risk for problems having long-term individual and societal consequences (President's New Freedom Commission on Mental Health, 2003). In addition, nearly 3 million U.S. students ages 6–21 years have diagnosed learning disabilities (U.S. Department of Education, 2004). The high prevalence of children's behavioral and learning disorders is exacerbated by the number of youths who do not receive the treatment they need. For example, in a given year, only 20–30% of those children with recognized behavioral disorders receive mental health care. This scenario worsens for youths from low-income families, those in the juvenile justice system, and those with substance abuse problems, as well as ethnic minority youths (Masi & Cooper, 2006).

The types of difficulties encountered by many children and adolescents are diverse and stem from a broad array of factors, such as poverty, victimization, limited social competencies, and poor motivation. Such issues often have a ripple effect in the school context because they can potentially lead to heightened levels of disruptive behavior, anxiety, risk-taking behavior, suicide, and other emotional vulnerabilities (U.S. Public Health Service, 2001). Fortunately, when schools provide prevention- and intervention-focused school-based psychological service delivery, the critical mental health and behavioral needs of their students can be addressed. However, the quality of school-based mental health services often hinges on the capacity of school psychologists and other key mental health providers (e.g., social workers, counselors) to select appropriate interventions.

Despite the pivotal role of intervention selection in school-based mental health and special needs service delivery, the field of school psychology continues to grapple with how to best facilitate the application of research-based evidence to everyday practice with real students in real schools. One of the first barriers is to address the practice gap regarding what school psychologists value and what they do on a daily basis. In a recent study, school psychologists working in an urban district indicated prevention and intervention as the most valued activities and ones for which they most desired professional development, yet they rated traditional assessment as their most predominant activity (Stoiber & Vanderwood, 2008). In addition, several authors have argued that a viable research-to-practice agenda needs to reflect the diverse ecological and complex qualities of schools, ones that often cannot be captured through the use of "traditional" laboratory-like procedures and methodologies (Meyers, Meyers, & Grogg, 2004; Stoiber, 2002; Stoiber & Kratochwill, 2000; Stoiber

& Waas, 2002). The multiple factors and reasons for youths' psychosocial and educational difficulties make the task of selecting and implementing interventions more complex. In light of the complexities surrounding both school contexts and providing services for children with difficulties, we have created a framework for understanding and implementing effective intervention service delivery within a social–ecological model (as illustrated in Figure 13.1).

In this model, the knowledge, skills, understandings, and decision making of school-based practitioners interface with resources available in the school. These distal and proximal socioeconomic–cultural factors vary in the degree to which they affect the ways interventions are selected and applied, both at the individual and systems levels. At a proximal level, school psychologists typically hold a direct role in intervention selection. However, other influences, such as the child's family and teachers, educational philosophies and values, and community–district–school resources all can affect how an intervention is derived and whether it is applied effectively. For example, teacher acceptance and commitment to a program

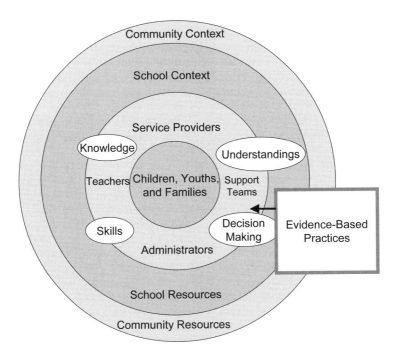

FIGURE 13.1. Model of contextual factors that affect evidence-based practices.

or an intervention strategy, as well as site-based administrative support, are among the most potent determiners of high-quality and sustained use of evidence-based practices (Gettinger & Stoiber, 2006; Kratochwill & Hoagwood, 2006). In applying research-based interventions to the real world of schools, it is useful to examine which features of intervention studies are necessary for the designation of "evidence-based." Various sources and types of evidence can be drawn on when selecting interventions; thus it is important to determine the features of the research base, as well as the resulting evidence, that matter most.

The role of science, or research, is to inform educational policy and practices. Intervention research has been evident since the early 1900s; however, interest in translating research findings into effective instructional and intervention practices has been particularly invigorated with the evidence-based practice (EBP) movement in the United States, Canada, the United Kingdom, Australia, and other countries (see American Psychological Association Presidential Task Force on Evidence-Based Practice, 2006; Gibbs, 2002; Kratochwill, 2006; Kratochwill & Stoiber, 2000; Shavelson & Towne, 2002; Stoiber & Kratochwill, 2000; Stoiber & Waas, 2002). Although there were virtually no citations in Medline or PsycINFO on EBP between 1900 and 1995, there has been a marked rise in citations since 1995 (Hoagwood & Johnson, 2003).

Evidence-Based Standards and Criteria for Evaluating Intervention Research Studies

One of the most significant activities related to the evidence-based practices movement is that various professional groups within the field of psychology, including school psychology, have developed criteria and published information regarding evidence-based interventions (e.g., see Kratochwill & Stoiber, 2002; Lonigan, Elbert, & Johnson, 1998; Masia-Warner, Nangle, & Hansen, 2006). The American Psychological Association has approved and posted criteria for evaluating treatment standards or guidelines (*www.apa.org/practice/guidelines/treatcrit.html*). A major task related to the evidence-based practice movement in school psychology has

been the construction of a manual (Kratochwill & Stoiber, 2002), titled *Procedural and Coding Manual for the Review of Evidence-Based Interventions* (hereafter called the *Procedural and Coding Manual*). The purpose of the *Procedural and Coding Manual* is to describe the procedures developed by the Task Force on Evidence-Based Interventions in School Psychology (Kratochwill & Stoiber, 2002) to identify, review, and code studies of psychological and educational interventions for various academic, social–emotional, and health and mental health concerns experienced by school-age children and their families. In addition, other groups, such as the Promising Practices Network (*www.promisingpractices.net*) and the federally funded initiative What Works Clearinghouse (WWC; *www.whatworks.ed.gov*), have followed the initiatives established in the fields of medicine, such as the University of Oxford's Centre for Evidence-Based Medicine (*www.cebm.net*), and psychology (Nathan, 1998; Weisz & Hawley, 1999). For example, WWC has begun the process of reviewing academic and behavioral programs for implementation in the schools; evidence ratings on the level of research to support practices on a variety of topics (e.g., dropout prevention, reducing behavior problems in the elementary school classroom, improving adolescent literacy, effective literacy and English language instruction for English learners) are available at the WWC website. Several books also have been published on evidence-based interventions and treatments for children and adolescents (e.g., Barrett & Ollendick, 2004; Burns & Hoagwood, 2005; Kazdin & Weisz, 2003).

The purpose of evidence-based practice guidelines that have been developed by various professional organizations is to educate mental health and health-care professionals, including school psychologists, in criteria that should be considered for evaluating interventions and to promote their implementation of effective practices. One of the major assumptions or rationales for establishing evidence-based practice guidelines is that they will help standardize treatment approaches and reduce practice variation. In general, evaluations of the evidence base supporting an intervention focus on whether reliable and valid methods were applied and whether the intervention led to successful outcomes. Such review efforts have been based on criteria used for the designation of "evidence-based." Another way to think about such guidelines is that they help individuals determine how well a particular intervention works through the process of systematically finding, appraising, and using research findings as the basis for selecting and implementing interventions.

Interestingly, most review efforts aimed at establishing "evidence-based interventions" have placed an emphasis on outcomes stemming from multiple studies involving randomized controlled trials, or RCTs, as "evidence" (Weisz, Jensen-Doss, & Hawley, 2006). That is, RCTs are viewed as the "gold standard" in substantiating that a treatment is efficacious or proven to work. As the name suggests, RCTs involve the random allocation (or assignment) of participants to different interventions or treatment conditions. RCTs are the scientific standard for drawing causal inferences about the effects of interventions. It is important to resist concluding, however, that those interventions not yet studied in controlled trials are ineffective. Instead, these should simply be considered as untested to date (American Psychological Association Presidential Task Force, 2006). The term *treatment efficacy* denoted the effects of a given intervention compared with either no treatment or an alternative intervention in a controlled clinical context. The primary purpose of evaluating efficacy is to document whether a beneficial effect of the intervention can be demonstrated scientifically. In addition, multiple research designs can be useful in developing evidence-based practice guidelines, with different research designs viewed as appropriate for different research questions. Greenberg and Newman (1996) offer some of the following uses for various research designs:

- Clinical observation, including individual case studies, to provide unique sources of innovation and scientific discovery regarding hypotheses
- Qualitative research for descriptive purposes (e.g., how an individual responds to an intervention strategy)
- Systematic case studies to compare one set of individuals with another with similar characteristics

- Single-participant experimental designs to establish causal relationships as they occur within an individual
- Public health and ethnographic research to examine treatment availability, utilization, and acceptance
- Field-based effectiveness research to assess the ecological validity and application of interventions
- Meta-analysis to synthesize results from multiple studies, test hypotheses, and measure quantitatively the size of effects.

Evidence from all of these types of research is important for developing conclusions about the effectiveness of intervention practices. In general, however, the more sophisticated research methodologies, including quasi experiments and randomized controlled studies and their equivalent, are viewed as a more stringent way to evaluate specific interventions. That is, the degree of contribution to conclusions about efficacy is linked to the type of research in ascending order, starting with clinical observation and consensus among recognized experts and moving up a hierarchical ladder to RCTs, which are most powerful because they rule out threats to internal validity in a single experiment.

In addition to the features of RCTs (which within the educational setting typically means including at least one experimental treatment group and one control group), an extensive set of research criteria has been considered pertinent in evaluating the effectiveness of an intervention. A brief description of categories of criteria, along with the reasons for their inclusion, follows. For the purposes of conceptual clarity, the criteria are grouped into four sets. These sets of criteria or guidelines for evaluating research evidence do not reflect all of the possible criteria that may be considered, nor the possible organizing schemes to categorize them. For example, the American Psychological Association (2002) has endorsed 21 different types of criteria, with some criteria having five or more subcriteria. Using the American Psychological Association guidelines (2002), 68 criteria must be considered in evaluating an intervention. Such a large number of criteria may present more details than most practitioners have the time or desire to examine.

Guidelines and Criteria
for Examining Research Support

Table 13.1 presents four categories or sets of considerations that are recommended to examine the evidence base to support a prevention or intervention program or strategy. The four categories are: scientific basics, key features, clinical utility aspects, and feasibility and cost-effectiveness. These categories correspond closely to those established by the School Psychology Task Force on Evidence-Based Interventions (Kratochwill & Stoiber, 2002) and reflect the belief that good guidelines for selecting interventions should be flexible and sensitive to realities of schools and school-based practice (Stoiber, Lewis-Snyder, & Miller, 2005). Scientifically mindful practitioners should consider not only these guidelines but also, to maximize their effectiveness, should take into consideration their own characteristics and the unique characteristics of the individual student or system within which they are working. Intervention success does not hinge solely on qualities of the intervention. Rather, intervention success is most likely to occur when comixed with a strong therapeutic relationship and a mutual expectation for positive change between the practitioner and the individual(s) targeted in the intervention. Such a position is apparent in the American Psychological Association Policy Statement of Evidence-Based Practice in Psychology (EBPP),[1] which was approved as policy by the American Psychological Association's Council of Representatives during its August 2005 meeting (American Psychological Association, 2006):

> Evidence-based practice in psychology (EBPP) is the integration of the best available research with clinical expertise in the context of patient characteristics, culture, and preferences.[2] ... Psychological services are most effective when responsive to the patient's specific problems, strengths, personality, sociocultural context, and preferences. Many patient characteristics, such as functional status, readiness to change, and level of social support, are known to be related to therapeutic outcomes. ... Some effective treatments involve interventions directed toward others in the patient's environment, such as parents, teachers, and caregivers. A central goal of EBPP is to maximize patient

choice among effective alternative interventions. (p. 284)

Given these parameters for evidence-based practice and those set forth by the School Psychology Task Force on Evidence-Based Interventions (Kratochwill & Stoiber, 2002), the following four sets of criteria are intended to provide an organizational framework for (1) examining intervention research qualities and (2) selecting evidence-based interventions and/or practices for application within school settings. In general, due to the extensive nature of criteria, more than one study is usually needed to confirm that a prevention or intervention program meets the highest criteria of being "evidence based." That is, a prevention or intervention program can be rated on a scale ranging from strong to weak evidence. Based on such a rubric, evidence ratings would be based on the following research support:

1. Strong support: several high-quality studies with consistent results (i.e., further research is very unlikely to change reported outcomes) or one multiple-site high-quality study
2. Moderate support: Either one high-quality study or several studies with some limitations
3. Low or no support: indicated by (a) several studies with severe limitations, (b) expert opinion, (c) no direct research evidence (see, e.g., the Institute of Education Science levels of evidence at *www. ies.ed.gov.ncee/wwc*).

Many education and psychology researchers agree, however, that much of the most advanced research (such as studies incorporating RCTs) that is available to synthesize findings does not address some of the most important issues being faced in real-world educational settings (American Psychological Association, 2006; Stoiber & Kratochwill, 2000). In situations in which available research is limited, it is especially helpful for researchers and practitioners to be knowledgeable about the guidelines presented in this chapter for evaluating and selecting prevention or intervention programs or strategies. With knowledge of the guidelines presented in this chapter, real-world practi-

TABLE 13.1. Evidence-Based Indicators for Evaluating Prevention and Intervention Studies

Indicator	Example of evidence to consider
I. Scientific basics—general characteristics	
Empirical/theoretical basis	• Empirical studies underlie basis of intervention • Theoretical basis of intervention provided
General design characteristics	• Randomized control group (experimental) or quasi-experimental design • Pre- and post-intervention assessment • Length of intervention specified • Treatment integrity assessed
Statistical treatment/data analysis	• Appropriate use of statistical methods • Sufficient sample size to measure effects (e.g., 30 in both treatment and comparison group)
Type of intervention program	• Target of program or strategy (e.g., risk prevention, family support, parent education)
Outcome improved	• Outcome improved (e.g., academic, mental health, or behavioral improvement)
II. Key features	
Internal validity controls	• Control threats to internal validity (e.g., maturation or development of participants, history, statistical regression)
Measurement procedures	• Appropriate assessment procedures • Psychometrically sound measures
Comparison group	• Type of comparison group (no treatment, wait-list only, alternative treatment) • Participant matching • Equivalent dropout rate
Primary/secondary outcomes are statistically significant	• At least one outcome is statistically significant at .05 level
Educational/clinical/cultural significance	• Results indicate actual benefit to the target group
Identifiable intervention components	• Information indicating which intervention components produced which outcomes
Implementation fidelity/ integrity	• Demonstration of procedures measuring and documenting that intervention was implemented as expected
Follow-up assessment conducted	• Assessed outcomes beyond the implementation period (e.g., 6 months, 1 year) • Evidence of durability of effects
III. Clinical utility aspects	
Participant factors	• Random selection of participants • Diversity of participants • Age/development of participants (e.g., disability status) • Gender of participants • Social–economic status
Characteristics of site of implementation	• Type of setting (clinic, school) • Type of community locale • Applicability to school setting or real-world educational context

(cont.)

TABLE 13.1. *(cont.)*

Indicator	Example of evidence to consider
Length of intervention	• Reasonable length of intervention to demonstrate effects
Intensity/dosage	• Reasonable intensity and/or frequency of intervention • Specify sessions required for effects
Characteristics of the intervenor	• Training requirements and/or qualifications for intervenor • Specifications regarding ethnicity and gender
Replication	• Information provided regarding likelihood of replication
IV. Feasibility and cost-effectiveness	
Treatment acceptability	• Information on treatment acceptability (e.g., clients, implementers, parents)
Cost-analysis data	• Information on cost of implementation • Information on cost analysis per participant, classroom, or other unit
Training and support resources	• Cost of materials • Amount of training required • Amount of personnel support required
Context match and feasibility	• Match to actual school or educational setting or to available personnel

tioners can apply evidence-based criteria to select interventions that have not yet been reviewed by an expert panel or group.

The guidelines aim to assist readers in understanding (1) qualities and aspects of empirical research used to determine empirically supported principles and to determine whether a prevention or intervention program or strategy has a strong evidence base, (2) intervention program aspects to consider when selecting an intervention program or intervention strategies, and (3) research parameters that should be included when designing and conducting high-quality intervention studies. In this respect, the guidelines can assist both practitioners and researchers in making decisions using the best research evidence. There are multiple types of research evidence—such as efficacy, effectiveness, cost-effectiveness, treatment acceptability, and context generalizability—that can contribute to effective selection of intervention programs and practices (American Psychological Association, 2006). The process of determining whether a particular prevention or intervention program is research- or evidence-based might begin by reviewing individual studies based

on an established set of criteria, such as the four guidelines presented in this chapter. To examine the effects of a particular prevention or intervention program or strategy, the best available research (either a single study or multiple studies) is coded based on such criteria (see Kratochwill & Stoiber, 2002; Lewis-Snyder, Stoiber, & Kratochwill, 2002) to document its "evidence base."

As shown in Table 13.1, the first set of considerations used in evaluating intervention research relates to scientific basics—*the empirical/theoretical basis, general design qualities*, and *statistical treatment* of the prevention or intervention under review. These criteria provide a context for understanding what was done and why. The primary question is: Does the study seem relevant and purposeful in dealing with the area of concern? For example, an examination of the theoretical and/or empirical basis for a study may indicate theoretical evidence such as the role of cognitive-behavioral theory in procedures used to intervene with children who bully and have peer relations problems. The appropriate use of methodological and statistical procedures includes examining issues such as whether an appropriate unit of analysis is adopted, whether statistical error rate is controlled, and whether a sufficient sample size is recruited to test for effects.

The type of design employed is examined within the category of general design characteristics, including whether a randomized control group was employed. As randomized controlled experiments are not always feasible (or ethical) in the school environment, qualities of quasi experiments also should be examined. Quasi experiments do not involve random assignment of students to treatment conditions but include other qualities aimed at reducing threats to internal validity. In evaluating the study design, systematized clinical observation would be weighted more heavily than unsystematized observation methods; consensus or agreement in results among recognized experts would be more compelling than individual observation. Carefully controlled studies and appropriate methodology may include systematized clinical case studies and clinical replication series whereby an intervention is examined with a series of students who exhibit a similar disorder or problem behavior. It is important to note that even randomized controlled experiments are only definitive when all aspects of the design and methodology, including the population of study participants, are fully represented. Other general design considerations include whether the intervention occurred for a reasonable length of time and whether researchers measured treatment integrity (intervention implemented as intended). Statistical treatment also is considered in the first category of scientific basics. Here it is important to examine whether: (1) the researchers employed appropriate statistical methods, (2) the study included a sufficient sample size to measure effects, and (3) there were significant positive effects on appropriate outcomes (e.g., improved reading comprehension, school attendance, attitude toward school, compliance with teacher directions).

A second set of criteria, key features, incorporates a focus on *internal and construct validity criteria* (see Table 13.1). Internal validity occurs when a researcher controls all extraneous variables, or the "noise" influencing the results of a study. In this way he or she ensures that the variable being manipulated by the researcher is indeed the one affecting the results. Internal validity means

that one has evidence that the intervention treatment or program caused what one has observed (i.e., the outcome) to happen. Construct validity refers to whether what one observes was what one wanted to observe. Thus, whereas construct validity is relevant in most observational or descriptive studies, internal validity is not relevant in such studies. However, for studies that examine the effects of prevention or intervention programs, internal validity may present as a primary consideration. Internal validity is relevant for assessing interventions because it is desirable to be able to conclude that the program of interest made a difference (i.e., is the cause of observed results) as opposed to other possible causes. There are several threats to internal validity that researchers attempt to control, including: maturation of participants, testing, history, and statistical regression. One of the most difficult aspects to grasp about internal validity is that it is relevant only to the specific study in question.

The second set of criteria takes into consideration the treatment conditions being compared. First, a determination should be made as to whether the treatment group attained better results than "doing nothing," such as when an assessment-only or wait-list control group is used. Comparisons with "no treatment" inform us as to whether the intervention has efficacy and also whether it has adverse effects. The next level of comparison offers information as to whether there are qualities in the intervention that create change, and thus an alternative intervention is used. Incorporating an alternative intervention, such as a discussion group that does not employ active components, helps investigate whether positive results may be due to such features as a therapeutic relationship or may result from "nontherapeutic" components, such as focused time and attention. The strongest recommendations stem from results showing the intervention under consideration to be more effective than alternative interventions that are known to produce effective results (American Psychological Association Presidential Task Force, 2006).

Importantly, to discern whether positive effects are due to the intervention being evaluated, individuals in the no-treatment group or alternative-treatment group should be comparable or equivalent in demonstrating the same level of performance or problem area prior to treatment (often referred to as participant matching). In examining the equivalence of participants, one should also check for equivalent research dropout rates for participants. Other key study features related to internal and/or construct validity include: (1) whether key outcomes are statistically significant and ideally specify clinical significance (actual benefit to the target population); (2) identifiable components that indicate which aspects of the intervention produced which outcomes; (3) evidence of intervention fidelity or integrity; and (4) evidence of durability of effects. In examining indicators of internal and construct validity, clearly some types of problem behaviors or difficulties lend to well-controlled experiments better than others. In addition, short-term focused treatments can be researched more easily than longer term treatments aimed at more multifaceted concerns (American Psychological Association Presidential Task Force, 2006). Importantly, even an intervention that is well supported based on group-level results may not necessarily produce positive results for an individual student. Some students are simply more resistant to change. Also keep in mind that all intervention studies involve some level of subjective judgment, which influences decision making regarding who received the intervention, how the intervention was implemented, and the manner in which change was measured (American Psychological Association Presidential Task Force, 2006). Thus a study may result in statistically significant change but may not represent clinically significant change such that the type or level of change mattered (i.e., made a difference for an individual participant's functioning or mental health).

The third category of criteria for designating an evidence base includes information that consumers, including practitioners, should consider when evaluating the appropriateness of an intervention for their specific needs (see Table 13.1). These criteria address the *clinical utility* of a treatment (American Psychological Association Presidential Task Force, 2006). Clinical utility speaks to the acceptability of an intervention to stakeholders, as well as to the range of applicability. To examine the clinical utility of a study, it is useful to consider character-

istics typically known as external validity indicators. External validity refers to the likelihood of generalizability of effects to other treatment participants, other contexts, or other intervenors, regardless of the efficacy that may have been established in the research setting (American Psychological Association Presidential Task Force, 2006). To make a determination as to whether the intervention will likely produce positive effects in the actual context being considered, participants should be described in sufficient detail to permit other researchers and interventionists to determine both the conditions under which participants were drawn (e.g., whether they were selected randomly) and under which the intervention occurred to examine the likely generalizability to intended participants.

Information included within the third set of criteria address the question: To what extent is it likely that the intervention will be applied effectively in my particular school, or with a particular child, given the current surrounding conditions? Emphasis is placed on the importance of the intervention program being replicated across investigators and, in particular, across diverse participants as evidence for its use with minority youths and families. Examinations of clinical utility pose such specific questions as: What are the age, development, ethnic and cultural backgrounds of participants? How much training is required for interventionists to implement it? How many sessions are necessary for long-term change to occur? Intervenors who have developed a specialized skill set may be successful in producing outcomes, but other, less experienced professionals may not. Interventions that demonstrate efficacy with one ethnic, cultural, or linguistic group may not be equally appropriate and productive with a different group. Comas-Díaz (2006) found that culturally insensitive intervention approaches can lead intervenors to unknowingly select goals or embrace values that reflect the culture and background of the therapist rather than that of the child or family. Researchers have found that sound, evidence-based interventions are generally effective for ethnic minorities (Weisz et al., 2006), but that it is beneficial when treatment occurs in their native language and in a context that reflects the values of the minority group (Griner & Smith, 2006). As research is translated or applied for the purpose of selecting interventions, it is important for practitioners to consider particular aspects of the research study that suggest a good fit to their own particular circumstances. An examination of characteristics of the study permits practitioners to judge whether an intervention will produce intended outcomes for their targeted population.

Responses to questions regarding clinical utility do not easily fall into "Yes" or "No" categories or even ratings of the level of support (e.g., strong support, potential support, no support). Nevertheless, information regarding clinical utility will provide a fuller picture of whether and how an intervention worked, for whom, and under what conditions. In this regard, the third set of criteria may be the most useful for school psychologists working in educational contexts. The notion that "one size does not fit all" pertains to the expectation that student demographic factors play an important role in determining the clinical utility of an intervention. Although a particular intervention may have a strong evidence base, it may not be helpful for a particular student because the student does not have the necessary prerequisite cognitive or behavioral competencies to be responsive to it; or the child may live in a community with high rates of violence and crime, which, in turn, have an impact on the child's levels of resiliency and/or motivation to change. As another example, a child who experiences anxiety related to academic performance would likely require a different intervention and would be expected to respond differently from a child who is anxious and also experiences serious depression and social isolation. Thus the context of the child and surrounding factors and circumstances should be considered, including severity of the problem, comorbidity, and external stressors.

The fourth set of selection guidelines regards evidence for feasibility and cost-effectiveness across types of settings. Regardless of how effective an intervention is, if teachers, school psychologists, or other school-based service providers are reluctant or refuse to deliver an intervention, the evidence to support it does not hold much utility. Similarly, the level of training or clinical skill required to optimally perform the intervention may interfere with whether it is readily applied. Although the feasibility and cost-effectiveness criteria are especially relevant for schools during tight budgetary times, they should be separated from scientific evidence of the effectiveness of an intervention. In the real world of schools, costs related to implementing an intervention are typically explored and weighed in selecting an intervention. When costs become the primary consideration, they supersede other criteria. However, good guidelines take nonmonetary costs, such as reducing the need for special education and the stigma of having a disability or improving one's functional competence, into account.

The fourth set of guidelines is especially applicable for school-based providers, as researchers have found that approximately 70% of children with both a diagnosis and impaired functioning received services from the schools. Furthermore, the public schools emerged as the sole provider of mental health services for nearly half of children with severe emotional disturbance, and they are viewed as the primary provider of mental health services for children (Burns et al., 1995; Hoagwood & Erwin, 1997). Another issue regarding the need to select the most feasible intervention in the school setting is the lack of follow-through for outpatient treatment, with 40–60% of individuals who begin outpatient treatment attending only a few sessions (Harpaz-Rotem, Leslie, & Rosenheck, 2004). Factors that affect service utilization and whether treatment is continued include individual and family characteristics and satisfaction with the intervention (Weisz, Jensen-Doss, & Hawley, 2005). For example, poverty status has been associated with both the tendency to discontinue interventions and shorter duration of treatment. As a group, Hispanic/Latino and African American children are more likely to leave mental health services prematurely than are white children (Bui & Takeuchi, 1992). Families from various cultural backgrounds have been found to differ in the degree to which they view child emotional and behavioral difficulties as disturbed and as to whether these problems are likely to improve without professional therapeutic support (President's New Freedom Commission on Mental Health, 2003; Weisz et al., 2005). Thus efforts to promote continued involvement should focus on whether and how the intervention is responsive to the child's and the family's needs and expectations. For example, although several distinct types of intervention approaches have been shown to be effective in treating youths with disruptive or antisocial problems (e.g., multisystemic therapy [MST], functional family therapy [FFT], and multidimensional foster care), certain components of a treatment modality may fit better to a particular student and family than others (Chambers, Ringeisen, & Hickman, 2005; Stoiber, Ribar, & Waas, 2004). In this respect, school psychologists need to be aware of and sensitive to the research evidence base both for decision making in their own practices and in their referrals for outside intervention service delivery.

In summary, the four categories of criteria presented in this chapter are intended to provide both researchers and practitioners with a comprehensive, but not exhaustive, set of guidelines for designing and evaluating evidence-based interventions. The guidelines incorporate criteria that may be applied to examine whether a particular intervention program or strategy is empirically supported based on available research. However, as noted previously, evaluations of the evidence in support of an intervention program or strategy typically involve research evidence that has accrued from multiple studies, so as to evaluate such factors as generalizability, feasibility, and cost-effectiveness. The following section demonstrates the application of these suggested guidelines to evidence-based selection of interventions by comparing the types and levels of evidence for two intervention programs that target a similar issue and treatment population.

Applying Evidence-Based Criteria in Selecting Interventions

Two interventions designed to target externalizing behavior in children, parent–child interaction therapy (PCIT; Brinkmeyer & Eyberg, 2003) and the Incredible Years series (Webster-Stratton & Reid, 2003), are examined based on the four sets of criteria presented in Table 13.1. By applying these criteria, the two interventions are compared in terms of research support, along with other important features that may influence decision making when selecting interventions, including clinical utility features and feasibility and cost factors.

The PCIT program incorporates child-directed interaction (CDI) in its first phase, which is based on attachment theory and focuses on developing positive, nurturing interactions between parent and child (Herschell, Calzada, Eyberg, & McNeil, 2002). In the CDI stage, the parent is taught to engage in play led by the child, or nondirective play, while offering praise, reflecting the child's statements, imitating the child's play, describing the child's behavior, and being enthusiastic (Eyberg, 1988). The second stage of PCIT is parent-directed interaction (PDI), which is based on social learning theory (Eyberg et al., 2001). In this stage, parents are taught to ignore inappropriate behaviors and provide positive attention in response to their child's appropriate behavior (Eyberg, 1988).

PCIT involves two didactic training sessions whereby CDI and PDI are introduced to the parent through modeling (Eyberg, 1988), followed by weekly 1-hour sessions at which each parent interacts individually with the child in a playroom as he or she is observed through a one-way mirror by the therapist and the other parent. A bug-in-ear device is often used to provide the parent with immediate feedback and suggestions. At the end of each session, progress is discussed with parents. Homework involves practicing CDI and PDI daily, and treatment length is typically between 10 and 16 sessions (Herschell et al., 2002).

Research support for PCIT has been strong. One study demonstrated the superiority of PCIT to a wait-list control in reducing child problem behaviors, such that children in the treatment group were in the normal range on a measure of child problem behaviors following PCIT, whereas those in the wait-list group remained in the clinical range (Eyberg, Boggs, & Algina, 1995). In another study, a treatment group was compared with a group of normal classroom controls and a group of untreated deviant classroom controls (McNeil, Eyberg, Eisenstadt, Newcomb, & Funderburk, 1991). Not only did PCIT result in child improvements in home behavior following treatment, but also home improvements were related to school improvements. Finally, an independent research team replicated previous findings of the effectiveness of

PCIT, showing that children receiving PCIT demonstrated significant improvement over those in a wait-list control group and that treated children could not be distinguished from normal children at 6-month follow-up (Nixon, Sweeney, Erickson, & Touyz, 2003). PCIT has led to documented improvements in the quality of parent–child interactions (Eyberg et al., 1995; Hood & Eyberg, 2003), and parents report significantly lower levels of parental stress and significantly greater feelings of competence in parenting ability (Nixon et al., 2003).

Research has suggested that gains made by families throughout the course of PCIT are maintained over time. One study suggested that maternal ratings of posttreatment child behaviors strongly predicted child behaviors 3–6 years later (Hood & Eyberg, 2003). In this sample, three-fourths of children showing clinically significant improvement at posttreatment maintained these gains at follow-up. In a study of 1- or 2-year maintenance, children's behavior problems remained at posttreatment levels at follow-up according to maternal reports, and 54% of children continued to score in the normal range on measures of disruptive behaviors (Eyberg et al., 2001). In a study aimed at determining the maintenance of school effects at 12- and 18-month follow-ups, children were found to maintain posttreatment scores on problem behavior and compliance at 12 months (Funderburk et al., 1998). Although scores on compliance measures were maintained at 18 months, scores on all other school behavior measures fell toward pretreatment levels. Meanwhile, home behavior remained within normal limits. Overall, home gains are maintained over time, whereas school generalization was not maintained beyond 1 year.

The Incredible Years series is the second intervention that we review. The Incredible Years series was designed for parents and/ or teachers of high-risk children ages 2–10 years or children with behavioral problems. Incredible Years is based on the theoretical notion that a number of factors contribute to behavioral problems, including ineffective parenting, family factors, child risk factors, and school risk factors (Incredible Years, 2008; Webster-Stratton, 2001; Webster-Stratton & Reid, 2003). Early intervention is considered most effective because conduct

disorder becomes increasingly more difficult to treat over time.

The Incredible Years program includes parent, teacher, and child intervention components. All of the components utilize videotape modeling, role play, practice, and live feedback in training methods (Webster-Stratton & Reid, 2003). The purposes of the parent program are to improve parent–child relationships and parenting practices, to replace negative disciplinary strategies with more positive strategies, to improve parent problem-solving skills, to increase family support networks, to increase home–school collaboration, and to increase parent involvement in child academic activities (Webster-Stratton, 2001; Webster-Stratton & Reid, 2003). The parent programs include a BASIC–Early Childhood program (twelve to fourteen 2-hour weekly sessions targeting children 2–7 years), which is the core component, an ADVANCE (14 weeks targeting children 4–10 years), and a SCHOOL (4–6 sessions for children 5–10) program. The teacher training program uses the book *How to Promote Children's Social and Emotional Competence* (Webster-Stratton, 1999) and consists of a 32-hour workshop presented over four days. All parent programs are based on videotape vignettes and intended for groups of 8–12 parents. The child program is a 22-week program intended for groups of six children meeting for 2 hours per week.

Extensive outcome studies have been conducted on the parent, teacher, and child components of the Incredible Years program. Webster-Stratton and Reid (2003) reported that, when compared with a wait-list control group, the BASIC–Early Childhood parent training component resulted in significant improvements in parent attitudes and parent–child interactions and significant reductions in negative discipline strategies and child conduct problems. Other researchers compared mothers in the BASIC parent-training group with control mothers and found that the BASIC participants reported significantly fewer problem and negative behaviors in their children (Scott, Spender, Doolan, Jacobs, & Aspland, 2001; Taylor, Schmidt, Pepler, & Hodgins, 1998), In addition, a component analysis conducted by Webster-Stratton demonstrated that the combination of group discussion, trained therapist, and videotape modeling produced more lasting results than treatments that included only one of the components (Webster-Stratton & Reid, 2003). Further, Webster-Stratton and Reid (2003) reported that ADVANCE resulted in significantly more prosocial solutions to problems among children than did BASIC alone, and parents reported significantly greater consumer satisfaction than those receiving only BASIC.

The teacher training (TT) program resulted in teachers being significantly less critical, harsh, and inconsistent and significantly more nurturing than control teachers (Webster-Stratton, 2001). Another study demonstrated significantly higher parent–teacher bonding in experimental than in control classrooms (Webster-Stratton & Reid, 2003). Overall, the studies on the teacher program replicated the findings from the parent and child programs, and the teacher training resulted in improved classroom management skills. Teacher effects were maintained at 1-year follow-up (Webster-Stratton & Reid, 2003).

In studies examining the child training components, child training (CT) and parent training (PT) alone were compared with the combination of CT and PT, and all three treatment conditions (i.e., combined PT + CT + TT) were compared with a control group (Webster-Stratton & Reid, 2003). Treated children in all three groups displayed significantly improved behavior compared with the control group. CT and the combination child and parent training resulted in significant improvements in problem-solving and conflict-management skills. PT alone and in combination with CT resulted in significantly more positive interactions between parents and children than did CT alone. All significant changes were maintained at 1-year follow-up, and child conduct problems had significantly decreased over the period. However, the greatest reductions were noted for children in the combined child and parent training condition. Further, preliminary evidence suggests that the addition of the teacher training component to child and parent training may result in even greater change in conduct problems at home with parents and in school when compared with a control group and that only this combination (PT + CT + TT) of treatment resulted in significant change in children's social competence with

their peers (Webster-Stratton, Reid, & Hammond, 2004). However, because the effects of other program components (ADVANCE, CT, TT) were combined with the BASIC parent training component, no conclusions can be made with regard to the respective contributions of each component alone in altering participants' outcomes. Despite the lack of strong conclusions regarding some components of the Incredible Years series, a study by Beauchaine, Webster-Stratton, and Reid (2005) supports the effectiveness of the parent training component in treating children with early-onset conduct problems. Beauchaine et al. (2005) additionally reported that children's age and gender did not predict or moderate program outcomes.

The two interventions, PCIT and the Incredible Years series, target similar behaviors and incorporate components directed at both parents and children. Choosing between two similar interventions that address the same problem can be difficult. The four sets of guidelines are used to demonstrate some of the factors considered in intervention selection (see Table 13.2). First, it should be noted that both intervention programs have a strong theoretical base and that, although there are some differences, both emphasize behavioral principles, including increasing caregiver attention to positive behaviors and providing consequences for inappropriate behaviors. Studies examining effects for both programs have employed appropriate research designs and statistical procedures.

Second, in terms of internal validity considerations, both interventions have identifiable components and produced statistically significant key outcomes, and both interventions are manualized to promote adherence to a specified set of procedures. Further, both PCIT and Incredible Years have been compared with some type of control group and have been evaluated by independent research teams, thus strengthening their evidence base. However, whereas PCIT has been compared only with waiting-list control groups, component analyses have been conducted on the Incredible Years program by comparing the program as designed to a group discussion treatment component and a treatment involving exposure to the videotapes without a facilitator. Although the comparison to various components does not completely fulfill the requirement that the

TABLE 13.2. Application of Selection Criteria to Two Intervention Programs

Criteria	Subcriteria	Parent–child interaction therapy	Incredible Years series
Empirical and theoretical basis, general design qualities, statistical treatment	• Theoretical basis	• Attachment and social learning theories	• Multifactor
	• Statistical treatment	• Strong evidence	• Strong evidence
	• General design qualities	• Strong evidence	• Strong evidence
Internal and construct validity	• Treatment versus wait-list control	• Strong evidence	• Strong evidence
	• Treatment versus alternative treatment	• No	• Some evidence from component analysis
	• Statistically significant key outcomes	• Significant improvements in home and school behavior	• Significant improvements in home and school behavior
Clinical utility	• Diversity of participants	• Limited	• Limited
	• Training required for implementation	• Yes	• Yes
	• Applicability to school settings	• Potential	• Yes
Feasibility and cost-effectiveness	• Feasibility in school setting	• Potential	• Potential
	• Cost-effectiveness	• High cost	• Moderate cost

Incredible Years program be compared with other active treatments, it does provide evidence that the parent-training program and combined program (PT + CT + TT) are more effective than its other various components. Research on the benefits of PCIT program components has not been provided. Thus for the second set of criteria the evidence in support of the Incredible Years is slightly stronger.

The third set of criteria focuses on clinical utility and requires examining whether the sample children in efficacy studies have characteristics that compare to the demographics for one's particular circumstances. In this regard, the limited application of either program with ethnic minorities is noteworthy. Although there is evidence of the Incredible Years showing positive outcomes with at risk populations and with parents from more disadvantaged backgrounds (Reid, Webster-Stratton, & Baydar, 2004) and although it has been implemented in multiple states and international sites (e.g., Australia, Canada, England, New Zealand, and

Sweden), few replication studies have been conducted with ethnically diverse children. Similarly, a few researchers have begun to investigate the effects of implementing the PCIT program with ethnically diverse children and families (Brinkmeyer & Eyberg, 2003; Matos, Torres, Santiago, Jurado, & Rodriguez, 2006).

Overall consideration of the two interventions provided thus far suggests that the Incredible Years has somewhat stronger research evidence than PCIT; however, feasibility and cost factors could affect intervention selection at a particular practice site. Both interventions require training, but the cost and required training for the Incredible Years program is far greater. The PCIT program requires attending a 5-day workshop costing $3,000 plus the cost of necessary materials and equipment (University of Florida, 2008). In contrast, Incredible Years requires 9 days of group leader training costing $1,200 plus the cost of the relevant kits, which could be as low as $3,700 (for the child, parent, and teacher program) but would likely cost more, as this covers the costs of kits for just one age range and as most school psychologists typically work with a wider age range than is covered in one kit. Despite the greater startup costs for the Incredible Years program than for PCIT, Incredible Years is more cost-effective because it is administered in a group format, whereas PCIT only serves one child and family at a time. Whichever intervention is chosen, the limited application of either intervention program with diverse populations and contexts suggests the need for, and benefit of, school-based professionals conducting evaluative procedures in conjunction with implementing a selected intervention program.

There are a number of factors that have an impact on intervention selection. Although level of empirical support should emerge as the most important factor, it would be naïve to minimize the role of clinical utility factors, including student and setting characteristics, cost, and feasibility. Nonetheless, when selecting interventions, professionals should weigh and balance the potential advantages of stronger empirical support with site characteristics, required resources, and costs needed to implement an intervention program. The illustration comparing PCIT and Incredible Years demonstrates the need for school psychologists to function as evidence-based practitioners who apply evaluation procedures in conjunction with intervention implementation, as many "proven" intervention programs may not have been investigated with participants or settings similar to those surrounding the setting in which it will be applied.

Emergence of Evidence-Base-Applied-to-Practices Approach

As several researchers and scholars have argued for the urgency of improving educational outcomes for children and families, support is emerging for a "practitioner as researcher" or evidence-base-applied-to-practices (EBAP) approach (Kratochwill & Hoagwood, 2006; Meyers et al., 2004; Stoiber et al., 2005). Within this agenda is recognition that different schools reflect diverse ecological and complex qualities, ones that often cannot be captured through laboratory-like procedures and methodologies.

EBAP approaches have broader application in actual classrooms, as they include *intervention strategies based on scientific principles and empirical data*. In this regard, particular strategies with a strong theoretical base may be evaluated using data-based decision making. In an EBAP framework, a scientific basis informs practice, and practice outcomes inform ongoing and future decision making. As such, practitioners function as researchers by applying data-based approaches for systematic planning, monitoring, and evaluating outcomes of their own service delivery (Stoiber & Kratochwill, 2002; Stoiber, 2004). As educators witness the positive outcomes associated with their scientifically and data-informed practice, they are more likely to sustain it. Meyers et al. (2004) and Stoiber and associates (Stoiber, 2002; Stoiber et al., 2005; Stoiber & Waas, 2002) argued that such an approach is indicated due to a general lack of evidence for using particular interventions with particular children in particular contexts (i.e., situated knowledge).

The integration of research and practice is the foundation of EBAP in intervention selection. EBAP is based on the assumption that scientific knowledge should be drawn on in designing and implementing effective prevention and intervention services for a particular student, group of students, classroom, or system. EBAP is broader than evidence-based interventions (EBI) or evidence-based treatments (EBT), which generally refer to prevention or intervention programs for which there exists a strong empirical base (Kratochwill & Stoiber, 2002; Kratochwill, 2006; Kratochwill & Hoagwood, 2006). The concept of EBAP acknowledges the importance of integrating science and practice but also recognizes the challenges inherent in this integration. An EBAP approach incorporates forms of evidence stemming from diverse methodologies and sources. These sources include data from one's own application of the intervention, as well as data from clinical observations, qualitative approaches, process outcome studies, single-participant designs, RCTs, quasi-experimental program evaluation, and summary meta-analyses. Importantly, the 2006 American Psychological Association Presidential Task Force on Evidence-Based Practice report emphasizes the essential role of clinical judgment and clinical expertise across the steps of evidence-based practice, including assessment and diagnosis, case formulation, intervention design and implementation, monitoring of progress, and decision making.

In adopting an EBAP model, school-based practitioners hold a central role in determining the effectiveness of interventions used in their own practice. The term *treatment effectiveness* typically refers to demonstration of positive outcomes in real-world settings, such as schools (American Psychological Association Presidential Task Force, 2006). Given the constraints of directly applying programs and practices based on efficacy studies to the school setting, it is especially important for school psychologists to formulate, monitor, and evaluate interventions that fit into the school context and are acceptable to students and families (American Psychological Association Presidential Task Force, 2006; Stoiber & Waas, 2002; Stoiber, 2004). An EBAP model of service delivery would incorporate a scientific basis to inform intervention decision making both for selecting and for evaluating the effects and utility of an intervention. An EBAP model naturally includes a data-based problem-solving approach, which is particularly applicable for teachers and educators to use in monitoring and examining a child's response to the intervention.

Controversies and Considerations in Applying Guidelines for Selecting Interventions

For school-based practitioners to apply evidence-based criteria in selecting interventions, considerable improvements in the quality and quantity of intervention research are needed. For example, recent separate examinations of education intervention studies (in learning disabilities, early childhood, and autism) indicated that less than 15% measured treatment integrity (Snyder, Thompson, McLean, & Smith, 2002; Wolery & Garfinkle, 2002). There is a dearth of intervention studies involving school-age students as participants, especially within classroom contexts, which is likely due to several obstacles that present important limitations to the documentation and use of evidence-based interventions. One documented issue regards teacher resistance toward implementing innovative strategies (Gettinger & Stoiber, 2008). Similarly, school administrators are rarely open to the random assignment of students to classrooms for experimental purposes, especially for an extended period of time (Gettinger & Stoiber, 2006). Attrition presents another problem in that children may change classrooms and even schools during the intervention. Perhaps the greatest obstacle to research-to-practice applications pertains to issues of acceptance, feasibility, and sustainability (Gettinger & Stoiber, 2009; Stoiber & Kratochwill, 2000; Stoiber, 2002). As discussed earlier, regardless of the research-based effects shown for an intervention, school administrators will likely assess the cost–benefit ratio to make sure that the intervention is practical to implement. Questions regarding a range of costs, such as those for materials, time, and training, often rise to the top of the list in intervention decision making. For schools and staff to "buy in," such costs must be balanced against the expected payoffs of the intervention.

Response to Intervention and EBAP

For effective response-to-intervention (RTI) implementation, evidence-based practices and the use of EBAP are necessary. First, the school-based practitioner or team must be able to reliably document that the child has received high-quality instruction and scientifically based intervention. In light of the current knowledge base on evidence-based interventions and programs, identifying such strategies and ensuring that they were implemented as intended is no small challenge. Several researchers have noted advantages of initially applying less intrusive interventions at the school and class level and moving to more comprehensive and intensified interventions as needed (Gettinger & Stoiber, 2009; O'Shaughnessy, Lane, Gresham, & Beebe-Frankenberger, 2003). Constructing such hierarchies of intensity requires an understanding of instructional procedures, with those strategies that require less teacher support or fewer modifications tried early in the sequence (Barnett, Daly, Jones, & Lentz, 2004).

Stoiber (2004) has suggested that in determining the focus of the intervention it is important to target high-priority academic or behavioral concerns. In designing the intervention, the following should be considered: (1) incorporate goals for changing behavior that the child is capable of learning or adapting; (2) focus on developing "key" competencies that likely have powerful effects on adjustment or on "access" behaviors that allow entry to beneficial environments; (3) make sure chosen interventions correspond to the child's needs as opposed to the practitioner's intervention preferences or biases; (4) emphasize simplicity, as it usually promotes intervention integrity and efficiency; and (5) work toward getting all involved adults to scaffold and support the behavior. Finally, in constructing individual positive support plans for targeting challenging behavior, research has supported the use of comprehensive interventions that include different types of strategies. These include a three-pronged "prevent–teach–respond," or PTR, approach designed to (1) prevent or eliminate setting conditions or triggers that set off the prioritized concern (*prevention strategies*); (2) teach competencies that serve as alternatives to the prioritized concern (*teaching strategies*); and/or (3) alter responses that have been maintaining the prioritized concern (*alternative response strategies*; Gettinger & Stoiber, 2006; Stoiber, 2004; Stoiber, Gettinger, & Fitts, 2007). Importantly, interventions aimed at children with externalizing behaviors should attempt to teach new skills such as self-control, flexibility, frustration tolerance, and group and peer cooperation rather than only reduce challenges.

Once the intervention is selected based on the four guidelines and criteria for evaluating programs and strategies, the school psychologist or intervention team should establish socially and empirically valid outcomes that can be measured repeatedly and reliably across the duration of the intervention. This step requires the practitioner and/or team to know and understand educational benchmarks that are validated in relation to long-term outcomes. For example, if a norm-referenced indicator, such as reading comprehension at the 35th percentile, is selected as the outcome, it should be known whether this constitutes the level of proficiency a child needs to effectively function in current and future general education classrooms (Denton, Vaughn, & Fletcher, 2003; Kratochwill & Stoiber, 2002). Obviously, establishing appropriate benchmarks for the social-behavioral domain can be more difficult because grade-level standards are less available. For this reason, practitioners may benefit from resources such as the Functional Assessment and Intervention System (Stoiber, 2004), which includes benchmarks for social-behavioral goals that have been socially validated by educators.

To apply RTI principles in determining need for special education, it also is useful to define the level of intervention intensity required for the child to improve or perform at expected levels. With an RTI model, a child is identified as having a disability when (1) pre- and postintervention performance has not changed significantly despite implementation of a validated intervention or (2) intensive intervention was required for the child to respond at an expected level of performance (Barnett et al., 2004; National Association of State Directors of Special Education [NASDSE], 2005). Intensive interventions or instruction differs significantly from regular education in terms of the resources and support needed, time required, amount of professional involvement beyond the classroom teacher, and other factors necessary for facilitating progress. Implementation of RTI should mean real change in the services a child receives as part of the decision-making and, ultimately, education process. However, such change can occur only through the combined efforts of researchers, practitioners, university educators, and policymakers. Although many compelling reasons have been given for rethinking eligibility decision making, most essential is the failure of traditional methods to be linked to effective, ongoing schoolwide and individual intervention planning and thus to produce positive outcomes in students (Barnett et al., 2004). Decision-making models based on RTI use the quality and degree of student response to intervention as key criteria for determining student need and/or disability. Successful implementation of RTI will require integration with general education, a reallocation of resources, and new educational research and training initiatives.

EBAP and No Child Left Behind

In addition to EBAP approaches setting the stage for prioritizing scientifically minded approaches to selecting and implementing interventions, they are connected closely to the current federal focus on No Child Left Behind (NCLB, 2001). The NCLB legislation was partly a reaction to the observation that education as a field was publishing very few articles reflecting well-designed and scientifically credible (e.g., incorporating strong psychometric qualities and random assignment of participants to experimental groups) methodologies (Shavelson & Towne, 2002). NCLB specifies that students must undergo effective instruction (i.e., scientifically- or evidence-based programs and interventions) for the purpose of educational accountability and for improving outcomes for all students.

Although the NCLB educational initiative relies on scientific or research-based practices, there are indications of fewer educational intervention studies today than were conducted in the 1970s and 1980s (Hsieh et al., 2005). Several researchers have criticized the quantity and quality of studies in important areas that affect student educational outcomes, such as reading (Troia, 1999), early childhood (Snyder et al., 2002), emotional disturbance (Mooney, Epstein, Reid, & Nelson, 2003), learning disabilities (Tunmer, Chapman, Greaney, & Prochnow, 2002), and special education (Seethaler & Fuchs, 2005). For example, Seethaler and Fuchs (2005) reviewed five prominent special education journals and documented that only 5% of all articles included a focus on mathematics or reading interventions. Seethaler and Fuchs' (2005) results are especially noteworthy because interventions targeting early literacy development and reading comprehension emerge as among those considered most needed and as potentially most effective for improving long-term student outcomes (Denton et al., 2003).

Conclusion

In education, interventions are developed typically to alter and often improve student functioning and outcomes. School psycholo-

gists hold an essential role in the selection of interventions that target a broad range of student performance, including those in cognitive, behavioral, and affective areas. Intervention research is designed to test the effectiveness of programs, practices, and policies for youths and families, frequently by comparing some new, improved, or alternative method with regard to the outcome of interest. The dissemination and implementation of efficacious interventions has been targeted as a critical next step by which evidence-based interventions can occur in natural school settings. Practitioner-as-researcher and other EBAP approaches hold considerable promise, as they target several important barriers to the dissemination of educational interventions, including issues of (1) acceptability, or the degree to which consumers find the intervention procedures and outcomes acceptable in their daily lives; (2) feasibility, or the degree to which intervention components can be implemented in naturalistic contexts; and (3) sustainability, or the extent to which the intervention can be maintained without support from external agents. As school psychologists collaborate with regular education and special education teachers, EBAP initiatives have the potential to result in widespread improvement in instructional practices, such as the implementation of RTI and compliance with NCLB. In this regard, researchers, school psychologists, school-based educators, and parents may together promote success in all children—which is the primary intent of applying guidelines for evidence-based practice in selecting interventions.

Notes

1. An expanded discussion of this policy statement including the rationale and references supporting it may be found in the Report of the Presidential Task Force on Evidence-Based Practice, available online at *www.apa.org/practice/ebpreport.pdf.*
2. To be consistent with discussions of evidence-based practice in other health care fields, the Task Force on Evidence-Based Practice used the term *patient* to refer to child, adolescent, adult, older adult, couple, family, group, organization, community, or other populations receiving psychological services. However,

the Task Force on Evidence-Based Practice recognized that in many situations there are important and valid reasons for using such terms as *client*, *consumer*, or *person* in place of *patient* to describe the recipient of services. In schools, the term *student* may be the most appropriate.

References

American Psychological Association. (2002). Criteria for evaluating treatment guidelines. *American Psychologist, 57,* 1052–1059.

American Psychological Association Presidential Task Force on Evidence-Based Practice. (2006). Evidence-based practice in psychology. *American Psychologist, 61,* 271–285.

Barnett, D. W., Daly, E. J., Jones, K. M., & Lentz, F. E. (2004). Response to intervention: Empirically based special service decisions from single-case designs of increasing and decreasing intensity. *Journal of Special Education, 38,* 66–79.

Barrett, P. M., & Ollendick, T. H. (Eds.). (2004). *Handbook of interventions that work with children and adolescents: Prevention and treatment.* Hoboken, NJ: Wiley.

Beauchaine, T. P., Webster-Stratton, C., & Reid, M. J. (2005). Mediators, moderators, and predictors of one-year outcomes among children treated for early-onset conduct problems: A latent growth curve analysis. *Journal of Consulting and Clinical Psychology, 73,* 371–388.

Brinkmeyer, M. Y., & Eyberg, S. M. (2003). Parent–child interaction therapy for oppositional children. In A. E. Kazdin & J. R. Weisz (Eds.), *Evidence-based psychotherapies for children and adolescents* (pp. 204–223). New York: Guilford Press.

Bui, K., & Takeuchi, D. T. (1992). Ethnic minority adolescents and the use of community mental health care services. *American Journal of Community Psychology, 20,* 403–417.

Burns, B. J., Costello, E. J., Angold, A., Tweed, D., Stangl, D., Farmer, E. M., et al. (1995). Children's mental health service use across service sectors. *Health Affairs, 14*(3), 147–159.

Burns, B. J., & Hoagwood, K. E. (2005). Evidence-based practice: Effecting change. *Child and Adolescent Psychiatric Clinics of North America, 14*(2), xv–xvii.

Chambers, D. A., Ringeisen, H., & Hickman, E. E. (2005). Federal, state, and foundation initiatives around evidence-based practices. *Child and Adolescent Mental Health, 14,* 307–327.

Comas-Díaz, L. (2006). Cultural variation in the therapeutic relationship. In C. D. Goodheart, A. E. Kazdin, & R. J. Sternberg (Eds.), *Psy-*

chotherapy: Where practice and research meet (pp. 81–105). Washington, DC: American Psychological Association.

Denton, C. A., Vaughn, S., & Fletcher, J. M. (2003). Bringing research-based practice in reading intervention to scale. *Learning Disabilities Research and Practice, 18,* 201–211.

Eyberg, S. (1988). Parent–child interaction therapy: Integration of traditional and behavioral concerns. *Child and Family Behavior Therapy, 10,* 33–46.

Eyberg, S. M., Boggs, S. R., & Algina, J. (1995). New developments in psychosocial, pharmacological, and combined treatments of conduct disorders in aggressive children. *Psychopharmacology Bulletin, 31,* 83–91.

Eyberg, S. M., Funderburk, B. W., Hembree-Kigin, T. L., McNeil, C. B., Querido, J. G., & Hood, K. K. (2001). Parent–child interaction therapy with behavior problem children: One- and two-year maintenance of treatment effects in the family. *Child and Family Behavior Therapy, 23*(4), 1–20.

Funderburk, B. W., Eyberg, S. M., Newcomb, K., McNeil, C. B., Hembree-Kigin, T., & Capage, L. (1998). Parent–child interaction therapy with behavior problem children: Maintenance of treatment effects in the school setting. *Child and Family Behavior Therapy, 20*(2), 17–38.

Gettinger, M., & Stoiber, K. C. (2008). Applying a response-to-intervention model for early literacy development among low-income children. *Topics in Early Childhood and Special Education, 27,* 198–213.

Gettinger, M., & Stoiber, K. C. (2009). Effective teaching and effective schools. In T. Gutkin & C. Reynolds (Eds.), *Handbook of school psychology* (4th ed., pp. 769–790). Hoboken, NJ: Wiley.

Gettinger, M., & Stoiber, K. C. (2006). Functional assessment, collaboration, and evidence-based treatment: An experimental analysis of a team approach for addressing challenging behavior. *Journal of School Psychology, 44,* 231–252.

Gibbs, S. (Ed.). (2002). Educational psychology and evidence [Special issue]. *Educational and Child Psychology, 19*(3 & 4).

Greenberg, L. S., & Newman, F. L. (1996). An approach to psychotherapy change process research: Introduction to the special section. *Journal of Consulting and Clinical Psychology, 64,* 435–438.

Griner, D., & Smith, T. B. (2006). Culturally adapted mental health intervention: A meta-analytic review. *Psychotherapy: Theory, Research, Practice, Training, 43,* 531–548.

Harpaz-Rotem, I., Leslie, D. L., & Rosenheck, R. A. (2004). Treatment retention among children entering a new episode of mental health care. *Psychiatric Services, 55*, 1022–1028.

Herschell, A. D., Calzada, E. J., Eyberg, S. M., & McNeil, C. B. (2002). Parent–child interaction therapy: New directions in research. *Cognitive and Behavioral Practice, 9*, 9–16.

Hoagwood, K., & Erwin, H. D. (1997). Effectiveness of school-based mental health services for children: A 10-year research review. *Journal of Child and Family Studies, 6*, 435–451.

Hoagwood, K., & Johnson, J. (2003). School psychology: A public health framework: 1. From evidence-based practices to evidence-based policies. *Journal of School Psychology, 41*, 3–21.

Hood, K. K., & Eyberg, S. M. (2003). Outcomes of parent–child interaction therapy: Mothers' reports of maintenance three to six years after treatment. *Journal of Clinical Child and Adolescent Psychology, 32*, 419–429.

Hsieh, P., Acee, T., Chung, W., Hsieh, Y., Kim, H., Thomas, G. D., et al. (2005). Is educational intervention research on the decline? *Journal of Educational Psychology, 97*, 523–529.

Incredible Years: *Parents, teachers, and children training series.* (2008). Retrieved July 18, 2008, from *www.incredibleyears.com/*.

Kazdin, A. E., & Weisz, J. R. (Eds.). (2003). *Evidence-based psychotherapies for children and adolescents.* New York: Guilford Press.

Kratochwill, T. R. (2006). Evidence-based interventions and practices in school psychology: The scientific basis of the profession. In R. F. Subotnik & H. J. Walberg (Eds.), *The scientific basis of educational productivity* (pp. 229–267). Greenwich, CT: Information Age.

Kratochwill, T. R., & Hoagwood, K. E. (2006). Evidence-based interventions and system change: Concepts, methods, and challenges in implementing evidence-based practices in children's mental health. *Child and Family Policy and Practice Review, 2*, 12–17.

Kratochwill, T. R., & Stoiber, K. C. (2000). Empirically supported interventions in school psychology: Conceptual and practice issues: Part 2. *School Psychology Quarterly, 15*, 233–253.

Kratochwill, T. R., & Stoiber, K. C. (2002). Evidence-based intervention in school psychology: Conceptual foundations of the Procedural and Coding Manual of Division 16 and the Society for the Study of School Psychology Task Force. *School Psychology Quarterly, 17*, 314–389.

Lewis-Snyder, G., Stoiber, K. C., & Kratochwill, T. R. (2002). Evidence-based interventions in school psychology: An illustration of the task force coding criteria using group-based research design. *School Psychology Quarterly, 17*, 423–465.

Lonigan, C. J., Elbert, J. C., & Johnson, S. B. (1998). Empirically supported psychosocial interventions for children: An overview. *Journal of Clinical Child Psychology, 27*(2), 138–145.

Masi, R., & Cooper, J. L. (2006). *Children's mental health: Facts for policymakers.* New York: National Center for Children in Poverty, Mailman School of Public Health, Columbia University.

Masia-Warner, C., Nangle, D. W., & Hansen, D. J. (2006). Bringing evidence-based child mental health services to the schools: General issues and specific populations. *Education and Treatment of Children, 29*, 165–172.

Matos, M., Torres, R., Santiago, R., Jurado, M., & Rodriguez, I. (2006). Adaptation of parent–child interaction therapy for Puerto Rican families: A preliminary study. *Family Process, 45*, 205–222.

McNeil, C. B., Eyberg, S., Eisenstadt, T. H., Newcomb, K., & Funderburk, B. (1991). Parent–child interaction therapy with behavior problem children: Generalization of treatment effects to the school settings. *Journal of Clinical Child Psychology, 20*, 140–151.

Meyers, J., Meyers, A. B., & Grogg, K. (2004). Prevention through consultation: A model to guide future developments in the field of school psychology. *Journal of Educational and Psychological Consultation, 15*, 257–276.

Mooney, P., Epstein, M. H., Reid, R., & Nelson, R. J. (2003). Status and trends in academic intervention research for students with emotional disturbance. *Remedial and Special Education, 24*, 273–287.

Nathan, P. E. (1998). Practice guidelines: Not yet ideal. *American Psychologist, 53*, 290–299.

National Association of State Directors of Special Education. (2005). *Response to intervention: Policy considerations and implementation.* Alexandria, VA: Author.

Nixon, R. D. V., Sweeney, L., Erickson, D. B., & Touyz, S. W. (2003). Parent–child interaction therapy: One- and two-year follow-up of standard and abbreviated treatments for oppositional preschoolers. *Journal of Abnormal Child Psychology, 32*, 263–271.

No Child Left Behind Act of 2001, Pub. L. No. 107-110 (2001).

O'Shaughnessy, T. E., Lane, K. L., Gresham, F. M., & Beebe-Frankenberger, M. E. (2003). Children placed at risk for learning and behavior difficulties. *Remedial and Special Education, 24*, 27–35.

President's New Freedom Commission on Mental Health. (2003). *Achieving the promise: Transforming mental health care in America.* Washington, DC: Author.

Reid, M. J., Webster-Stratton, C., & Baydar, N.

(2004). Halting the development of conduct problems in Head Start children: The effects of parent training. *Journal of Clinical Child and Adolescent Psychology, 33,* 279–291.

Scott, S., Spender, Q., Doolan, M., Jacobs, B., & Aspland, H. (2001). Multicentre controlled trial of parenting groups for child antisocial behaviour in clinical practice. *British Medical Journal, 323,* 1–5.

Seethaler, P. M., & Fuchs, L. S. (2005). A drop in the bucket: Randomized controlled trials testing reading and math interventions. *Learning Disabilities Research and Practice, 20,* 98–102.

Shavelson, R. J., & Towne, L. (2002). *Scientific research in education.* Washington, DC: National Academic Press.

Snyder, P., Thompson, B., McLean, M. E., & Smith, B. J. (2002). Examination of quantitative methods used in early intervention research: Linkages with recommended practices. *Journal of Early Intervention, 25,* 137–150.

Stoiber, K. C. (2002). Revisiting efforts on constructing a knowledge base of evidence-based intervention within school psychology. *School Psychology Quarterly, 17,* 460–476.

Stoiber, K. C. (2004). *Functional Assessment and Intervention System.* San Antonio, TX: Pearson.

Stoiber, K. C., Gettinger, M., & Fitts, M. (2007). Functional assessment and positive support strategies: Case illustration of process and outcomes. *Early Childhood Services, 1,* 165–179.

Stoiber, K. C., & Kratochwill, T. R. (2000). Empirically supported interventions and school psychology: Rationale and methodological issues. *School Psychology Quarterly, 15,* 75–105.

Stoiber, K. C., & Kratochwill, T. R. (2002). *Outcomes: Planning, monitoring, evaluating.* San Antonio, TX: Pearson.

Stoiber, K. C., Lewis-Snyder, G., & Miller, M. A. (2005). *Evidence-based interventions.* In S. Lee (Ed.), *Encyclopedia of school psychology* (pp. 196–199). New York: Sage.

Stoiber, K. C., Ribar, R., & Waas, G. (2004). Enhancing resilience through multiple family group interventions. In D. Catherall (Ed.), *Handbook of stress, trauma, and family* (pp. 433–451). New York: American Psychological Association Press.

Stoiber, K. C., & Vanderwood, M. L. (2008). Traditional assessment, consultation, and intervention practices: Urban school psychologists' use, importance, and competence ratings. *Journal of Educational and Psychological Consultation, 18,* 264–292.

Stoiber, K. C., & Waas, G. A. (2002). A contextual and methodological perspective on evidence-based intervention practices in school psychology in the United States. *Educational and Child Psychology, 19*(3), 7–21.

Taylor, T. K., Schmidt, F., Pepler, D., & Hodgins, H. (1998). A comparison of eclectic treatment with Webster-Stratton's Parents and Children Series in a children's mental health center: A randomized controlled trial. *Behavior Therapy, 29,* 221–240.

Troia, G. A. (1999). Phonological awareness intervention research: A critical review of the experimental methodology. *Reading Research Quarterly, 34,* 28–51.

Tunmer, W. E., Chapman, J. W., Greaney, K. T., & Prochnow, J. E. (2002). The contribution of educational psychology to intervention research and practice. *International Journal of Disability, Development, and Education, 49,* 11–29.

University of Florida. (2008). *Parent–child interaction therapy.* Retrieved July 18, 2008, from *pcit.phhp.ufl.edu/.*

U.S. Department of Education. Office of Special Education Programs. (2004). Status and trends in the education of racial and ethnic minorities: IDEA Database. Retrieved from *www.necs.ed.gov/pubs2007.*

U.S. Department of Education. (2003). *The high school leadership summit.* Retrieved from *www.ed.gov/about/offices/list/ovae/pi/hsinit/intex.html.*

U.S. Public Health Service. (2001). *Youth violence: A report of the Surgeon General.* Rockville, MD: U.S. Department of Health and Human Services Administration, National Institutes of Health, National Institute of Mental Health, Center for Mental Health Services.

Webster-Stratton, C. (1999). *How to promote children's social and emotional competence.* Thousand Oaks, CA: Sage.

Webster-Stratton, C. (2001). The incredible years: Parent, teacher and child training series. In D. S. Elliott (Ed.), *Blueprints for violence prevention: Book 11.* Boulder, CO: Regents of the University of Colorado, Institute of Behavioral Science.

Webster-Stratton, C., & Reid, M. J. (2003). The Incredible Years Parents, Teachers, and Children Training Series: A multifaceted treatment approach for young children with conduct problems. In A. E. Kazdin & J. R. Weisz (Eds.), *Evidence-based psychotherapies for children and adolescents* (pp. 224–240). New York: Guilford Press.

Webster-Stratton, C., Reid, M. J., & Hammond, M. (2004). Treating children with early-onset conduct problems: Intervention outcomes for parent, child, and teacher training. *Journal of Clinical Child and Adolescent Psychology, 33*, 105–124.

Weisz, J. R., & Hawley, K. (1999). *Procedural and coding manual for identification of beneficial treatments.* Washington, DC: American Psychological Association. Society for Clinical Psychology Division 12 Committee on Science and Practice.

Weisz, J. R., Jensen-Doss, A., & Hawley, K. M. (2005). Youth psychotherapy outcome research: A review and critique of the evidence base. *Annual Review of Psychology, 56*, 337–363.

Weisz, J. R., Jensen-Doss, A., & Hawley, K. M. (2006). Evidence-based youth psychotherapies versus usual clinical care: A meta-analysis of direct comparisons. *American Psychologist, 61*, 671–689.

What Works Clearinghouse. (2008). WWC procedures and standards handbook (Version 2.0). U.S. Department of Education, Institute of Education Sciences.

Wolery, M., & Garfinkle, A. N. (2002). Measures in intervention research with young children. *Journal of Autism and Developmental Disorders, 32*, 463–478.

Chapter 14

Proactive Strategies for Promoting Learning

Kenneth W. Howell
Joan Schumann

As the title indicates, this chapter offers strategies for promoting learning in the classroom. Take a minute to consider why you, a school psychologist, would want to know about ways to promote learning in a classroom. First, students without learning problems most likely will not be in need of such strategies (although these strategies would not harm them). However, those students who are not progressing through the curriculum at expected rates might need extra assistance. The problem is deciding who needs help and what help is needed. For school psychologists, there are two common ways to approach this problem-solving task: by focusing on explanations and causes for the problem and by concentrating on the search for effective strategies to improve learning. The third option is to do both; however, when a lack of resources and time restraints force a choice, the default should be a focus on strategies to improve learning.

In this chapter, we will (1) define learning problems, (2) describe recommended approaches to these problems and (3) delineate what we call "instructional strategies for promoting learning." We also provide two quick guides in Figures 14.1 and Figure 14.2 for the selection of instructional techniques aligned with this chapter's content. We hope that, by the end of this chapter, you will have a solid understanding of instruction that promotes learning, how it can be supported, and where to find additional information on the topic.

Learning Problems

Learning problems are often discussed in terms of psychodynamic functioning, perceptual or linguistic processing, and even neural damage. Sometimes it seems that the instructional paradigm is either ignored or treated superficially. To begin discussion, a clear image and definition of "learning problems" is needed.

To understand how educators recognize learning problems, we begin with the idea that learning is considered to be a *relatively permanent change in behavior brought about by instruction* (Schunk, 2008; Sternberg & Williams, 2002). Here, the term *instruction* includes any interaction with the environment, because the critical attribute of that definition is *a change in behavior*. Behavior change (even if expanded to include cognitive behavior) is traditionally used as the operational definition of learning. Students who fail to change after instruction are said to have learning problems. In school, the operational definition of a *learning problem* is failure to progress in regard to curricular expectations. One indicator of the severity of a learning problem is the size of performance discrepancies on these curricular objectives. Severity is also illustrated by a student's continued failure to progress through the curriculum at the expected rate, particularly after repeated use of otherwise effective instruction. This is referred to as "failure to respond."

Instruction is *how* a student is taught, and curriculum is *what* a student is taught (i.e., the organized body of objectives). Even the most strongly supported evidence-based instructional intervention will not work if it targets the wrong skill or segment of the curriculum (Odom et al., 2005). If a student is lacking in the prior knowledge (e.g., the prerequisite reading, math, or social skills) required by a task, the student will most likely need to learn those prerequisite skills before mastering more complex content areas. This means that learning problems can be corrected many times without even changing instruction, because what is needed is a temporary shift in curriculum focus or level. Instructional conditions do not always need to be changed to fill in missing knowledge. In this chapter, our primary focus is the description of instructional (not curriculum) interventions.

Alterable Variables

When we are trying to solve a learning problem or plan interventions for correction, the unit of analysis is not the learner. It is the interaction of instruction/assessment, curriculum, educational environment, and the learner (ICEL). Therefore, the evaluative question is not, What about this learner is causing the lack of progress? It is, What aspect(s) of the ICEL interaction need to be changed in order to improve the learner's progress? (Heartland Area Education Agency 11, 2007). Interventions to improve student learning involve change within the ICEL interaction. These alterable variables are the most productive targets of attention and inquiry within both evaluation and planning for educational changes (Bahr & Kovaleski, 2006). As a result, this chapter does not cover learner traits such as IQ, gen-

der, birth order, or processing preference. Similarly, it does not focus on environmental conditions such as school funding or class size. Although these factors may or may not be important in a student's life, each is generally viewed as "static" and considered beyond the influence of an individual student's instructional intervention (Sternberg & Hedlund, 2002).

Unfortunately, as school psychologists and special educators, we spend more time assessing the learner than we do assessing his or her instruction, curriculum, and educational environments. Also, great importance is typically attributed to variability among students. This includes variability revealed by measures designed to tap psychological, perceptual, and/or neurological constructs of factors that, relative to missing skills and strategies, account for smaller differences in student achievements (Duckworth & Seligman, 2005). Although debates about the relevance of perceptual and/or neurological constructs and factors such as IQ and learning style will apparently be with us forever (Fletcher, Coulter, Reschly, & Vaughn, 2004; Naglieri & Johnson, 2000), the illation based on these measures is grounded in unwarranted confidence and should have ceased long ago.

Discussions of unalterable variables can actually slow attempts to find the solutions to learning problems (Howell, Hosp, & Kurns, 2008). This is particularly true when the variables in question fall under the heading of *student ability*. The traditional concept of *ability* rests in distinction from the concept of *skill* as unalterable. It is typically not thought of as something to be changed through instruction (particularly short term). In distinction, *skills* and *knowledge* are taught and learned. By now, most educators have encountered presentations on the limitations and even risks of misusing the ability construct (Reschly, 2008). These include the conclusion that the measures typically utilized (e.g., IQ tests) are insufficiently informative or reliable. In addition, attempts to draw instructional recommendations from measures of cognitive and perceptual ability constructs, including aptitude-by-treatment interactions, have not been productive (Gresham, 2002; Reschly, 2008). Although there is no reason to repeat those findings here, there is even less reason to employ the procedures in practice (see Floyd, Chapter 4, this volume, for a more thorough discussion of this issue).

Learning Problems from an Instructional Perspective

The following discussion of learning difficulties takes a *learning/instructional perspective* that is grounded in educationally relevant and alterable variables. For convenience, we use reading for the example content for most of the presentation. However, the illustration applies across content areas.

As previously noted, we can recognize a student as having a learning problem when he or she is behind expectation in the academic and/or social curriculum. Lower than expected performance, progress, or both tells us the student needs support. It is the *need* for exceptional instruction, not a disability, that ultimately justifies a student's entitlement to special education (i.e., individuals with disabilities who do not need exceptional educational supports are not entitled to special education funding). Most often a performance deficit is the result of an enduring progress deficit (i.e., the student has not reached desired levels in the curriculum by the desired dates). Important to note is that performance deficits may also occur when a student changes schools (or classes) to one that uses different curricular sequences. Regardless of cause, when a student is behind in the curriculum (particularly in a basic skill such as reading), several factors compound and amplify the original deficit.

The first factor (assuming the example of reading) is that the student is denied access to information through reading. This limits acquisition of background knowledge required for future learning within areas aligned with and/or dependent on the content the student has not read. Also, because the reading deficit will cause the student's reading to be inaccurate and/or slow, he or she will have less actual engaged time with the task *even when he or she is working for the same amount of time* as successful students work. The issue here is not time on task; it is density of practice within a given unit of time. For example, a student who reads 60 words correctly in a minute reads three times as many words as a student who reads 20 words per minute in a given time period. So, in a 15-minute session, the faster

reader practices more reading. Over time, the cumulative disparity between the two readers multiplies exponentially.

Lack of access and low-density engagement commingle, regardless of content area, to produce Matthew Effects within aligned and/or dependent knowledge. The term *Matthew Effect* derives its name from a Christian biblical parable in the Gospel of Matthew. Basically it teaches that the rich will get richer and the poor will get poorer. Relative to academics, Matthew Effects begin when students who are successful receive greater benefits from work than their less competent peers. (For more information on the Matthew Effect, refer to Stanovich, 2000).

As time passes, a low-achieving student's lack of learning results in a lack of sufficient background and prior knowledge. Without prior knowledge, the student's problem becomes greater, as he or she is unprepared to learn within objectives aligned with and/or dependent on that background. As a consequence, tasks that are easy for others become increasingly difficult, because a major component of *task difficulty* is inadequate background knowledge (i.e., things seem hard when we do not know how to do them) and *cognitive load* increases as more tasks are introduced that the student is not ready to learn (i.e., missing prior knowledge makes the tasks too difficult; van Merriënboer & Sweller, 2005). Finally, *task-related difficulties* develop or increase. These include task avoidance behaviors and others that are typically mistaken for low motivation.

Obviously, the evolving image of a learning problem is grim. However, it becomes less hopeless when conceptualized as misalignment among the instruction, curriculum, educational environment, and learner (the ICEL components). Both effective instruction and learning problems occur within the context of these variables, and learning problems are corrected through changes in their arrangement. In a problem-solving paradigm, educators work to find the configuration of ICEL variables that will produce optimal change and learning for students. In contrast, fixed-ability models are incongruent with the application of problem-solving efforts that focus on the instructional context.

When low levels of performance, along with low rates of progress, indicate a learning problem, the pragmatic solution is accelerated progress in order to reach the target performance levels. The problem is how to accomplish that in the face of historically low progress (Access Center, 2005). Before we present the instructional interventions and problem-solving strategies required for the needed increase in progress, the ICEL domains need additional explanation.

Instruction's Role within ICEL

Changing and/or improving instruction is the most direct way to influence and accelerate the rate of student learning. However, like students, teachers come to classrooms with varying skills and resources. This *does not mean* that teachers cause all learning problems. However, a change in the teacher's behavior or teaching is often needed to fix a student's learning problem. For example, if the class does not allow sufficient time for practice to build a student's handwriting fluency, the problem will most likely be found through an analysis of the teacher's daily plans and time allocations (Hoadley, 2003), not through student test results.

Regardless of content, method, or materials, there are recognized sets of instructional actions (called *routines*) that can have a major influence on student learning. A successful routine can have many characteristics but four critical attributes must always be factored into planning. These are alignment, format, procedural fidelity, and dose. In the discussion that follows, a variety of instructional procedures related to these four attributes are presented. Others can also be found in Figure 14.1 (on pp. 240–241).

Alignment

Alignment refers to the coordinated arrangement of instruction/assessment, curriculum, educational environment, and learner need. It is accomplished by first establishing learning objectives that will take the student to acceptable levels of competence and self-sufficiency. These objectives represent the curriculum (i.e., the C component in ICEL). Alignment is established when all ICEL components coordinate with a student's needs (and with each other).

Format

Lesson plans can also have different types of *format*, sometimes called instructional routines. These formats can be thought of as templates designed to complement different categories of content or learning outcomes. Although all lessons should share certain components (e.g., the delivery of information, questioning, and activities), how these components are structured can vary. The way a teacher asks questions when teaching conceptual knowledge (e.g., photosynthesis) should be different from the way questions are asked during a lesson on factual knowledge (e.g., parts of a plant). Similarly, lessons targeting increases in fluency commonly employ routines that are different from those that target an increase in accuracy. Knowing about the various format templates allows one to quickly analyze, critique, or design lessons across multiple content domains.

Here is an example: When students' objectives specify increases in rate (e.g., rapid letter formation in writing or word recognition in reading), the fluency format or template is used to structure the lessons. Such lessons, regardless of content or age of the student, will generally utilize extensive drill and practice. They will have limited explanation and minimal error correction (because students should not be put into fluency building until they are reasonably accurate). In distinction, an accuracy-formatted lesson will provide considerable explanation and demonstration, as well as immediate and comprehensive correction. Lessons designed around the fluency template may not complement the needs of a student who is inaccurate, even if the lessons directly cover content the student needs to learn. Accuracy, fluency, and generalization outcomes are complemented by different types of lesson format.

As mentioned, lesson formats can also be aligned with categories of content (e.g., factual, conceptual, strategic). For example, in a class on academic survival skills, Dusty might have trouble learning to take notes if he does not understand the concept of main idea. *Concept* is a category of content (just as *fluency* is a category of proficiency). There are particular ways to teach factual, strategic, and conceptual information that complement each. Consequently, alignment is not limited to content.

There are times when school psychologists need to examine instruction and even to offer opinions and/or advice on how it is delivered. Although it may be unreasonable to expect school psychologists to know the specifics of every branch of curriculum and all instructional techniques, every lesson will have objectives, which themselves contain statements of behavior, condition, and criterion. Lessons can be built or aligned around any of those statements by selecting their complementary instructional formats. Here is a brief overview of formats based on the common objective components:

- Content is commonly categorized as *factual*, *strategic* and/or *conceptual*.
- Behavior and/or display is commonly categorized as *say*, *write*, *do* (*identify*, *produce*, and/or *generalize/apply*).
- Condition is commonly categorized as with or without assistance, in isolation or in context, in a familiar or in an unfamiliar setting.
- Proficiency/criterion is commonly categorized as *accuracy*, *fluency*, and/or *generalization/application*.

Each of these can be linked to instructional procedures and teacher actions. Figure 14.1 provides a summary and comparison of the formats. It can be used to guide analysis of lessons and to structure feedback on instruction.

Active participation is another important element of instructional format (Marks, 2000). Because it is widely acknowledged that learners benefit from the active use of information, it is just as widely accepted that lessons ought to include student activities. However, there is considerable confusion about the kind, or definition, of these activities. This confusion is easily removed by recalling the principle of alignment.

Learning academic information requires cognitive activity, and learning to climb a tree requires motor activity. But although the need for *cognitive activity* may seem obvious, it is remarkable how many educators routinely insist that students engage in time-consuming activities such as cutting, pasting, and illustrating to learn academics. Although many of these activities and projects are fun, they can be counterproductive if they supplant or redirect content-aligned cognitive activities. Drawing and other creative activities merit a valued position in the curriculum on the basis of their own worth; time spent on art should be allocated for improving art and not reading, vocabulary, science, or other nonaligned academic content areas. For students who are not learning to read, time is limited, and that which is spent illustrating a story needs to be judged in relation to the learning that might be missed in additional explanation, demonstration, or faster-paced practice (Hoadley, 2003; Marzano, Pickering, & Pollock, 2001).

For academic learning, "active" responding, engagement and/or practice results from *cognitive engagement*. For example, when a student points to the letter E during a reading lesson, we do not necessarily want to praise by saying "good pointing!" But that is often what happens. Saying "Yes, you've learned which letter is E" more directly addresses the thought process (i.e., the cognition) intended by the pointing activity (Walsh & Sattes, 2005).

Some activities, such as directing a student to *listen*, *follow along*, or *reflect*, introduce greater risk of cognitive *inactivity* than others. Saying "I want you to listen for the name of a tree frog and raise your hand when you hear one" is better, as the behavior (i.e., raising hand) verifies the desired cognition. Conversely, saying, "Be sure to remember to pay attention to all the frog names" might not prompt any form of engagement at all.

Questioning is often recommended for increasing active engagement (Harrop & Swinson, 2003; Walsh & Sattes, 2005). For example, it is usually best for a teacher to say, "Now I'm going to call on someone to tell me why Dubai is a center of commerce in the Middle East. And then I'll call on someone else to tell me if that answer was correct." This routine will get *all students* thinking about the question, not just the student called on. Another way to do this is to pause after a question and let all students think a while before requesting the answer from a particular student.

Procedural Fidelity

Research has identified both effective and ineffective procedures for presenting informa-

(text continues on page 244)

Technique/Level of proficiency	Information delivery	Teacher questions	Teacher responses	Related activities
Acquisition: 1. Prerequisite—mastery of aligned sub skills 2. Goal—accuracy	1. Extensive explanation and demonstration 2. Provide models and procedural prompts 3. Teach use of memory strategies	1. Ask about strategies and concepts 2. Do not emphasize answers 3. Emphasize *how to find* answers	1. Praise accurate use of procedures 2. Use elaborate correction procedures	1. Use only guided and controlled practice 2. Student completes partially worked items
Fluency: 1. Prerequisite—accuracy 2. Goal—to work at rate while maintaining accuracy	1. Ensure mastery of subskills 2. Review accuracy 3. Practice across contexts	1. Emphasize answers correct 2. Emphasize fluent answers but not unnecessary speed	1. Praise fluent work 2. Feedback on rate 3. No correction procedure for errors	1. Drill and practice 2. Independent practice
Generalization and transfer: 1. Prerequisite—Mastery of subskills 2. Goal—Use of skills across target settings	1. Teach related concepts and vocabulary 2. Explain how existing skills can be generalized and/or applied	1. Ask how existing skills can be modified 2. Practice in context	1. Use elaborate corrections when generalization or transfer fails to occur 2. Repeat item	1. Use "real world" examples 2. Deemphasize classroom-specific tasks
Factual	1. Terminology 2. Number statements 3. Tool skills 4. Items and answers 5. Rapid and accurate responding	1. Ask a lot of direct questions 2. Ask questions at a fast pace 3. Start with questions requiring only identification of the answer 4. Move to questions requiring production of the answer	**For correct work:** 1. Give frequent feedback on accuracy and rate 2. Give minimal praise required to maintain motivation **For errors:** 1. Give immediate feedback on errors or slow responses 2. No elaborate correction procedures 3. Repeat items missed	1. Learn and practice use of memory strategies 2. Short, intense lessons including drill and practice 3. Several short sessions rather than one long one 4. Make practice realistic 5. Vary the conditions and settings of the practice 6. Provide practice to fluency

Conceptual	1. Name the concept and use the same name during all initial lessons (use synonyms later); 2. Review relevant prior knowledge 3. Show multiple examples of the concept and point out the critical and noncritical attributes in each example 4. Use clear examples in early lessons and ambiguous examples in later lessons 5. Work with the student to prepare a diagram (map) of the concept 6. Demonstrate how an example can be changed to a nonexample (and vice versa)	1. Ask the student to identify which things are, or are not, examples of the concept 2. Ask why something is or is not an example of the concept 3. Ask the student to identify things which are "always," "sometimes," or "never" attributes of the concept 4. Ask the student to supply examples and attributes 5. Intersperse questions throughout the delivery of information 6. Ask questions but do not "drill" the student	**For correct work:** 1. Give specific feedback by telling the student exactly what discrimination or information was correct 2. Periodically challenge correct answers 3. Ask students to support answers. **For errors:** 1. Use elaborate correction procedures during early lessons 2. Explain exactly why a response is wrong 3. Watch for and label examples of overgeneralization 4. Encourage students to judge and to correct their own work	1. Use activities that illustrate the range of concepts 2. Have the student sort items into categories 3. Have the student convert nonexamples into examples by changing the necessary attributes 4. Have the student "compare and contrast" examples and nonexamples 5. Use clear examples and nonexamples in early lessons and subtle ones in later lessons
Strategic	1. Name the strategy 2. Use explanations *and* demonstrations 3. Show recognition of problem 4. Work while talking aloud 5. Show recognition of alternative strategies; show self-monitoring and decision making 6. Show limits of the strategy and rules for its use 7. Leave a model if possible	1. Ask students to supply rules, steps, and procedures 2. Ask questions about how things are done—deemphasize finding the answers 3. Ask the student to predict the effect of an omitted or incorrect step 4. Ask, "What is the first thing you will do? What will you do next?"	**For correct work:** 1. Say, "Good, you did it correctly," not "Good, you got the right answer." 2. Say, "That's correct—now tell me how you got it." **For errors:** 1. Be sure the student has the skills needed to do the task 2. Ask students to recognize and correct their own errors 3. Repeat the item	1. Use guided practice (student thinks aloud, and teacher provides the feedback) 2. Have student act as teacher 3. Ask the student to recognize missing steps 4. Do not emphasize getting answers or finishing pages 5. Have the student practice recognizing when a strategy will or will not work

FIGURE 14.1. Instructional techniques by type of information and target proficiency.

Learning, Thinking, and Problem-Solving

Anderson, J. R., Greeno, J. G., Reder, L. M., & Simon, H. A. (2000). Perspectives on learning, thinking, and activity. *Educational Researcher, 29*(4), 11–13.

Azevedo, R., Cromley, J. G., & Seibert, D. (2004). Does adaptive scaffolding facilitate students' ability to regulate their learning with hypermedia? *Contemporary Educational Psychology, 29*, 344–370.

Bell, P., Barron, B., Reeves, B., & Sabelli, N. (2006). Learning theories and education: Toward a decade of synergy. In P. A. Alexander & P. H. Winne (Eds.), *Handbook of educational psychology* (2nd ed. pp. 209–244). Mahwah, NJ: Erlbaum.

Blackwell, L., Trzesniewski, K. H., & Sorich, C. (2007). Implicit theories of intelligence predict achievement across an adolescent transition: A longitudinal study and an intervention. *Child Development, 78*(1), 246–263.

Bransford, J., Stevens, R., Schwartz, D., Meltzoff, A., Pea, R., Roschelle, J., et al. (2000). Teachers' coaching of learning and its relation to students' strategic learning. *Journal of Educational Psychology, 92*, 342–348.

Higgins, S., Hall, E., Baumfield, V., & Moseley, D. (2005). A meta-analysis of the impact of the implementation of thinking skills approaches on pupils. In *Research Evidence in Education Library*. London: EPPI-Centre, University of London, Social Science Research Unit.

Mayer, R. E., & Wittrock, M. C. (1996). Problem-solving transfer. In D. C. Berliner & R. C. Calfee (Eds.), *Handbook of educational psychology*. New York: Macmillan.

Pintrich, P. R. (2002). The role of metacognitive knowledge in learning, teaching, and assessing. *Theory into Practice, 41*(4), 219–225.

Sternberg, R. J. (2003). Creative thinking in the classroom. *Scandinavian Journal of Educational Research, 47*(3), 325–338.

Attention

Barak, M., Lipson, A., & Lerman, S. (2006). Wireless laptops as means for promoting active learning in large lecture halls. *Journal of Research on Technology in Education, 38*, 245–263.

Memory

Access Center. Using mnemonic instruction to facilitate access to the general education curriculum. Retrieved November 9, 2005, from *www.k8accesscenter.org/training_resources/Mnemonics.asp*.

Hwang, Y., & Levin, J. R. (2002). Examination of middle-school students' independent use of a complex mnemonic system. *Journal of Experimental Education, 71*(1), 25–38.

Motivation

Covington, M. V. (2000). Goal theory, motivation and school achievement: An integrative review. *Annual Review of Psychology, 51*, 171–200.

Dweck, C. S. (2006). *Mindset: The new psychology of success.* New York: Random House.

Dweck, C. S. (2007). The perils and promises of praise. *Educational Leadership, 65*(2), 34–39.

Linnenbrink, E. A., & Pintrich, P. R. (2003). The role of self-efficacy beliefs in student engagement and learning in the classroom. *Reading and Writing Quarterly, 19*, 119–137.

Patrick, H., Anderman, L. H., Ryan, A. M., Edelin, K. C., & Midgley, C. (2001). Teachers' communication of goal orientations in four fifth-grade classrooms. *Elementary School Journal, 102*, 35–58.

Voke, H. (2002). *Student engagement: Motivating students to learn.* Alexandria, VA: Association for Supervision and Curriculum Development.

Academic Strategies

Deshler, D. D. (2005). Adolescents with learning disabilities: Unique challenges and reasons for hope. *Learning Disability Quarterly, 28*(2), 122–124.

DiPerna, J. C., Volpe, R., & Elliott, S. N. (2005). A model of academic enablers and mathematics achievement in the elementary grades. *Journal of School Psychology, 43*, 379–392.

(cont.)

FIGURE 14.2. Resources pertaining to improved classroom learning.

McLaughlin, M., McGrath, D. J., Burian-Fitzgerald, M. A., Lanahan, L., Scotchmer, M., Enyeart, C., et al. *Student content engagement as a construct for the measurement of effective classroom instruction and teacher knowledge*. Washington, DC: American Institutes for Research.

Swanson, L. H., & Deshler, D. (2003). Instructing adolescents with learning disabilities: Converting a meta-analysis to practice. *Journal of Learning Disabilities, 36*(2), 124–145.

Wolpow, R., & Tonjes, M. (2005). *Integrated content literacy*. Dubuque, IA: Kendall/Hunt.

English Language Learners

Kinsella, K. (2000, Fall). Reading and the need for strategic lexical development for secondary ESL students. *California Social Studies Review.*

Kinsella, K. (2006, October). Structured "academic talk" for English learners: A key to narrowing the verbal gap in K–12 classrooms. Paper presented at Office of English Language Acquisition Celebrate Our Rising Stars Summit, Washington, DC.

Walqui, A. (2003). What makes reading difficult for adolescent English learners? *Teaching English as a second language to adolescent English learners.* San Francisco: WestEd.

Computation

Clarke, B., Baker, S., Smolkowski, K., & Chard, D. J. (2008). An analysis of early numeracy curriculum-based measurement: Examining the role of growth in student outcomes. *Remedial and Special Education, 29*, 46–57.

Fuchs, L. S., Fuchs, D., Prentice, K., Burch, M., Hamlett, C. L., Owen, R., et al. (2003). Enhancing third-grade students' mathematical problem solving with self-regulated learning strategies. *Journal of Educational Psychology, 95*(2), 306–315.

Hosp, J., & Ardoin, S. (2008). Assessment for instructional planning. *Assessment for Effective Intervention, 33*(4), 69–77.

Kelley, B., Hosp, J., & Howell, K. (2008). Curriculum-based evaluation and math: An overview. *Assessment for Effective Intervention, 33*(4), 250–256.

Reading

Deshler, D. D., Schumaker, J. B., Lenz, B. K., Bulgren, J. A., Hock, M. F., Knight, J., et al. (2001). Ensuring content-area learning by secondary students with learning disabilities. *Learning Disabilities Research and Practice, 16*(2), 96–108.

Fung, I., Wilkinson, I. A., & Moore, D. W. (2003). L1-assisted reciprocal teaching to improve ESL students' comprehension of English expository text. *Learning and Instruction, 13*, (1), 1–31.

Gersten, R., Fuchs, L. S., Williams, J. P., & Baker, S. (2001). Teaching reading comprehension strategies to students with learning disabilities: A review of research. *Review of Educational Research, 71*, 279–320.

Klingner, J. K., Vaughn, S., Arguelles, M. E., Hughes, M. T., & Leftwich, S. A. (2004, September/October). Collaborative strategic reading: "Real-world" lessons from classroom teachers. *Remedial and Special Education, 25*, 291–302.

Written Expression

Harris, K. R., Graham, S., & Mason, L. H. (2006). Improving the writing, knowledge, and motivation of young struggling writers: The effects of self-regulated strategy development with and without peer support. *American Educational Research Journal, 43*, 295–340.

Zimmerman, B. J., & Kitsantas, A. (2002). Acquiring writing revision and self-regulatory skill through observation and emulation. *Journal of Educational Psychology, 94*(4), 660–668.

Classroom Behavior

Mitchem, K. J. (2005). Be proactive: Including students with challenging behavior in your classroom. *Intervention in School and Clinic, 40*(3), 188–191.

FIGURE 14.2. *(cont.)*

tion, demonstrating, questioning, correcting errors, giving feedback, and managing common classroom tasks. These procedures are often specified within particular instructional programs or sets of materials. Others are associated more generally with effective instruction (Subotnik & Walberg, 2006; Vaughn & Fuchs, 2003). It is likely that almost any procedure seen in a typical classroom has been investigated. Obviously, those instructional routines and procedures with empirical support should be used, but to do so means using them as they were employed during validation. It is not enough to use a validated procedure. It needs to be implemented with fidelity (Lane, Bocian, MacMillan & Gresham, 2004; see also Noell, Chapter 30, this volume, for a more in-depth discussion of this issue).

Dose Factor

Related to procedural fidelity is the idea of adequate instructional *dose*. *Dose factor* (or dosage) means the same thing in instructional delivery that it means in a pharmacy. If an intervention is employed exactly as it should be, but not in the same amount (e.g., for only half the required time), the desired rate of learning might not be obtained. There are few guidelines for setting optimal dosage except for the obvious: The correct dose is the amount needed for effective learning. Time is an important element of instruction (Gettinger, 1984), but it is not the only element. Increasing time in the math support class from 30 to 60 minutes per week may represent only a 15-minute increase if the student will spend half that time illustrating a story. Student progress must be monitored to fine-tune dosage (or any of the other components of interventions).

Curriculum's Role within ICEL

When we say a student is "behind," we mean "behind in the curriculum." In curriculum-based and problem-solving models, the most likely reason for a student's poor performance on a given task is assumed to be missing prior/background knowledge. Because this prerequisite knowledge resides at lower levels of the curriculum, evaluators and teachers need to be familiar with the curriculum and the aligned measures needed to find that correct level for instruction. Knowledge of the subject area being taught and/or evaluated is an extraordinarily important consideration when working to solve learning problems (Nelson & Machek, 2007). However, the curriculum has more dimensions than most educators realize.

As explained earlier, the curriculum is *what* is taught, and instruction is *how* it is taught. The curriculum is commonly divided into subject areas within which objective sequences are produced. *Objectives* are specified learning outcomes and are expected to include statements of *content*, specifying what will be taught; *behavior*, specifying what the student must do (i.e., do, write, or say) to display knowledge of the content; *conditions*, specifying the context or circumstances under which the student will work (e.g., during an assignment, with or without assistance); and *criterion*, specifying the quality of performance (i.e., expected accuracy, fluency, or quality). For example, "*Emily will write* [behavior] *question marks* [content] *with 100% accuracy* [criterion] *during the history test* [condition]."

Whereas goals are typically general statements covering large segments of curriculum, behavioral/performance objectives operationally specify the behavior(s) students will be prepared to perform when instruction is finished. Having clearly defined objectives is necessary for targeted evaluation and direct, explicit instruction. Although instructors *teach to objectives*, they do so by directing instruction to their students' thought processes and knowledge, not necessarily to the task utilized as the display mechanism or behavior selected to give that knowledge an operational definition. Improved performance on measures aligned with the objectives is taken as the necessary *indicator* of changes in knowledge and thought process (because knowledge and thought processes are themselves covert).

Within any subject area (e.g., multiplication, Civil War history, punctuation), the same content may include different *types of knowledge*. Various theories and taxonomies for structuring and subdividing knowledge have been suggested over the years. The idea behind these taxonomic systems is that information can be categorized and possibly sequenced in instructionally beneficial ways (often without consideration of the behavior–criterion–condition components associated with the objectives). Of these, Bloom's taxonomy of outcomes is the most familiar to teachers, although not necessarily the most functional (Anderson & Krathwohl, 2001).

In some cases, templates for categorizing and organizing the subdivisions of curriculum can help guide our planning and decision making. For instance, a simple *know*-and-*apply* sequence is functional for planning and evaluating most early-grade outcomes because it forces consideration of *application*, as well as *knowledge*. For example, "Jim will *know how to* write question marks with 100% accuracy during the history test" followed by "Jim will *apply his knowledge* of question marks with 100% accuracy during the history test." Another common taxonomic format uses *fact*, *concept*, and *strategy* (sometimes called *know*, *understand* and *do*). For example: "Jenny Mae will display knowledge of the *factual information* required to complete multiplication problems" followed by "Jenny Mae will display knowledge of the *concepts* required to complete multiplication problems" followed by "Jenny Mae will display knowledge of the *strategies* required to apply information in order to complete multiplication problems."

Aligning Curriculum and Instruction

Teaching a student to be accurate may require different instruction from that used to build fluency or application. Similarly, the ways to teach facts, concepts, and strategies are not the same. Even within the same content, teaching and evaluative approaches often need to be adjusted or aligned according to the emphasis on facts, concepts, or strategies (as well as accuracy, fluency, or application). Alignment requires instructors to match the conditions of instruction and evaluation with objectives. Once this has been accomplished, standard evaluation formats and instructional routines can be utilized, making lesson planning both efficient and comprehensive. Some routines for teaching facts, concepts, and strategies to the proficiency levels of accuracy, fluency, and generalization/maintenance are presented in Figure 14.1. A review of this figure

should give readers an image of the differences among the formats. The figure can also provide a quick source of information about the intervention attributes required to teach particular types of content or to reach particular outcomes. This information can be used to ensure alignment of instruction with intended outcomes.

The reader should be aware that techniques and terminology presented in Figure 14.1 are not uniformly defined across instructional levels, paradigms, and content. Also, instructors will vary in skill at using them. Consequently, it is always a good idea for a school psychologist to talk over the information with his or her audience. Before assuming a recommendation will be employed as expected, the school psychologist should always ask these questions: Can the teacher (1) Discriminate correct from incorrect use of the technique? (2) Correctly explain how to use the technique? (3) Correctly demonstrate how to use the technique?

Educational Environment's Role within ICEL

The important thing to remember relative to the educational environment is the word *educational*. Without minimizing the importance of the world outside the classroom, educators sometimes need to be reminded that what is going on out there is largely *unalterable* (as the term *unalterable* has been defined earlier) and relatively distal to class instruction and learning interactions. Some of the alterable variables of greatest importance within the educational environment are: knowledgeable and skilled staff; clearly articulated objectives and instructional plans; routine benchmark monitoring of all students; effective and intense time utilization (i.e., available, allocated, engaged, and academic time); availability of aligned and high-quality (i.e., empirically supported) instructional materials; continuous curriculum-based progress monitoring accompanied by data-based decision making for students who have problems learning; and appropriate and flexible grouping options (Johnson, 2002; Williams et al., 2005; Walqui, 2000).

The student/learner is intentionally placed last in the ICEL discussion because students are usually the first thing considered in the search for the cause of a problem. In addition, the focus on student variables has often led educators away from useful information. Attributing learning problems to unalterable, noncurricular student or environment characteristics can detract us from more obvious explanations for student learning problems.

The most immediate and likely reason for a student not performing or learning a particular skill is that he or she does not know how to do it (i.e., the student is lacking the prior background knowledge needed to perform and/or learn; Marzano, 2004). Educators provide students with that needed prior background knowledge through instruction. Therefore, when a student is failing to progress through the objectives of the curriculum, the first course of action should be to determine whether she or he is missing needed prerequisite (background) skills. Consider the following as examples:

- Question: "Why might Dustin struggle to read words with silent *e*?"
- Answer: "He has never been taught the silent *e* rules."
- Question: "Why might Claire be challenged by multiple-digit addition problems?"
- Answer: "She has yet to master her addition facts."

As the old saying goes, "Sometimes the best step forward is one step back." Time spent teaching missing background knowledge can be recaptured by drastically improving the rate and quality of future student learning (Howell, Hosp, & Kurns, 2008; Marzano, 2004).

Teaching Learning Strategies and Promoting Their Use in the Classroom

Students learn about more than subject matter at school. Most of them also learn *how to learn* within the academic context. And, once equipped with that knowledge, they learn additional subject matter faster. These skills are variously referred to as *academic strategies*, *learning strategies*, *task-related skills*, *academic enablers*, and *study and test-taking strategies*. They fall into the category of *tacit knowledge*, representing what we might think of as a student's know-how

or academic "with-it-ness" (Sternberg & Hedlund, 2002). Sometimes they are explicitly taught; however, many educators and most students remain relatively unfamiliar with the content of effective study and learning. In the context of this content and its instruction, the concept of a learning problem shifts its definition. It moves from being an information-processing problem to being a curriculum-and-instruction problem, and, in so doing, helps resolve the questions, What does education have to offer psychology? and What does psychology have to offer education? (Mayer, 2001).

Academic strategies are commonly taught to promote the application of adaptive attention, memory, and motivation, as well for study and academic work. Many of these strategies are content-specific (i.e., their application is limited to certain tasks), whereas others are more "general" in their utility (Ericsson, 2006). For example, Bhattacharya (2006) documented positive outcomes for learning science content by teaching a strategy for use of syllable-based morphological information to understand science terminology. The findings were consistent with the conclusions of other studies showing that similar strategies can have a remarkably positive impact on student learning across content-area classes in the higher grades (Mayer, 2001; Pashler et al., 2007; Reed, 2008). However, past experience suggests the need for both clarity and caution when discussing evaluation or instruction of learning strategies. School psychology and special education both have unfortunate histories of attempts to assess and teach various hypothesized cognitive and perceptual processes (Arter & Jenkins, 1979; Fletcher et al., 2004; Torgesen, 2002).

Strategic knowledge, unlike factual knowledge, is not about answers but rather about *how to arrive at answers*. The emphasis is on the *process* of completing work, not getting the task itself completed. For example, because there are both correct and incorrect ways to complete computations, an instructor focusing on strategies should be focused on *how* a student solved 20 + 25 = 45, not just the fact that the student gets the answer right (the *right* answer could have been copied off another student's paper—a common maladaptive strategy). Often there may be more than one strategy for doing the same thing correctly. For example, when teaching students to rearrange numbers for borrowing (i.e., regrouping) within subtraction, one could teach the student this rule: "borrow when there isn't a sufficient quantity to allow subtraction." As an alternative one can also teach this task-monitoring strategy (called the "BBB" strategy): "When the big number is on the bottom, we borrow" (Stein, Kinder, Silbert, & Carnine, 2006).

There are many academic strategies that can be applied to a variety of content areas (e.g., reading, math, social skills). Highly successful learners use them regularly. However, all students do not simply pick up their correct use. Perhaps unfortunately, there is nothing approaching an agreed-on set of academic learning skills composing the "accepted curriculum" of academic strategies. This means that students moving among schools and districts may be behind (i.e., remedial), corrective (i.e., having a patchwork of skills) or even ahead depending on what was taught in the schools they came from and what is expected in the schools they go to.

Academic strategies are not uniformly addressed, as both good and bad programs exist to teach them. Although almost every student gets some advice about studying and test taking, some are taught very specific approaches to acquiring, processing, and displaying knowledge, and others are not. In schools in which these techniques are taught, the students should be expected to employ them in all of their subsequent classes (DiPerna, Volpe, & Elliott, 2005). Part of this instruction often includes teaching students to stop using *erroneous* strategies. This can be difficult because, even though an erroneous strategy is not working, the student continues to practice it each time he or she uses it. (Students can practice incorrect strategies, as well as correct ones, to high levels of "proficiency.") Another important goal of strategy instruction is teaching students when and when not to employ a particular strategy (Hamman, Berthelot, Saia, & Crowley, 2000).

Students fail to use strategies correctly when they: (1) do not know the process; (2) do not know when to employ the process; (3) do not recognize when the process being used is not working; and/or (4) simply prefer another strategy. All readers of this chapter are utilizing some combination of both reading task and self-monitoring strategy use. These are obviously difficult functions for students who are missing prerequisite knowledge of a task (Hamman et al., 2000).

In the absence of a predefined curriculum, one could consider the preceding problems 1–4 to see which apply to tasks of concern for a particular student. The problems can then be converted into objectives.

Strategy Instruction

It is always important to provide both guided and independent practice during strategy acquisition. As many academic strategies are cognitive and covert, these demonstrations and examples often need to be provided through verbal mediation or self-talk (Baker, Gersten, & Scanlon, 2002; Hamman et al., 2000; Wolgemuth, Cobb, & Alwell, 2008). This practice should also include examples of error recognition, as it is a precondition for self-correction (Kirschner, Sweller, & Clark, 2006). One way to increase the utility of instruction or recommendations is to ask or to advise teachers to ask the following four questions (using the example of how to teach *asking for assistance in class instead of interrupting a presentation*). The goal would be to plan the lesson so that, once it is finished, one can answer "Yes" to each of these questions:

1. Does the student know the appropriate steps to asking for assistance?
2. Can the student tell when it is appropriate to ask?
3. Can the student catch a mistake in asking if he or she makes one?
4. Does the student find asking preferable to interrupting?

Additionally, educators often will need to teach across a variety of contexts in order to ensure generalizing to multiple environments. This will be increasingly true in the upper grades (one might also need to provide multiple practice opportunities throughout the day). Finally, support and guidance will eventually need to be reduced as the student moves to independent success through practice and high levels of proficiency. When there are errors, remember that replacement strategies always need to be more effective and efficient ways of *solving the same problems* and *completing the same tasks* for which an erroneous strategy is employed. This is particularly true if the student is expected to use this strategy over time and across settings (Ericsson, 2006).

Attending

The topic of attention illustrates widespread confusion of skill and ability. First, notwithstanding the general controversies regarding causation, syndromes, and categorization it has inspired, the term *attention deficit* is most unfortunate in a very connotative way. As indicated earlier, implying that attention is a capacity can encourage fixed-ability thinking. For many, attention has come to suggest a substance *that can somehow evaporate* (e.g., "Most of my kids have 8 pounds of attention, but poor Cheryl only has 4!")

Interventions and/or adaptations for students with trouble attending fall roughly into three categories: psychopharmacological, behavioral, and instructional. Classroom-based approaches emphasize behavioral and instructional interventions (Harlacher, Roberts, & Merrell, 2006). However, recommended instructional interventions (e.g., peer tutoring, small group size, short lessons, and computer use) are often advanced for their utility at reducing activity and class disruptions, not for their effectiveness at increasing learning (although peer tutoring *is* very effective). As every reader is most likely aware, there is no guarantee that a nonactive student in a calm class will either attend or learn. Many interventions are valued mainly for providing *windows of instructional opportunity*, not for promoting focus or increasing vigilance. Teachers will be disappointed in *attention interventions* if they do not know how to use good instructional techniques to focus the student on the critical components of lessons and tasks. Attentive nonlearners do not remain attentive for long.

Lessons intended to teach attending skills may focus on adaptive strategies for self-monitoring, self-evaluation, increasing task perseverance, and selective attention. Selective attention is particularly important. During instruction, attention has two pertinent

components: arousal and focus. Although there is a tendency to think of students with "attention problems" as *overaroused*, during instruction it is more productive to think and instruct for focus or *selection* (although arousal gets more press because of the association of *attention deficit* with *hyperactivity*). Selective attention refers to the allocation and maintenance of attention to central/critical information (not to irrelevant/noncritical information). Instructional approaches to attention may either teach content-specific skills or target more general attention skills.

General academic attention strategies are those that can be applied across a variety of academic tasks and/or settings. For example, teaching students how to recognize, select, and underline key terms in texts would be considered *general*, as the underlining strategy is not limited to social studies or science texts. (Again, generalization of any strategy to another context can be facilitated by training across context and situations [Deshler & Swanson, 2003].) But in addition, Gettinger and Seibert (2002) suggest that students be taught that strategies can be modified and tailored to meet their own needs.

Securing and Directing Attention

Teachers can effectively secure student attention and use any of several techniques to direct it. This is especially important early in skill acquisition. Here are three ways in which an instructor can initially secure or redirect student attention: (1) Use novelty, change, and surprise; (2) conversely, use uniform presentation routines, signals, and visuals to reduce uncertainty in presentations (allows student to focus on the content of the lesson, not the way it will be taught); and (3) provide and use consistent labels for the things students will work with routinely.

When an instructor directs attention, he or she shifts it to the critical information of a given task or concept. A nonexample of directing attention would look like this: The instructor holds up a square and says "This is a square." Then the instructor holds up a triangle and says, "This is a triangle." An example of correctly directing attention would look like this: The instructor holds up a square and a triangle next to each other and says: "This is a square, notice that a square has four corners. You count the corners as I point to them." In this task, the critical information is the number of sides and corners a shape contains. By directing student attention to the important information, the instructor in the second example is illustrating the attributes while modeling how to select and focus on the appropriate stimuli. In addition, the instructor is also contrasting the square and triangle to show what a square is *not*. This is critical; one cannot teach what something *is* without also teaching what it is *not*. One cannot teach a student what to focus on without teaching what *not* to focus on.

Here are some other ways instructors can direct student attention: (1) Ask students to label or indicate the relevant attributes of a task (do not use the terminology *relevant attributes* unless it is skill appropriate); (2) modify relevant attributes through elaboration (e.g., adding color or size); (3) do this only during initial instruction as needed; (4) attenuate the additions as the student's skills improve; and/or (5) use precorrection by asking questions about critical aspects of a task before the student begins to work (or make errors).

This last technique, use of precorrection, can also be accomplished by using lead questions. Lead questions guide the student through the task. For example, "In a minute I'm going to show you some shapes. I'll want you to tell them apart and name them. Can you tell me one thing you can look for to find the answers?" If the student says, "How many sides they have," the instructor would say, "You've remembered one way to tell shapes. Can you give me another thing to look for?" Then the instructor would show the shapes and have the student carry out the task. Additional options for promoting attention and teaching adaptive attending skills are provided in Figure 14.1.

Storage and Recall

Memory involves both storage and recall of information. Students who are successful at memory tasks find ways to connect new information to existing knowledge. Like attention, memory includes a set of active skills that educators can improve through instruction (Wolgemuth et al., 2008). As with attention, monitoring is important for successful use of memory strategies. Students who are not successful at storing and retrieving information often have unrealistic ideas about how much information they can or cannot store and retrieve. This is part of understanding task difficulty. Until students can monitor task demands and their own attention and memory skills, they have no basis for figuring out on their own which things will or will not require the use of any mnemonics they have learned.

There is another explanation for failures to recall and store information, which, although obvious, always needs to be emphasized. If the student does not understand information, it probably will not be remembered. Basically, that makes effective instruction the most fundamental of all aids to memory.

Promoting Storage

Given that combining prior and novel information is at the core of learning, activities centered on that intersection can be particularly useful. For example, strategies for storage of information can include both active preview and review. Previewing activities evoke a student's background knowledge before the presentation of new material; this provides a foundation for processing new messages. Reviewing allows the learner to reconstruct and re-form existing information. As a result, teaching strategies for both activities can help with the combining of existing and future knowledge, as well as organized storage (Marzano, 2004; Schunk, 2008). In practice, this can involve the teacher reviewing previous learning and previewing or introducing new lesson objectives in one coordinated presentation. That practice can also highlight key concepts while alerting students to portions of the current lesson that should be remembered.

To close the link between preview and review, instructors can also give a learning goal for the lesson by saying: "By the end of this lesson, you will know ... " and then reviewing by asking, "Now, what is it you are going to remember?" The aligned preview and review statements used in that context can later be turned into aligned questions and/or practice exercises (e.g., "Today we learned that all _____ ").

Promoting Recall

Creating meaningful organizational structures or sequences for the presentation of content is important for recall. Teaching students the steps in a process while having them actually carry it out will elaborate otherwise rote practice routines. Also, multiple opportunities for active student responding during instruction can improve recall.

Teaching Memory Skills

Teachers can provide instruction on a variety of strategies to promote the effective use of storage and recall. These include strategies such as: (1) mnemonic techniques for discrete and factual information (Wolgemuth et al., 2008); (2) note taking and other complex rehearsal procedures; (3) information organizing procedures; and (4) approaches to summarizing, such as merging notes around the structure of key concepts.

Effective instructors teach students how to remember material as they teach the material ("Do you recall what the 'BBB strategy' is used for and what it means?"). An ineffective instructor may simply fail to offer strategies for remembering information, provide no logical sequence or structure for lessons, and/or overwhelm students with objectives requiring prerequisite knowledge that they have yet to acquire (all established pedagogical procedures for ensuring that the information will be forgotten).

Motivation and Perseverance

Students who are seen as motivated persevere in the face of task difficulty (and, for that matter, all other forms of difficulty). Those considered unmotivated do not (Blackwell, Trzesniewski, & Dweck, 2007). The prevailing explanation for these differences can be found in the studies of students' implicit theories of intelligence and work (Dweck, 2006). The students who are less successful

describe themselves as helpless and attribute their unsuccessful outcomes to nonalterable and/or external causes such as stupidity, task difficulty, luck, poor teachers, or even bad days. For a student with this helpless explanatory set, it is completely rational to give up in the face of perceived difficulty. In distinction, for students who see failures and accomplishments as resulting from things that can be controlled, such as their own effort and the quality of their work, difficulty becomes the signal to work longer and better (Dweck, 2006, 2007). Interestingly, nonadaptive attributions of success (e.g., "I got an A because I'm smart") can be as detrimental to motivation as nonadaptive attributions of failure (e.g., "I got an F because I'm dumb"). Therefore, it is more important to praise *effort* and *improved performance* (i.e., progress) than talent, intelligence, or even high performance. Here are some attribution examples:

Event	Student statement	Type of attribution
Fails assignment.	"I'm too dumb to do this!"	• *Nonadaptive*: Internal *ability* attribution to a nonalterable cause. • *Correct to*: Internal effort.
Fails assignment.	"The test was too hard!"	• *Nonadaptive*: External *task difficulty* attribution to a nonalterable cause. • *Correct to*: Internal effort.
Fails assignment.	"I didn't study the material!"	• *Adaptive*: Internal *effort* (lack of effort) attribution (alterable).
Passes assignment.	"I'm really smart!"	• *Nonadaptive*: Internal *ability* attribution to a nonalterable cause. • *Correct to*: Internal effort.
Passes assignment.	"I really worked hard for that grade!"	• *Adaptive*: Internal effort (alterable). • *Praise for*: Effort and progress.

Summary

In conclusion, this chapter presented an overview of learning problems as understood within an instructional paradigm (as opposed to a student-centered deficit/disability model). Within that discussion the point was made that this view is no less *psychological*; it simply operates on the basics and research of learning and instruction, not disability and incapacity.

Considerable space was allocated to a general discussion of instructional routines and the delivery of lessons for different categories of content. The focus was not on content, under the assumption that classroom teachers will be best prepared in those areas. Instead, an attempt was made to provide generic routines for various instructional actions and goals. Also, recommended approaches to improving and teaching attention, memory, and motivation were presented within skill sets, which can be directly influenced by instruction. These were also treated as crucial areas in regard to improving student learning on a general level, as they extend across all content areas.

Accelerating the rate of student learning (our primary task) is accomplished primarily by improving the students' prior knowledge and teachers' instructional actions. As professionals, we encourage you to concentrate on instructor behaviors in order to maximize student learning of critical content and academic strategy knowledge. By providing students with opportunities to acquire general learning strategies, educators can empower students and accelerate their progress through the curriculum. The goal, of course, is to prepare them with the skills required to obtain the same degree of success as their classmates.

References

Access Center. (2005). *Strategies to improve access to the general education curriculum.* Retrieved September 1, 2008, from *www.k8accesscenter.org/training_resources/strategies_to_improve_access.asp.*

Anderson, L. W., & Krathwohl, D. R. (Eds.). (2001). *A taxonomy for learning, teaching, and assessing: A revision of Bloom's educational objectives.* Boston: Allyn & Bacon Pearson Education.

Arter, J. A., & Jenkins, J. R. (1979). Differential diagnosis prescriptive teaching: A critical appraisal. *Review of Educational Research, 49,* 517–555.

Bahr, M. W., & Kovaleski, J. F. (2006). The need for problem-solving teams. *Remedial and Special Education, 27*(11), 2–5.

Baker, S., Gersten, R., & Scanlon, D. (2002). Procedural facilitators and cognitive strategies: Tools for unraveling the mysteries of comprehension and the writing process, and for providing meaningful access to the general curriculum. *Learning Disabilities Research and Practice, 17*(1), 65–77.

Bhattacharya, A. (2006). Syllable-based reading strategy for mastery of scientific information. *Remedial and Special Education, 27*(2), 116–123.

Blackwell, L. S., Trzesniewski, K. H., & Dweck, C. S. (2007). Implicit theories of intelligence predict achievement across an adolescent transition: A longitudinal study and an intervention. *Child Development, 78,* 246–263.

Deshler, D., & Swanson, H. L. (2003). Instructing adolescents with learning disabilities: Converting a meta-analysis to practice. *Journal of Learning Disabilities, 36*(2), 124–135.

DiPerna, J. C., Volpe, R., & Elliott, S. N. (2005). A model of academic enablers and mathematics achievement in the elementary grades. *Journal of School Psychology, 43,* 379–392.

Duckworth, A. L., & Seligman, M. E. P. (2005). Self-discipline outdoes IQ in predicting academic performance of adolescents. *Psychological Science, 16,* 939–944.

Dweck, C. S. (2006) *Mindset: The new psychology of success.* New York: Random House.

Dweck, C. S. (2007). The perils and promises of praise. *Educational Leadership, 65*(2), 34–39.

Ericsson, K. A. (2006). The influence of experience and deliberate practice on the development of superior expert performance. In K. A. Ericsson, N. Charness, P. J. Feltovich, & R. R. Hoffman (Eds.), *The Cambridge handbook of expertise and expert performance* (pp. 685–705). Cambridge, UK: Cambridge University Press.

Fletcher, J. M., Coulter, W. A., Reschly, D. J., & Vaughn, S. (2004). Alternative approaches to the definition and identification of learning disabilities: Some questions and answers. *Annals of Dyslexia, 52*(2), 304–331.

Gettinger, M. (1984). Measuring time needed for learning to predict learning outcomes. *Exceptional Children, 53*(1), 17–31.

Gettinger, M., & Seibert, J. K. (2002). Contributions of study skills to academic competence. *School Psychology Review, 31*(3), 350–365.

Gresham, F. M. (2002). Responsiveness to intervention: An alternative approach to the identification of learning disabilities. In R. Bradley, L. Danielson, & D. Hallahan (Eds.), *Identification of learning disabilities: Research to practice* (pp. 467–519). Mahwah, NJ: Erlbaum.

Hamman, D., Berthelot, J., Saia, J., & Crowley, E. (2000). Teachers' coaching of learning and its relation to students' strategic learning. *Journal of Educational Psychology, 92,* 342–348.

Harlacher, J. E., Roberts, N. E., & Merrell, K. W. (2006). Class-wide interventions for students with ADHD. *Teaching Exceptional Children, 39*(2), 6–12.

Harrop, A., & Swinson, J. (2003). Teachers' questions in the infant, junior and secondary school. *Educational Studies, 29*(1), 49–57.

Heartland Area Education Agency 11. (2007). *Program manual for special education.* Johnston, IA: Author.

Hoadley, U. (2003). Time to learn: Pacing and the external framing of teachers' work: I. *Journal of Education for Teaching: International Research and Pedagogy, 29*(3), 265–277.

Howell, K. W., Hosp, J. L., & Kurns, S. (2008) Best practices in curriculum-based evaluation. In A. Thomas & J. Grimes (Eds.), *Best practices in school psychology* (5th ed., pp. 344–362). Bethesda, MD: National Association of School Psychologists.

Johnson, R. S. (2002). *Using data to close the achievement gap: How to measure equity in our schools.* Thousand Oaks, CA: Corwin Press.

Kirschner, P. A., Sweller, J., & Clark, R. (2006). Why minimal guidance during instruction does not work: An analysis of the failure of constructivist, discovery, problem-based, experiential, and inquiry-based teaching. *Educational Psychologist, 41*(2), 75–86.

Lane, K., Bocian, K. M., MacMillan, D. L., & Gresham, F. M. (2004). Treatment integrity: An essential—but often forgotten—component of school-based intervention. *Preventing School Failure, 48,* 36–43.

Marks, H. (2000). Student engagement in instructional activity: Patterns in the elementary, middle and high school years. *American Educational Research Journal, 37,* 153–184.

Marzano, R. J. (2004). *Building background knowledge for academic achievement: Research on what works in schools.* Alexandria, VA: Association for Supervision and Curriculum Development.

Marzano, R. J., Pickering, D. J., & Pollock, J. E. (2001). *Classroom instruction that works: Research-based strategies for increasing student achievement.* Alexandria, VA: Association for Supervision and Curriculum Development.

Mayer, R. E. (2001). What good is educational psychology? The case of cognition and instruction. *Educational Psychologist, 36*(2), 83–88.

Naglieri, J. A., & Johnson, D. (2000). Effectiveness of a cognitive strategy intervention in improving arithmetic computation based on the PASS theory. *Journal of Learning Disabilities, 33,* 591–597.

Nelson, J. M., & Machek, G. R. (2007). A survey of training, practice, and competence in reading assessment and intervention. *School Psychology Review, 36*(2), 311–327.

Odom, S. L., Brantlinger, E., Gersten, R., Horner, H. H., Thompson, B., & Harris, K. R. (2005). Research in special education: Scientific methods and evidence-based practices. *Council for Exceptional Children, 71*(2), 137–148.

Pashler, H., Bain, P., Bottge, B., Graesser, A., Koedinger, K., McDaniel, M., et al. (2007). *Organizing instruction and study to improve student learning: A Practice Guide* (NCER 2007-2004). Washington, DC: U.S. Department of Education, Institute of Education Sciences, National Center for Education Research. Retrieved November 18, 2008, from *ncer.ed.gov/ncee/wwc/pdf/practiceguides/20072004.pdf.*

Reed, D. K. (2008). A synthesis of morphology interventions and effects on reading outcomes for students in grades K–12. *Learning Disabilities Research and Practice Institute of Education Sciences, 23*(1), 36–49.

Reschly, D. J. (2008). School psychology paradigm shift and beyond. In A. Thomas & J. Grimes (Eds.), *Best practices in school psychology* (5th ed., pp. 3–16). Bethesda, MD: National Association of School Psychologists.

Schunk, D. H. (2008). *Learning theories: An educational perspective.* Upper Saddle River, NJ: Pearson Education.

Stanovich, K. E. (2000). *Progress in understanding reading: Scientific foundations and new frontiers.* New York: Guilford Press.

Stein, M., Kinder, D., Silbert, J., & Carnine, D. W. (2006). *Designing effective mathematics instruction: A direct instruction approach* (4th ed.). Upper Saddle River, NJ: Pearson/Merrill/Prentice Hall.

Sternberg, R. J., & Hedlund, J. (2002). Practical intelligence, *G*, and work psychology. *Human Performance, 15,* 143–160.

Sternberg, R. J., & Williams, W. M. (2002). *Educational psychology.* Boston: Allyn & Bacon.

Subotnik, R., & Walberg, H. (Eds.). (2006). *The Scientific Basis of Educational Productivity.* Greenwich, CT: Information Age.

Torgesen, J. (2002). Empirical and theoretical
support for direct diagnosis of learning disabilities by assessment of intrinsic processing
weaknesses. In R. Bradley, L. Danielson, & D.
Hallahan (Eds.), *Identification of learning disabilities: Research to practice* (pp. 565–613).
Mahwah, NJ: Erlbaum.

van Merriënboer, J., & Sweller, J. (2005). Cognitive load theory and complex learning:
Recent developments and future directions.
Educational Psychology Review, 17, 147–
177.

Vaughn, S., & Fuchs, L. S. (2003). Redefining
learning disabilities as inadequate response
to instruction: The promise and potential
problems. *Learning Disabilities Research and
Practice, 18,* 137–146.

Walqui, A. (2000). *Access and engagement: Program design and instructional approaches
for immigrant students in secondary school.*
McHenry, IL: Delta Systems.

Walsh, J. A., & Sattes, B. D. (2005). *Quality
questioning: Research-based practice to engage every learner.* Thousand Oaks, CA: Corwin Press.

Williams, T., Kirst, M., Haertel, E., et al. (2005).
Similar students, different results: Why do
some schools do better? Mountain View, CA:
EdSource.

Wolgemuth, J. R., Cobb, R. B., & Alwell M.
(2008). The effects of mnemonic interventions
on academic outcomes for youth with disabilities: A systematic review. *Learning Disabilities Research and Practice, 23*(1), 1–10.

Chapter 15

Proactive Strategies for Promoting Social Competence and Resilience

Kenneth W. Merrell
Verity H. Levitt
Barbara A. Gueldner

The need to provide effective support for children and adolescents with behavioral, social, and emotional problems has never been greater. This increased need exists due to a combination of factors, including changing family structures, the increasing percentage of children who are born into and grow up in poverty, shifting cultural practices regarding child rearing and the development of appropriate behavior, the multiple and complex demands placed on educators, and the sometimes toxic effects of media and popular culture aimed at our children and youth (e.g., Children's Defense Fund, 1997; Garbarino, 1995; Ringeisen, Henderson, & Hoagwood, 2003). In short, because of these varied and complex risk factors, many students in our nation's schools have not developed adequate social competence, and many lack the resilience to cope effectively with the difficult experiences they may face during their formative years.

Because the promotion of social competence and social–emotional resilience among students in school settings is the focus of this chapter, it is worthwhile to establish some basic definitions of these constructs, at least as we refer to them in this work. *Social competence* is a very broad construct, one that is inclusive of both social skills and peer rela-

tions and that includes summary judgments by others regarding how socially competent one is (see Merrell & Gimpel, 1998, and Merrell, 2008a, for a more detailed exploration of this topic). Social competence has been conceptualized as a complex, multidimensional construct that consists of a variety of behavioral and cognitive characteristics and various aspects of emotional adjustment, which are useful and necessary in developing adequate social relations and obtaining desirable social outcomes. *Resilience*, on the other hand—at least as it is applied to human social–emotional behavior—refers to the process of positive adaptation to significant adversity. In defining this construct, Luthar (2000) emphasized that it comprises two critical conditions: exposure to significant threat or adversity and the achievement of positive adaptation "despite major assaults on the developmental process" (p. 543). For purposes of this chapter, we consider social–emotional resiliency as the ability to "bounce back" and cope effectively in the face of difficulties that might otherwise lead to significant social and emotional problems such as depression, anxiety, social withdrawal, and peer problems.

This chapter, like all the chapters in this volume, is aimed at focusing on practical solutions to everyday problems faced by school psychologists and their professional peers, solutions that are consistent with the problem-solving orientation espoused by the editors. Within this chapter, an additional major emphasis is on delivering proactive or preventative strategies for social competence and resilience through the use of the increasingly well-known *three-tiered model* for developing and implementing interventions for various achievement and behavior problems. The basis of the three-tiered model (also referred to as the "triangle of support"), which is derived from the field of public health, is detailed in many other sources, including the U.S. Department of Education's Center for Positive Behavioral Interventions and Supports website at *www.pbis.org*. Because the three-tiered approach to prevention is detailed extensively by Ervin, Gimpel Peacock, and Merrell (Chapter 1, this volume) and Hawkins, Barnett, Morrison, and Musti-Rao (2, this volume), we have chosen not to restate this information in this chapter. Readers who desire to better integrate this chapter content on social and emotional learning with the three-tiered prevention model are encouraged to review Chapters 1 and 2 and to refer to an article by Merrell and Buchanan (2006).

In addition to the preventative framework of positive behavior support, a variety of strategies, techniques, and interventions have been developed to assist educators and mental health professionals in promoting social competence and resilience among children and adolescents. In addition to such general strategies as effective behavior management and the use of individual and small-group counseling, some previous efforts have been aimed directly at our constructs of interest. Social skills training, for example, has been a staple of school-based social–emotional intervention for at least three decades, often with mixed results. Our view is that structured social skills training interventions are a necessary, although not always sufficient, tool for promoting social competence of students in school settings. A wide array of packaged social skills training programs is available for use in general and special education settings in schools. Because there are so many similarities across these programs in both content and approach, we have chosen not to describe or compare specific packaged

programs in this area but to include some comments about the general characteristics of this type of intervention.

Two of the editors of this volume (G.G.P., K.W.M.) have authored a previous work that provides a basic summary and guide to the essential aspects of conceptualizing, assessing, and treating social skills deficits (Merrell & Gimpel, 1998). That work detailed a "synthesized" model of the essential principles of effective instruction in social skills training. These essential principles included the components of social skills training interventions that were most common across various packaged programs, that were theoretically based, and that were consistent with the research literature on effective instructional and behavior-change principles. Table 15.1 illustrates these eight core features for effective social skills instruction and provides details regarding how the essential steps would be implemented in practice.

Although traditional structured social skills training interventions have been shown to produce small but often meaningful short-term gains in many studies (e.g., Kavale & Forness, 1995; Maag, 2005), these interventions often are plagued with a disconnection between the training situation and the "real world," where the skills must be used on a day-to-day basis. Comprehensive reviews of the social skills training research, such as those conducted by Gresham and colleagues (e.g., Gresham, 1997, 1998; Gresham, Cook, Crews, & Kern, 2004), have verified the notion that social skills training interventions as they are routinely practiced in schools may produce short-term gains but have room for significant improvement. Social validity, or the extent to which the social skills training program is valued by teachers and students, is one aspect that, Gresham noted, has often been lacking in these interventions. For example, we have observed that many well-intentioned social skills training programs suffer from a lack of authenticity or "street cred" in how children are taught to engage in challenging social situations. For example, teaching a socially inept and anxious child to respond to taunting from peers by mouthing the well-practiced platitude, "Please stop teasing me; I don't like it when you do that!" will seldom stop the peer harassment and may even lead to further rejection and alienation of the socially inept stu-

TABLE 15.1. A Synthesized Model of Principles for Effective Instruction in Social Skills Training

Introduction and problem definition

- Group leader presents problem situations, assists participants in defining the problem.
- Group leader assists participants in generating alternatives and problem solving.

Identification of solutions

- Specific instructions engaging in the desired social behavior are presented by group leader to participants.
- Group leader assists participants in identifying social skill components.

Modeling

- Group leader models the desired social behavior for participants.
- Both cognitive/verbal rehearsal component and behavioral enactment component are modeled by group leader.

Rehearsal and role playing

- Participants are verbally guided through steps in enacting the desired social behavior.
- All participants are asked to perform the desired social skill through realistic and relevant role-play situations.

Performance feedback

- Participants are reinforced for correct enactment of desired social behavior in role-play situation.
- Corrective feedback and additional modeling is provided when participants fail to enact desired social behavior in role-play situation.
- If corrective feedback was provided, participants are given additional opportunity for rehearsal and role-playing until desired social behavior is correctly enacted.

Removal of problem behaviors

- Problem behaviors interfering with acquisition and performance of social skills are eliminated through reinforcement-based and/or reductive procedures.

Self-instruction and Self-evaluation

- Participants are asked to "think aloud" during training, modeled by group leader.
- Self-statements reflecting distorted thinking or belief systems are modified.
- Training sessions include a gradual shift from overt instruction and appraisal to self-instruction and appraisal.

Training for generalization and maintenance

- Throughout training, situations, behaviors, and role players are made as realistic to natural social situations as possible.
- Appropriate homework assignments are given.
- Classroom teachers and parents are enlisted to monitor homework, encourage practice of skills, and provide feedback to participants.

Note Adapted from Merrell and Gimpel (1998). Copyright 1998 by Lawrence Erlbaum Associates. Adapted by permission.

dent. Such a response is simply not the way most kids talk to each other in the real world but sounds more like a script generated by a well-meaning but out-of-touch adult. As a result of problems such as these, the positive aspects of many social skills training efforts are sometimes canceled out because of problems with social validity, maintenance, and generalization (see Merrell, 2008b, and Merrell & Gimpel, 1998, for more thorough discussions of this issue).

It is now generally accepted that to be most effective, interventions to promote social competence and resilience should be (1) well-planned, (2) coordinated, (3) articulated across settings, (4) conducted with sufficient training and administrative support, (5) long enough in duration to have an impact on the problem areas, (6) research based, and (7) inclusive of progress and outcome evaluation data (Elias, Zins, Graczyk, & Weissberg, 2003; Greenburg, Domitrovich, & Bumbarger, 2001). For interventions with children whose social competence and resiliency deficits are severe, we would hasten to add that multicomponent or multisystemic interventions are desirable if at all possible. In addition, we believe that whatever interventions are used to promote these aims should have social validity, should be sufficiently easy to use and maintain, and should be of reasonable cost so that they are not limited to externally funded efforts (Merrell & Buchanan, 2006).

In the rest of this chapter we provide a discussion of some effective strategies to promote social competence and resilience at each of the three levels or tiers of support: primary or universal; secondary, or targeted; and tertiary, or indicated. We have not attempted to include all possible interventions at these levels, an effort that would be laudable but is well beyond the constraints of a single brief chapter such as this one. Rather, we have selected examples of interventions that we believe readers will find to be illustrative and useful. For more comprehensive discussions of interventions to promote social competence and resilience, readers are referred to more extensive treatments of the topic, such as works by Forness, Kavale, Blum, and Lloyd, 1997; Maag, 2004; Merrell and Gimpel, 1998; and O'Neill et al., 1997. The chapter concludes with a discussion on developing a true continuum or cascade of services in school settings and on working toward developing systems in which the meaningful implementation of the three-tier model is a reality.

Primary or Universal Strategies

Without a systematic and coordinated approach to prevention, schools often implement short-term, fragmented initiatives that neither address the needs of their students nor create environments that encourage and support student learning across a variety of contexts (Greenberg, et al., 2003; Payton et al., 2000; Zins, Bloodworth, Weissberg, & Walberg, 2004). A comprehensive model of school-based social and behavioral supports begins with a primary or universal prevention component targeting *all* students within a school. The main goal of universal prevention strategies is to promote health and resilience on a schoolwide and classwide basis so that students are less likely to become at risk for learning or social-behavioral problems (Walker et al., 1996). The proactive nature of universal prevention efforts allows schools to maximize their resources by reducing the

number of students in need of intensive social and behavioral supports.

Key features of universal strategies for promoting social-behavioral competence include both the prevention of youth problem behavior and the simultaneous teaching of prosocial skills to promote youth resilience. In order to prevent children from developing problem behavior, schoolwide preventive interventions focus on strengthening children's social and behavioral skills while enhancing the school climate, creating environments conducive to learning and positive growth. Implementation efforts for universal prevention programming involve the consistent use of research-based effective practices both schoolwide and classwide, ongoing monitoring of these practices and student outcomes, staff training, and professional development.

School-related risk and protective factors that affect student success should guide universal prevention programs. According to Hawkins, Catalano, and Miller (1992), several school-related risk and protective factors can significantly affect a student's overall success and healthy development. Research findings indicate that key risk factors for future problem behavior include early and persistent antisocial behavior, academic failure in elementary school, and a lack of attachment to school. Conversely, there are a host of school-related protective factors, such as the encouragement and development of prosocial skills, that can prevent students from diverting toward a path of academic failure, antisocial behavior, and mental health problems. By combining both risk-reduction and skill-building efforts for all students within a school, universal programming may have a significant impact on preventing students from developing academic, social, or emotional problems.

Social and Emotional Learning

Social and emotional learning (SEL) is an umbrella term often used for universal prevention programming that integrates the development of students' academic, behavioral, and emotional skills and provides a comprehensive framework for promoting social competence and resilience. As defined by the Collaborative for Academic, Social, and Emotional Learning (CASEL; 2007),

SEL focuses on creating safe, well-managed, and positive learning environments for all students, as well as providing social competence instruction within five domains. The five person-centered social competency domains within SEL are presented in Table 15.2. These core SEL competencies include cognitive, affective, and behavioral skills that are critical to promoting positive behaviors across a range of contexts.

Integrating systematic social and emotional instruction within a positive and nurturing environment provides students with a foundation from which they can successfully develop social competence and increase their academic success despite environmental and personal adversity. There is a wealth of evidence indicating the link between SEL and increased academic and social outcomes for students. Much of the research has shown that evidence-based SEL programming incorporating safe and well-managed learning environments with social competency classroom instruction results in greater school attachment and a reduction in high-risk behavior (Zins, Weissberg, Wang, & Walberg, 2003; Greenberg, Kusche, & Riggs, 2004; Hawkins, Smith, & Catalano, 2004). Additionally, Zins et al. (2003) reported that students who exhibited social and emotional competency skills had higher academic performance than their peers who did not exhibit those same skills.

Universal SEL programs that are designed to both explicitly teach SEL skills and reinforce the application of those skills across contexts are more likely to result in long-term benefits (Greenberg et al., 2003). Several subsequent key elements of quality SEL programs enhance the long-term benefits for children and youths. Programs should have a clear design incorporating research-based principles of effective teaching strategies, as well as a consistent lesson format for feasibility and ease of implementation. To enhance the effectiveness of programs for all students, these programs should span multiple years and developmental stages and begin as early as the primary grades (Greenberg et al., 2003). Integrating both the environment-centered and person-centered components of SEL will reinforce prosocial skills and provide a safe and healthy environment for positive student growth. To ensure that quality SEL preventive programming meets the needs of *all* students, it is critical to consider cultural adaptations that may be appropriate. Last, using a data-based decision framework, including the screening and monitoring of student progress is essential to determining the needs of individual students and ensuring that each student receives the appropriate dosage and intensity of SEL intervention (Lopez & Salovey, 2004; Greenberg et al., 2003; Greenberg et al., 2001; Payton et al., 2000).

TABLE 15.2. Five Core Competencies within Social–Emotional Learning

Competency domain	Definition and examples
Self-awareness	Accurately assessing one's feelings, interests, values, and strengths; maintaining a well-grounded sense of self-confidence
Self-management	Regulating one's emotions to handle stress, control impulses, and persevere in overcoming obstacles; goal setting; expressing emotions appropriately
Social awareness	Ability to empathize with and take the perspective of others; recognizing and appreciating individual and group similarities and differences
Relationship skills	Establishing and maintaining healthy and rewarding relationships; preventing, managing, and resolving interpersonal conflict; seeking help when needed
Responsible decision making	Making decisions based on consideration of safety concerns, appropriate social norms, respect for others, and likely consequences of various actions; applying decision-making skills to academic and social situations

The Strong Kids Programs

One example of a universal SEL intervention that incorporates the essential characteristics of quality research-based programming is the *Strong Kids* curricula. We include this discussion on Strong Kids as an example of a well-designed and practical social–emotional learning curriculum but add that it is not possible to go into more depth on the topic within the constraints of this chapter. Readers who desire more in-depth coverage of this topic are referred to the several references provided in this section. The Strong Kids curriculum, consisting of five related but developmentally unique components (Merrell, Carrizales, Feuerborn, Gueldner, & Tran, 2007a, 2007b, 2007c; Merrell, Parisi, & Whitcomb, 2007; Merrell, Whitcomb, & Parisi, 2009) is a universal SEL program designed for youths from preschool through grade 12. These curricula were designed to prevent the development of mental health problems, as well as to promote social and emotional health, by addressing the five pathways to wellness advocated by Cowen (1994), including: (2) forming early wholesome attachments, (2) acquiring age-appropriate competencies, (3) having exposure to settings that favor wellness outcomes, and (4) coping effectively with stress. These five pathways have guided much of the research on prevention of mental health problems and the promotion of psychological wellness and social and emotional resilience.

The Strong Kids programs each contain 10–12 lessons incorporating elements of behavioral, affective, and cognitive principles to aid in both teaching and mastering of key concepts and skills. Although there is some similarity in content across the five versions of the curriculum, the number and length of lessons, as well as the specific content focus of the programs, are somewhat unique and focused across the five age- and grade-level breakdowns that are addressed: preschool, grades K–2, grades 3–5, grades 6–8, and grades 9–12. Table 15.3 provides an outline of the contents and lesson structure of the Strong Kids and Strong Teens versions of these curricula, those programs that extend from grade 3 through grade 12. These programs were designed as brief, low-cost

TABLE 15.3. **Program Structure and Lesson Content of the Strong Kids and Strong Teens Social–Emotional Learning Curricula**

Lesson	Title	Description
1	About Strong Kids: Emotional Strength Training	Overview of the curriculum
2	Understanding Your Feelings: Part 1	Introduction to emotions Identify emotions as comfortable or uncomfortable
3	Understanding Your Feelings: Part 2	Discussion of appropriate and inappropriate ways of expressing emotions
4	Dealing with Anger	Recognizing triggers to anger Practicing ways to change inappropriate responses
5	Understanding Other People's Feelings	Identifying others' emotions by using clues
6	Clear Thinking: Part 1	Recognizing negative thought patterns
7	Clear Thinking: Part 2	Challenging these thought patterns to think more positively
8	The Power of Positive Thinking	Promoting optimistic thinking
9	Solving People Problems	Conflict resolution strategies
10	Letting Go of Stress	Stress reduction and relaxation exercises
11	Behavior Change: Setting Goals and Staying Active	Increasing time spent in enjoyable activities and meeting goals
12	Finishing Up!	Review of the lessons

programs requiring minimal professional training and resources for implementation. Teachers or other school staff can easily incorporate the lessons into the general or special education curriculum. The program design integrates research-based teaching practices illustrated by the sequencing, pacing, and structure of each lesson. In addition, the program includes a leader's manual to enhance ease of implementation and evaluation tools designed to measure students' social and emotional outcomes related to the overall goals of the Strong Kids program.

Several research studies conducted to date using various versions of the Strong Kids curriculum have demonstrated the effectiveness of these programs (e.g., Castro-Olivo, 2006; Feuerborn, 2004; Gueldner & Merrell, 2008; Merrell, Juskelis, Tran, & Buchanan, 2008; Tran, 2007). All of these studies have shown positive results in terms of significant increases in students' knowledge of SEL concepts. Some studies have shown significant reductions in internalizing problem symptoms (but not externalizing problems), as well as meaningful increases in students' perceptions of their social–emotional assets and resilience characteristics. Additionally, some of these studies have measured the social validity of the programs from both teacher and student perspectives. These studies have all shown a high amount of satisfaction and confidence in the programs by both students and teachers.

Each lesson of the Strong Kids curriculum has a similar layout, and the components of each lesson are semiscripted for ease of implementation. Included are activities designed to promote the generalization and maintenance of new skills learned across a variety of settings (e.g., home, community, other school settings). Suggestions for instructors to support and promote the acquisition of new skills are provided in each lesson. For example, lesson 4 of the Strong Kids and Strong Teens components, "Dealing with Anger," teaches students skills to help them manage their anger in healthy ways. Students are taught a six-step sequential "anger model" to improve their ability to recognize anger emotions and four specific skills to help them manage their anger. Figure 15.1, a student handout and instructor overhead transparency from Strong Kids for grades 6–8, displays and defines the

components of this six-step model. Lesson 9, "Solving People Problems," is designed to promote awareness of useful strategies for resolving conflict between and among peers. Interpersonal conflict is one of the primary contributing factors to mental health issues such as depression, anxiety, and negative thinking patterns. Therefore, learning appropriate and effective methods for resolving interpersonal conflicts may be a strong preventive measure against social and emotional problems (Merrell et al., 2007). Figure 15.2, also from Strong Kids for grades 6–8, presents the four-step social problem-solving model described to students as a way to solve problems or disagreements.

The Strong Kids curriculum programs are one example of a research-based SEL program aimed at promoting social and emotional resilience and preventing social-behavioral problems. Universal SEL programs such as Strong Kids are not designed to address the behavioral and emotional needs of *all* students within a school. Some students may require more intensive services to prevent them from developing severe social, behavioral, or academic problems. For these students, secondary or tertiary prevention strategies are utilized to provide targeted or individualized support to prevent serious behavioral or emotional problems from developing. However, universal preventative efforts that are implemented with sufficient resources allocated and reasonable fidelity and follow-through are designed so that there may be a significant reduction in the number of students at risk for serious problem behavior.

Secondary or Targeted Strategies

For those students who do not respond to universal interventions, more intensive secondary approaches may be necessary to prevent problems from worsening. Secondary preventive interventions address the needs of students who are at risk for chronic emotional or behavioral problems and show early signs of maladjustment (Durlak & Wells, 1998). Students who are at risk for behavioral or emotional problems generally do not require highly intensive individualized services, but they require interventions that target their specific risk factors. Secondary

⊠ STRONG KIDS. Definitions of the Anger Model

Trigger

Any situation that results in your feeling angry

Interpretation

The process of thinking about what has happened to you and deciding what it means

Emotional reaction (anger)

What you feel after interpreting a situation or trigger

Decision

Making a choice about the action you will take

Behavior

Acting out the decision that you made

Consequence

The direct results of your behavior

STRONG KIDS
LESSON 4

FIGURE 15.1. Student handout illustrating the six-step anger management model, from the Dealing with Anger lesson of Strong Kids for Grades 6–8. From Merrell, Carrizales, Feuerborn, Gueldner, and Tran (2007b). Copyright 2007 by Paul H. Brookes Publishing. All rights reserved. Reprinted by permission.

STRONG KIDS. Problem-Solving Model

Step 1—Identify the problem

Have the other person state his or her wants and feelings.

Use empathy and active listening skills.

Read the other person's body language.

Describe your wants and feelings using "I" statements.

Describe how you feel.

Summarize both people's wants and feelings.

Step 2—Brainstorm solutions

Each person should generate at least two solutions.

Step 3—Choose a solution

Does it work for all involved?

Is it a win–win situation?

Is someone willing to compromise?

If no agreement can be reached, go back to the previous step.

Step 4—Make an agreement

All people must accept the terms of the solution and formalize the solution with a handshake or a written contract.

STRONG KIDS
LESSON 9

FIGURE 15.2. Student handout of four-step problem-solving model from the Solving People Problems lesson of Strong Kids for Grades 6–8. From Merrell, Carrizales, Feuerborn, Gueldner, and Tran (2007b). Copyright 2007 by Paul H. Brookes Publishing. All rights reserved. Reprinted by permission.

prevention strategies, therefore, can address the needs of students with similar risk factors either individually or in small-group interventions aimed at preventing the onset of emotional or behavioral disorders (Kutash, Duchnowski, & Lynn, 2006).

As part of a continuum of prevention services, secondary strategies play a crucial role in promoting the healthy development of youths by preventing social and behavioral disorders from developing. Universal screening for behavior or emotional problems (see McIntosh, Reinke, & Herman, Chapter 9, this volume) can be used to identify students who are at risk for serious problems. After students are screened and identified, schools can then provide appropriate targeted or secondary supports based on each student's level of need. This data-based process enables schools to determine the intensity of intervention necessary to prevent emotional and behavioral disorders.

Children at risk for either externalizing or internalizing disorders often have deficits in social and problem-solving skills, as well as a heightened propensity for making *cognitive distortions* (i.e., hostile or maladaptive attribution biases in the way they think about things; Greenberg, Domitrovich, & Bumbarger, 2000). These social and cognitive factors can significantly affect children's abilities to develop and maintain normative peer and adult relationships and to achieve academically. Therefore, social, cognitive, and academic skills encompass possible targets for secondary preventative interventions. Secondary intervention selection depends on the severity of a child's problem behavior and the internalizing or externalizing nature of the behavior. There are numerous research-based secondary prevention programs aimed at reducing the risk factors and increasing the protective factors for children at risk for serious emotional and behavioral problems. The following sections present several programs used to address either externalizing or internalizing problem behavior through the instruction of prosocial skills and emotional competencies.

Secondary Prevention Programs for Externalizing Problems

The school context requires students to make certain interpersonal adjustments to ensure successful peer and teacher relationships. Children who are behaviorally at risk often engage in maladaptive interpersonal behaviors with their teachers and peers that significantly affect their school adjustment and overall school success. Conversely, children who exhibit adaptive social behavior patterns tend to have more positive social and academic outcomes (Sprague & Walker, 2005). Many secondary preventive interventions focus on reducing children's social skills deficits, allowing them to effectively adapt to their school environment. For example, the Social Relations Intervention Program (Lochman, Coie, Underwood, & Terry, 1993) is an intervention designed to address children's adjustment difficulties related to their peer social context. Developed for children ages 9–12, the Social Relations Intervention Program combines key elements of social skills training and cognitive-behavioral training to decrease students' aggressive behavior and adjustment difficulties and improve students' social competence. The program consists of four components: (1) social problem solving (teaching students a plan for dealing with day-to-day social interaction challenges), (2) positive play training (modeling and training appropriate positive play behaviors), (3) group-entry skill training (how to join a group of peers in an ongoing activity), and (4) anger control training (self-analysis and self-management of volatile situations involving anger arousal). Through a series of 34 sessions, students learn how to solve interpersonal conflicts appropriately, reduce their impulsive behavior, and effectively engage with their peers. This intervention was evaluated by Lochman and colleagues with a sample of low-income inner-city youths with very positive results. Participants in the program demonstrated significantly less aggressive behavior and significantly more prosocial behavior, not only at completion of the intervention but also at a follow-up 1 year later.

Another example, the First Step to Success Program (Walker, Stiller, Severson, Feil, & Golly, 1998), is an early-intervention secondary prevention program aimed at improving the behavioral trajectory of young children exhibiting patterns of problem behavior. The First Step program consists of two intervention modules (school-based and home-based) that are implemented in unison to provide at-risk students with the social-behavioral skills needed to successfully meet the academic and social demands of the school environment. The program begins with a universal screening procedure in which behaviorally at-risk students are identified as needing to receive the intervention. Designed to be incorporated into the existing academic curriculum, the classroom-based component focuses on teaching the target children adaptive behaviors that foster academic and social success. Behavioral criteria are set each day, and the student is rewarded for reaching each behavioral criterion. The program typically requires 2 months, or 30 program days, for implementation, as students are required to meet their daily behavioral criterion to proceed in the program. In conjunction with the classroom-based component, a 6-week home-based intervention provides students with additional behavioral monitoring and reinforcement for school success. A First Step consultant visits the student's home once a week for approximately 45–60 minutes and provides parents with activities to help build their child's social-behavioral competence. The lessons for this component involve guides and parent–child games and activities. Consultants emphasize ways in which parents can help their child with communication and sharing, cooperation, limit setting, problem solving, friendship skills, and confidence. The evidence base in support of First Step is both extensive and impressive. In summarizing several studies conducted to evaluate intervention efficacy of this program, Conroy, Hendrickson, and Hester (2007) noted, "there is ample evidence to support the positive effects of the First Step to Success early intervention program. As the research indicates, the First Step to Success program has been implemented across a number of children and classrooms, resulting in positive gains. In addition, it appears that these positive gains maintain for a period of time, and some teachers are likely to continue to implement the intervention following training" (p. 213).

Secondary Prevention Programs for Internalizing Problems

Unlike students at risk for externalizing problems, students at risk for developing internalizing problems often go unnoticed with respect to these problems at school and sometimes at home, as well. However, research on childhood internalizing disorders indicates that the majority of children who experience significant anxious or depressive symptoms are at increased risk for the development of clinical depression, anxiety, or substance use disorders (Kendall, Aschenbrand, & Hudson, 2003). Based on this research, there is a great need for effective preventative interventions targeting children at risk for internalizing problems.

The Coping with Stress course (Clarke & Lewinsohn, 1995) is a secondary preventative intervention for adolescents experiencing elevated depression symptoms but who do not yet have a diagnosable major depressive disorder or "clinical depression." The intervention is an adaptation of the Adolescents Coping with Depression course (Clarke, Lewinsohn, & Hops, 1990), a program that is designed to be used to treat youths diagnosed with major depressive disorder. The Coping with Stress course consists of 15 group sessions, 45–50 minutes each, designed to teach adolescents effective coping strategies and to enhance their emotional resilience to prevent the development of clinical depression or other mood disorders. The program incorporates cognitive-behavioral techniques that teach adolescents to recognize and challenge irrational thought patterns that contribute to the development of depression. Each lesson utilizes role plays, cartoons, and group discussions tailored to the developmental level of the participants. The program sessions can be implemented in a school setting; however, trained school psychologists or mental health counselors typically lead the intervention groups. A major focus of this intervention is to teach participants effective and adaptive ways of coping with stress. Education regarding affect, cognition, and the link between these two spheres is perhaps the primary focus of the program. Randomized clinical trial research conducted by Clarke and colleagues (1990) demonstrated impressive reductions in depression symptoms in the treatment groups, not only at the conclusion of the intervention but also at 1 year postintervention. The U.S. Department of Health and Human Services' Substance Abuse and Mental Health Services Administration (SAMSHA) lists the

Coping with Stress program on the National Registry of Evidence-Based Programs and Practices, giving it a "promising program" designation.

The Penn Resiliency Project (PRP; Gillham, Reivich, Jaycox, & Seligman, 1996) is a collection of school-based primary and secondary interventions designed to prevent depression and anxiety by teaching adaptive coping skills and building resilience. The program focuses on the promotion of optimistic thinking as a manner of responding to daily life stressors. PRP comprises 12 group lessons, 90 minutes each, designed for use with 10- to 13-year-olds. The curriculum teaches cognitive-behavioral and social problem-solving skills as techniques to both challenge negative or irrational beliefs and utilize effective coping strategies when faced with adversity. As part of the program, children also learn adaptive relaxation, assertiveness, and negotiation techniques for healthy relationship management. The PRP has expanded in recent years to include interventions that go beyond the initial 12-lesson intervention, but this component is a core part of the project. Researched with funding from the National Institutes of Health, the PRP is considered to be an evidence-based intervention. Gillham et al.'s (1996) study of the PRP included a 2-year follow-up of late elementary-and middle-school-age students who were at risk for depression, using a randomized treatment–control design. The gains found with the treatment group were very impressive, showing that, in effect, participation in the PRP cut risk for developing major depression in half.

Of course, in addition to the interventions described in this section—all of which have significant empirical support—for addressing social-behavioral concerns at a secondary level of prevention, many other effective interventions, techniques, and packaged programs are available. Readers who wish to identify more in-depth reviews and discussions of secondary-level interventions for students with internalizing problems are referred to more extensive treatments of this topic, such as works by Doll and Cummings (2008), Kratochwill and Morris (2007), and Merrell (2008b). We encourage practitioners to select interventions for use at this level and other levels of prevention based not only on proven efficacy and effectiveness but also on consideration of the practical needs and realities of the school environments in which the interventions will be used and taking into account aspects of the program's usefulness in addition to proven effectiveness, such as the reach, potential for adoption, implementation ease, and maintenance probability (Merrell & Buchanan, 2006).

Tertiary or Indicated Strategies

There are many students who are in need of immediate and often long-term attention because of serious mental health and social-behavioral problems. These students may benefit from the types of primary and secondary prevention strategies that have previously been described in this chapter, but the reality is that their intense needs may require a much more concentrated and potent intervention plan than is typically available through primary or secondary strategies. By definition, tertiary prevention involves the care of an individual who has a well-established problem or deficit. The individual may or may not have a specific disorder or disability; the diagnosis and classification aspect of the tertiary level is less important than the intensity of the individual's need. The intent of services at the tertiary level is to restore the person to his or her highest function, to minimize the negative effects of the disorder, and to prevent complications. In other words, tertiary intervention services seek to reduce the gap between current functioning and desired functioning and to curtail or prevent negative outcomes and a worsening of the problem. For children and adolescents who have developed mental health and social-behavioral disorders and who are currently experiencing severe problems, intense and coordinated intervention strategies are often necessary to manage major problems and to maintain functional mental health, as well as to prevent future occurrences of severe symptoms.

Necessity of Tertiary Efforts in Schools

Although a legitimate argument can be made that tertiary prevention of mental health disorders is not the primary responsibility or mission of schools, we should consider the somewhat stark reality of the situation, which argues otherwise. In most cases, schools have become *de facto* mental health service centers, and many students who have significant emotional and behavioral problems will receive mental health services in the schools or not at all (Hoagwood & Johnson, 2003). Even in communities that have ample resources for mental health services outside of school settings, the initial impetus for seeking such services may need to be instigated by school personnel, who may need to be involved in some way in follow-up care or progress monitoring after outside treatment is provided. Our position is that educators and school-based mental health specialists should become as knowledgeable and skilled as possible in tertiary approaches to mental health and social-behavioral issues. We think this need is especially true for tertiary approaches that involve partnering and collaboration with community-based medical and mental health providers. Refusing to acknowledge or address the problem is shortsighted and unhelpful, and it may even be unethical and potentially harmful to children.

Schools are in a strategic position to support students who have tertiary-level problems. Whether the focus is on remedying and rehabilitating a student who is experiencing a serious mental health problem or on teaching social competence and resilience skills to youths who are at risk, these tasks are filled with challenges and barriers that may seem immovable. Weist (2005) described today's school mental health movement addressing universal through tertiary mental health issues as "young and tenuous" (p. 735), in which evaluation, consultation, and treatment services are commonly in short supply but an invaluable part of supporting students. Our work in schools, providing services and inquiring about these issues, undeniably supports the notion that teachers believe that the mental health of students is absolutely necessary to their academic and overall success, but the skills possessed and the resources available to implement such services may be limited (Buchanan, Gueldner, Tran, & Merrell, in press).

Examples of Tertiary Service Models

Despite whatever barriers may exist in serving the mental health needs of tertiary-level students, dedicated professionals have made progress in developing and offering such services. Grants and research-supported initiatives may provide some schools with the financial resources to train and support school personnel in implementing interventions and finding ways to maintain these services over time (Weist, 2005). School-based health clinics, although not currently the norm in U.S. schools, are expanding, and they provide a venue from which students can obtain immediate and ongoing treatment from professionals having medical and mental health training (e.g., nurse practitioners, social workers, psychologists, psychiatrists). One of the primary concerns in many of these settings is teaching social competence and promoting resilience. The challenge is that many schools experience multiple obstacles that limit their capacity to acquire needed resources that would assist children and families with acute and chronic problems. Additionally, many of the problems students experience fall outside the scope of practice for many school-based clinicians. As a result, students and their families typically are encouraged to access mental health services in the community, and the path from the identified problem to an effective solution is frequently fraught with difficulties.

There are many ways in which school personnel can adequately respond to the need to promote social competence and resilience among students who are experiencing significant mental health problems. Schools typically have at least one professional who is trained to respond to mental health issues, including crises. Responding often includes referring students to community-based professionals who are trained and who have the capacity to provide appropriate services. Many schools exist in areas with very limited access to community mental health, especially psychiatry services. With this barrier in mind, we must consider ways in which students with tertiary-level problems can be supported within the ability and resources available in the school and in the community. Where community resources are more abundant, it is beneficial for school professionals to initiate and foster ongoing relationships with community agencies such as family and pediatric medicine clinics; psychiatric service providers, including teaching hospitals that may have low-fee clinics; social service agencies; and community-based mental health programs. These connections can provide a potentially rich array of supports to students, enhance the efficiency with which community-based services are accessed, and foster collaborative partnerships among school, community, and home that promote an ecological approach to assessment and intervention. Of course, school districts nationally have a wide variety of policies that guide the decision to refer students experiencing mental health problems to a community agency, so it is vital to understand such guidelines prior to doing so (and perhaps to work toward changing these policies when they are not in the best interests of students).

"Wraparound" Services

One of the more promising recent innovations in this area has been the articulation and delivery of student mental health services under the "wraparound" model. The term *wraparound service* does not denote a specific intervention or model of intervention. Rather, it is a general concept or a "big idea" that is based on the notion of providing individualized, community-based intervention services to children and youths, both in their homes and in schools (Brown & Hill, 1996; Furman & Jackson, 2002; VanDenBerg & Grealish, 1996). Various states and communities have adopted, and in some cases mandated, wraparound services for children who have significant mental health concerns. In some cases, the expansion of the wraparound approach has been facilitated by expansions in the authorizing legislation for Medicaid, and in other cases, it has been initiated due to developments in social policy analysis and activism. Although there is relatively little empirical evidence to either support or refute the wraparound approach, it has intuitive appeal because it tends to formalize the process and facilitate communication among professionals and families as plans are made and services delivered to high-needs students.

Wraparound services, like other forms of intervention that involve collaboration between schools and other community agencies, often involve referrals from school personnel to mental health, social service, and medical professionals. Generally, referrals to professionals outside of the school setting are appropriate when (1) students experience problems that are severe and/or chronic, (2) daily functioning is impaired, (3) the safety of the student or others is of concern, (4) interventions provided at school do not appear to be effective, or (5) the student would most likely benefit from an intervention not provided at school (Merrell, 2008b). Primary care clinics and emergency departments are often the first community resources that are accessed when students and families are in serious crisis situations. More commonly, families seek the advice of their primary care physicians to obtain a referral to a mental health agency and, sometimes, an evaluation to determine whether medical interventions such as mental health medications could be helpful.

Community Agency Collaboration: A Critical Role for School Psychologists

The assistance that a school-based practitioner can provide during times of transition between the school and community mental health or medical agencies is typically both influential and appreciated. For the best impact on the student's academic success and school adjustment, we cannot emphasize enough the importance of a school-based practitioner's having some form of direct communication with community-based providers. Many families attend a medical appointment unsure of how to describe the extent or complexity of the problem. A brief letter written by the school-based mental health practitioner can support the student and family through this process and assist the physician to better understand the nature of the problem and its impact on home and school functioning. Such proactive engagement in a collaborative process between education and medicine ultimately benefits the student in improving mental health. Phone conversations with community mental health providers can provide similar benefits. Of course, legal and ethical confidentiality and privacy requirements must be observed when communicating with nonschool professionals, and many families do not wish to have highly personal issues shared with the school, nor is this type of information relevant or appropriate in many cases. However, most students and families welcome the opportunity for schools to share information with community treatment providers with the intention of coordinating services in both settings. Our view is that this process of supporting the social competence and resilience development of students with tertiary-level needs is best facilitated through a problem-solving process that focuses on remedying deficits with assets and competencies.

Tertiary-Level Services Require a Comprehensive Approach

In a previous work, Merrell and Walker (2004) described some of the essential components of effective services for students with intensive needs in the area of social–emotional behavior, or those who are considered to be at the "top of the triangle." These critical pieces are worth reviewing in this section to add some perspective to our discussion on promoting social competence and resilience for students with intense needs. One of the key ideas we wish to emphasize in this vein is that tertiary-level services are more than just a collection of specific interventions. Rather, effective support for students with intense social–emotional problems and deficits requires a comprehensive approach that ranges from appropriate ongoing screening and assessment processes to careful follow-up, progress monitoring, and communication with partners in community agencies outside of schools.

In terms of identifying and evaluating students with intense needs, it is often necessary to move beyond basic screening procedures, which may be useful in identifying students who may have a problem but are typically less helpful in understanding the details of the problem and then developing a plan to dramatically reduce the distance between what is happening and what is expected or desired (Merrell, Ervin, & Gimpel Peacock, 2006). Such assessment is usually individual rather than group based. For the assessment to be helpful in planning interventions, possible functions of behavioral problems should be considered to the greatest extent possible (Watson & Steege, 2003). Two other elements to consider in assessing students with significant deficits in social competence and resilience are (1) evaluating the students' assets and strengths, as well as their deficits and problems; and (2) incorporating a multimethod, multisource, multisetting design for gathering information (Merrell, 2008a), so that the important contexts and persons within a student's life can be considered in planning the interven-

tion. Readers interested in more details on social–emotional assessment and evaluation procedures are referred to Miller, Chapter 11, this volume, which includes additional treatment of this topic.

Another important issue to consider in delivering tertiary-level preventative intervention services for students with behavioral, social, and emotional problems is that the assessment and intervention-planning process should involve a careful matching of the intervention with the identified problem of deficit (Merrell, 2008a; Peacock Hill Working Group, 1991) and should be connected to the presumed function of the behavior to the greatest extent possible. All too often, the assessment and problem-identification phase of intervention planning results in vague and overly general recommendations for intervention selection. For example, through careful observation and data gathering, it may be demonstrated that a particular student exhibits significant deficits in social skills related to showing appropriate self-management and impulse control within social contexts with peers, which leads to alienation of other students and ultimately to social rejection by peers. In a case such as this, an intervention recommendation or plan to provide "social skills training" is overly vague and does not get at the heart of the matter or help the intervenor support the student in any meaningful way. An intervention recommendation such as this one is akin to a health care professional's conducting a careful medical evaluation on a child who is found to have bronchial pneumonia and then recommending that the child should be provided with "medical treatment for respiratory problems." Although the recommendation may be technically correct, it is not particularly helpful because it is not matched closely enough with the identified problem. Going back to our example of the student with specific social skills deficits, a recommendation for social skills training that focuses on teaching the student to delay impulsive reactions in social settings and to use appropriate self-management and self-monitoring tools within peer interaction contexts will prove to be much more useful than the generic social skills training recommendation.

In summary, some of the key elements to consider in developing and implementing tertiary-level interventions for students who have intense needs related to social skills deficits and a lack of resilience skills include:

- Effective screening measures to identify existence of problems.
- Multisource, multisetting, multimethod assessment procedures that are aimed at considering the scope and intensity of problem or deficit across contexts.
- Function-based analysis of problems and intervention selection.
- Careful matching of interventions to problems or deficits.
- Selecting and using evidence-based interventions that have been proven to be useful for students who have intense needs.
- Providing sufficient time and intensity for indicated interventions; such interventions for students with intense needs will likely require more time and practice than interventions for students with less severe needs.
- Making interventions part of a comprehensive overall plan for supporting the student, considered within the context of academic, behavioral, and social–emotional support.
- Considering wraparound services involving support for students with intense needs that extends beyond the school day; involving community partners as appropriate.

In terms of some specific interventions that may be useful within a Tier 3 or tertiary system of support, we again wish to emphasize that tertiary intervention requires a comprehensive approach to service rather than simple reliance on specific interventions. That said, this volume includes several chapters that provide coverage of specific interventions that may be useful for students who have intense needs and deficits related to social competence and resilience. For example, Chapter 19 by MacKay, Andreou, and Ervin, describes peer-mediated interventions, a collection of techniques that have proven to be useful for students with a variety of needs and varied levels of deficits. Hoff and Sawka-Miller, in Chapter 20, detail the use of self-management interventions, a collection of procedures and tools that have a long history of success for students with significant academic and social–emotional needs. Chapter 25, by Bushman and Gimpel Peacock, promotes the use of problem-

solving skills training, an intervention focus that may be useful across the three levels in the three-tiered model of service delivery. In addition, Chapter 26, by Swearer, Givens, and Frerichs, details the use of cognitive-behavior therapy for youths with anxiety and depression, a treatment approach that has an impressive evidence base for prevention, early intervention, and treatment of significant internalizing problems. In Chapter 27, Kern, Benson, and Clemens address severe behavior problems of children and youths, a topic that is a natural extension of promoting social competence and resilience. Again, we emphasize that the specific intervention itself is only one component of tertiary support; just as important is the overall comprehensive system of care and management that must be in place in order for students with extremely intense needs to receive adequate support.

Providing a Continuum of Supports for All Students

Incorporating a three-tiered prevention approach with an ongoing problem-solving process for determining and meeting students' needs is a potentially efficient method for delivering preventive interventions in school settings, whether the focus is on promoting social competence and resilience or any other basic approach to academic, behavioral, and social–emotional needs.

As our examples in this chapter have shown, universal preventative interventions may be aimed at the whole school population, but they are not necessarily designed to meet the complete behavioral and emotional needs of all students within a school. By utilizing initial screening and ongoing formative assessment of students' social and emotional progress, schools can provide individual students with the appropriate level and intensity of intervention in a timely manner. This screening and formative assessment component of the primary (or universal) level of the three-tiered model connects well with the first phase of problem solving described by Merrell et al. (2006) and discussed by Gimpel Peacock et al. in Chapter 1 of this volume as reflecting the question, *What is the problem?*

Students identified as being at additional risk after universal screening and universal supports are provided belong in the secondary tier of the three-tiered model, which is considered to reflect a targeted rather than a universal approach to prevention. We believe that the problem-solving model espoused within this volume and the four primary questions that are used within this model are appropriate within each of the three tiers of the "triangle" of support that we also advocate. That said, within Tilly's (2002) discussion of problem solving, providing services to Tier 2 or targeted students especially involves not only the *What is the problem?* question, but in many cases the second question, *Why is it occurring?*, a query that may be answered through additional screening and brief assessment, such as the use of teacher rating scales and a brief functional assessment.

The third and fourth questions within the problem-solving model, namely *What should be done about it?* and *Did it work?* reflect the process of developing specific intervention plans and then monitoring and evaluating the effect of the intervention to determine whether it has achieved the intended goals. Again, these two questions are applicable across all three tiers of the triangle support, but they often have specific salience at the top tier of the three-tiered model. In fact, in delivering tertiary-level (or indicated) preventive services, these two questions are usually considered to be critical core components. The *What should be done about it?* question is usually addressed following a comprehensive individualized assessment that takes into account the student's current level of functioning, assets, and problems and also considers what is desired as an outcome. Our experience is that this particular problem-solving question is almost always a crucial issue when considering the students with the most intense needs, even if the practitioners working with these students are not using best-practice assessment and intervention methods. However, the question *Did it work?* is regrettably overlooked in many instances, despite its essential contribution to solving the problem. In our experience, even the majority of cases in which school-based interventions are implemented with intense-needs students, this fourth question is often the aspect that is missing and that keeps many well-intentioned efforts from rising to the level of a true problem-solving approach. Because this question requires follow-up

evaluation, answering it may require a fundamental or systematic shift in approach for many practitioners who are working in the mode of diagnosis and prescription but who seldom take (or have) the opportunity to engage in comprehensive follow-up to see whether the intervention effort was implemented with integrity and whether or not it produced the desired outcome (Merrell, 2008b).

If a true continuum or cascade of services is to be provided to students, whether the focus is on social competence and resilience or any other academic or mental health need, then certain conditions must be in place within a school system. In many cases, arriving at the point at which *all* students are provided with appropriate and effective services may require a fundamental shift in the ways that we think about services and in the ways that our systems are organized with respect to allocating resources and then requiring accountability for these resource allocations (Merrell et al., 2006).

In our view, one of the essential features required to move our systems ahead in this manner is *effective administrative leadership*. Although individual teachers and student support professionals may accomplish a great deal by trying to implement a problem-solving three-tiered approach to serving all students, these individual efforts will be difficult and of limited impact if they are not championed and institutionalized by principals, superintendents, directors of special education services, and other key leaders within the school system. It is difficult to overestimate the importance of enthusiastic and visionary administrative leadership in helping to establish systems of support for students in which a true continuum of services is available.

In many cases, supporting students in this comprehensive and preventative manner might require a reallocation of resources, both in terms of staff time expectations and of how limited funds are spent. For example, we have met many school psychologists who are regrettably stuck in an archaic test-and-place mode who would like to use their skills to make a more varied and broad impact in providing support to students but who feel unable to move out of their current limited roles because of expectations, job descriptions, budget allocations, or their own view of their role and function. Even with a supportive administrator in place, a continuum of mental health services for students with social–emotional problems will be difficult to achieve if the personnel who are the best trained to develop effective support plans are unavailable to do so because of other priorities.

Finally, we propose that parent involvement and home–school partnerships may be another key feature of moving from a crisis-oriented approach to promoting social competence and resilience through a comprehensive and systematic approach in which the needs of *all* students are considered. Although it is sometimes difficult to obtain parental involvement when developing plans to support students who have mental health needs and are lacking in resilience, the prevailing view is that effective home–school collaborations may be an important, if not critical ingredient in this process (Pianta & Walsh, 1998). Particularly when students' needs are at the secondary (Tier 2) or tertiary (Tier 3) levels of support, it may be beneficial, if not essential, to involve parents in order to maximize the social competence and resilience gains of students who have significant mental health needs.

References

Brown, R. A., & Hill, B. A. (1996). Opportunity for change: Exploring an alternative to residential treatment. *Child Welfare, 75,* 35–57.

Buchanan, R., Gueldner, B. A., Tran, O. K., & Merrell, K. W. (in press). Social and emotional learning in classrooms: A survey of teachers' knowledge, perceptions, and practices. *Journal of Applied School Psychology.*

Castro-Olivo, S. M. (2006). *The effects of a culturally adapted social–emotional learning curriculum on social–emotional and academic outcomes of Latino immigrant high school students.* Unpublished doctoral dissertation, University of Oregon, Eugene.

Children's Defense Fund. (1997). *Rescuing the American dream: Halting the economic freefall of today's young families.* Washington, DC: Author.

Clarke, G. N., & Lewinsohn, P. M. (1995). *Instructor's manual for the Adolescent Coping with Stress course.* Unpublished manual, Oregon Health Sciences University, Portland.

Clarke, G. N., Lewinsohn, P. M., & Hops, H. (1990). *Instructor's manual for the Adolescent Coping with Depression course.* Eugene, OR: Castalia Press.

Collaborative for Academic, Social, and Emotional Learning. (2003). *Safe and sound. An educational leaders' guide to evidence-based social and emotional learning (SEL) programs.* Chicago, Author.

Conroy, M. A., Hendrickson, J. M., & Hester, P. P. (2007). Early identification and prevention of emotional and behavioral disorders. In R. B. Rutherford, M. M. Quinn, & S. R. Mathur (Eds.), *Handbook of research in emotional and behavioral disorders* (pp. 204–220). New York: Guilford Press.

Cowen, E. L. (1994). The enhancement of psychological wellness: Challenges and opportunities. *American Journal of Community Psychology, 22*(2), 149–179.

Doll, B., & Cummings, J. A. (Eds.). (2008). *Transforming school mental health services: Population-based approaches to promoting the competency and wellness of children.* Thousand Oaks, CA: Corwin Press/National Association of School Psychologists.

Durlak, J. A., & Wells, A. M. (1998). Evaluation of indicated preventive intervention (secondary prevention) mental health programs for children and adolescents. *American Journal of Community Psychology, 26*(5), 775–802.

Elias, M. L., Zins, J. E., Graczyk, P. A., & Weissberg, R. P. (2003). Implementation, sustainability, and scaling up of social–emotional and academic innovations in schools. *School Psychology Review, 32*(3), 303–319.

Feuerborn, L. L. (2004). *Promoting emotional resiliency through instruction: The effects of a classroom-based prevention program.* Unpublished doctoral dissertation, University of Oregon, Eugene.

Forness, S. R., Kavale, K. A., Blum, I., & Lloyd, J. (1997). A mega-analysis of meta-analyses: What works in special education and related services. *Teaching Exceptional Children, 13*(1), 4–9.

Furman, R., & Jackson, R. (2002). Wrap-around services: An analysis of community-based mental health services for children. *Journal of Child and Adolescent Psychiatric Nursing, 15*(3), 121–141.

Garbarino, J. (1995). *Raising children in a socially toxic environment.* New York: Wiley.

Gillham, J. E., Reivich, K. J., Jaycox, L. H., & Seligman, M. E. P. (1996). Prevention of depressive symptoms in schoolchildren: Two-year follow-up. *Psychological Science, 6,* 343–351.

Greenberg, M. T., Domitrovich, C., & Bumbarger, B. (2000). *The prevention of mental disorders in school-age children: A review of the effectiveness of prevention programs.* University Park, PA: Pennsylvania State University,

College of Health and Human Development, Prevention Research Center for the Promotion of Human Development. Retrieved August 10, 2007, from *www.prevention.psu.edu/pubs/docs/CMHS.pdf.*

Greenberg, M. T., Domitrovich, C., & Bumbarger, B. (2001). The prevention of mental disorders in school-aged children: Current state of the field. *Prevention and Treatment, 4,* 1–48.

Greenberg, M. T., Kusche, C. A., & Riggs, N. (2004). The PATHS curriculum: Theory and research on neurocognitive development and school success. In J. E. Zins, R. P. Weissberg, M. C. Wang, & H. J. Walberg (Eds.), *Building academic success on social and emotional learning: What does the research say?* New York: Teachers College Press.

Greenberg, M. T., Weissberg, R. P., O'Brien, M. U., Zins, J. E., Fredericks, L., Resnik, H., et al. (2003). Enhancing school-based prevention and youth development through coordinated social, emotional, and academic learning. *American Psychologist, 58,* 466–474.

Gresham, F. M. (1997). Social competence and students with behavior disorders: Where we've been, where we are, and where we should go. *Education and Treatment of Children, 20,* 233–249.

Gresham, F. M. (1998). Social skills training with children. In T. S. Watson & F. M. Gresham (Eds.), *Handbook of child behavior therapy* (pp. 475–497). New York: Plenum Press.

Gresham, F. M., Cook, C. R., Crews, S., & Kern, L. (2004). Social skills training for students with emotional and behavioral disorders: Validity considerations and future directions. *Behavioral Disorders, 30,* 32–46.

Gueldner, B. A., & Merrell, K. W. (2008). *Evaluation of a social–emotional learning intervention using performance feedback to teachers in a structured consultation model.* Manuscript submitted for publication.

Hawkins, J. D., Catalano, R. F., & Miller, J. Y. (1992). Risk and protective factors for alcohol and other drug problems in adolescence and early adulthood: Implications for substance abuse prevention. *Psychological Bulletin, 112*(1), 64–105.

Hawkins, J. D., Smith, B. H., & Catalano, R. F. (2004). Social development and social and emotional learning. In J. E. Zins, R. P. Weissberg, M. C. Wang, & H. J. Walberg (Eds.), *Building academic success on social and emotional learning: What does the research say?* New York: Teachers College Press.

Hoagwood, K., & Johnson, J. (2003). School psychology: A public health framework: I. *Journal of School Psychology, 41,* 3–21.

Kavale, K. A., & Forness, S. R. (1995). *Social skills deficits and training: A meta-analysis of the research in learning disabilities* (Vol. 9, pp. 116–196). Greenwich, CT: JAI Press.

Kendall, P. C., Aschenbrand, S. G., & Hudson, J. L. (2003). Child-focused treatment of anxiety. In A. E. Kazdin & J. R. Weisz (Eds.), *Evidence-based psychotherapies for children and adolescents.* New York: Guilford Press.

Kratochwill, T. R., & Morris, J. R. (2007). *The practice of child therapy* (4th ed.). New York: Taylor & Francis/Routledge.

Kutash, K., Duchnowski, A. J., & Lynn, N. (2006). *School-based mental health: An empirical guide for decision makers.* Tampa, FL: University of South Florida, Louis de la Parte Florida Mental Health Institute, Department of Child and Family Studies, Research and Training Center for Children's Mental Health.

Lochman, J. E., Coie, J. D., Underwood, M. K., & Terry, R. (1993). Effectiveness of a social relations intervention program for aggressive and nonaggressive rejected children. *Journal of Consulting and Clinical Psychology, 61*(6), 1053–1058.

Lopez, P. N., & Salovey, P. (2004). Toward a broader education: Social, emotional, and practical skills. In J. E. Zins, R. P. Weissberg, M. C. Wang, & H. J. Walberg (Eds.), *Building academic success on social and emotional learning: What does the research say?* New York: Teachers College Press.

Luthar, S. (2000). The construct of resilience: A critical evaluation and guidelines for future work. *Child Development, 71*(3), 543–562.

Maag, J. W. (2004). *Behavior management: From theoretical implications to practical applications* (2nd ed.). Belmont, CA: Wadsworth/Thomson Learning.

Maag, J. W. (2005). Social skills training for youth with emotional and behavioral disorders and learning disabilities: Problems, conclusions, and suggestions. *Exceptionality, 13,* 155–172.

Merrell, K. W. (2008a). *Behavioral, social, and emotional assessment of children and adolescents* (3rd ed.). New York: Erlbaum/Taylor & Francis.

Merrell, K. W. (2008b). *Helping students overcome depression and anxiety: A practical guide* (2nd ed.). New York: Guilford Press.

Merrell, K. W., & Buchanan, R. S. (2006). Intervention selection in school-based practice: Using public health models to enhance systems capacity of schools. *School Psychology Review, 35,* 167–180.

Merrell, K. W. (with Carrizales, D., Feuerborn, L., Gueldner, B. A., & Tran, O. K.). (2007a). *Strong kids—Grades 3–5: A social and emotional learning curriculum.* Baltimore: Brookes.

Merrell, K. W. (with Carrizales, D., Feuerborn, L., Gueldner, B. A., Tran, O. K.). (2007b). *Strong kids—Grades 6–8: A social and emotional learning curriculum.* Baltimore: Brookes.

Merrell, K. W., Carrizales, D., & Feuerborn, L., Gueldner, B. A., Tran, O. K. (2007c). *Strong teens—Grades 9–12: A social and emotional learning curriculum.* Baltimore: Brookes.

Merrell, K. W., Ervin, R. A., & Gimpel Peacock, G. A. (2006). *School psychology for the 21st century: Foundations and practices.* New York: Guilford Press.

Merrell, K. W., & Gimpel, G. A. (1998). *Social skills of children and adolescents: Conceptualization, assessment, treatment.* Mahwah, NJ: Erlbaum.

Merrell, K. W., Juskelis, M. P., Tran, O. K., & Buchanan, R. (2008). Social and emotional learning in the classroom: Evaluation of strong kids and strong teens on students' social–emotional knowledge and symptoms. *Journal of Applied School Psychology, 24,* 209–224.

Merrell, K. W., Parisi, D., & Whitcomb, S. (2007). *Strong start for grades K–2: A social and emotional learning curriculum.* Baltimore: Brookes.

Merrell, K. W., & Walker, H. M. (2004). Deconstructing a definition: Social maladjustment versus emotional disturbance and moving the EBD field forward. *Psychology in the Schools, 41,* 899–910.

Merrell, K. W., Whitcomb, S., & Parisi, D. (2009). *Strong start for preschool: A social and emotional learning curriculum.* Baltimore: Brookes.

O'Neill, R. E., Horner, R. H., Albin, R. W., Sprague, J. R., Storey, K., & Newton, J. S. (1997). *Functional assessment and program development for problem behavior: A practical handbook* (2nd ed.). Pacific Grove, CA: Brookes/Cole.

Payton, J. W., Wardlaw, D. M., Graczyk, P. A., Bloodworth, M. R., Tompsett, C. J., & Weissberg, R. P. (2000). Social and emotional learning: A framework for promoting mental health and reducing risk behavior in children and youth. *Journal of School Health, 70*(5), 179–185.

Peacock Hill Working Group. (1991). Problems and promises in special education and related services for children and youth with emotional or behavioral disorders. *Behavioral Disorders, 16,* 299–313.

Pianta, R. C., & Walsh, D. J. (1998). Applying the construct of resilience in schools: Cautions from a developmental systems perspective. *School Psychology Review, 27,* 407–417.

Ringeisen, H., Henderson, K., & Hoagwood, K. (2003). Context matters: Schools and the "research to practice gap" in children's mental health. *School Psychology Review, 32,* 153–168.

Sprague, J. R., & Walker, H. M. (2005). *Safe and healthy schools: Practical prevention strategies.* New York: Guilford Press.

Tilly, D. (2002). Best practices in school psychology as a problem-solving enterprise. In A. Thomas & J. Grimes (Eds.), *Best practices in school psychology* (4th ed., Vol. 1, pp. 21–36). Bethesda, MD: National Association of School Psychologists.

Tran, O. K. (2007). *Promoting social and emotional learning in schools: An investigation of massed versus distributed practice schedules and social validity of the Strong Kids curriculum in late elementary aged students.* Unpublished doctoral dissertation, University of Oregon, Eugene

VanDenBerg, J. E., & Grealish, M. E. (1996). Individualized services and supports through the wrap-around process. *Journal of Child and Family Studies, 5,* 7–21.

Walker, H. M., Horner, R. H., Sugai, G., Bullis, M., Sprague, J. R., Bricker, D., et al. (1996). Integrated approaches to preventing antisocial behavior patterns among school-age children and youth. *Journal of Emotional and Behavioral Disorders, 4*(4), 194–209.

Walker, H., Stiller, B., Severson, H. H., Feil, E. G., & Golly, A. (1998). First Step to Success: Intervening at the point of school entry to prevent antisocial behavior patterns. *Psychology in the Schools, 35,* 259–269.

Watson, T. S., & Steege, M. W. (2003). *Conducting school-based functional behavioral assessments: A practitioner's guide.* New York: Guilford Press.

Weist, M. D. (2005). Fulfilling the promise of school-based mental health: Moving toward a public mental health promotion approach. *Journal of Abnormal Child Psychology, 33*(6), 735–741.

Zins, J. E., Bloodworth, M. R., Weissberg, R. P., & Walberg, H. J. (2004). The scientific base linking social and emotional learning to school success. In J. E. Zins, M. C. Wang, & H. J. Walberg (Eds.), *Building academic success on social and emotional learning: What does the research say?* New York: Teachers College Press.

Zins, J. E., Weissberg, R. P., Wang, M. C., & Walberg, H. J. (Eds.). (2003). *Building academic success on social and emotional learning: What does the research say?* New York: Teachers College Press.

Chapter 16

Evidence-Based Reading Instruction

Developing and Implementing Reading Programs at the Core,
Supplemental, and Intervention Levels

Sylvia Linan-Thompson
Sharon Vaughn

Among the recent changes in education, one of the most significant has been the renewed focus on the prevention of learning difficulties. Compared with previous reform attempts, the current efforts have been bolstered by the research in beginning reading that has emerged in the past 15 years (e.g., National Reading Panel, 2000; Snow, Burns, & Griffin, 1998) and the systematic use of curriculum-based measurement (CBM) to monitor students' progress in reading. Perhaps one of the key elements of the current reform in reading instruction is the notion of implementing a preventive approach.

Central to a preventive approach is the belief that providing students with a learning environment characterized by systematic, explicit, and differentiated instruction can prevent many learning difficulties, particularly those associated with lack of educational opportunity and with living in poverty. Moreover, a preventive approach can minimize the degree of difficulty experienced by students by providing them intensive instruction at the onset of their formal educational experience. In the past, many students would experience years of failure before receiving appropriate instruction (Fletcher, Coulter, Reschly, & Vaughn, 2004). Prevention requires early identification of students

at risk or likely to be at risk; a flexible and responsive instructional program that addresses the learning needs of a wide range of children, as well as providing intervention for students at risk; and continuous progress monitoring to adjust instruction.

A major challenge is the ongoing implementation of screening and assessment practices, as well as providing flexible instruction in response to the assessment data. Educators often dutifully implement measures of early reading, though the data are often underutilized due to lack of understanding of how to effectively use it to make systemic changes at the school or district level. The degree of change required varies with teacher knowledge, practice, and beliefs and should be considered when planning and implementing a prevention model. The greater the change required in teachers' practices and beliefs, the more likely there is to be resistance and lack of integrity in implementation (Gresham, 1989). Even when teachers are willing to embrace the changes, there is uncertainty about what type of instruction is appropriate and how to determine when interventions provided are effective and when students require special education.

Evidence of the critical role that core intervention plays in reducing learning difficulties is accumulating. It is now clear that to successfully prevent reading difficulties, core intervention has to be the strongest link in the continuum of services. The use of research-based curricular materials implemented with integrity and of multiple grouping formats can strengthen primary instruction, contributing to increased success in the development of reading for most students and reserving supplemental and intensive interventions for those students whose difficulties cannot be addressed by a comprehensive core intervention.

In this chapter, we identify elements of effective reading instruction and intervention within early reading (kindergarten through third grade). We address implementation from the perspective of a multi-tiered instructional framework considering classwide or core instruction, as well as interventions for students at risk for reading difficulties and those with reading disabilities.

Multi-Tiered Instruction

In a multi-tiered model, instruction is differentiated within and across tiers in response to student need (see also Ervin, Gimpel Peacock, & Merrell, Chapter 1, and Hawkins, Barnett, Morrison, & Musti-Rao, Chapter 2, this volume). When a multi-tiered model is applied to a specific content area such as reading or mathematics, core intervention refers to the instruction provided classwide to all students. The purpose of core instruction is to provide students with grade-appropriate content in the general education classroom. Typically, instruction is provided by the classroom teacher for 90–120 minutes a day. Major components include universal screening to determine students' skill levels on key tasks, flexible grouping to maximize instructional time and student time on task, and the use of a research-based reading program. Furthermore, instruction is differentiated for those students who may need additional learning opportunities or, conversely, may need instruction and practice in more advanced skills. This component is often overlooked during core instruction, as many educators believe that the provision of subsequent instructional tiers *is* the mechanism for differentiating instruction. Though supplemental and intensive interventions

certainly have an important role, those interventions are not meant to supplant comprehensive primary instruction.

Secondary intervention is for students for whom core intervention alone is not likely to be sufficient. These students are identified based on screening scores or progress monitoring scores that indicate that they are not making adequate progress. The goal of secondary intervention is to provide these students with additional focused instruction and purposeful practice with corrective feedback (McMaster, Fuchs, Fuchs, & Compton, 2005). The programs and procedures used for secondary intervention should supplement and enhance the instruction provided during primary intervention.

Secondary reading intervention is exemplified by focused, intensive instruction delivered to small, homogeneous groups (e.g., 2–6 students) by a trained intervenor four to five times a week. Secondary interventions that have been effective in improving student outcomes last approximately 30 minutes, though interventions for younger students may be as short as 15 minutes (O'Connor, 2000). Participation in supplemental instruction increases students' engaged time and their opportunities to practice and receive feedback in the most critical areas. Thus this instruction is most effective if it is provided *outside* core reading instruction. Many students, though not all, will reach grade-level expectations with this level of support (Linan-Thompson, Vaughn, Prater, & Cirino, 2006; Mathes & Denton, 2003; McMaster et al., 2005; Vaughn, Linan-Thompson, & Hickman-Davis, 2003; Vellutino & Scanlon, 2002). Students who do not make adequate progress with this level of support receive an even more intensive intervention. This tertiary intervention may be provided before referral. If they are still not making adequate progress, they will continue to receive tertiary intervention during the referral and placement process for special education. Students receiving this level of support require extensive modifications to the learning environment and specifically designed instruction. Tertiary intervention is characterized by longer intervention sessions and a smaller group size, often one-on-one, to provide more time on task and additional opportunities for student–teacher interactions. Both secondary and tertiary interventions can be provided by a number of different personnel, from paraprofessionals to certified teachers, increasing the flexibility a school or district has in staffing these positions (Scammacca, Vaughn, Roberts, Wanzek, & Torgesen, 2007).

Movement in and out of the tiers of intervention is based on students' ability to meet grade-level expectations and to demonstrate progress on specified measures. Though sometimes treated as a succession of steps that must be completed in order to identify students for special education, the real goal in a prevention approach is to maximize opportunities for students to succeed in the general education classroom. When implemented correctly, a multi-tiered instructional model provides a framework for seamless delivery of instruction based on student need (see Tilly, Niebling, & Rahn-Blakeslee, Chapter 34, this volume, for an in-depth discussion of this issue).

Components of Effective Multi-Tiered Interventions

Harn, Kame'enui, and Simmons (2007) identified the following four elements as variables that had a significant impact on tertiary intervention: performance monitoring, purposeful instructional design and delivery, prioritized content, or *use of the content that has the greatest impact on student learning*, uninterrupted instructional time and grouping. As general principles of instruction they promote efficiency in teaching and, as such, are also important in primary and secondary interventions. In the following sections we discuss each in relation to each tier of intervention.

Assessment

Universal screening, the two to three screenings a year of all children in a class, is the initial step in targeting students who require additional instruction in the classroom (see VanDerHeyden, Chapter 3, this volume). In addition to screening, progress monitoring through CBM, as well as other measures, can assist teachers in determining students' progress so that appropriate instruction can be provided. Students' scores on these measures are used to form instructional groups for small-group instruction, to pair students

for structured pair work, and to effectively differentiate instruction during core reading instruction.

Data from screening measures also have a role in the identification of students who need intervention. Entry and exit criteria for intervention serve to determine who is provided intervention and how intensive (e.g., time, group size) an intervention is provided. In some models, students who score significantly below their peers will receive tertiary instruction, whereas those students who are less deficient will receive secondary instruction as early as kindergarten (Harn et al., 2007). In other models, all students who are below benchmark will receive secondary interventions initially and will receive tertiary interventions only if they fail to make adequate progress with secondary interventions (Vaughn, Wanzek, Woodruff, & Linan-Thompson, 2007).

Screening measures vary by grade level and assess the most pertinent and predictive skills for that stage of reading development (Fuchs & Fuchs, 2007; Good, Simmons, & Kame'enui, 2001). To be effective, the measures must be valid, reliable, and available in multiple parallel forms (Fuchs & Fuchs, 1998; Good & Kaminski, 2003). For their use to be sustainable, measures must also be quick to administer and score and must provide information about students' academic skills that is useful in planning instruction (Fuchs & Fuchs, 2007). To be valuable in a multi-tiered model, the data have to be used. Teachers must learn to analyze and use the data provided by CBM. A list of screening measures for kindergarten through third grade can be found in Table 16.1.

In using data to make instructional decisions, it is important to identify the percentage of students who do not meet the benchmark on each measure, to determine whether the deficit can be addressed with primary instruction or whether secondary intervention is needed, and to identify the instructional components to be taught. For example, in a first-grade class, 25% of the students did not meet the benchmark on a phonemic awareness fluency measure, and 40% did not meet the benchmark on a letter–sound correspondence measure at the beginning of the year. Because phonemic awareness is often readily mastered through appropriate instruction, these students may benefit from targeted sec-

TABLE 16.1. Screening Measures Typically Used, by Grade Level

Grade	Skill	Measures
Kindergarten	• Knowledge of letter names • Knowledge of letter sounds • Ability to segment sounds in words	• Letter-naming fluency • Letter-sound fluency • Phonemic awareness fluency
First grade	• Ability to segment sounds in words • Ability to associate sounds with letters and use that knowledge to read words or non-words • Ability to automatically read words in connected text	• Phonemic awareness fluency • Non-word-reading fluency • Fluent word reading • Oral reading fluency
Second grade	• Ability to associate sounds with letters and use that knowledge to read words or non-words • Ability to automatically read words in connected text • Reading for understanding	• Non-word-reading fluency • Fluent word recognition • Oral reading fluency • Maze passages
Third grade	• Ability to automatically read words in connected text • Reading for understanding	• Oral reading fluency • Maze passages

Note. Data from Fuchs and Fuchs (2007) and Good, Simmons, & Kame´enui (2001).

ondary intervention with focused instruction in the phonemic awareness skills of blending and segmenting words at the phoneme level. The 40% of students who did not meet benchmark on the letter–sound correspondence measure would benefit from focused small-group instruction as part of primary intervention. This is a skill that many first-grade students are still developing, and these students may make adequate progress with this level of intervention. If they do not, then secondary intervention should be provided. Of course, if these same skills were very low in older students (e.g., middle- to end-of-year first or second graders), then it is likely to be appropriate to provide secondary intervention in both areas immediately.

Additionally, periodic assessment to measure students' progress on grade-appropriate measures is necessary to determine which students are responding to instruction (Vellutino, Scanlon, & Lyon, 2000). It is essential to monitor the progress of students receiving secondary interventions one to two times a month and those receiving tertiary interventions two to four times a month. After groups are formed following initial screening, progress monitoring provides teachers with the information needed to adjust instruction, regroup students, and determine the need for more intensive instruction. A more thorough discussion of reading assessment can be found in Marcotte and Hintze, Chapter 5, this volume.

The role of assessment is critical in a multi-tiered model. The value of CBM lies in the data that it provides on which concepts and skills students have and have not acquired. Teachers can then use the information to make instructional decisions in a timely manner before students fall further behind. In this proactive approach, teachers use the baseline data to begin instruction at the point and with the intensity needed by each student. The progress-monitoring data provide the teacher feedback on the accuracy of those decisions. The cyclical nature of this process provides a means for verifying the efficiency and impact of instruction.

Research-Based Reading Instruction

Across the three intervention tiers, well-designed, effective programs have several common characteristics. They include clear, direct teaching of reading skills and strategies with understandable directions and explanations combined with adequate modeling and feedback. In teaching students to blend the sounds of words to read the word, the teacher should first tell students what they will be doing explicitly. Next, the teacher should give them step-by-step directions, then model what he or she wants them to do—"first I say the sound of each letter, then I read the whole word"—while pointing to each letter, saying the sound and sweeping his or her finger under the word and reading the word aloud. If students make an error during practice, the teacher models again to ensure that students are practicing the task correctly.

Introduction of skills is followed by multiple opportunities to practice. All students, particularly those struggling to read, need ample opportunity to practice the new skills they are acquiring, first with guidance and, eventually, independently. For example, after modeling how to blend the sounds of a word to read it, the teacher should ask students first to say the sounds of a word while pointing to each letter then should ask them to read the word while moving his or her finger under the word. After students have had an opportunity to practice with several words, the teacher should ask individual children to complete the task. In planning instruction, use of systematic, coordinated instructional sequences maximize learning opportunities. An initial letter sequence for the preceding example would include at least one vowel and two to three consonants to increase the number of words that can be created and practiced.

Additionally, students will need opportunities to use these newly acquired skills with a range of materials. Students can first practice reading words in isolation; then, as they become more fluent, they learn to use the sounds of letters to decode unknown words they encounter in text. Opportunities for practice can be built in through the use of flexible grouping. After initial whole-group instruction, students can practice decoding words with a partner, with a small group of students during teacher-led instruction, or while working with peers in a learning center.

Programs that include principles of direct instruction such as these in their design and delivery are most effective for beginning readers, particularly those at risk for reading failure due to lack of opportunity to learn (Chard & Kame'enui, 2000; Foorman, Francis, Fletcher, & Schatschneider, 1998).

Primary Intervention

Primary intervention involves a complex set of instructional practices adjusted to meet the needs of a range of learners and includes all of the critical elements associated with improved outcomes for that developmental level in reading. Core reading programs are the basis for primary instruction and have an impact on the effectiveness of primary intervention (American Institutes for Research, 1999). The recent versions of most commercial basal programs include instruction in the five basic components of reading instruction: (1) phonemic awareness, an awareness that words are composed of sounds and that those sounds can be manipulated; (2) he alphabetic principle, the correspondence between letters and sounds; (3) automaticity with the code, the ability to read text effortlessly and accurately; (4) vocabulary development, learning new words and their meanings; and (5) comprehension development, the use of strategies to understand text. There are, however, differences among programs in the degree of explicitness and systematicity of each component. (The basic components of reading instruction are described in more detail in the next section, on secondary intervention.) Another variable is the degree to which programs focus on high-priority skills in each component. Providing detailed guidance on primary instruction is beyond the scope of this chapter; however, specific details about instructional practices for each grade level are available (e.g., Vaughn & Linan-Thompson, 2004).

Secondary Intervention

Secondary intervention provides increased instructional time for adjusting those elements of reading instruction that are most likely to improve outcomes for students, relating directly to their reading-level and grade-level expectations. For example, for many students, word study—instruction in spelling patterns and the structure of language—is needed to build automaticity. Automatic, fluent reading is less effortful, and students can concentrate on understanding and learning from print. In a well-designed program, the instructional focus shifts over time. At the very beginning stages of reading acquisition, the focus is on the development of phonemic awareness and letter-naming skills. Phonemic awareness, the ability to hear and manipulate sounds in words, is an essential foundational skill in the acquisition of reading skills and is important in kindergarten. Students are given instruction and practice in (1) isolating phonemes ("What is the first sound in *sat*?"), (2) blending ("What word do you have if you blend /b/ /i/ /t/?"), (3) segmenting ("Tell me all the sounds in *cat*"), and (4) manipulating phonemes ("What do you have if you take the /p/ from *pat*?"). Beyond kindergarten, phonemic awareness skills are best developed when they are linked to print, and the focus shifts to the alphabetic principle and phonics. *Alphabetic principle* refers to the principle that the letters in words are represented by sounds. At this point, students are taught the sounds of the letters, that some sounds are represented by more than one letter, and that some letters have more than one sound. *Phonics* refers to the process of teaching students to use sound–letter relationships to decode words. Once students can decode some words, instruction can focus on building automaticity through multiple opportunities to read text of increasing difficulty. Additionally, students learn to read words that are not decodable, such as *was*, *his*, or *the*. Instruction in the use of comprehension strategies is an ongoing element that receives additional focus as students read connected text. Comprehension strategies are those processes that successful readers use before,

during, and after reading to organize new information and to incorporate it into existing schemas or to develop new schemas. Students learn to predict what they will read about, to monitor their own comprehension while reading, and to identify the main idea of the text after reading. The time allotted to each component reflects the impact on the development of basic reading skills. For first-grade students, more time is allotted to phonics and word study initially. As students become proficient readers, the time allotted for each component can shift to provide more instruction and practice in reading text of increasing difficulty and in improving comprehension skills. Examples of content for secondary and tertiary interventions can be found in Table 16.2.

Comprehensive secondary interventions include all the components of reading in each session, but there are examples of effective interventions in which instruction is targeted. Targeted interventions focus on one or two skills, and additional skills are integrated as others are mastered. Targeted interventions are more responsive to individual student needs and may be more expedient in that the additional instructional time is spent on those high-priority skills in

TABLE 16.2. Examples of Content for Secondary and Tertiary Interventions

Time	Component	Description
Comprehensive secondary intervention		
15 minutes	Phonics and word recognition	Instruction in letter–sound knowledge, reading of phonetically regular words, sight-word reading, reading of multisyllabic words, and spelling
5 minutes	Fluency building	Instruction to increase rate and accuracy when reading in connected text
10 minutes	Passage reading and comprehension	Instruction in the use of comprehension strategies before, during, and after reading
Comprehensive tertiary intervention		
1–2 minutes	Sound review	Instruction in letter–sound correspondences
20–25 minutes	Phonics and word recognition	Instruction in reading of phonetically regular words, sight-word reading, reading of multisyllabic words, and spelling
5 minutes	Fluency building	Instruction to increase rate and accuracy when reading in connected text
15–20 minutes	Passage reading and comprehension	Instruction in the use of comprehension strategies before, during, and after reading

which the student is experiencing the most difficulty. This intensive instruction may result in quicker development of necessary basic skills, allowing students to participate in more complex reading tasks (O'Connor, 2007).

In determining which type of intervention to use, comprehensive or targeted, consider the needs of the students, the number of students requiring secondary intervention, and the resources available. If there are few students in need of secondary interventions, or if students have very distinct needs, consider a targeted intervention. If there are clusters of students who are deficient in similar areas or in multiple areas, a comprehensive intervention may be more suitable.

Regardless of the content included, comprehensive or targeted, programs should include instruction that integrates explicit language, systematic instructional sequences, and incremental introduction of skills. A systematic instructional sequence will include an explicit introduction of the lesson, including the purpose of the lesson. The teacher will model that task and provide guided practice prior to asking students to practice independently. With the introduction of each new skill, sufficient instruction and modeling, opportunity to practice, and review are needed (Carnine, Silbert, Kame´enui, & Tarver, 2004; Torgesen, 2002). These practices are beneficial in primary instruction but essential in secondary interventions.

Another decision in the implementation of secondary intervention is related to the model of intervention that will be provided. There are two common types (Batsche et al., 2006), though many implementation practices are possible. The first, standard protocol, refers to interventions in which students receive the same predetermined intervention. Though the starting point may vary among groups of children as a result of their beginning skill, in general students move through the intervention in a sequential manner and stay in the intervention for a prescribed length of time. The second, a problem-solving approach, is more responsive to individual needs of students, both in the length of the intervention and the content. Although this model is more responsive, it also may be more resource-intensive and may require more expertise than may be

available in the district. In reality, these two models are not incompatible. As Tilly, Niebling, and Rahn-Blakeslee (Chapter 34, this volume) point out, the standard protocol approach is a form of problem solving applied to a larger unit of analysis—the school. The advantage of the standard protocol approach is its efficiency. By the same token, use of a standard protocol approach will not eliminate the need for problem solving within tiers. Therefore, both are compatible and necessary.

Tertiary Intervention

Unlike secondary intervention, in which both standard and problem-solving protocols are effective, a problem-solving protocol may be best for tertiary interventions, as the needs of students vary along many dimensions (Denton, Fletcher, Simos, Papanicolaou, & Anthony, 2007; Harn et al., 2007). A synthesis of tertiary interventions indicated that large effects were associated with instruction in phonemic awareness, decoding, and word study, with guided and independent practice in progressively more difficult text, with use of comprehension strategies while reading, and with writing exercises (Wanzek & Vaughn, 2007). The focus of instruction in phonemic awareness, decoding, and word study is to ensure that students develop the foundational skills needed to read words effortlessly. As students develop these word-level skills, they apply them to text reading. Initially, the texts are often decodable ones, with controlled vocabulary that allows students to apply the decoding skills they are learning. Gradually, they will move to less controlled text that includes more sight words and longer words that require more advanced word-reading strategies by students. Writing exercises such as practice spelling and dictation allow students to apply letter–sound correspondences to their writing. Interventions also address the development of more complex reading skills, such as the use of comprehension strategies. Comprehension strategies help students organize information as they read to facilitate comprehension. Activities such as monitoring one's own understanding of the text, predicting and verifying predictions, and summarizing key points while reading help students comprehend what they read.

However, to ensure that the intervention is tailored to students' needs, the instructional content, delivery, level of intensity, and duration of instruction should vary. To determine the best match between learner and intervention, Marston, Muyskens, Lau, and Canter (2003) propose a four-step problem-solving model that includes defining the problem, developing a hypothesis of the problem and identifying an intervention, monitoring student progress, and making adjustments as appropriate (see also Ervin et al., Chapter 1, and Tilly et al., Chapter 34, this volume). Within the context of tertiary intervention, this process allows highly individualized instruction for each student who needs it. However, to be feasible in most schools, this level of individualization must be reserved for those students with the most difficult-to-remediate reading problems. Descriptions and examples of reading interventions can be found at *texasreading.org*.

Grouping for Intervention

Flexible grouping refers to the use of multiple grouping formats to deliver instruction. During core reading instruction, the use of flexible grouping provides a means of differentiating instruction, of using time more efficiently, and of providing students opportunities to be members of more than one group. Formats commonly used include whole class, heterogeneous small groups, homogeneous small groups, pairs, and individual instruction. Whole-class and homogeneous small-group formats are most effective for delivering new instruction, whereas the remaining formats are best used for providing students with additional practice.

Whole-group instruction is necessary for introducing new information, for modeling, and for class discussions. Further, it gives all students access to general instruction. However, this format may have many limitations, such as insufficient instruction in and review of high-priority skills, lack of active participation, and limited opportunities to practice, particularly for students with learning difficulties. Therefore, follow-up with small groups is necessary to reinforce and review the skills and concepts taught to the whole group and to compensate for those missed opportunities. Small-group instruction in primary intervention is differentiated based

on student needs and is closely aligned with the content of the core curriculum.

To enhance the teaching of reading, homogeneous small groups of three to five students can be used to provide focused reading instruction that reinforces skills and provides additional practice. Instruction provided three to five times a week to same-ability groups can provide the additional instruction needed by some students to reach benchmarks within the context of primary intervention.

Students will need multiple opportunities to practice the skills they will be acquiring. Structured-pair work is easily integrated into core instruction because it engages all the students in the class in meaningful tasks while the teacher monitors. Structured-pair work also provides same-age peers within a class with opportunities to engage in reciprocal tutoring activities. Practices embedded in structured-pair work that are beneficial to struggling readers are modeling, targeted practice, and immediate error correction. Examples of targeted tasks that students can practice during structured-pair work include letter naming, sound identification, word reading, passage reading, spelling, vocabulary, and comprehension. Regardless of the task, the more able student in the pair would first model the task—name the letters, read the passage, and so forth. The second student in the pair would then complete the task. If at any time the student makes an error, the more able partner would provide corrective feedback. In this process, the students would stop, the task would be modeled correctly, and the student would be asked to repeat that particular element before moving on. In a letter-naming task, the first student would begin by naming all the letters in a row. The second student would then name the letters in the same row. If a letter were named incorrectly, the correct name would be provided.

Further, instructional tasks are differentiated by pairs and are targeted to the needs of the less able student in the pair. This does not mean that the teacher must prepare different materials for each pair, because it is likely that multiple pairs will be practicing the same tasks. Structured-pair work has been used successfully to reinforce a variety of reading skills, from basic letter naming and phonics to comprehension strategies

(Greenwood & Finney, 1993; Greenwood, Maheady, & Delquadri, 2002; Mathes, Fuchs, Fuchs, Henley, & Sanders, 1994).

The use of various grouping formats during primary intervention allows for maximum instructional flexibility. When and how each format is used will depend on the needs of students. They are not meant to be static but rather responsive to the learning demands and environment.

Secondary and tertiary interventions are best provided to students in homogeneous small groups or one-on-one to better focus instruction (Vaughn, Linan-Thompson, Kouzekanani, et al., 2003). To maintain the level of intensity needed by students to accelerate learning, students are regrouped as needed.

Treatment Integrity

In addition to ensuring that core programs address the critical areas of reading instruction and incorporate practices of effective instructional design, programs must be implemented with integrity. Treatment integrity refers to the degree to which an intervention is implemented as planned (Gresham, 1989). A complete discussion of this topic is provided by Noell, in Chapter 30, this volume. Failure to document integrity of implementation may lead to erroneous conclusions about the benefit of interventions for individual children or groups of children (Gresham, 1989), which could result in the perpetuation of the practice of placing children in special education due to lack of adequate educational opportunity.

Components of the intervention that may be compromised include the level of specificity and explicitness of the language used by the teacher, the number and range of models, the instructional pace, student–teacher interactions, and the completeness with which content is covered. If intervenors fail to implement even one or two of these components, the consequences for students could be detrimental.

Gresham (1989) identified the five factors that may weaken treatment integrity: (1) treatments are too complex; (2) they require too much time; (3) they require materials that are not easily accessible; (4) they are not perceived as effective by those who must implement the treatment; and (5) the imple-

TABLE 16.3. Systemic Decisions

District level

- Develop a plan for universal screening.
  - Determine purpose of universal screening.
  - Determine which measure to use.
  - Establish entry and exit criteria for supplemental instruction.
- Choose a program that has strong evidence of effectiveness.
  - Examine program for completeness.
  - Identify areas that need to be strengthened.
  - Examine other resources for secondary and tertiary interventions.
  - Identify personnel to provide secondary and tertiary intervention.
- Provide professional development.
  - Identify needs related to the implementation of a universal screening system.
  - Identify needs related to the implementation of research-based reading programs at each tier.

School level

- Ensure treatment integrity at all tiers.
  - Provide professional development.
  - Provide clarity and specificity of the intervention steps.
  - Develop plan for observations.
  - Provide performance feedback. Systematically measure the percentage of correctly implemented intervention steps in a protocol or provide information to the teacher about the degree to which the intervention was correctly implemented.
- Use assessment data.
  - Use screening data to group students and plan reading instruction.
  - Use progress monitoring data to make subsequent decisions about student placement.

Note. Data from Gresham (1989); Harn, Kame'enui, and Simmons (2007); and Torgesen (2002).

menter is not motivated to use the treatment. Each of these threats to integrity can be addressed with careful planning, clear communication of expectations, and appropriate professional development. Strategies for improving systematic implementation of multitiered models appear in Table 16.3.

Professional Development

If we agree that a significant goal of reading instruction is to ensure that all students develop the skills needed to be efficient readers in a timely manner, then we have to commit to providing the most effective instruction to students as soon as they enter school. To achieve this, teachers must avail themselves of the latest research. Though not always easy given the rate at which new research is emerging, ongoing systematic professional development is an effective means for identifying areas in need of strengthening.

Garet, Porter, Desimone, Birman, and Yoon (2001) found that professional development activities that included the following six features promoted better self-reported outcomes for teachers than other professional development activities.

1. *Focus on content.* The degree to which activities focus on improving and deepening educators' content knowledge of a subject matter. In reading, this would include a focus on building teachers' knowledge of the instructional components of reading, including specific strategies for teaching each. In other instances, the focus might be on general teacher practice, such as classroom management.

2. *Promotion of active learning.* The degree to which professional development offers opportunities to become actively engaged in meaningful analysis of teaching and learning. In a study with kindergarten teachers (Vaughn et al., 2008), teachers had opportunities to observe and to be observed, to receive feedback, and to plan implementation during grade-level meetings either with the guidance of a member of the research team or on their own.

3. *Coherence.* The degree to which activities are part of a coherent program of teacher learning and to which connections are evident among the intervention and the teachers' goals and activities. When the content of professional development is aligned with the educational standards that teachers are expected to implement, then teachers are more likely to implement and sustain new practices.

4. *Reform-type activity.* The degree to which the activity (e.g., study group, teacher network, mentoring relationship, or individual research project) is organized to facilitate change. Teacher professional development that includes multiple delivery formats, such as large-group workshops, individual coaching or mentoring, and small-group teacher collaborative groups, allow teachers to integrate new practices as they build new knowledge and skills.

5. *Collective participation.* The degree to which the professional development activity emphasizes collaboration among groups of teachers from the same school, department, or grade level, as opposed to participation of individuals from many schools. To increase implementation, all teachers in a grade level were part of the project. In addition, as new grades were added, teachers across grades were encouraged to share lessons learned to facilitate implementation and to develop school-based plans to organize aspects of the new practices, such as screening students or providing tutoring (Vaughn et al., 2008).

6. *Duration.* The degree to which the total number of contact hours spent in an activity and the time span over which the activity takes place are sufficient to achieve the activity's goals. To facilitate the integration of new knowledge and practices, Vaughn et al. (2008) provided short (2.5 hours) professional development sessions to small groups of teachers over the year. A new component was introduced and practiced in each session. The sessions were followed by classroom visits to observe or model as needed by individual teachers.

Specifically, professional development that emphasizes content knowledge, active learning, and coherence leads to teachers' reporting enhanced knowledge and skills and changes in actual teaching practices. In addition, activities that have longer duration (both number of hours and span of time) and that encourage collective participation of teachers are effective because they tend to place more emphasis on content, provide more opportunities for active learning, and provide more coherent professional development (Birman, Desimone, Porter, & Garet, 2000; Garet et al., 2001).

Participation of kindergarten teachers in a year-long professional development program that incorporated many of these practices as part of primary intervention (Vaughn et al., 2008) resulted in improved outcomes for students in two areas—word reading and phoneme segmentation. Further, teachers self-reported changes in their practice and knowledge in identifying students who needed additional instruction.

During the first year of the study, all kindergarten students were screened, and those identified as at risk were tested in January, in May, and then again in the fall of first grade. Neither teachers nor their students were provided intervention. In the second year, the students of these same kindergarten teachers were screened and were randomly assigned by teachers to one of two interventions: Tier 1 (professional development for teachers with occasional in-class support) plus Tier 2 (researcher provided intervention for students) or Tier 1 for teachers with typical school services for students.

To determine the effectiveness of professional development with occasional in-class support (Tier 1) on the reading performance of kindergarten students at risk for reading problems, Vaughn et al. (2008) compared student performance with that of students from the previous year when teachers were not provided with professional development.

Researchers provided kindergarten teachers with five professional development sessions throughout the school year. All were held for 2.5 hours, with the exception of the first one, which was 6 hours long. The first three sessions were held with all 23 kindergarten teachers together, and the remaining three were held with teachers from two schools at one time to make group sizes smaller and allow more teacher interaction. The five professional development sessions focused on content knowledge, general teacher practice, and a particular curricular material. Topics focused on content knowledge included phonological awareness, the use of Dynamic Indicators of Basic Early Literacy Skills (DIBELS; Good & Kaminski, 2003) for progress monitoring, using assessment information to group students for instruction, and follow-up of DIBELS training. Classroom behavior management was the only general teacher practice topic, and implementation of Kindergarten Peer-Assisted Learning Strategies (K-PALS; Mathes, Torgesen, & Clancy-Menchetti, 2001) was the particular curricular material introduced.

The professional development was of sufficient span and duration, focused on content, and included opportunities for collective participation. Additionally, the in-class follow-up promoted active learning and coherence across training and expected practice. This level of support resulted not only in change in teacher practice but also in improved outcomes for children. This level of investment may be necessary to ensure treatment integrity only when initiating change. It is possible that as practices become integrated, the level of support can be diminished without adverse consequences for student learning.

Conclusion

As school personnel are challenged to meet the instructional needs of the highly diverse population of students in a changing environment, new models of intervention that incorporate research-based practices are needed. A preventive multi-tiered model differs from more traditional approaches to instruction in that it is fluid and responsive to student needs. A broad range of instructional support of varying degrees of intensity is available, and students access the support as needed. There is empirical support for the critical components of a multi-tiered model, ongoing assessment, comprehensive, explicit, and systematic reading instruction, and the use of multiple tiers. Although questions remain about specific variations in the implementation of a multi-tiered model, the success of the model in increasing outcomes for students should increase educators' confidence in the benefit of implementing structured reading instruction and intervention programs.

References

American Institutes for Research. (1999). *An educator's guide to schoolwide reform*. Arlington, VA: Educational Research Service.

Batsche, G., Elliott, J., Graden, J. L., Grimes, J., Kovaleski, J. F., Prasse, D., et al. (2006). *Response to intervention: Policy considerations and implementation*. Alexandria, VA: National Association of State Directors of Special Education.

Birman, B. F., Desimone, L., Porter, A. C., & Garet, M. S. (2000). Designing professional development that works. *Educational Leadership, 57*, 28–33.

Carnine, D. W., Silbert, J., Kame'enui, E. J., & Tarver, S. G. (2004). *Direct instruction reading* (4th ed.). Upper Saddle River, NJ: Pearson.

Chard, D. J., & Kame'enui, E. J. (2000). Struggling first-grade readers: The frequency and progress of their reading. *Journal of Special Education, 34,* 28–38.

Denton, C. A., Fletcher, J. M., Simos, P. G., Papanicolaou, A. C., & Anthony, J. L. (2007). An implementation of a tiered intervention model. In D. Haager, J. Klingner, & S. Vaughn (Eds.), *Evidence-based reading practices for response to intervention* (pp. 107–135). Baltimore: Brookes.

Fletcher, J. M., Coulter, W. A., Reschly, D. J., & Vaughn, S. (2004). Alternative approaches to the definition and identification of learning disabilities: Some questions and answers. *Annals of Dyslexia, 54,* 304–331.

Foorman, B. R., Francis, D. J., Fletcher, J. M., & Schatschneider, C. (1998). The role of instruction in learning to read: Preventing reading failure in at-risk children. *Journal of Educational Psychology, 90,* 37–55.

Fuchs, L. S., & Fuchs, D. (1998). Treatment validity: A unifying concept for reconceptualizing the identification of learning disabilities. *Learning Disabilities Research and Practice, 13,* 204–219.

Fuchs, L. S., & Fuchs, D. (2007). The role of assessment in the three-tier approach to reading instruction. In D. H. Haager, J. Klingner, & S. Vaughn (Eds.), *Evidence-based reading practices for response to intervention (pp. 29–42).* Baltimore: Brookes.

Garet, M. S., Porter, A. C., Desimone, L., Birman, B. F., & Yoon, K. S. (2001). What makes professional development effective? Results from a national sample of teachers. *American Education Research Journal, 38,* 915–945.

Good, R. H., III, & Kaminski, R. A. (2003). *DIBELS: Dynamic Indicators of Basic Early Literacy Skills* (6th ed.). Longmont, CO: Sopris West.

Good, R. H., III, Simmons, D. C., & Kame'enui, E. J. (2001). The importance of decision-making utility of a continuum of fluency-based indicators of foundational reading skills for third-grade high-stakes outcomes. *Scientific Studies of Reading, 5,* 257–288.

Greenwood, C. R., & Finney, R. (1993). Monitoring, improving, and maintaining quality implementation of the classwide peer tutoring program using behavioral and computer technology. *Education and Treatment of Children, 16,* 19–47.

Greenwood, C. R., Maheady, L., & Delquadri, J. (2002). Class-wide peer tutoring. In G. Stoner, M. R. Shinn, & H. M. Walker (Eds.), *Interventions for academic and behavior problems* (2nd ed., pp. 611–649). Bethesda, MD: National Association of School Psychologists.

Gresham, F. M. (1989). Assessment of treatment integrity in school consultation and prereferral intervention. *School Psychology Review, 18,* 37–50.

Harn, B. A., Kame'enui, E. J., & Simmons, D. C. (2007). The nature and role of the third tier in a prevention model for kindergarten students. In D. H. Haager, J. Klingner, & S. Vaughn (Eds.), *Evidence-based reading practices for response to intervention* (pp. 161–184). Baltimore: Brookes.

Linan-Thompson, S., Vaughn, S., Prater, K., & Cirino, P. T. (2006). The response to intervention of English language learners at risk for reading problems. *Journal of Learning Disabilities, 39,* 390–398.

Marston, D., Muyskens, P., Lau, M., & Canter, A. (2003). Problem-solving models for decision making with high-incidence disabilities: The Minneapolis experience. *Learning Disabilities Research and Practice, 18,* 187–200.

Mathes, P. G., & Denton, C. A. (2003). "Slow responders" in early literacy interventions. In B. R. Foorman (Ed.), *Effective preventions and interventions for children at-risk of reading difficulties or with identified reading disabilities* (pp. 38–52). Baltimore: York Press.

Mathes, P. G., Fuchs, D., Fuchs, L. S., Henley, A. M., & Sanders, A. (1994). Increasing strategic reading practice with Peabody classwide peer tutoring. *Learning Disabilities Research and Practice, 9,* 233–243.

Mathes, P. G., Torgesen, J. K., & Clancy-Menchetti, J. (2001). *K-PALS kindergarten peer-assisted learning strategies.* Frederick, CO: Sopris West.

McMaster, K. L., Fuchs, D., Fuchs, L. S., & Compton, D. L. (2005). Responding to nonresponders: An experimental field trial of identification and intervention methods. *Exceptional Children, 71,* 445–463.

National Reading Panel. (2000). *Teaching children to read: An evidence-based assessment of the scientific research literature on reading and its implications for reading instruction* (NIH Publication No. 00-4754). Washington, DC: National Institute of Child Health and Human Development.

O'Connor, R. (2000). Increasing the intensity of intervention in kindergarten and first grade. *Learning Disabilities Research and Practice, 15,* 43–54.

O'Connor, R. E. (2007). Layers of intervention that affect outcomes in reading. In D. Haager, J. Klingner, & S. Vaughn (Eds.), *Evidence-based reading practices for response to intervention* (pp. 139–157). Baltimore: Brookes.

Scammacca, N., Vaughn, S., Roberts, G., Wanzek, J., & Torgesen, J. K. (2007). *Extensive reading interventions in grades k–3.*

From research to practice. Portsmouth, NH: RMC Research Corporation, Center on Instruction.

Snow, C. E., Burns, M. S., & Griffin, P. (Eds.). (1998). *Preventing reading difficulties in young children*. Washington, DC: National Academic Press.

Torgesen, J. K. (2002). The prevention of reading difficulties. *Journal of School Psychology, 40,* 7–26.

Vaughn, S., & Linan-Thompson, S. (2004). *Research-based methods of reading instruction: Grades K–3*. Alexandria, VA: Association for Supervision and Curriculum Development.

Vaughn, S., Linan-Thompson, S., & Hickman-Davis, P. (2003). Response to instruction as a means of identifying students with reading/learning disabilities. *Exceptional Children, 69,* 391–410.

Vaughn, S., Linan-Thompson, S., Kouzekanani, K., Bryant, D. P., Dickson, S., & Bloniz, S. A. (2003). Reading instruction grouping for students with reading difficulties. *Remedial and Special Education, 24,* 301–315.

Vaughn, S., Linan-Thompson, S., Woodruff, A. L., Murray, C., Wanzek, J., Scammacca, N., et al. (2008). Effects of professional development on improving at risk students' performance in reading. In C. R. Greenwood, R. R. Kratochwill, & M. Clements (Eds.), *School-wide prevention models: Lessons learned in elementary schools* (pp. 115–142). New York: Guilford Press.

Vaughn, S., Wanzek, J., Woodruff, A. L., & Linan-Thompson, S. (2007). Prevention and early identification of students with reading disabilities: A research review of the three-tier model. In D. H. Haager, J. K. Klingner, & S. Vaughn (Eds.), *Evidence-based reading practices for response to intervention* (pp. 11–28). Baltimore: Brookes.

Vellutino, F. R., & Scanlon, D. M. (2002). The interactive strategies approach to reading intervention. *Contemporary Educational Psychology, 27,* 573–635.

Vellutino, F. R., Scanlon, D. M., & Lyon, G. R. (2000). Differentiating between difficult-to-remediate and readily remediated poor readers: More evidence against the IQ–achievement discrepancy definition of reading disability. *Journal of Learning Disabilities, 33,* 223–238.

Wanzek, J., & Vaughn, S. (2007). Research-based implications from extensive early reading interventions. *School Psychology Review, 36,* 541–561.

Chapter 17

Evidence-Based Math Instruction

Developing and Implementing Math Programs at the Core, Supplemental, and Intervention Levels

David J. Chard
Leanne R. Ketterlin-Geller
Kathleen Jungjohann
Scott K. Baker

Much of what we enjoy and understand about the modern world can be attributed, in part, to humanity's development and use of numbers. Anthropologists, archeologists, and historians have documented the use of numbers in all organized societies, from early antiquity to modern day (Cohen, 2005). The use of mathematics to measure, document, assess, model, analyze, and innovate can be seen in architecture, engineering, sport, business, government, religion, academics, and daily life. The importance of mathematics to the development of technologies to solve existing and future problems cannot be overestimated. The late I. Bernard Cohen, in his book *The Triumph of Numbers* (2005), chronicled numerous examples of how mathematical knowledge served to improve people's lives. Today, however, there is growing concern that the need for mathematical knowledge is more important than ever and that generations of individuals are not becoming mathematically proficient.

Arguably, many individuals have been able to live independent and successful lives with rudimentary mathematics skills. However, phenomena that we encounter every day (e.g., business reports, personal financial information, scientific findings, and varied statis-

tics) increasingly are reported numerically in charts and graphs that require our informed interpretation. Much as strong literacy skills are critical in an information-based society, basic mathematical proficiency is necessary for individuals to live independently. Further, if individuals are interested in pursuing postsecondary degrees and professional careers, knowledge of algebra and statistics is essential to advancement. Failure to prepare students who can pursue advanced degrees has implications for individuals, as well as for society in general.

In many countries, attention has turned to the substandard achievement of students in mathematics and to concerns about the failure of public educational systems to prepare professionals in fields such as science and engineering who will use mathematical knowledge and skills in their work. However, their concerns are not new. For example, flagging mathematics achievement has been a source of concern in the United States for more than 50 years. The persistence of the challenge to improve mathematics outcomes punctuates the need for innovative thinking in solving the low-achievement problem. Evidence from the National Assessment of Educational Progress (NAEP; National Center for Education Statistics, 2007) suggests that there is some improvement in school mathematics achievement. However, American students continue to demonstrate poor performance compared with national standards and in international comparisons (Mathematics Learning Study Committee, 2001). Persistent problems in mathematics achievement are particularly troubling given that the achievement gap faced by students from low-income and minority backgrounds, as well as students with disabilities, is significant (NAEP, 2007). This evidence and the general perception that U.S. students need better mathematical preparation for college has resulted in heightened standards and greater attention to the way teachers teach mathematics and the way it is assessed.

In 1995, U.S. students generally performed poorly in mathematics compared with other countries, as reported in the Trends in International Mathematics and Science Study (TIMSS; Gonzales et al., 2004). In 2003, although performance of U.S. fourth graders did not show measurable improvement over their 1995 performances, trends began to change for U.S. eighth graders, as they demonstrated a significant improvement relative to the 1995 performance and international comparisons. Overall, longitudinal results are encouraging in some areas and disconcerting in others. U.S. performance on the TIMSS still falls short of many industrialized nations, though scores in general have improved somewhat in the past 15 years.

Unfortunately, although overall mathematics achievement has improved over the years, improvements have not been noted across student groups. For example, students with disabilities are not experiencing similar rates of improvement. Additionally, mathematics achievement for other subpopulations (e.g., Latinos, African Americans, and Native Americans) remains considerably lower than achievement rates for white and Asian/Pacific Island students. These disparities suggest that more needs to be done to make mathematics instruction more effective and accessible for all students. This means that, if we are to reverse the trends, significant changes are needed in the ways schools conceptualize and deliver educational services. School psychologists can help in revolutionizing and integrating these services into existing systems.

The Role of the School Psychologist

The role of the school psychologist in improving mathematics achievement for all learners can be separated into two specific components. The first is the consulting role the school psychologist plays in assisting teachers to address the instructional needs of students in academic areas, including mathematics. The second role is that of assessment and measurement expert. School psychologists must continue to exercise their knowledge of assessment principles in the selection and administration of assessments and measures for determining which students need the most support, the nature of that support, and the progress of students' mathematical development. In action, however, these roles are not separable and should complement each other.

In the remainder of this chapter, we discuss how school psychologists can think about their role in supporting instruction in mathematics for all students in a contemporary model for service delivery, particularly students with mathematical disabilities or other characteristics that may impede their mathematical achievement. We begin by providing an overview of ways in which school psychologists can support the improvement of mathematics learning and achievement overall. We then shift to discussing how different types of assessment can inform instruction, with implications for providing consultation to classroom teachers and other support personnel. Additionally, we detail how school psychologists can use recent innovations and research findings on assessment in mathematics to support students by helping their teachers to make good instructional decisions.

General Considerations
for Improving Mathematics Instruction

As consultants to classroom teachers, school psychologists should understand the needs teachers have in terms of enhancing their own understanding of mathematics, as well as the tools at their disposal for improving their instruction. In this section we describe some of the primary challenges teachers face in changing their knowledge and practice. Subsequently, we detail specific materials and tools that school psychologists can access in order to assist teachers in their professional development and their instructional effectiveness.

Pedagogical and Mathematical Knowledge

A school psychologist can be an integral resource to teachers who have not had sufficient opportunity to develop their own mathematical content knowledge for teaching. Efforts to improve mathematics instruction have frequently called attention to the need for teachers to have robust mathematical knowledge for teaching precisely and rigorously (e.g., Ball, Hill, & Bass, 2005; Ma, 1999). The concern about the adequacy of teachers' mathematical knowledge has led to a line of research focused on the types of knowledge necessary to teach mathematics effectively. It turns out that it is not quite as simple as knowing mathematics.

Some scholars suggest that one of the major challenges in improving mathematics instruction is ensuring that elementary and middle school teachers have adequate knowledge of mathematical content (Ma, 1999; Milgram, 2005; Wu, 1997). Milgram (2005) contends that teachers often do not understand the precise nature of mathematics, which results in their teaching concepts and principles in a manner that reinforces inaccurate ideas and poor skill development. Moreover, without this precision, teachers are often unable to teach their students to pose and solve important problems. Wu (1997) argued that the lack of mathematical knowledge in teachers, combined with efforts to redefine mathematics as a result of educational reforms, would lead to difficulties in graduating students with mathematical proficiency. His decade-old predictions seem to have been accurate.

Hill, Rowan, and Ball (2005) suggest that effective teaching requires more than just teachers who possess their own mathematical knowledge, however. Hill et al. (2005) introduced the construct of *mathematical knowledge for teaching*. This type of knowledge refers to "knowledge of mathematical ideas, skills of mathematical reasoning and communication, fluency with examples and terms, and thoughtfulness about the nature of mathematical proficiency" (p. 17). With this knowledge teachers are able to analyze

students' errors to understand how to proceed with instruction, to develop multiple illustrative representations of mathematical concepts, and to sequence examples to guide students' thinking to increasingly sophisticated levels. For example, in teaching fractions, teachers demonstrate mathematical knowledge for teaching by selecting a range of appropriate conceptual models, such as area models or number line models, and sequence instruction in a way that reasonably supports students' understanding (e.g., teaching set models of fractions using money followed by teaching area models). Additionally, when students make errors, teachers are able to identify the source of their misunderstanding. For example, in multidigit multiplication, students sometimes fail to accommodate place value, resulting in incorrect answers.

The previous examples of the knowledge required to teach mathematics may seem self-evident to master mathematics teachers, but until recently there was no evidence that this knowledge was related to student outcomes. In an attempt to understand the relationship between mathematical knowledge for teaching and student outcomes, Hill et al. (2005) assessed 700 first- and third-grade teachers and their almost 3,000 students. While controlling for student socioeconomic status (SES), absenteeism, teacher credentials and experience, and average length of mathematics lessons, they found that teachers' performance on an assessment of mathematical knowledge, both general and specialized, significantly predicted the size of student gain scores. Importantly, in their follow-up analyses, Hill et al. (2005) reported that the effect of teacher knowledge on student gains was similar to the effect of students' SES on students' gains. This finding suggests that teacher's mathematical knowledge of content for teaching may mediate the widening achievement gap for disadvantaged students.

School psychologists can use this information about effective instruction and mathematical knowledge for teaching to support teachers and encourage them to pursue professional development in mathematics. There is a growing list of resources that may be useful for supporting teachers in enhancing their knowledge of mathematics and mathematics for teaching, including the

U.S. Department of Education's Center on Instruction (*www.centeroninstruction.org/index.cfm*) and the website for the National Council of Teachers of Mathematics (*www.nctm.org*). We also highly recommend efforts by Milgram (2005) and the Center for Proficiency in Teaching Mathematics at the University of Michigan (*cptm.soe.umich.edu/um-colloquia.html*). Additionally, we think that in some cases it may be necessary for teachers, and perhaps school psychologists, to enroll in courses, seminars, or study sessions that focus intensively on mathematics knowledge of both types to enhance the effectiveness of their teaching.

School psychologists should also be familiar with the tools that are available to teachers who are responsible for providing core instruction in mathematics. These tools include national and state standards for mathematics learning, including standards and guidance documents from the National Council of Teachers of Mathematics (NCTM), commercially published curricular materials, and content and pedagogical knowledge necessary for ensuring that students progress toward mathematics proficiency. Each of these tools is briefly described next.

Standards and Expectations

The NCTM (1989), the largest professional organization for mathematics educators, published a set of mathematical standards almost 20 years ago, leading a standards movement that has changed the very nature of U.S. education. NCTM has since revised the standards (2000) and offered more focused guidance in how to interpret and use the standards during planning and classroom instruction. The greatest value of the NCTM standards may be that they started the conversation about what is expected in mathematics education and guided states to establish standards that are aligned with national and international expectations. We fully anticipate that the NCTM will continue to evaluate the standards and will be responsive to stakeholder communities (e.g., mathematicians, educators, business owners, college professors) in determining how to revise the expectations of students over time.

In the context of low achievement described earlier, many teachers find themselves overwhelmed by the breadth of topics identified in the standards and in published curricular materials. In an effort to promote curriculum coherence and to help teachers focus on the most critical topics necessary for mathematics success, the NCTM (2006) published *Curriculum Focal Points*. *Focal Points* focuses on "a small number of significant mathematical 'targets' for each grade level" and "offers a way of thinking about what is important in school mathematics that is different from commonly accepted notions of goals, standards, objectives, or learning expectations" (NCTM, 2006, p. 1).

Standards and guidance documents such as *Focal Points* play a key role in helping to identify which students need support beyond the core instruction and which students may need special education services. Because the standards serve as the primary source of learning objectives for mathematics, they set up expectations that become a reference for determining which students are on track and which students are not in light of the instruction provided. Nationwide efforts have been undertaken to ensure that teachers are knowledgeable about their state's standards in mathematics, can design and modify instruction aligned with the standards, and can recognize proficient performance at each grade level. School psychologists should familiarize themselves with the NCTM standards and with *Focal Points*, as well as with the standards for mathematics instruction in their states, to ensure that, as they consult with teachers on specific instructional modifications, they are aware of the grade-level expectations in mathematics and that the modifications they recommend are aligned with the standards. For example, in the following third-grade mathematics standard from the State of California, the student is expected to be able to use division to determine unit cost of an item:

2.7 Determine the unit cost when given the total cost and number of units.

In consultation with a teacher whose student is having difficulty in math, a school psychologist might work with the teacher to improve the ways he or she demonstrates how to solve a problem, such as using repeated addition to estimate the answer. This advice could take advantage of the student's background knowledge and help him or her see the relationship between multiplication and division. Ultimately, however, it is expected that the student would learn how to divide the total cost by the number of units to determine the precise unit costs.

Familiarity with the standards and the concomitant grade-level expectations alone is not likely to result in instruction that maximizes student learning. In many cases, teachers will need to connect their understanding of mathematics with their knowledge of student cognition and development in order to design and modify instruction to assist their students to achieve important learning outcomes (Carpenter et al., 2004). Instructional design expertise also requires an intimate knowledge of curricular materials available to teachers for teaching mathematics. School psychologists should also be very familiar with these curricular materials. In some school districts, these are commercially available textbooks. In others, curricular materials can range from online interventions to teacher-created materials.

Curricular Materials

The development of curricular materials, including textbooks and supplemental materials and programs, was once only market driven. Increasingly, developers must also reflect the available research on learning in a given domain. Unfortunately, there is less research on mathematics educational tools and their relative efficacy than there is on reading instructional materials. However, as a result of the NCTM standards (1989, 2000), there has been a shift from materials that focused singularly on either computation and procedural fluency *or* conceptual understanding to those that build procedural fluency *while* ensuring conceptual understanding of a particular area of mathematics and ultimately providing students with an opportunity to integrate their understanding of foundational mathematical concepts into strategic problem solving.

A perennial criticism of commercially available curricular materials is that they provide an equal focus on each area set out in national and state standards. This is a problem for teachers who are already trying to address a wide range of academic domains in a fixed time period. In such cases,

the aforementioned NCTM (2006) *Curriculum Focal Points* can be useful in providing teachers with a clear understanding of which foundational areas need to be most heavily emphasized and at which grade level. For example, in the primary grades, ensuring that students develop mastery of early number concepts and operations must become the highest priority, even if it means sacrificing a focus on other mathematical content. The areas that were outlined by the NCTM *Focal Points* authors include:

- Number and operations (e.g., base-10 numeration, place value)
- Geometry (e.g., finding the perimeter of an area)
- Measurement (e.g., finding the volume of a 3-dimensional figure)
- Algebra (e.g., solving for unknown variables in an equation)
- Data analysis, probability, and statistics (e.g., finding the mean of a set of data)

As noted in *Focal Points*, the document serves to guard against the fragmenting of expectations and standards and focuses curricula and instruction on key areas that form the foundation of mathematical learning.

As we have described, improving instruction in mathematics requires attention to multiple facets, including teachers' pedagogical and content knowledge, tools, and principles of effective instruction. However, even when knowledgeable teachers implement well-designed curricular tools in an effective manner, some students will need additional support. The remainder of this chapter focuses on how school psychologists can support differentiated instruction in mathematics through the implementation of a multi-tiered model of instructional support.

Mathematics in a Multi-Tiered Model of Instructional Support

Dissatisfaction with instructional effectiveness for the wide range of students in schools has led to the development of multi-tiered models of differentiated instructional support. Typically, these multi-tiered models consist of three tiers of support, with Tier 1 representing core instruction in general education and Tiers 2 and 3 representing increased levels of support based on student need (Schaughency & Ervin, 2006; Greenwood, Kratochwill, & Clements, 2008). Multi-tiered models are one way that has been proposed for implementing response-to-intervention (RTI; Individuals with Disabilities Education Improvement Act 2004, 20 USC 1400; Vaughn & Fuchs, 2003; see also Ervin, Gimpel Peacock, & Merrell, Chapter 1, and Hawkins, Barnett, Morrison, & Musti-Rao, Chapter 2, this volume). Although many individuals perceive of RTI primarily as an alternative means of determining who should receive special education services as a result of having a learning disability, we are of the opinion that it offers a rich opportunity to reconceptualize the method that schools employ for delivering instructional supports to all students. This view of RTI takes a preventive approach to providing support for all students while acknowledging that some students are not likely to benefit from general education instruction alone, no matter how well it is designed and implemented (Chard et al., 2008). For students who need additional support to ensure their success, informed and tailored group or individual interventions are necessary to making adequate progress.

We also believe that operating in a multi-tiered model of instructional support offers us an opportunity to reconceptualize the relationship between school psychologists, teachers, and other support personnel. This new relationship would employ the knowledge and skills that school psychologists possess to help teachers enhance the impact of their teaching by seeing it as part of a system of curriculum, instruction, and assessment that, when fully integrated, inform one another for optimal effect. Tier 1 instruction, typically provided in the general educational classroom to the widest range of students, involves teaching mathematics as outlined in state content standards. To address the needs of students in the general classroom, teachers must employ instructional design and delivery techniques that maximize student engaged time, advance students' conceptual understanding, and help all students to make adequate progress in computational fluency and problem solving. However, as in other academic areas, such as reading, the

context of a large classroom and standardized instructional content almost ensures that some students will need additional support in order to reach benchmark expectations. Knowing which students will need extra support in mathematics requires an integrated system of instruction and assessment. The system of assessments includes (1) screening to determine students' current levels of understanding, (2) diagnostic assessments to identify areas in need of additional instruction, and (3) progress monitoring to gauge the effectiveness of current instruction. School psychologists, with their assessment and measurement knowledge, can assist teachers in understanding principles of measurement and assessment to enable them to select and design assessments that provide meaningful information for valid decision making. In the next section, we describe tools that school psychologists have at their disposal to assist teachers teaching mathematics in the general education classroom and that can be used to identify and provide instructional supports for students who are likely to need additional support to ensure success.

Instructional Decision Making in Tier 1

School psychologists have traditionally become involved with instruction and assessment only after a teacher refers a student for support. In a multi-tiered support model, school psychologists support the general education teacher in an effort to prevent problems by using the tools and knowledge we described earlier. In addition to helping teachers to recognize and develop mathematical knowledge for teaching and to focus their instruction on essential learning objectives, school psychologists play a role in helping to identify students who may be at risk for failure in the domain of mathematics. Assessment expertise is required to interpret test scores for these classification, or screening, decisions.

Screening is the process of using test results to identify students' current domain-specific knowledge and skills for the purposes of predicting future performance on an outcome goal. Typically, the outcome goal is performance on a general measure of mathematics achievement, such as the state accountability test. Scores on the screener test are classified into one of three categories corresponding to the projected level of risk of not meeting expectations on the outcome measure. Placement into a particular tier is based on comparing students' scores with a predetermined performance level that corresponds with the proposed amount of instructional support a student might need in order to meet the outcome goal. Tier 1 placement indicates that the student is expected to reach the outcome goal with high-quality core instruction. Students in Tier 2 are at some risk of not reaching the outcome goal, and, therefore, instruction should be designed to address the students' knowledge and skill levels with appropriate structures and scaffolds to ensure success. Tier 3 classification indicates that the student is at greater risk of not meeting the expectations and needs individualized instruction. To provide appropriate support in a timely manner, screening tests are typically administered three times per year.

School psychologists can not only help teachers with interpretation of screening results but can also provide guidance on test selection. Teachers readily have access to results from classroom-based assessments such as end-of-chapter tests or teacher-made tests, statewide achievement tests, and other district- or school-level tests. School psychologists have the expertise to help teachers understand that although results from these tests might be appropriate for making some instructional decisions, these tests are not useful for making screening decisions within a multi-tiered instructional support model. They lack the technical qualities of assessment systems designed for predicting future outcomes and monitoring student learning over time. Rather, a screening test should represent the breadth and depth of content expected on the outcome measure (see Burns & Klingbeil, Chapter 6, this volume, for a detailed discussion of this issue).

Tier 2: Differentiating Instruction for Struggling Learners

Differentiation of instruction begins with attention to critical features of mathemat-

ics instructional tools and materials that enhance teachers' effectiveness in working with a wide range of learners. For example, some authors have provided guidelines on selecting or creating materials that would serve teachers in their efforts to teach all students as effectively as possible (e.g., Chard & Jungjohann, 2006; Kinder & Stein, 2006). Although these guidelines may be most useful for program developers, they can also assist school psychologists by providing them with a clear understanding of how instructional materials often fall short of scaffolding instruction or providing sufficient review for struggling learners. With this knowledge, school psychologists can assist teachers in modifying their instruction to address the needs of children who typically cannot access the general education curriculum without added support provided in Tier 2. Modifying instruction requires that teachers understand students' needs in relation to their mathematical development. Providing teachers with resources to support their pedagogical, mathematical, and developmental knowledge can enable them to ensure that a wide range of students can be successful in mathematics.

Understanding Diverse Learners' Needs

For students who do not meet the cut score that predicts success on grade-level expectations, instructional modifications are necessary. For many teachers, making instructional modifications to address diverse learning needs in a classroom of learners may be overwhelming. To reduce teachers' anxieties, we suggest that school psychologists encourage them to think about the needs of diverse learners who are slightly below grade level as falling into just four major categories: (1) memory and conceptual difficulties, (2) background knowledge deficits, (3) linguistic and vocabulary difficulties, and (4) strategy knowledge and use (Baker, Simmons, & Kame'enui, 1995). Helping teachers to understand these common learner characteristics will help them address the needs of learners who require Tier 2 support. Each area of need is briefly described next, and the implications for instructional modifications are discussed. In addition, each area is also summarized in Table 17.1.

TABLE 17.1. Common Instructional Modifications to Meet Student Needs

Description of learner need	Instructional modification	Examples
Difficulty remembering new and abstract mathematical ideas	Enhancing memory and conceptual understanding	• Teach new concepts and principles in a sequence from simple to complex. • Use concrete manipulatives and mathematical models. • Demonstrate examples and nonexamples of concepts. • Provide regular review of new and previously taught concepts.
Gaps in prerequisite knowledge of mathematics (e.g., number sense, vocabulary, and fluency with basic facts)	Fill gaps in background knowledge	• Preteach prerequisite knowledge and skills. • Assess background knowledge to identify gaps. • Differentiate instruction and practice.
Difficulties with the language of mathematics (e.g., precise terms, symbols)	Support mathematical vocabulary	• Define and use mathematical symbols precisely in a wide variety of contexts. • Describe and develop vocabulary precisely. • Encourage the use of mathematical vocabulary in classroom discourse. • Provide opportunities for students to talk mathematically and provide feedback on their use of terminology.
Difficulties learning and applying problem-solving strategies	Teach strategies explicitly	• Model important problem-solving strategies. • Teach why and when to apply strategies, as well as how. • Teach midlevel strategies that are problem specific rather than just teaching generic problem-solving approaches.

Memory and Conceptual Difficulties

Students with memory and conceptual difficulties experience problems remembering key principles or understanding the critical features of a particular concept. Moreover, they often attend to irrelevant features of a concept or problem. For example, in a word problem, extraneous information provided by the problem's author to challenge students to sort relevant from irrelevant information to reach a solution poses particular difficulties for some students. Teachers need to give students practice in analyzing problems and identifying the relevant information needed to reach a solution.

Many students, but especially those with memory and conceptual difficulties, benefit from instruction that initially introduces concepts and principles with a high degree of clarity and continues to reinforce the most significant topics. Part of this initial clear instruction involves ensuring that the knowledge being taught is relevant to the learner. Mathematics becomes relevant, and thus "learned," when descriptions and examples go beyond procedural application to include *why* we do what we do mathematically. Therefore, in helping teachers to plan effective and differentiated instructional lessons, school psychologists should encourage teachers to consider the following questions:

1. Are the examples of concepts, principles, and strategies thoroughly and clearly developed to avoid confusion? For example, when introducing the concept of equality,

does the teacher give multiple examples using concrete and graphic examples?

2. Is the gradual development of knowledge and skills moving from simple to complex? For example, do single-digit operations precede double-digit ones?

3. Where appropriate, are negative examples of concepts, principles, and strategies included to illustrate the relevant mathematical features? For example, when teaching the concept of equality, does the teacher present examples of expressions in which the two sides of a number sentence are not equal and make it clear to students why the equal sign should not be used?

4. Is a well-planned system of review implemented? Is there an explicit attempt to ensure that newly taught concepts are reviewed and reinforced to enhance student retention and fluency?

Background Knowledge Deficits

Students with background knowledge deficits experience a wide range of problems in learning complex mathematics. These deficits might stem from a lack of number sense typically garnered in early childhood or from inadequate teaching and learning of skills and strategies fundamental to later mathematics learning. For example, many students struggle to understand rational numbers and how operations with rational numbers differ from whole-number operations. These differences depend on the strength of the learners' facility with whole-number operations. When observing teachers' instruction, school psychologists may want to ask themselves:

1. Is the teacher using preteaching opportunities to ensure that students will be successful with new content? For example, if the lesson objective is problem solving with fractions, does the teacher review or preteach fraction concepts and operations to ensure that the students have the tools to solve the lesson's problems?

2. Has there been an assessment of background knowledge to assist the teacher in planning? For example, does the teacher prime students' mathematical vocabulary related to the lesson objective?

3. Is the instruction and practice differentiated to scaffold learning? For example, does the teacher provide additional examples of how to translate a word problem to a number sentence while allowing students to move on to practice independently if they are comfortable?

Linguistic and Vocabulary Difficulties

Students with linguistic and vocabulary difficulties may be challenged at two levels. First, they often struggle to distinguish important symbols in mathematics that represent key concepts and principles, such as the symbols for addition and multiplication or the square root symbol. Additionally, many students are challenged by unique mathematical vocabulary. This occurs, in large part, because of an underdeveloped knowledge of morphemes and/or of strong word recognition skills. When helping teachers who are working with students with linguistic and vocabulary challenges, school psychologists may want to ask:

1. Is explicit attention paid to defining and using mathematical symbols in a wide variety of contexts and with a high degree of precision?

2. Is careful attention paid to the description and development of vocabulary knowledge?

3. Does the teacher encourage the use of mathematical vocabulary in classroom discourse?

4. Are there opportunities for students to talk mathematically and receive feedback regarding their use of terminology?

Strategy Knowledge and Use

Many students, even typically developing learners, experience difficulties with strategic learning. Consequently, problem solving poses inordinate challenges, as good problem solvers engage in self-talk and persist in finding a solution despite repeated failure. Not only do many students experience difficulties working through the steps of a strategy, but also they often do not understand which strategy to apply and when. As teachers work on developing strategy knowledge in their students, school psychologists may want to ask:

1. Does the teacher model important problem-solving strategies?
2. Is the teacher teaching why and when to apply strategies, as well as how?
3. Is the teacher teaching midlevel strategies that are problem specific rather than just teaching generic problem-solving approaches?

As with any cognitive strategy, modeling requires the use of "think-alouds" to make overt for students how to solve problems.

Monitoring Students' Learning Progress

Monitoring students' progress is important in all three tiers of the multi-tiered model, but teachers must be particularly vigilant with students who are receiving Tiers 2 and 3 support. Progress monitoring is ongoing analysis of performance data on specifically designed progress monitoring measures to make decisions about students' progress toward the outcome goals. Progress monitoring involves gathering baseline data, establishing performance goals, collecting samples of performance over time, and evaluating the alignment between students' observed and anticipated growth rates given the goal. Because students' scores are compared with their own prior performances over time, an empirical database is created that can be used to design and modify instructional programs that are responsive to students' learning needs (Stecker & Fuchs, 2000).

In monitoring progress, students' rates of growth are evaluated to determine whether they are progressing at an appropriate rate that will promote goal attainment. This information is often extrapolated to evaluate whether or not a specific instructional strategy was successful for a student.

School psychologists can help organize a progress monitoring system to support progress monitoring decisions. Several features of the measurement system need to be carefully analyzed in order to adequately monitor growth over time. Multiple parallel forms of the progress monitoring measures are necessary to track changes over time. Alternate forms must be comparable in order to infer that changes in scores are the result of changes in knowledge and/or skill and not

of variability in the measures. Additionally, progress monitoring tests should be sensitive enough to detect small to large changes in students' knowledge and skills over time. A more extensive discussion of these issues is given by Burns and Klingbeil, Chapter 6, this volume.

For some students, supplemental instruction may not produce sufficient changes in the growth trajectories to affect their risk status. For these students, individualized instruction may be necessary. The next section describes the assessments and instructional principles that can be applied in the Tier 3 level of support.

Tier 3: Individualized Interventions

Once students are identified as needing significant support, it is necessary to administer diagnostic assessments in order to determine the specific focus of intervention that can be used for grouping and intervention selection or development. In this chapter we associate diagnostic assessment with Tier 3 and individualized interventions. However, we are aware that in some schools resources are available for the use of diagnostic assessments even with students receiving Tier 2 support. In most instances, schools do not have sufficient resources to utilize diagnostic data on large numbers of students, and, therefore, administering diagnostic assessments may not be the best use of time.

Diagnostic assessments are used in a multitiered model to determine areas in which students demonstrate persistent difficulties in domain-specific knowledge and skills. In this context, diagnosis results in a better understanding of the student's mathematical misconceptions or deficits in student thinking. Diagnostic tests are most frequently administered only to those students who are identified through screening tests as being at risk for failure in mathematics. Because these students often have enduring deficits that are not easily remedied by typical classroom instruction, diagnostic assessments are essential for designing instructional interventions that are aligned with students' learning needs. The reader is referred to Burns and Klingbeil, Chapter 6, this volume, for further discussion of these issues.

Features of Effective Interventions

Multi-tiered support models accommodate students who do not respond to core instruction by providing more intensive intervention support. Tier 3 interventions target the needs of students who (1) enter school with very limited knowledge of number concepts and counting procedures, (2) received inadequate instruction in previous years of schooling and fell behind their peers, or (3) continue to experience problems regardless of motivation, quality of former mathematics instruction, number knowledge, and number sense when entering school. As a result of effective interventions, some of these students may quickly catch up to their peers, necessitating a move to a lower level of support. However, for students who need Tier 3 interventions, it is important that the interventions reflect the evidence based on effective intervention strategies.

Evidence about the features of mathematics interventions is emerging. In this section, we provide a summary of the major findings from three syntheses of research on effective practices for students with mathematics difficulties, including mathematics disabilities, that include more than 50 empirical studies (Baker, Gersten, & Lee, 2002; Gersten et al., in press; Kroesbergen & Van Luit, 2003). Knowledge of this research can provide school psychologists with the information needed to help intervenors or special education teachers to design interventions that are based on research findings.

The basic index of effect size used in these meta-analyses was Cohen's d, defined as the difference between the experimental and comparison group means divided by the pooled standard deviation. According to Cohen (1988), 0.80 is considered a large effect, 0.50 a moderate effect, and 0.20 a small effect. Positive effects were reported for (1) systematic and explicit instruction (d = 1.19 and 0.58 for special education students and low-achieving students, respectively); (2) student think-alouds (d = 0.98 for special education students); (3) visual and graphic depictions of problems (d = 0.50 for special education students); (4) peer-assisted learning (d = 0.42 and 0.62 for special education students and low-achieving students, respectively); and (5) formative assessment (ongoing) data provided to teachers (d = 0.32 and 0.51 for special education students and low-achieving students, respectively) or students (d = 0.33 and 0.57 for special education students and low-achieving students, respectively).

In sum, students who are struggling with mathematics benefit from explicit instruction in how to use specific skills and multistep strategies. Explicit instruction refers to teachers modeling the behaviors they expect students to use when solving mathematics problems. So, if a teacher is explicitly teaching fraction addition with like denominators, she or he would demonstrate the following steps.

Step 1: Check to see if the denominators are the same. If they are, then you can add the two fractions.
Step 2: Add the numerators.
Step 3: Use the same denominator in your sum as was in the two fractions you added.

This modeling is supported by teaching students to verbalize the steps in solving the problem and, when necessary, to use visuals in representing problems. Additionally, students benefit when their teachers receive feedback from formative assessments to inform and modify their instruction. Finally, peer-assisted learning opportunities in which students focus on problem details, observe models of proficient students' problem solving, or are guided by more proficient peers result in improved mathematics performance for struggling learners (see MacKay, Andreou, & Ervin, Chapter 19, this volume, for more on the topic of peer-mediated interventions).

Tier 3 interventions must be aligned with the findings of this emerging research. However, they must also be responsive to student need. Tier 3 interventions in mathematics are not yet common, so what we describe here is based mostly on our experiences in special education. Teachers who are providing intensive intervention must address the content standards that are expected of students mathematically while constantly evaluating whether the learner is prepared to progress forward. In other words, they must carefully control the instructional pace. Because progress in learning mathematics is dependent on one's previously learned knowledge and skills, it is critical that the teacher pace instruction based on the learner's demonstrating mastery over critical prerequisite knowledge. For example, if a student has not demonstrated an understanding of place value (e.g., being able to describe 13 as 10 and 3), then teaching the skill of multidigit addition is only procedural and fruitless in terms of advancing the students' mathematical learning.

In addition to controlled instructional pacing, students needing Tier 3 intervention benefit from smaller instructional groups. There is little research to support this assertion. However, it is reasonable to assume that with smaller groups teachers are able to guide student practice more closely, provide more immediate feedback to students' responses, and ensure that they have students' attention when teaching new content. Smaller instructional groups also allow teachers to respond to students' growth during instruction so that they can accelerate or slow down through problem types based on their responses to previous problems. We also believe that the ability to adjust instructional pacing and to closely monitor student learning provides the teacher with the opportunity to teach students self-questioning skills to guide their problem solving. These skills are often not explicitly demonstrated and nurtured in struggling students, yet they are critical to adaptive reasoning when solving problems. Examples of these questions include: What am I being asked to find here? Is there information given to me that I don't need? How can I rewrite this problem into a math sentence? Questions of this type have not traditionally been used to support student learning.

Conclusion

Our intent in this chapter was to provide school psychologists with practical, logical, and research-based ways in which to support enhanced mathematics instruction in elementary schools. Low achievement and insufficient learning in school mathematics is a pervasive and long-term problem that requires an innovative, systemic, and complex set of solutions. School psychologists can provide valuable support to teachers as they identify areas of improvement they need to make in their own mathematics knowledge and in their instruction. We believe that strengthening mathematics instruction will include identifying effective professional tools, enhancing teachers' general and specialized mathematical knowledge, and assisting teachers in making their instruction more accessible to a wide range of learners.

We also propose that schools seriously consider an alternative model of instructional support, such as the multi-tiered model we have described here. Successful implementation of a multi-tiered model of mathematics instructional support completely depends on schools evaluating their core mathematics instruction and taking steps to strengthen instruction for all students. School psychologists will be vital to this effort as they use their assessment expertise and knowledge of instructional research to support decision making.

References

Baker, S., Gersten, R., & Lee, D. (2002). A synthesis of empirical research on teaching mathematics to low-achieving students. *Elementary School Journal, 103,* 51–73.

Baker, S. K., Simmons, D. C., & Kame'enui, E. J. (1995). *Vocabulary acquisition: Synthesis of the research* (Technical Rep. No. 13). Eugene: University of Oregon, National Center to Improve the Tools of Educators.

Ball, D. L., Hill, H. C., & Bass, H. (2005, Fall). Knowing mathematics for teaching. *American Educator,* 14–46.

Carpenter, T. P., Blanton, M. L., Cobb, P., Franke, M. L., Kaput, J., & McClain, K. (2004). *Scaling up innovative practices in math and science.* Madison, WI: University of Wisconsin, National Center for Improving Student Learning and Achievement in Math and Science.

Chard, D. J., Harn, B., Sugai, G., Horner, R., Simmons, D. C., & Kame'enui, E. J. (2008). Core features of multi-tiered systems of reading and behavioral support. In C. R. Greenwood, T. R. Kratochwill, & M. Clements (Eds.), *Schoolwide prevention models: Lessons learned in elementary schools* (pp. 31–58). New York: Guilford Press.

Chard, D. J., & Jungjohann, K. (2006, Spring). Scaffolding instruction for success in mathematics learning. *Intersection: Mathematics educators sharing common ground.* Houston, TX: Exxon Mobil Foundation.

Cohen, I. B. (2005). *The triumph of numbers: How counting shaped modern life*. New York: Norton.

Cohen, J. (1988). *Statistical power analysis for the behavioral sciences* (2nd ed.). Hillsdale, NJ: Erlbaum.

Gersten, R., Chard, D. J., Baker, S. K., Jayanthi, M., Flojo, J. R., & Lee, D. S. (in press). Experimental and quasi-experimental research on instructional approaches for teaching mathematics to students with learning disabilities: A research synthesis. *Review of Educational Research.*

Gonzales, P., Guzman, J. C., Partelow, L., Pahlke, E., Jocelyn, L., Kastberg, D., et al. (2004). *Highlights from the Trends in International Mathematics and Science Study (TIMSS) 2003*. Washington, DC: National Center for Education Statistics.

Greenwood, C. R., Kratochwill, T. R., & Clements, M. (2008). *Schoolwide prevention models: Lessons learned in elementary schools.* New York: Guilford Press.

Hill, H. C., Rowan, B., & Ball, D. L. (2005). Effects of teachers' mathematical knowledge for teaching on student achievement. *American Educational Research Journal, 42,* 371–406.

Kinder, D., & Stein, M. (2006). Quality mathematics programs for students with disabilities. In M. Montague & A. K. Jitendra (Eds.), *Teaching mathematics to middle school students with learning difficulties* (pp. 133–153). New York: Guilford Press.

Kroesbergen, E. H., & Van Luit, J. E. H. (2003). Mathematics intervention for children with special educational needs. *Remedial and Special Education, 24,* 97–114.

Ma, L. (1999). *Knowing and teaching elementary mathematics: Teachers' understanding of fundamental mathematics in China and the United States*. Mahwah, NJ: Erlbaum.

Mathematics Learning Study Committee. (2001). *Adding it up*. Washington, DC: National Academy Press.

Milgram, R. J. (2005). *The mathematics preservice teachers need to know*. Palo Alto, CA: Author.

National Center for Education Statistics. (2007). *National Assessment of Educational Progress: The nation's report card*. Washington, DC: U.S. Department of Education.

National Council of Teachers of Mathematics. (1989). *Principles and standards for school mathematics*. Reston, VA: Author.

National Council of Teachers of Mathematics. (2000). *Principles and standards for school mathematics*. Reston, VA: Author.

National Council of Teachers of Mathematics. (2006). *Curriculum focal points for prekindergarten through grade 8 mathematics: A quest for coherence*. Reston, VA: Author.

Schaughency, E., & Ervin, R. (2006). Building capacity to implement and sustain effective practices to better serve children. *School Psychology Review, 35,* 155–166.

Stecker, P. M., & Fuchs, L. S. (2000). Effecting superior achievement using curriculum-based measurement: The importance of individual progress monitoring. *Learning Disabilities Research and Practice, 15,* 128–134.

Wu, H. (1997). *On the education of mathematics teachers*. Retrieved November 15, 2007, from *math.berkeley.edu/~wu*.

Chapter 18

Evidence-Based Written Language Instruction

Developing and Implementing Written Language Programs
at the Core, Supplemental, and Intervention Levels

Merilee McCurdy
Stephanie Schmitz
Amanda Albertson

The importance and impact of writing is prominent in today's society. Writing plays a major role in informing and influencing the public through such media as books and short stories, popular music, politics, and advertisements. Writing skills also are of great importance in the work environment. For example, the over 90% of recently surveyed midcareer professionals recognized the importance of writing in their careers, citing the "need to write efficiently as a skill of great importance in their day-to-day work" (National Commission on Writing in America's Schools and Colleges, 2003, p. 11). Further, survey findings from 120 major American corporations indicated that half of the responding companies use writing as one of their criteria when making such personnel decisions such as hiring and promoting (National Commission on Writing in America's Schools and Colleges, 2004). All careers and jobs do not require the same sophistication of writing. However, writing will be required at some point in almost all types of employment. For example, a construction employee may be asked to write a short note to the boss explaining a medical absence, an athlete may be asked to write a biographical statement for the local newspaper, or a public school bus driver may have to write a discipline report following a fight. In each situation, the employee may be evaluated based on the quality of the written statement.

Similarly, students engage in writing activities for many reasons (Barone & Taylor, 2006). For example, students may be instructed to write a story for the purpose of informing others, of entertaining the audience, of convincing the target audience of a particular thought or action, of demonstrating knowledge and understanding of a particular topic, or of reflecting on information or on their own thoughts. Multiple types of writing may be required in one product. Therefore, proficient writing skills are necessary to demonstrate mastery of different writing styles. Unfortunately, development of these skills may not occur naturally for all students.

Historically, schools have provided a less than adequate amount of time, effort, and resources to assist students in becoming proficient writers (National Commission on Writing, 2003). However, national examinations of writing performance conducted by the National Assessment of Educational Progress (NAEP) indicate that student writing is improving (National Center for Education Statistics, 2003). The evaluation of fourth-grade writing performance in 2002 indicated a significant improvement in basic writing skills over the 1998 assessment. Specifically, an increase from 84 to 86% at or above the basic level was found, with 28% of these students performing at or above the proficient level. Results from the 2007 National Writing Assessment administered to both 8th- and 12th-grade students (National Center for Education Statistics, 2008) indicated some improvement in basic writing skills from the 2002 assessment for both 8th and 12th graders. Specifically, over the course of a decade, the number of 8th-grade students at or above the basic level increased from 84 to 88%, with 33% of these students performing at or above the proficient level. Additionally, an increase from 78 to 82% was found in the number of 12th-grade students at or above the basic level, with 24% of these students at or above the proficient level.

Although most students are writing at or above the basic level, indicating that they have mastered the basics of writing, few are writing at the proficient level or are able to compose meaningful text. The data from NAEP indicate that, when students are asked to transfer their thoughts into written language, most produce a fairly basic and common composition that includes average content, organization, and mechanics. Although these students can produce a written product that can be understood by readers, most students cannot write at a level that meets the expectations and demands that will continue to be placed on them throughout their educational careers, in the work environment, and in society (National Commission on Writing in America's Schools and Colleges, 2003).

Children who experience difficulty writing perform at lower levels in the areas of writing mechanics (e.g., spelling, punctuation, capitalization). In addition, these students are not adept at planning or revising a written product, and they produce fewer ideas and less text than skilled writers (Graham & Harris, 1997). Poor writers have also been found to have a lack of knowledge about the writing process itself and will write sequentially about a familiar topic rather than tell a detailed, organized story (Graham, Harris, MacArthur, & Schwartz, 1991). Therefore, writing produced by students with learning disabilities is often plagued by poor story development, inadequate revision, decreased text production, and multiple grammatical errors.

Consider the writing sample in Figure 18.1. This student is a 12-year-old female in the fifth grade. Based on previous testing, she is of low average intelligence and reads on grade level. However, written language testing indicates performance in the borderline range. For this assessment, the student was provided a picture of children playing basketball. She was given 1 minute to think about her story and 3 minutes to write it. She wrote (spelling corrected for understanding): "I love b-ball so was shooting with the guys at my school me and the guys so I ask if I can play No Ha Ha just kidding Yes and we were happy." For many readers, the quality of this writing sample may be surprising given the student's age. However, this student makes many mistakes common to children with writing concerns. In this writing sample, punctuation is used once at the end of the story, multiple words are misspelled, handwriting is poor, and the story explains sequential facts but does not tell a thorough story.

For skilled writers, the process of writing is comprehensive and encompasses numerous skills. Although writing is often associated with mechanics and grammar, it should instead be thought of as an activity that "requires students to stretch their minds, sharpen their analytical capabilities, and make valid and accurate distinctions" (National Commission on Writing in America's Schools and Colleges, 2003, p. 13). Proficient writers can convey messages, engage in storytelling, and expand their own knowledge.

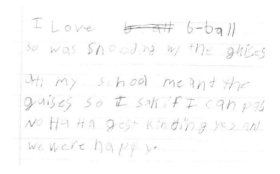

FIGURE 18.1. Sample of student writing.

For many people, the development of writing skills is a complex process that continues into adulthood.

The main purpose of this chapter is to provide information on evidence-based instruction and intervention that should be used to target multiple writing skill areas. To present a broad view of written language deficits and skill areas, this chapter first describes the theory behind instruction in writing. The chapter continues by discussing the developmental stages of writing and specific writing process target areas, including planning, writing production, and revising. Finally, mechanics, spelling, and motivation are discussed as specific writing skills that may require additional, focused instruction.

Definition and Application of the Cognitive-Process Theory of Writing

Flower and Hayes (1981) developed a cognitive-process theory of writing in which the main components are basic mental processes that have a hierarchical structure (see Figure 18.2). The process model is in contrast to the stage model, in which the writing process is described as a "linear series of stages, separated in time, and characterized by the gradual development of the written product" (Flower & Hayes, 1981, p. 367). In a stage model, a writer would focus attention on each phase of the writing process but not intermix the phases. Therefore, a writer would not be taught to return to the planning process during the writing or revising stage. In contrast, the cognitive-process theory of writing is based on four key points: (1) the writing process is "best understood as a set of distinctive thinking processes" that writers use while composing text; (2) these processes are organized in a hierarchical structure in which any of the processes can overlap or be embedded within another; (3) the writing process is directed by the writer and is dependent on his or her goals for the written product; and (4) writers create their own goals either by developing both primary and supporting goals that fulfill the writer's purpose or by modifying or creating new goals based on what the writer has learned while engaged in the writing process (Flower & Hayes, 1981, p. 366). Both models iden-

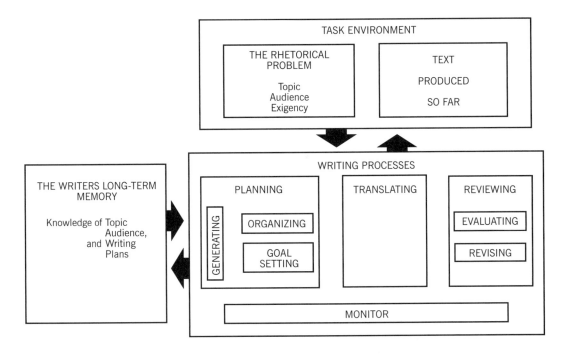

FIGURE 18.2. Theory of writing instruction developed by Flower and Hayes (1981). Copyright by the National Council of Teachers of English. Reprinted by permission.

tify stages of the writing process (i.e., planning, translating, and reviewing). However, the process model allows the writer to rely on his or her own goals to direct the writing. In addition, the process model understands that the writing stages are not distinct but may be used at any time during the writing process.

According to this theory, the act of writing involves three major elements: (1) the task environment, which includes all of those things outside of the writer that influence written work; (2) the writer's long-term memory, which contains knowledge of the writing topic, the audience, and a variety of writing plans; and (3) the three writing processes of planning, translating, and reviewing (Flower & Hayes, 1981). With regard to the task environment, the most important component at the beginning of the composing process is the provided topic; at this point, the writer considers the situation, the target audience, and the writer's own goals for writing (Flower & Hayes, 1981). The writer's ability to define and represent the identified topic is an important part of the writing process. A second component of the task environment is the written text. As writing proceeds, the writer becomes more limited in what can be stated. Just as the title limits the content of a written product and a topic sentence defines a paragraph, each written word both determines and limits the writer's options of what content should follow so as to produce meaningful text. As the written product continues to expand, more demands are placed on both the writer's time and attention while he or she is writing. These demands constantly compete with the retrieval of knowledge from the writer's long-term memory, as well as with the writer's plan for handling the identified problem (Flower & Hayes, 1981).

The second element in the cognitive-process model, the writer's long-term memory, contains knowledge about the topic and the target audience, as well as important information about various writing plans and formats (Flower & Hayes, 1981). One problem associated with long-term memory is the retrieval of information, or finding the exact prompt or cue that is necessary to release the needed information. A second problem facing the writer is the need to adapt the information retrieved from long-term memory to correspond with the identified topic (Flower & Hayes, 1981). Specifically, the writer may have successfully retrieved information about a particular topic from long-term memory but might have been unable to organize the information in such a way that it is understandable to the reader.

The third element in the cognitive-process model, and the element addressed most frequently by schools, consists of the writing processes of planning, translating, and reviewing. Planning is a critical part of the writing process and is typically viewed as the act of generating and organizing content (Flower & Hayes, 1980; Graham, 2006). In the Flower and Hayes (1980) model, planning is broken down into three different activities. First, students must be able to develop goals for their writing. These goals should be continuously modified to address the task and writing style (e.g., narrative, persuasive, informative). Next, students must generate ideas for their writing. Finally, students must select from the available ideas to accomplish the goals identified in the first step.

Translating is defined as the process of transferring ideas into written or visible language (Flower & Hayes, 1981). This process requires the writer to simultaneously deal with the multiple demands required of written language (e.g., syntax, grammar, spelling, letter formation). Whereas skilled writers perform such tasks automatically, translating ideas into text may overwhelm the inexperienced writer. If the writer needs to devote conscious attention to these demands, then the act of translating ideas to written language can interfere with the generation and organization of ideas (Flower & Hayes, 1981). Based on previous research, Berninger and Swanson (1994) proposed a modification to the translation process to include two components that are important for beginning or novice writers. These components are text generation, which involves the generation of ideas, and transcription, which describes the ability to produce written text (Berninger & Swanson, 1994). Beginning writers or students with learning disabilities may have difficulty with the transcription component of the writing process, as seen through such skills as forming clearly written letters or producing adequate amounts of text. Deficits in these areas will negatively affect the overall quality of the written product and may affect the writer's ability to focus on other areas of the writing process.

The reviewing process involves reading through one's text either to expand on or revise the text produced during the translating process or to evaluate and/or revise the original plan for the written product (Flower & Hayes, 1981). The reviewing process can be a planned or unplanned event. When reviewing is planned, it frequently leads to additional planning and translating. However, reviewing can also occur spontaneously as the writer is evaluating either the current text or his or her own detailed plan. Further, reviewing may occur at any time during the writing process (Flower & Hayes, 1981). It is not uncommon for writers to interrupt planning and translating activities with the purpose of reviewing the written product or plan and making modifications.

Given all that is known about the process of writing and the importance of strong writing skills, it is disconcerting that educational systems do not allocate resources and provide additional teacher professional development toward the improvement of writing instruction practices. Several challenges exist that may inhibit schools' ability to provide the necessary resources to promote quality writing instruction. For example, educators are pulled in many different directions, and adequate time for writing may not be a stated school priority. Additionally, the assessment of student writing skills is a complex matter, and reliable and valid measures may not be available to measure progress and results in a way that is acceptable to educators (see Gansle & Noell, Chapter 7, this volume). Finally, teachers will require support and assistance to enhance their understanding of what constitutes "good" writing and how to teach students to become proficient writers (National Commission on Writing in America's Schools and Colleges, 2003). Barone and Taylor (2006) also note several issues that arise in the area of writing instruction. Specifically, strong instruction should balance mechanics (e.g., grammar, spelling, handwriting) with writing quality (e.g., ideas, organization, style). However, many curricula and instructional practices do not stress the integration of the two approaches and may emphasize one over the other. Strong writers must demonstrate mastery of the mechanics

of writing while producing a quality written product made up of organized topics, structured paragraphs, and informative statements. A second issue with writing instruction is related to the assessment of writing skills. Researchers must discover techniques for assessing and evaluating student writing, not only to determine ongoing student progress but also to identify future instructional needs. Given the multiple skills required of proficient writers, educators need assessment tools that can guide their instructional decision making. A final concern emphasizes the need to establish which teachers hold the instructional responsibility for writing instruction. Students are required to write in most classrooms. Unfortunately, most teachers neglect to provide students with feedback regarding their writing performance. Until all teachers take on this responsibility, many students will make minimal progress in becoming proficient writers.

Developmental Stages of Writing

Learning to write is similar to learning to read. In fact, the two skills are highly connected (Shanahan, 1984; Tompkins, 2002). Strong readers are usually strong writers. However, this is not always the case. As with reading, students learn to write by progressing through a series of developmental stages (Levine, 1987). In each stage, students are expected to master different skills. Information learned in one stage is necessary for successful completion of the following stages. All students will not progress through each stage and develop mastery of the skills. However, proficient writers will demonstrate mastery of the skills at each stage.

One of the most commonly accepted and frequently cited models of the developmental stages of writing was proposed by Levine (1987). In the first stage of this model, Imitation, preschool and first-grade students are becoming familiar with the concept of print. They are learning to form letters and numbers and may begin to write small words or simple sentences. In the next stage, Graphic Presentation, first- and second-grade students master letter writing, use invented spelling techniques, become overconcerned with the appearance of their writing, and are introduced to the basic rules of writing (e.g., capitalization, punctuation). In late second grade through fourth grade, students are in the Progressive Incorporation stage of writing. During this period, students become more adept at following the rules of writing, start using cursive writing, and begin using revising techniques. Student writing is not sophisticated, as students are focused on writing mechanics and are not using planning techniques prior to writing. As students advance to the fourth through seventh grades, they are in the Automatization stage of writing. Students begin to realize that writing is a process that requires planning, multiple drafts, and various revising practices. Students are expected to be more independent in their writing and to monitor their own performances. The final two stages of writing development are Elaboration in seventh to ninth grades and Personalization–Diversification in the ninth grade and beyond. In both of these stages, student writing becomes a communication tool. Basic writing skills are more automatic for the student, and writing is now used to communicate ideas and to persuade or educate the reader. Students begin to use more complex writing styles specific to the goals of the written product and to use an advanced vocabulary. Overall, their writing is more sophisticated and creative.

Characteristics of Quality Core Instruction

Writing has been part of American education for some time, yet there does not seem to be complete agreement on how to teach it (Barone & Taylor, 2006). This conflict may be due, in part, to the fact that both teachers and students have varying ideas as to what constitutes writing instruction. Specifically, although writing instruction has been described as lessons in spelling, vocabulary, grammar, and handwriting, it has also been perceived as having value for creative expression and as an assessment or evaluation tool for various subjects and content areas (Barone & Taylor, 2006). What, then, are important instructional components or aspects that should be included as part of writing instruction? The fundamental discussion in research and applied practice concerns the product or process approach to teaching written language. Teaching specific writing skills (e.g., grammar, spelling, mechanics) is considered a product approach to writing, whereas an instructional focus on the writing process as a whole (e.g., planning, forms of writing, audience) constitutes the process approach to teaching writing (Bromley, 1999). Historically, instruction has focused on one approach over the other. In the current age of test readiness, the focus is on the mastery of basic writing skills, and instruction is focused on separate writing stages. However, the most effective teachers emphasize both the product and process approaches in their classrooms and rely on a balanced approach to writing instruction.

Meta-Analyses of Writing Instruction

In the past, investigators have attempted to make sense of the research on written language instruction. In doing so, they have used meta-analyses as useful quantitative syntheses of research on techniques educators can use to improve student writing product and process skills (Graham & Perin, 2007; Graham, 2006; Graham & Harris, 2003; Gersten & Baker, 2001; Hillocks, 1986). In one meta-analysis, three general categories of teaching components were identified: explicit teaching of the three basic stages of the writing process (i.e., planning, writing, and revising), awareness of different text structures used for various writing tasks (such as essay writing or personal narratives), and peer or teacher feedback on the overall quality of the written product (Gersten & Baker, 2001). This research was a starting point for future meta-analyses examining writing instruction. Although Gersten and Baker (2001) identified essential instructional techniques, the methodology examined two types of writing (expository and narrative writing) in 13 studies from 1963 to 1997. Additional investigations were needed to update the findings, and they include a more thorough review of the research on writing instruction. More recently, an extensive meta-analysis reviewed 123 documents to examine a variety of instructional strategies used to teach written language to students in 4th–12th grades (Graham & Perin, 2007). Based on the results, 10 instructional recommendations were made to educators. The six recommendations with effect sizes at or above 0.50 can be found in Table 18.1 and are provided in order based on effect size: strategy instruction (0.82); explicit teaching of text summarization (0.82); peer assistance (0.75); setting product goals (0.70); word processing (0.55); and sentence combining (0.50). Several of these recommendations are discussed either individually or in relation to other interventions later in this chapter.

Although the meta-analyses point to many research-supported instructional practices, the job of implementing these practices is still left to the teacher, as these strategies are not always included in a school's writing curriculum. Writing curricula should incorporate these strategies to be considered well rounded, making sure that such strategies are developmentally appropriate for the ages and/or grades for which they are intended. Therefore, it is important to determine the adequacy of the writing program or curriculum chosen for use in the classroom.

Researchers have learned much about writing instruction. They have informed the field through meta-analyses and by providing instructional recommendations. However, research has not adequately addressed the amount of instruction that is necessary for writing improvements to occur in students with written language concerns, though some general recommendations have been made. Christenson, Thurlow, Ysseldyke, and McVicar (1989) put it best when they stated, "Quality instruction requires a certain quantity of time" (p. 227). Unfortunately, not all students are exposed to high-quality writing instruction, and even those who are may have difficulty mastering and generalizing the taught skills. It is up to educators to determine why a student is not a successful writer and to determine what writing skills would benefit from further, more intensive instruction. To make these judgments, educators should rely on a problem-solving model employing data-based decision making.

The Problem-Solving Model and Student Writing Concerns

In many cases, teachers provide high-quality, research-supported classroom instruction in written language. Yet some children still do not respond to instruction. It is important to determine whether the difficulties of struggling writers are due to an inadequate core writing curriculum or to a lack of high-quality instruction. After examining the core writing curriculum to determine developmental appropriateness and inclusion of appropriate instructional targets addressing the writing product and writing process, one must evaluate the quality of instruction. In any academic area, high-quality instruction will include direct teaching of a specific skill and modeling of that skill. In addition, students should have the opportunity to practice accurate use of that skill with immediate and direct feedback from the teacher. When 80% of students in a classroom or in a school are performing below grade-level expectations, it is an indicator that problems exist with the core curriculum or with the quality of instruction being provided.

However, some students will continue to struggle and perform below grade level in the area of writing even with the use of an adequate core writing curriculum and in the presence of high-quality instruction. These

---

TABLE 18.1. Top 6 Instructional Recommendations for Teaching Writing

1. Teach students to use strategies during each stage of writing (i.e., planning, writing, and revising). The self-regulated strategy development program is an example of an effective instructional model.

2. Teach students to summarize previously written material (e.g., readings from textbooks). Learning this skill improves students' ability to concisely organize written material.

3. Allow students to assist each other in the development and revision of their writing. When peers work together, the result is higher quality written products.

4. Identify product goals for the specific writing required. These goals may be focused on the purpose of the paragraph or type of paragraph, amount of specific information, or number of story elements.

5. Students should have a word processor or computer available to use when writing.

6. Teach students to create more complex and sophisticated sentences through combining two or more basic, or simple, sentences into a single sentence.

Note. Data adapted from Graham and Perin (2007).

students will require further, more specific instruction in one or more skill areas. When the problem-solving process in the context of a multi-tiered prevention–intervention model (e.g., response to intervention [RTI]), schools can use data-based decision making to identify student skill deficits and to identify an empirically based intervention to supplement the core curriculum. The problem-solving model, which can be organized into a series of four steps (see Ervin, Gimpel Peacock, & Merrell, Chapter 1, this volume), should be used to assist in determining the amount and type of intervention that might be most effective for a student based on his or her area of individual need. Within this four-step model, a problem is identified and analyzed, goals are set, and a plan is implemented and evaluated. Through the use of this process, data are gathered at each step to assist in making instruction more effective and in selecting appropriate programs and techniques to help struggling students.

When using a problem-solving approach in the area of written language, the problem-identification and problem-analysis steps should inform identification of the target skills and appropriate intervention. This evaluation should occur on an individual-child level based on assessments of students' writing accuracy, writing production, knowledge of the writing process, and motivation level. Schools using a data-based problem-solving approach can provide targeted supplemental instruction to students not responsive to the core curriculum. These supplemental programs and techniques can assist student learning by providing additional instruction in a skill or set of skills not mastered by the student.

Areas for Targeted Supplemental Instruction

The following sections provide information on instructional practices recommended for each stage of the writing process. However, a comprehensive approach to instruction that includes all writing stages is necessary at the core level. These specific strategies and instructional practices can assist educators with students who are experiencing deficits in a specific area. A more robust core curriculum will target multiple skills simultaneously.

Planning

Planning is typically viewed as the process of generating and organizing content (Flower & Hayes, 1980; Graham, 2006; Vallecorsa, Ledford, & Parnell, 1991). Although planning has been identified as a fundamental skill for effective writing (De La Paz & Graham, 2002; Vallecorsa et al., 1991), it is apparent that the planning process is not emphasized in the writings of school-age children (McCutchen, 1995). Additionally, even when prompted to plan, students' plans are often weak and unsophisticated (Berninger, Whitaker, Feng, Swanson, & Abbott, 1996). Given the complexity and importance of planning, it is imperative that instructional practices be strengthened to ensure skill development in this area. The most researched planning instruction program to date is Self-Regulated Strategy Development (SRSD; Danoff, Harris, & Graham, 1993; Graham & Harris, 1989a; Lienemann, Graham, Leader-Janssen, & Reid, 2006; Reid & Lienemann, 2006; Saddler, 2006; Saddler, Moran, Graham, & Harris, 2004; Sawyer, Graham, & Harris, 1992).

Self-Regulated Strategy Development

Instruction in SRSD emphasizes an interactive learning style between teachers and students in which students' responsibility for employing instructed strategies is gradually increased. SRSD includes six instructional stages: Develop Background Knowledge, Discuss It, Model It, Memorize It, Support It, and Independent Performance (Graham & Harris, 1999; Graham, Harris, & MacArthur, 2006). These stages are described in Table 18.2.

SRSD can be taught using a variety of strategies that are explicitly taught to students and are used to prompt students as they write. For example, students might be taught a five-step strategy that includes instructions to (1) look at the picture, (2) let your mind be free, (3) write down the mnemonic for the story parts, (4) write down story-part ideas for each part, and (5) write your story, use good parts, and make sense (Graham & Harris, 1989a; Sawyer et al., 1992). Additionally, a common three-step strategy used includes instructions to (1) think, Who will read this, and why am I writing this? (2)

TABLE 18.2. Stages of Instruction in the Self-Regulated Strategy Development Model

Stage	Description
Develop background knowledge	Students are taught any background knowledge needed to use the strategy successfully.
Discuss it	The strategy ands its purpose and benefits are described and discussed.
Model it	The teacher models how to use the strategy and introduces the concept of self-instruction.
Memorize it	The student memorizes the steps of the strategy.
Support it	The teacher supports or scaffolds student mastery of the strategy.
Independent use	Students use the strategy with little or no supports.

Note. From Graham, Harris, and MacArthur (2006). Copyright 2006 by SAGE Publications. Reprinted by permission.

plan what to say using the mnemonic, and (3) write and say more (Graham & Harris, 1989b; Sexton, Harris, & Graham, 1998).

In addition to the strategies described in the previous paragraph, the objectives of SRSD are generally accomplished through the use of mnemonics that incorporate the story or essay elements that should be included in different types of student writing. These mnemonics are explicitly taught to students to help them remember the necessary story elements required in their writing. Students then memorize these mnemonics so they can use them even when the mnemonics are not present. The use of these strategies provides students with a way to self-monitor their writing quality and quantity. Examples of mnemonics used during the instruction of written language planning strategies can be found in Tables 18.3 and 18.4.

SRSD has demonstrated success for a wide variety of students. Specifically, improvements in writing were found for students experiencing multiple disabilities and learning difficulties (Lienemann et al., 2006; Saddler et al., 2004), as well as for students who were considered high achieving (De La

Paz, 1999). Additionally, students in the 2nd grade (Harris, Graham, & Mason, 2006; Lienemann et al., 2006; Saddler et al., 2004; Saddler, 2006), as well as students in the 10th grade (Chalk, Hagan-Burke, & Burke, 2005), improved their writing performances through instruction that focused solely on planning and writing. A strength of the SRSD evaluation research is the inclusion of a comparison group. This type of controlled research provides clear support for the inclusion of instruction in planning techniques. Specifically, studies examining the differences between students who received instruction in planning and those in comparison groups who received typical classroom writing instruction indicated increases in number of elements included, planning time, length of composition, quality of composition, and coherence of the story (De La Paz & Graham, 1997; Graham & Harris, 1989a; Graham, Harris, & Mason, 2005; Graham, MacArthur, Schwartz, & Page-Voth, 1992; Harris et al., 2006; Sawyer et al., 1992; Troia, Graham, & Harris, 1999), as well as maintenance of all of these variables (Graham & Harris, 1989b; Graham et al., 1992), for students in the instructional groups, whereas students in the comparison groups did not demonstrate such gains.

Text Structure Instruction

Although SRSD is well researched and found to be effective, other strategies have research support. Instructing students in the structure of texts as a method for planning compositions has been found effective in improving student story planning. Text structure functions as a cuing system that demonstrates logical connections in text and illustrates the linkage between ideas (Meyer, Brandt, & Bluth, 1980). Additionally, effective text comprehension and production is facilitated by the ability to search for and utilize different text structures (Englert & Hiebert, 1984).

Previous research has found instruction in text structure to be an effective planning tool (Vallecorsa & deBettencourt, 1997; Gambrell & Chasen, 1991). Using this technique, students are taught to identify as many as eight story elements (i.e., main characters, locale, time, starter event, goals, actions, ending, and characters' reactions)

TABLE 18.3. Mnemonics for Narrative Writing

W-W-W-What = 2, How = 2
Danoff, Harris, & Graham (1993); Graham & Harris (1989a);
Sawyer, Graham, & Harris (1992)

W	Who is the main character; who else is in the story?
W	When does the story take place?
W	Where does the story take place?
What	**What** does the main character want to do?
What	**What** happens when he or she tries to do it?
How	**How** does the story end?
How	**How** does the main character feel?

POW
Lienemann, Graham, Leader-Janssen, & Reid (2006); Reid &
Lienemann (2006); Saddler (2006); Saddler, Moran, Graham, &
Harris (2004)

P	Pick my ideas
O	Organize my notes
W	Write and say more

SPACE
Troia & Graham (2002); Troia, Graham, & Harris (1999)

S	Setting
P	Problems
A	Actions
C	Consequences
E	Emotions

TABLE 18.4. Mnemonics for Essay Writing

DARE
Chalk, Hagan-Burke, & Burke (2005); De La Paz & Graham (1997)

D	Develop a position statement
A	Add supporting arguments
R	Report and refute counterarguments
E	End with a strong conclusion

STOP and LIST
Troia & Graham (2002); Troia, Graham, & Harris (1999)

S	Stop
T	Think
O	Of
P	Purposes
L	List
I	Ideas
S	Sequence
T	Them

by examining previously written stories. Specifically, the story elements are explicitly taught by first identifying the elements within stories, then fitting the elements into a story structure outline that reflects all eight story elements. Students are then taught to use a story structure planning outline as a guide for composing stories. Instruction is typically characterized by teacher modeling, teacher guidance, verbal prompting, and direct questioning, followed by gradual movement toward independent practice. When using text structure instruction, students produced more story elements following instruction than prior to instruction. Additionally, students receiving text structure instruction wrote more complex, goal-based stories (Vallecorsa & deBettencourt, 1997; Gambrell & Chasen, 1991).

Writing Production

Translating, or writing production, is the creation of text on a page to communicate thoughts and ideas. Although planning techniques may help increase student writing production, planning does not guarantee that writing production will improve. Often, specific instruction and motivation strategies are necessary for students to engage in actual writing. Students experiencing writing difficulty do not produce adequate amounts of written text, and this affects the quality of their writing practice (Troia, 2006). When students do not write, they do not generate text sufficient for teacher feedback, nor do they capitalize on their opportunities to respond (Skinner, 1998). Increasing opportunities to respond (i.e., practice) is an important element when teaching any skill, as practice increases student familiarity with the task at hand. Only through repeated practice can students master the skills required for writing proficiency.

The time students with learning disabilities spend writing has been examined. Although writing time varies across classrooms, average student writing time has been documented at approximately 25 minutes per day (Christenson, Thurlow, Ysseldyke, & McVicar, 1989). Although it is possible that the amount of time that students with learning disabilities spent engaged in writing since the publication of this study may have increased, this meager amount of writing time should cause concern among educators, especially considering that the total writing time documented by these researchers included all writing activities for the day (e.g., mathematics problems, fill-in-the-blank tasks, and copying activities). More recent evidence indicates that approximately 97% of elementary students spend 3 hours or less per week on writing tasks and that approximately 49% of high school students report that they are asked to complete a paper of three or more pages once or twice per month in English (National Commission on Writing in America's Schools and Colleges, 2003). The lack of classroom time devoted to writing instruction is concerning. Students must have adequate time to translate their thoughts, ideas, and opinions to paper. Further, time must be allotted for teachers to teach writing skills and for students to learn and master the skills necessary to become competent writers (National Commission on Writing in America's Schools and Colleges, 2003). However, allocating time to writing instruction is not enough for students to develop writing skills. Teachers must use quality writing instruction and teaching strategies for classroom writing time to be useful.

SRSD has demonstrated effectiveness in increasing the amount of text produced by students writing both narrative stories (Danoff et al., 1993; Graham et al., 2005; Harris et al., 2006; Lienemann et al., 2006; Reid & Lienemann, 2006; Saddler, 2006; Saddler et al., 2004; Troia et al., 1999) and essays (Chalk et al., 2005; De La Paz, 1999; De La Paz & Graham, 1997; Graham et al., 1992; Sexton et al., 1998). Additionally, SRSD has shown that these increases can be maintained up to 6 weeks following instruction (Reid & Lienemann, 2006; Saddler, 2006; Saddler et al., 2004).

In addition to SRSD, the use of performance feedback on writing quantity has demonstrated effectiveness in increasing writing production. In one of the earliest uses of performance feedback, the combined use of explicit timing, public posting of the greatest number of words written, and instructions for students to exceed their highest score resulted in substantial increases in writing production, as well as writing quality, for second- and fifth-grade students

(Van Houten, Morrison, Jarvis, & McDonald, 1974). More recently, similar increases in production and quality were found when fourth-grade students graphed the number of words they wrote, counted the number of words written in each other's compositions, proofread their own stories, and shared their stories with the class (Kasper-Ferguson & Moxley, 2002). Thus, not only can performance feedback on student writing performance increase student writing production, but it can also improve the quality of student writing.

The saying that "practice makes perfect" is true for writing. If students do not practice writing skills, they will not become proficient writers. However, practice alone is not enough, and quality instruction is needed. As described earlier, students must receive instruction in planning techniques. In addition, students will require instruction in revision strategies and writing mechanics, but they also must be motivated to use all instructed skills.

Revising

The terms *revising* and *editing* are often used synonymously in the field of written language. However, the two terms represent different forms of the writing process. In each, the original written product is modified or changed with the goal of improving it. Differences lie in what occurs during each process. While revising, students should examine the overall paper to ensure that the goals for writing the paper have been met and that the audience is appropriately addressed. Revision occurs at the topic, paragraph, and sentence levels, and the revision process could require an extensive amount of time. In contrast, editing involves a thorough proofreading of the paper to locate and correct typographical and grammatical errors. Editing is often the final stage of the writing process and is used to perfect minor flaws in a paper. This section focuses on strategies to improve the revision skills of students.

Students with learning disabilities do not use effective revising strategies (Troia, 2006). These students will make a cursory review of their papers, making superficial changes. Examinations of student revising techniques found that most students spend little time revising, edit errors in writing mechanics only (e.g., punctuation, handwriting, capitalization), and often harm more than help the quality of their writing (Graham, 1997; McCutchen, 1995). Often students with writing disabilities will exchange one similar word for a previously written word or will erase and rewrite the same word. True revising techniques are not used.

Instruction in revision techniques should provide students with strategies that can be used during the revising process to prompt the accurate use of techniques. Although many students use these strategies effectively and quickly, students with learning disabilities find revising strategies difficult. The underlying issue with revising is that students with learning disabilities have difficulty identifying mistakes in their writing and will indicate that their written products are well produced (Graham, 1997). Because these students cannot identify flaws in their own writing, revision is very difficult. Therefore, the identification of written errors is the first step toward success in the revising process.

Two strategies have been found to help students locate writing errors, and these strategies may result in an increase in their ability to improve the written product. When students with learning disabilities are asked to read passages containing errors, they are more likely to locate errors if they read the passage aloud (Espin & Sindelar, 1988). Educators should ask students to read their written stories aloud to increase the chance that they will find errors in their writing.

The second strategy is to use peer assistance and feedback to help students with learning disabilities locate writing errors or areas requiring elaboration. In some cases, written peer feedback has been found as effective as or even more effective than teacher feedback for students' writing quality. In one study, students served as peer editors (Karegianes, Pascarella, & Pflaum, 1980) by providing peer feedback to other students in the classroom. In addition, students relied on peer feedback to enhance their own writing. Results indicated that students in the peer-feedback group benefited more than students in the teacher-feedback group. When teachers provide feedback, students may be minimally engaged in the location of errors. Instead, they become reliant on teacher feedback to identify their writing errors. In contrast, the act of providing peer feedback serves to teach students the editing process. When students are actively engaged in providing feedback to their peers, they learn more about the editing process and the use of classroom scoring rubrics. Similar results can be found in the peer-tutoring literature, as academic skills improve for both the tutors and tutees. The act of tutoring or providing peer feedback often improves the tutor's skills, as well as the skills of the student receiving the tutoring (Medcalf, Glenn, & Moore, 2004).

A secondary and important benefit to using peer feedback and revising is the release of teacher time spent engaged in these processes, thereby allowing teachers to spend more time assisting individual students or a small number of students each day. One common concern for all teachers is the amount of time required to provide students with quality feedback on a written product. Teachers spend 94.1% of their feedback time correcting basic writing mechanics (Lee, 2008) and much less time assisting students with more advanced writing skills, such as generation of ideas or elaboration of topics. In addition, an analysis of teacher editing marks indicated that 91.4% of teacher feedback identified writing weaknesses and not strengths (Lee, 2008). Because teachers view their editing techniques as superficial and ineffective, they are less likely to engage in more advanced editing procedures. Teacher time spent in the feedback process is a valid concern. Consider the typical classroom today. If a teacher has 25–30 students in the classroom, she or he could spend 3 to 4 hours reading student papers and providing feedback. Of course, longer papers require more time, and shorter assignments require less time. However, the time requirement is substantial.

In summary, the act of planning, translating, and revising requires the use of many specific skills. In addition, students are expected to write using appropriate mechanics, including spelling. Explicit instruction in mechanics, including the basic rules of grammar, sentence construction, and spelling, may be necessary.

Specific Writing Skills Requiring Instruction

Instruction in Mechanics

The mechanics of writing, such as grammar, punctuation, and capitalization, are basic skills often not mastered by students. Because these skills are expected of even beginning writers, inappropriate use of these basic skills can affect the reader's opinion of the writer's abilities. These skills can be explicitly taught using programs and interventions that employ the teaching strategies of direct instruction in specific skills, increased amounts of writing practice, performance feedback, and motivation. Past research has demonstrated the effects of these strategies on students' use of appropriate writing mechanics (McCurdy, Skinner, Watson, & Shriver, 2008). As part of this study, a treatment package of combined teaching strategies was used in three special education classrooms, in which students were taught to write in complete sentences, include adjectives, and use compound sentences. In each classroom, students met the predetermined goal and demonstrated variable maintenance of the writing skills.

Additional studies have found direct instruction to improve writing skills in students, but again the research is sparse in this area (Walker, Shippen, Alberto, Houchins, & Cihak, 2005). Direct instruction uses immediate and corrective feedback and comprises a structured sequence of lessons that follow a specific set of instructional stages. Specifically, teachers first model the information to be learned by independently providing the correct response, then lead the students in providing the correct response as a group, and finally test the students on their mastery of the information through the administration of both immediate and delayed task probes. Direct instruction has been effective for poor writers with learning disabilities and behavior disorders (Keel & Anderson, 2002), as well as with students identified as gifted (Ginn, Keel, & Fredrick, 2002). In each study, the Reasoning and Writing program (Engelmann & Grossen, 1995) was used for a brief amount of time (i.e., 6 weeks for students with learning disabilities and behavior disorders and 10 weeks for gifted students). The Reasoning and Writing program uses direct instruction principles, provides a wide range of writing genres, such as narratives, expository texts, and essays, and requires students to follow the stages of the writing process for each genre (Walker et al., 2005). Data from norm-referenced testing indicated significant improvements for most students based on the Spontaneous Writing subtest of the Test of Written Language—Third Edition (TOWL-3; Hammill & Larsen, 1996). A second program using principles of direct instruction, Expressive Writing (Engelmann & Silbert, 1983), has been found to improve the writing quality of high school students with learning disabilities. The Expressive Writing program is similar to the Reasoning and Writing program except that it provides only a narrative writing genre when instructing students in the stages of the writing process (Walker et al., 2005). Using single-case experimental methodology and pre–post comparisons on the TOWL-3, three students improved their writing skills following 50 sessions of instruction in this program. In addition, gains were found to maintain 2, 4, and 6 weeks after termination of instruction.

One large concern regarding these two programs is the time required for intervention sessions. Each program, Reasoning and Writing and Expressive Writing, requires approximately 50 minutes per instructional session. When using a problem-solving model, such as RTI, schools are searching for supplemental interventions that can be used in a small-group format within a relatively short period of time. It may be difficult for schools to find 50 minutes three to four times a week to pull students from core instruction. However, these programs have the strongest evidence base, suggesting that intensive interventions are probably necessary for children with learning disabilities. When teaching a skill as complex as written language, schools may need to devote extra time to writing to improve students' skills.

Spelling

Many children with and without writing concerns are poor spellers. At this point, some teachers and parents question the need for direct spelling instruction. In the age of computer spelling checkers, it seems that children can achieve in a school setting with poor spelling skills. However, due to the need for paper-and-pencil writing in many places of employment, lack of spelling skills may harm those interested in professional careers in which mastery of spelling rules is necessary.

Spelling instruction can take on several different forms (Simonsen & Gunter, 2001), such as phonemic, whole-word, and morphemic approaches. In each, spelling instruction is based on principles of direct instruction and skills are explicitly taught. However, spelling is taught differently across programs. Using phonemic approaches to spelling instruction, students are taught to identify the sounds that correspond to written letters. An example of this approach includes the Spelling Mastery program (Dixon & Engelmann, 1999), which provides instruction in letter–sound relationships throughout the course of the program. Whole-word spelling instruction is based on memorization of spelling words. Examples of this technique include the Add-a-Word program (Pratt-Struthers, Struthers, & Williams, 1983) and Cover, Copy, Compare (Nies & Belfiore, 2006). In each, students are asked to review a model of a word spelled correctly and to independently write the targeted spelling word. If the word is not spelled accurately, repeated practice writing the word correctly is required. The morphemic approach teaches students the common rules when using prefixes, suffixes, and roots of words. The Spelling Through Morphographs (Dixon & Engelmann, 2001) program is an example of this approach to spelling instruction.

The examples provided include only a few of the spelling instruction programs and interventions found to be effective. In fact, spelling may be one of the most researched areas of written language. As is the case with all supplemental instruction, each approach to spelling instruction will not be effective for all children. The educator or psychologist should conduct assessments to determine the most effective program for an individual student (see Daly, Hofstadter, Martinez, & Andersen, Chapter 8, this volume).

Motivation

Based on our personal experience, students with learning disabilities in written language find writing aversive. In fact, most children will not state a preference to engage in writing tasks. Writing may not be motivating for all students. The writing process is difficult to master, and for students with writing concerns, it is even more so. Research on response effort indicates that as effort on a task increases, preference for that task decreases (Friman & Poling, 1995). With academic tasks, response effort can be viewed as ease of task completion (Neef, Shade, & Miller, 1994). Therefore, the more difficult the task, the higher the required response effort and the lower the task engagement. For students who can write fluently (i.e., accurately and quickly), response effort is reduced. For students who have difficulty writing, response effort is increased. Based on this concept of response effort, educators should modify writing tasks to ensure an appropriate instructional level for students with writing disabilities. Once fluent skills are acquired, task difficulty level can be increased. By modifying tasks, response effort is reduced, and the probability that students will engage in the task should increase.

The discrete-task hypothesis (Skinner, 2002) is another motivational theory that is relevant to understanding why some students might not be motivated to write. According to the discrete-task hypothesis, completion of discrete tasks within a larger task serves as a conditioned form of reinforcement. For example, completion of a math worksheet requires the completion of several individual math problems. Assuming that the completion of the entire worksheet is reinforcing, completion of each math problem also is reinforcing. This example is similar to the reinforcing effect of checking an item off a "to do" list. Crossing off each item represents completion of a discrete task and is reinforcing for that person. However, writing is a process that does not include obvious discrete tasks. Therefore, a high amount of intermediate reinforcement is not available during completion of a written paper. It may be possible to include discrete tasks in writing assignments by including headings or varying page size. The impact of these modifications on student motivation has not yet been investigated.

Eventually, and following improvement in writing skills, students may develop the in-ternal motivation to write. Until internal motivation develops (Bruning & Horn, 2000), external motivation is necessary. Skinner, Williams, and Neddenriep (2004) point out that rewards are not frequently used by schools to improve academic performance. However, rewards provide students with the motivation that may otherwise be lacking for them to perform their best. Group contingencies can be independent, interdependent, or dependent (Kelshaw-Levering, Sterling-Turner, Henry, & Skinner, 2000). Examples of group contingencies using mystery motivators (Moore, Waguespack, Wickstrom, & Witt, 1994; Kelshaw-Levering et al., 2000), the Good Behavior Game (Tingstrom, Sterling-Turner, & Wilczynski, 2006; Barrish, Saunders, & Wolf, 1969), and the marble jar program have been found to be effective in classrooms. Each reward program relies on principles of group contingencies and serves to motivate the behavior of a small or large group. In addition, mystery motivators, chart moves and grab bag rewards (Jenson & Sloane, 1979), and basic rewards (e.g., privileges, edibles, or tangibles) provided contingent on appropriate learning behavior can motivate individual students. Specifically, in the area of written language, students should be motivated to use newly instructed skills, to produce accurate writing, and to produce adequate amounts of text. Further, using group contingencies to reduce negative student behaviors and to increase appropriate classroom or small-group behaviors (e.g., in seat, task engagement) is also effective.

Summary

Writing is a very complex process composed of multiple dependent skills. For students to be successful writers, they must master numerous skills associated with planning, transcribing, and revising. In addition, students must be internally and externally motivated to write. Unfortunately, educators may not have the background knowledge or ongoing professional development needed to assist students in their classrooms. Differing approaches to written language instruction can be confusing for those without knowledge of the empirical research base for each approach, program, and intervention.

The problem-solving approach to academic skills problems should help to alleviate some of these difficulties. Using the problem-solving approach with an RTI model of service delivery, schools should begin to evaluate the quality and effectiveness of the core curriculum endorsed by school districts or state education agencies to address all aspects of the writing process. Additionally, schools should begin a critical review of the research on supplemental writing programs, several of which are mentioned in this chapter. Data collected during this process will assist educators in the detection of students experiencing writing concerns, in the identification of specific skill deficits, and in the provision of empirically based supplemental interventions. Only though professional development in the areas of writing development, quality writing instruction, and supplemental writing programs will schools systems begin to improve student writing skills.

References

Barone, D. M., & Taylor, J. (2006). *Improving students' writing, K–8: From meaning-making to high stakes!* Thousand Oaks, CA: Corwin Press.

Barrish, H. H., Saunders, M., & Wolf, M. M. (1969). Good behavior game: Effects of individual contingencies for group consequences on disruptive behavior in a classroom. *Journal of Applied Behavior Analysis, 2*, 119–124.

Berninger, V. W., Whitaker, D., Feng, Y., Swanson, L., & Abbott, R. (1996). Assessment of planning, translation, and revising in junior high students. *Journal of School Psychology, 34*, 23–52.

Berninger, V. W., & Swanson, H. L. (1994). Modifying Hayes and Flower's model of skilled writing to explain beginning and developing writing. In E. C. Butterfield (Ed.), *Children's writing: Toward a process theory of the development of writing skill* (pp. 57–83). Greenwich, CT: JAI Press.

Bromley, K. (1999). Key components of sound writing instruction. In L. B. Gambrell, L. M. Morrow, S. B. Neuman, & M. Pressley (Eds.), *Best practices in literacy instruction* (pp. 152–174). New York: Guilford Press.

Bruning, R., & Horn, C. (2000). Developing motivation to write. *Educational Psychologist, 35*, 25–37.

Chalk, J. C., Hagan-Burke, S., & Burke, M. D.

(2005). The effects of self-regulated strategy development on the writing process for high school students with learning disabilities. *Learning Disability Quarterly, 28*, 75–87.

Christenson, S. L., Thurlow, M. L., Ysseldyke, J. E., & McVicar, R. (1989). Written language instruction for students with mild handicaps: Is there enough quantity to ensure quality? *Learning Disability Quarterly, 12*, 219–229.

Danoff, B., Harris, K. R., & Graham, S. (1993). Incorporating strategy instruction within the writing process in the regular classroom: Effects on the writing of students with and without learning disabilities. *Journal of Reading Behavior, 25*, 295–322.

De La Paz, S. (1999). Self-regulated strategy instruction in regular education settings: Improving outcomes for students with and without learning disabilities. *Learning Disabilities Research and Practice, 14*, 92–106.

De La Paz, S., & Graham, S. (1997). The effects of dictation and advanced planning instruction on the composing of students with writing and learning problems. *Journal of Educational Psychology, 89*, 203–222.

De La Paz, S., & Graham, S. (2002). Explicitly teaching strategies, skills, and knowledge: Writing instruction in middle school classrooms. *Journal of Educational Psychology, 94*, 687–698.

Dixon, R. C., & Engelmann, S. (1999). *Spelling Mastery*. Columbus, OH: SRA/McGraw-Hill.

Dixon, R. C., & Engelmann, S. (2001). *Spelling Through Morphographs*. Columbus, OH: SRA/McGraw-Hill.

Engelmann, S., & Grossen, B. (1995). *Reasoning and writing, level F*. Columbus, OH: SRA/McGraw-Hill.

Engelmann, S., & Silbert, J. (1983). *Expressive writing: I*. Desoto, TX: SRA/McGraw-Hill.

Englert, C. S., & Hiebert, E. H. (1984). Children's developing awareness of text structures in expository materials. *Journal of Educational Psychology, 76*, 65–75.

Espin, C., & Sindelar, P. (1988). Auditory feedback and writing: Learning disabled and nondisabled students. *Exceptional Children, 55*, 45–51.

Flower, L. S., & Hayes, J. R. (1981). A cognitive process theory of writing. *College Composition and Communication, 32*, 365–387.

Flower, L. S., & Hayes, J. R. (1980). The dynamics of composing: Making plans and juggling constraints. In L. W. Gregg & E. R. Steinberg (Eds.), *Cognitive processes in writing* (pp. 31–50). Hillsdale, NJ: Erlbaum.

Friman, P. C., & Poling, A. (1995). Making life easier with effort: Basic findings and applied research on response effort. *Journal of Applied Behavior Analysis, 28,* 583–590.

Gambrell, L. B., & Chasen, S. P. (1991). Explicit story structure instruction and the narrative writing of fourth- and fifth-grade below-average readers. *Reading Research and Instruction, 31,* 54–62.

Gersten, R., & Baker, S. (2001). Teaching expressive writing to students with learning disabilities: A meta-analysis. *Elementary School Journal, 101,* 251–272.

Ginn, P. V., Keel, M. C., & Fredrick, L. D. (2002). Using Reasoning and Writing with gifted fifth-grade students. *Journal of Direct Instruction, 2,* 41–47.

Graham, S. (1997). Executive control in the revising of students with learning and writing difficulties. *Journal of Educational Psychology, 89,* 223–234.

Graham, S. (2006). Strategy instruction and the teaching of writing: A meta-analysis. In C. A. MacArthur, S. Graham, & J. Fitzgerald (Eds.), *Handbook of writing research* (pp. 187–207). New York: Guilford Press.

Graham, S., & Harris, K. R. (1989a). Components analysis of cognitive strategy instruction: Effects on learning disabled students' compositions and self-efficacy. *Journal of Educational Psychology, 81,* 353–361.

Graham, S., & Harris, K. R. (1989b). Improving learning disabled students' skills at composing essays: Self-instructional strategy training. *Exceptional Children, 56,* 201–214.

Graham, S., & Harris, K. R. (1997). It can be taught but it doesn't develop naturally: Myths and realities in writing instruction. *School Psychology Review, 26,* 414–424.

Graham, S., & Harris, K. R. (1999). Assessment and intervention in overcoming writing difficulties: An illustration from the self-regulated strategy development model. *Language, Speech, and Hearing Services in Schools, 30,* 255–264.

Graham, S., & Harris, K. R. (2003). Students with learning disabilities and the process of writing: A meta-analysis of SRSD studies. In L. H. Swanson, K. R. Harris, & S. Graham (Eds.), *Handbook of learning disabilities* (pp. 383–402). New York: Guilford Press.

Graham, S., Harris, K. R., & MacArthur, C. (2006). Explicitly teaching struggling writers: Strategies for mastering the writing process. *Intervention in School and Clinic, 41,* 290–294.

Graham, S., Harris, K. R., MacArthur, C. A., & Schwartz, S. (1991). Writing and writing instruction for students with learning disabilities: Review of a research program. *Learning Disability Quarterly, 14,* 89–114.

Graham, S., Harris, K. R., & Mason, L. (2005).

Improving the writing performance, knowledge, and self-efficacy of struggling young writers: The effects of self-regulated strategy development. *Contemporary Educational Psychology, 30,* 207–241.

Graham, S., MacArthur, C., Schwartz, S., & Page-Voth, V. (1992). Improving the compositions of students with learning disabilities using a strategy involving product and process goal setting. *Exceptional Children, 58,* 322–334.

Graham, S., & Perin, D. (2007). A meta-analysis of writing instruction for adolescent students. *Journal of Educational Psychology, 99,* 445–475.

Hammill, D. D., & Larsen, S. C. (1996). *Test of Written Language—3 (TOWL-3).* Austin, TX: Pro-Ed.

Harris, K. R., Graham, S., & Mason, L. (2006). Improving the writing, knowledge, and motivation of struggling young writers: Effects of self-regulated strategy development with and without peer support. *American Educational Research Journal, 43,* 295–340.

Hillocks, G. (1986). *Research on written composition: New directions for teaching.* Urbana, IL: National Council of Teachers of English.

Jenson, W. R., & Sloane, H. N. (1979). Chart moves and grab bags: A simple contingency management system. *Journal of Applied Behavior Analysis, 12,* 334.

Karegianes, M. L., Pascarella, E. T., & Pflaum, S. W. (1980). The effects of peer editing on the writing proficiency of low-achieving tenth-grade students. *Journal of Educational Research, 73,* 203–207.

Kasper-Ferguson, S., & Moxley, R. A. (2002). Developing a writing package with student graphing of fluency. *Education and Treatment of Children, 25,* 249–267.

Keel, M., & Anderson, D. (2002). Using Reasoning and Writing to teach writing skills to participants with learning disabilities and behavioral disorders. *Journal of Direct Instruction, 2,* 48–55.

Kelshaw-Levering, K., Sterling-Turner, H., Henry, J. R., & Skinner, C. H. (2000). Randomized interdependent group contingencies: Group reinforcement with a twist. *Psychology in the Schools, 37,* 523–533.

Lee, I. (2008). Ten mismatches between teachers' beliefs and written feedback practice. *ELT Journal.* Retrieved March 7, 2008, from *doi:10.1093/elt/ccn010.*

Levine, M. D. (1987). *Developmental variation and learning disorders.* Cambridge, MA: Educators Publishing Service.

Lienemann, T. O., Graham, S., Leader-Janssen, B., & Reid, R. (2006). Improving the writing performance of struggling writers in second grade. *Journal of Special Education, 40,* 66–78.

McCurdy, M., Skinner, C. H., Watson, T. S., & Shriver, M. D. (2008). Examining the effects of a comprehensive writing program on the writing performance of middle school students with learning disabilities in written expression. *School Psychology Quarterly, 23,* 571–589.

McCutchen, D. (1995). Cognitive processes in children's writing: Developmental and individual differences. *Issues in Education: Contributions from Educational Psychology, 1,* 123–160.

Medcalf, J., Glenn, T., & Moore, D. (2004). Peer tutoring in writing: A school systems approach. *Educational Psychology in Practice, 20,* 157–178.

Meyer, B. J. F., Brandt, D. M., & Bluth, G. J. (1980). Use of top-level structure in text: Key for reading comprehension of ninth grade students. *Reading Research Quarterly, 16,* 72–103.

Moore, L. A., Waguespack, A. M., Wickstrom, K. F., & Witt, J. C. (1994). Mystery motivator: An effective and time-efficient intervention. *School Psychology Review, 23,* 106–118.

National Center for Education Statistics. (2003). *2002 writing report card for the nation and the states* (NCES Report No. 2003-529). Washington, DC: U.S. Department of Education.

National Center for Education Statistics. (2008). *The nations' report card: Writing 2007* (NCES Report No. 200-468). Washington, DC: U.S. Department of Education.

National Commission on Writing in America's Schools and Colleges. (2003). *The neglected "R": The need for a writing revolution.* New York: College Entrance Examination Board.

National Commission on Writing in America's Schools and Colleges. (2004). Writing: *A ticket to work … or a ticket out.* New York: College Entrance Examination Board.

Neef, N. A., Shade, D., & Miller, M. S. (1994). Assessing influential dimensions of reinforcers on choice in students with serious emotional disturbance. *Journal of Applied Behavior Analysis, 27,* 575–583.

Nies, K. A., & Belfiore, P. J. (2006). Enhancing spelling performance in students with learning disabilities. *Journal of Behavioral Education, 15,* 163–170.

Pratt-Struthers, J., Struthers, T. B., & Williams, R. L. (1983). The effects of the Add-A-Word Spelling Program on spelling accuracy during creative writing. *Education and Treatment of Children, 6,* 277–283.

Reid, R., & Lienemann, T. O. (2006). Self-regulated strategy development for written expression with students with attention-deficit/ hyperactivity disorder. *Exceptional Children, 73,* 1–16.

Saddler, B. (2006). Increasing story-writing ability through self-regulated strategy development: Effects on young writers with learning disabilities. *Learning Disability Quarterly, 29,* 291–305.

Saddler, B., Moran, S., Graham, S., & Harris, K. R. (2004). Preventing writing difficulties: The effects of planning strategy instruction on the writing performance of struggling writers. *Exceptionality, 12,* 3–17.

Sawyer, R. J., Graham, S., & Harris, K. R. (1992). Direct teaching, strategy instruction, and strategy instruction with explicit self-regulation: Effects on the composition skills and self-efficacy of students with learning disabilities. *Journal of Educational Psychology, 84,* 340–352.

Sexton, M., Harris, K. R., & Graham, S. (1998). Self-regulated strategy development and the writing process: Effects on essay writing and attributions. *Exceptional Children, 64,* 295–311.

Shanahan, T. (1984). Nature of the reading–writing relation: An exploratory multivariate analysis. *Journal of Educational Psychology, 76,* 466–477.

Simonsen, F., & Gunter, L. (2001). Best practices in spelling instruction: A research summary. *Journal of Direct Instruction, 1,* 97–105.

Skinner, C. H. (1998). Preventing academic skills deficits. In T. S. Watson & F. M. Gresham (Eds.), *Handbook of child behavior therapy* (pp. 61–82). New York: Plenum Press.

Skinner, C. H. (2002). An empirical analysis of interspersal research: Evidence, implications, and applications of the discrete task completion hypothesis. *Journal of School Psychology, 40,* 347–368.

Skinner, C. H., Williams, R. L., & Neddenriep, C. E. (2004). Using interdependent group-oriented reinforcement to enhance academic performance in general education classrooms. *School Psychology Review, 33,* 384–397.

Tingstrom, D. H., Sterling-Turner, H. E., & Wilczynski, S. M. (2006). The good behavior game: 1969–2002. *Behavior Modification, 20,* 225–253.

Tompkins, G. E. (2002). Struggling readers are struggling writers, too. *Reading and Writing Quarterly, 18,* 175–193.

Troia, G. A. (2006). Writing instruction for students with learning disabilities. In C. A. MacArthur, S. Graham, & J. Fitzgerald (Eds.), *Handbook of writing research* (pp. 324–336). New York: Guilford Press.

Troia, G. A., & Graham, S. (2002). The effectiveness of a highly explicit, teacher-directed strategy instruction routine: Changing the writing performance of students with learning disabilities. *Journal of Learning Disabilities, 35*, 290–305.

Troia, G. A., Graham, S., & Harris, K. R. (1999). Teaching students with learning disabilities to mindfully plan when writing. *Exceptional Children, 65*, 235–252.

Vallecorsa, A. L., & deBettencourt, L. U. (1997). Using a mapping procedure to teach reading and writing skills to middle grade students with learning disabilities. *Education and Treatment of Children, 20*, 173–189.

Vallecorsa, A. L., Ledford, R. R., & Parnell, G. G. (1991). Strategies for teaching com-position skills to students with learning disabilities. *Teaching Exceptional Children, 23*, 52–55.

Van Houten, R., Morrison, E., Jarvis, R., & McDonald, M. (1974). The effects of explicit timing and feedback on compositional response rate in elementary school children. *Journal of Applied Behavior Analysis, 7*, 547–555.

Walker, B., Shippen, M. E., Alberto, P., Houchins, D. E., & Cihak, D. F. (2005). Using the expressive writing program to improve the writing skills of high school students with learning disabilities. *Learning Disabilities Research and Practice, 20*, 175–183.

Chapter 19

Peer-Mediated Intervention Strategies

Leslie MacKay
Theresa Andreou
Ruth A. Ervin

The need to be needed is often more powerful than the need to survive.
—STEPHEN GLENN, *Raising Children for Success*

From a biological standpoint, human beings are social and require interaction with others to survive. Although not all of our social experiences with others are positive, working with our peers to accomplish tasks can be rewarding and can provide benefits beyond the task at hand. In attempts to capitalize on these potential benefits, teachers often create learning situations in which students work in cooperative groups or pairs. In this chapter, we discuss intervention strategies that use peers rather than adults as agents of change. Peers typically have some degree of equivalent standing or rank with others (e.g., similar age, grade, knowledge, status, ability or developmental level). The term *peer-mediated intervention* (PMI) has been used to describe all academic, behavioral, or social strategies that utilize fellow students, rather than adults, as direct or indirect agents of change (Hoff & Robinson, 2002).

In this chapter, we aim to provide readers unfamiliar with PMIs with foundational knowledge pertinent to the use of these interventions within a problem-solving process. First, we provide a rationale for involving peers as agents of change within the current context of school reform. Second, we discuss several potential reasons for choosing PMIs in school settings. Third, we describe a number of specific PMI strategies available in the empirical literature. We end with a discussion of special considerations when using PMIs in school settings.

General Rationale for Involving Peers as Agents of Change

There are several theoretical, developmental, and practical reasons for using PMIs. Early theories (e.g., Bandura, 1977; Piaget, 1965) noted the important role that peers play in child development and learning. According to Piaget (1965), for example, at a very young age children are socially influenced by one another and engage in a process of *symmetrical reciprocity*—that is, imitating the actions of other children. Piaget posited that peer interactions significantly contribute to the construction of social, moral, and intellectual capacities (DeVries, 1997). Social cognitive learning theory proposes that humans develop, adapt, and change through social experiences and observational learning (Bandura, 1977). According to Bandura

(1977), for example, the transmission of values, attitudes, and behavior occurs largely through the social relationships of peers. Beyond theoretical perspectives on the role of peers, a recent review of the developmental research on deviant peer influence suggests that peers can exert a powerful effect over the thoughts and behaviors of youths within a group (Gifford-Smith, Dodge, Dishion, & McCord, 2005). Given the evidence of the powerful influence that children have on each other, peers are logical and perhaps ideal candidates for facilitating change. PMIs can formally channel students' natural orientation to one another into positive social, behavioral, and cognitive engagement opportunities. Through the use of PMIs, teachers can capitalize on this natural resource in the classroom, harnessing the multidimensional factors of social learning to bring about positive changes.

From a practical standpoint, a potential advantage of PMIs is that teachers with limited time and resources can utilize these natural agents of change (i.e., peers) to reinforce, guide, and support student learning to maximize the instructional hours in a school day. Specifically, teachers can extend their instructional influence and coverage of basic skills via the utilization of peers, who are easily accessible across multiple settings. When a student needs extra guided practice or prompts to systematically apply steps and strategies to math activities, for example, peers can provide this supplemental instruction (Klingner & Vaughn, 1999; Kunsch, Jitendra, & Sood, 2007).

PMIs also fit within current practice guidelines, policies, and legislation within school settings. For example, within the United States, the President's Commission on Excellence in Special Education (2002) and recent revisions to the Individuals with Disabilities Act (IDEA) in 2004, practitioners are encouraged to act early and to intervene with evidence-based practices within the regular classroom to enable all learners to succeed (Gresham, 2006). Empirical studies have substantiated that PMIs can enhance student progress in both academic and social domains (e.g., Ginsburg-Block, Rohrbeck, & Fantuzzo, 2006; Rohrbeck, Ginsburg-Block, Fantuzzo, & Miller, 2003) for a variety of learners (e.g., Haring &

Breen, 1992; Rohrbeck et al., 2003) and across diverse real-life settings (e.g., Laushey & Heflin, 2000). Further, numerous meta-analytic studies have shown PMIs to be effective strategies (Johnson & Johnson, 2000; Rohrbeck et al., 2003).

PMI strategies can be applied at a system, classroom, or individual level (e.g., school-wide cross-age tutoring or peer mediation, classwide peer tutoring, one-on-one reciprocal teaching in math or reading), making them well suited to providing a continuum of services in a response-to-intervention (RTI) model. In addition, they make possible the alternative grouping arrangements or extra support often identified as necessary in the RTI process (O'Connor, Fulmer, Harty, & Bell, 2005) and can be utilized by classroom teachers as a vehicle to increase support for students with disabilities within the least restrictive environment (DuPaul & Henningson, 1993; Haring & Breen, 1992; Maheady, Harper, & Sacca, 1988).

Reasons for Choosing a PMI Strategy

Within a problem-solving model, it is important to select interventions that have empirical support and that also address the problem or issue at hand. For any given problem, there are many interventions from which a teacher or school psychologist can choose. In the following sections, we briefly describe 10 potential reasons that school psychologists might consider using a PMI. Five of these reasons relate to intended outcomes, and five relate to teacher preference or contextual fit issues. As with the selection of any intervention strategy, we recommend the use of a problem-solving process to guide decision making. Thus our list of potential reasons to utilize a PMI is presented primarily to summarize empirical literature on PMIs while illustrating some situations in which school psychologists might consider using a PMI. This section is not intended to be used as a template for matching interventions to specific problems.

Selecting PMIs to Produce Intended Outcomes

Within a problem-solving model, an intervention strategy might be selected because it will likely produce certain desired outcomes. For example, a school psychologist might want to improve students' active engagement in the learning process or improve a child's skills in a particular area such as reading. Within the research literature, PMI strategies have been associated with several important outcomes (e.g., Hoff & Robinson, 2002), and practitioners might consider the use of a PMI if they are interested in producing these outcomes.

Promoting Active Engagement

One major advantage of PMI is that it has been shown to increase students' active engagement in the learning process (Greenwood, Horton, & Utley, 2002; Greenwood, Maheady, & Delquadri, 2002) by creating more opportunities for the learner to make a response, seek clarification, ask questions, and provide and receive feedback (Hoff & Robinson, 2002; Mathes, Howard, Allen, & Fuchs, 1998). Studies of PMIs have resulted in increased academic engagement for students without disabilities in general education classrooms (e.g., Cushing & Kennedy, 1997), improved active learning time and reduced off-task behaviors in the classroom (e.g., Ginsburg-Block & Fantuzzo, 1997), and increased response opportunities for at-risk students and students with disabilities (e.g., Mathes et al., 1998).

For students with disruptive and inattentive behaviors, more rapid, individualized pacing and active participation can lead to improved academic and behavioral outcomes (DuPaul, Ervin, Hook, & McGoey, 1998; Greenwood, Delquadri, & Hall, 1989; Webb & Farivar, 1994). Spencer, Scruggs, and Mastropieri (2003) demonstrated how peer tutoring effectively led to increased achievement and on-task learning time for students with emotional and behavioral challenges. The benefits of enhanced peer interaction through reciprocal peer tutoring and smaller cooperative groupings has also been shown to increase the verbal engagement of English language learners (ELL) who in the past have been hesitant to respond (Greenwood, Arreaga-Mayer, Utley, Gavin, & Terry, 2001; Klingner & Vaughn, 1996). Some meta-analytic reviews examining the positive impact of cooperative learning and peer

tutoring on on-task learning behaviors have produced large (Johnson & Johnson, 1989) to moderate (Ginsburg-Block, Rohrbeck, & Fantuzzo, 2006) effect sizes.

Improving Academic Performance Outcomes

Exemplary PMI programs (e.g., classwide peer tutoring [CWPT], described in more detail in a later section of this chapter) have been instrumental in promoting academic success for all students in the classroom (Delquadri, Greenwood, Whorton, Carta, & Hall, 1986). For example, studies of CWPT applications in spelling, reading, and math have shown academic gains across ability groups of average students, low-achieving students, and students with learning disabilities (Burks, 2004; Fuchs, Fuchs, Mathes, & Simmons, 1997; Fuchs, Fuchs, Phillips, Hamlett, & Karns, 1995). In the following paragraphs, we briefly highlight some of the research supporting the use of various PMI strategies to improve academic performance in reading, math, writing, and content areas (e.g., social studies). Our review is provided to illustrate the breadth of research supporting the use of PMIs to improve academic performance. It is not exhaustive of all studies on academic gains using PMIs.

Extensive research has examined the use of PMIs to improve various aspects of reading development, including the effects on phonemic skills, decoding, reading fluency, sight-word identification, vocabulary acquisition, comprehension, and story elements (Mathes, Howard, Allen, & Fuchs, 1998; Barbetta, Miller, & Peters, 1991; Giesecke, Cartledge, & Gardner, 1993; Palincsar & Brown, 1984; Wheldall & Colmar, 1990). For example, in the areas of reading fluency and comprehension, paired reading and reciprocal teaching strategies have improved comprehension for students with learning disabilities and social-behavioral challenges (Palincsar & Brown, 1984). Also, collaborative strategic reading was noted to be effective as an instructional strategy in content areas at both the elementary and secondary levels (Klingner & Vaughn, 1999).

With respect to the domain of mathematics, there is empirical support for PMIs (Kunsch et al., 2007). Kunsch and colleagues (2007) conducted a research synthesis in the area of mathematics and concluded that peer-mediated interventions showed a strong effect for elementary students "at risk" for mathematical disabilities. Similarly, Franca, Kerr, Reitz, and Lambert (1990) reported favorable academic outcomes in their investigation of same-age peer tutoring in math for students with emotional–behavioral difficulties and found peer tutoring had a positive effect on students' correct responses and attitudes toward mathematics. CWPT reinforced by daily points and public display, has led to increased mastery of subtraction skills (Harper, Mallette, Maheady, Bentley, & Moore, 1995).

PMI strategies also have been shown to improve writing performance. For example, collaborative and highly structured peer-mediated prompting or scaffolding in writing produced significantly higher pre–post gains for children who wrote interactively as opposed to those in the control condition who wrote independently (Yarrow & Topping, 2001). Paired students also increased their self-esteem as writers (Yarrow & Topping, 2001). In another application, cross-age tutoring stimulated more critical thinking and discussions related to writing assignments for students in grades 3 and 4 (Schneider & Barone, 1997).

In addition to noted improvements in basic academic skill areas (i.e., reading, math, writing), PMI strategies have been associated with increased acquisition, retention, and application of factual information in the content areas of social studies, science, and art (Maheady et al., 1988; Rosenthal, 1994; Thurston, 1994). Studies of PMIs in health and physical education have also substantiated positive results (Anliker, Drake, & Pacholski, 1993; Block, Oberweiser, & Bain, 1995).

Improving Peer Interactions and Classroom Climate

Positive involvement with peers provides increased opportunities for children to engage in prosocial behaviors and may improve social acceptance (Hoff & Robinson, 2002). Research supports PMI strategies as being effective in increasing the frequency of prosocial behaviors of preschool and elementary-age students with disabilities (Odom & Strain, 1984; Strain & Odom, 1986). Peers with disabilities report improved interpersonal relations with typical peers outside of tutoring sessions (i.e., being viewed as more likeable, capable, and friendly by others; Maheady, Harper, Mallette, & Winstanley, 1991). Through the use of a PMI called positive peer reporting (PPR), for example, a number of studies have found an increase in positive peer interactions and acceptance ratings in the classroom setting (e.g., Bowers, McGinnis, Ervin, & Friman, 1999; Bowers, Woods, Carlyon, & Friman, 2000; Ervin, Miller, & Friman, 1996). In addition, structured peer interactions through a PMI called cooperative learning increased friendships between students with and without disabilities within and outside the classroom (Johnson & Johnson, 1986). In a large-scale study of 203 elementary students, peer-mediated activities that were designed to integrate students with autism into the classroom resulted in increased peer interactions (Kamps et al., 1998). In addition, the majority of the nontargeted peers reported enjoyment with the program and overall satisfaction in being friends and helpers to peers with autism, suggesting that PMIs can provide reciprocal benefits to students with and without disabilities. Peer partner strategies have been used successfully to increase positive social exchanges and decrease negative verbal interactions for students with behavior disorders and learning disabilities (Franca et al., 1990; Maheady et al., 1988). Interdependent group reward contingencies are a strategy for fostering interdependence among peers. Slavin (1990) found that, with respect to the impact on peer relations and academic outcomes, interdependent group reward contingencies (i.e., rewards provided to the group when all members met the preestablished criterion) were more effective than dependent group rewards (given to the group on the basis of particular students' performances) or independent rewards (given only to individuals who met a criterion). Cushing and Kennedy (1997) revealed that students without disabilities who were previously identified as having low levels of classroom participation and who served as peer supports for students with disabilities in a general education classroom improved their academic engagement, assignment completion, and grades. Similarly, within a sample of students with emotional–behavioral difficulties, Franca and colleagues (1990) found that same-age peer tutoring in math had positive effects on peer interactions and increased academic responding.

Encouraging Student Autonomy

When students are able to set their own goals and to monitor and assess their own learning, they may feel more autonomous and confident (Ginsburg-Block, Rohrbeck, & Fantuzzo, 2006; Rohrbeck et al., 2003). By allowing increased opportunities for self-directedness within the structure of the learning task and evaluation process, peer tutoring programs build feelings of self-efficacy and self-confidence (Ginsburg-Block, Rohrbeck, Fantuzzo, & Lavigne, 2006). More opportunities for student autonomy have been linked to increased academic outcomes (Rohrbeck et al., 2003).

Promoting Maintenance of Behavior Change and/or Generalization of Outcomes to Unprogrammed Settings or Situations

A primary challenge in special education is maintenance and generalization of target behaviors from the trained setting to natural settings. Strategies for promoting maintenance and generalization are incorporated into many PMI strategies, making them more conducive to facilitating lasting change (Stokes & Baer, 1977). For example, PMIs in the classroom can stimulate generalization of change outside the classroom to untrained and more common environments (e.g., the lunchroom, playground, or neighborhood) because peers are readily accessible in these various settings and can monitor or serve as cues (Hoff & Robinson, 2002). Not surprisingly, Haring and Breen (1992) found that peer interaction during structured activities translated into natural reinforcement beyond the classroom walls.

Selecting PMIs to Address Teacher Preference or Contextual Fit

As just discussed, PMIs may be selected to promote intended outcomes. In addition, PMI strategies might be chosen over other strategies because they match with a teacher's preference and/or fit the instructional context.

Differentiating Instructional Levels and Formats

A key advantage of PMIs is that teachers can structure PMIs to allow for heterogeneous groups of students in the same classroom as they move through the curriculum and learn at different rates (Fuchs, Fuchs, & Burish, 2000). A teacher can have students work together in a structured manner, simultaneously implementing different levels of curriculum and using different instructional procedures, accommodating a wide range of learners (Fuchs et al., 2000). For students, this means that instructional objectives, tasks, strategies, and materials can be tailored to meet their individual needs.

Flexibility and Adaptability

Findings from effectiveness research in the area of PMIs are encouraging because these strategies have broad applications and fit easily into instructional routines in the classroom (Maheady, Harper, & Mallette, 2001). They have been effectively applied with a broad range of students with disabilities (e.g., autism, learning disabilities, behavioral disorders, severe disabilities), with social concerns (e.g., peer rejection, social isolation), and with academic challenges. With increasing diversity among student populations come differing needs within classrooms. Fuchs and colleagues (1997) encouraged specialized adaptations with the use of a packaged version of CWPT in math peer-assisted learning strategies—math (PALS-M) by having different children simultaneously work on different math skills. Because pairs work together on individualized material, instructional time for all students is increased. Students provide necessary help, immediate feedback, and error correction to their partners. Through this restructuring, teachers successfully formulated adaptations and modified instruction when a student was identified as failing to make adequate progress.

Socially Valid Procedures

Classmates who serve as peer monitors may benefit significantly from their role (Dougherty, Fowler, & Paine, 1985). On surveys of social validity, both teachers and students report that they enjoy peer-mediated instructional approaches (Spencer et al., 2003; Barbetta et al., 1991). In fact, many studies have established the social validity of both didactic and group peer-mediated interventions (e.g., Cochran, Feng, Cartledge, & Hamilton, 1993; Franca et al., 1990; Greenwood et al., 2001; Spencer et al., 2003). Social interaction data and positive peer reports of a 5-year longitudinal study with elementary school children (n = 203) and participants with autism (n = 38) across multiple settings supports the contention that PMI strategies can facilitate meaningful integration and positive social outcomes for students with disabilities (Kamps et al., 1998). PMI strategies within this study included classwide or small-group peer tutoring, cooperative learning, special class buddies to assist with art and physical education, calendar activities, and play groups focused on social skill development. The majority of the typical peers interviewed reported that they enjoyed and benefited academically and/or socially from these programs. Overall, peer reflections indicated increased personal interest and satisfaction in working with or being friends with a classmate who has a disability (Kamps et al., 1998).

Cost Effectiveness, Practicality, and Ease of Implementation

Peer-mediated strategies not only produce meaningful results but have also been described as practical and cost-effective (Hoff & Robinson, 2002). Classroom peers are easily accessible and continuously present across multiple settings within the school day (transition times, restroom, lunch, or recess; Hoff & Robinson, 2002). A meta-analysis conducted by Ginsburg-Block, Rohrbeck, and Fantuzzo (2006) illustrates the cost-effectiveness of peer-assisted learning by showing that strategies targeting academic achievement also have a positive impact on social–emotional learning, thereby reducing the need for additional programs and resources. In fact, when compared with isolated social skills programs, PMIs with a primary focus on academic skills simultaneously produced comparable positive social outcomes (Ginsburg-Block, Rohrbeck, & Fantuzzo, 2006). Finally, Levin, Glass, and Meister (1987) found that peer tutoring was more cost-effective as a means of increasing academic achievement when compared with other instructional alternatives such as smaller class size, increased length of the school day, and computer-assisted instruction. These interventions are considered effective and low tech in that they require little time and resource expenditure for the results they produce (Heward, 1994).

Availability in Prepackaged or Manualized Format

A number of PMIs are available in packaged formats in which specific interventions with empirically demonstrated benefits are conveniently manualized. For example, Peer-Assisted Learning Strategies (PALS) is available in both reading (PALS-R) and math (PALS-M) formats (Fuchs & Fuchs, 1998). Teachers can follow the scripted manual to conduct the lessons and are given the necessary materials to implement weekly sessions in their classrooms. These materials help teachers save time by providing descriptions of established procedures and study guides and activities that outline structured peer interactions. PALS even provides specific curriculum-based procedures and computerized links for monitoring student progress (Ginsburg-Block, Rohrbeck, Fantuzzo, & Lavigne, 2006). The PALS teacher manual details implementation, rules, roles and responsibilities, awarding of points, and academic lessons (e.g., syllabication, decoding) and provides student assignment cards, correction procedures and forms, lesson sequence sheets, and written scripts to implement lessons. Having this manual readily accessible for consultants (school psychologists) and facilitators (teachers) may save time, increase procedural fidelity, and ease implementation, especially in the initial stages of setup.

Examples of Specific Evidence-Based PMIs

Within the research literature, there are many evidence-based PMI strategies from which to choose. Within this section we have selected several strategies to describe in more detail. These include: peer tutoring (i.e., CWPT, reciprocal peer tutoring, and PALS), peer monitoring, positive peer reporting, peer modeling, group contingencies, cooperative learning, peer education, and peer-mediated social skills training. Within each description, an overview of what the strategy looks like, its intended use, specific outcomes, empirical support, and links to additional resources are provided.

Peer Tutoring

Peer tutoring is an instructional strategy in which students work in dyads. Students can be paired in various ways (e.g., same-age, cross-age, high status with low status). Peer tutoring approaches can differ in terms of structure, setting, intensity, or targeted domain. Peer tutoring can involve "fixed" roles wherein students maintain their status of either tutor (instructor) or tutee (learner) throughout and/or across sessions or "role reciprocity," whereby students engage in both the tutor and tutee roles in one session. In general, peer tutoring facilitates high rates of responding, practice, feedback, and structured peer interactions. Two popular peer tutoring practices, CWPT and reciprocal peer tutoring (RPT), are discussed in this section, along with a packaged peer tutoring program, PALS.

Classwide Peer Tutoring

CWPT was developed by the researchers at the Juniper Gardens Children's Project of the University of Kansas (Greenwood et al., 1989). In CWPT, the teacher organizes the entire class into dyads. Dyads are assigned to one of two classroom teams for which they earn points. Students initially receive training on specific tutoring methods of reinforcement and error correction with feedback. The instructional format usually involves directed instruction and guided practice with a focus on mastery of a specific skill. During each tutoring session, the roles are switched, allowing students to participate as both the tutor and tutee. Together, dyads complete specific teacher-generated tasks and obtain reinforcement for their combined performance. Tutees earn points for correct responses, and teachers distribute bonus points to tutors for following procedures. At the end of the tutoring session, points are tallied for each team in the classroom. The winning team is applauded for their success, and the trailing team is applauded for their effort. The teacher monitors mastery of the

specific skill on a weekly basis using curriculum-based tests while also reinforcing appropriate tutorial procedures. Student pairs and classroom teams can change weekly.

CWPT has been successfully applied to a number of academic outcomes, such as passage reading (Greenwood, 1991), reading comprehension (Fuchs et al., 1997), mathematics (Greenwood et al., 1989), and spelling (Maheady et al., 1991). It has been implemented effectively in regular education and special education and with low-achieving students from kindergarten through high school levels. CWPT has improved literacy (spelling and vocabulary) in elementary-level ELLs (Greenwood et al., 2001). Improved academic outcomes have been found in students of low social economic status and those who are academically at risk (Greenwood et al., 1989). The immediate feedback in CWPT procedures has shown success with children with attention-deficit/hyperactivity disorder (ADHD; DuPaul et al., 1998; DuPaul & Henningson, 1993). CWPT as a longitudinal application has been found to be an effective instructional process (Greenwood, 1991). In addition, it is also a potential tool for preventing early school failure (Greenwood & Delquadri, 1995).

Reciprocal Peer Tutoring

Fantuzzo and colleagues developed RPT (Fantuzzo, Polite, & Grayson, 1990). Same-age student dyads of comparable ability level participate in two-way tutoring. Students are trained to complete specific RTP procedures, as well as to work in teams. The dyads work together in a two-part session. In the first session, the students alternate between peer teacher and student roles. The responsibility of the peer teacher is to help the student successfully solve problems by keeping him or her on task, giving instructional prompts, and providing praise and encouragement. The peer teacher presents flash cards in the selected skill area. The problem is presented on one side of the flash card, and the other side includes the answer and the steps to solve the problem. The peer teacher provides performance feedback and assistance. When the student answers a problem correctly, the peer teacher praises him or her and then presents the next problem. If the solution is incorrect, the peer teacher instructs the student to try the problem again in the box marked "try 2" on the worksheet. If the student is unable to answer the question on his or her own, the peer teacher provides assistance. Students then continue working on the problem in the space labeled "try 3." In the second session, individualized drill sheets are completed and scored within the student dyad. A team score is calculated based on the scores of the two team members. Previously selected team goals are compared with these scores to determine whether the team has met its goal and "won" for the day.

RPT can be used in reading (Sutherland & Snyder, 2007) and is commonly applied to mathematics instruction with elementary students (Fantuzzo, King, & Heller, 1992). Fantuzzo and colleagues (1992) evaluated the mathematics performance of fourth- and fifth-grade students who were at high risk for academic failure in an urban elementary school. Students who received both RPT and a reward displayed the highest levels of accurate mathematics computation.

Peer-Assisted Learning Strategies

PALS is a packaged version of CWPT, available from Vanderbilt Kennedy Center for Research on Human Development (1998), that was designed for grades 2–6 with a downward extension to kindergarten and an upward extension to the high school level in both math (PALS-M) and reading (PALS-R). PALS differs from CWPT in that the learning tasks for each student within the dyad are individually determined by curriculum-based assessments (Fuchs & Fuchs, 1998). In PALS-R the dyads are set up similarly to those in CWPT, though it is unique in its focus on phonological awareness, decoding activities, and comprehension strategies (Fuchs et al., 1997). During PALS-R, the tutor prompts the tutee to recall parts of the story using specific questions, to sum up the story in 10 words or less (paragraph shrinking), and to make a prediction about what will happen next. In the PALS-M, pairs practice specific problem-solving steps (Fuchs et al., 1995).

Low achievers with disabilities, low achievers without disabilities, and average achievers all improved more on fluency, accuracy, and comprehension with PALS than did a control group in a study done by Fuchs

and colleagues (1997). In a study on the sustainability of PALS-M with general education teachers who taught students both with and without disabilities, researchers found that teachers maintained an extremely high rate and quality of sustained use of PALS-M several years after the original research project ended (Baker, Gersten, Dimino, & Griffiths, 2004).

Peer Monitoring

In peer monitoring, peers are trained to observe and record targeted social or academic behaviors of specific students in collaboration with the teacher. In addition to monitoring, these trained peers often use prompts and provide positive reinforcements and consequences. Peer monitoring can be used to measure and track student behavior (e.g., time on task, work habits) and academic progress (McCurdy & Shapiro, 1992). First, the teacher identifies measurable behaviors in objective terms to be monitored and then selects an efficient monitoring system. Peers can observe a variety of social or academic behaviors (e.g., increased social participation, off-task academic performance; Henington & Skinner, 1998). To record the data, peer monitors can use a number of methods depending on the behavior. For example, peers can use narrative recording to provide written descriptions of observed events or event recording to record the frequency of each observed event.

Peer-monitoring programs have been conducted in a variety of settings with a variety of students. Carden-Smith and Fowler (1984) found that kindergarten-age children with serious behavior and learning problems were able to effectively manage their peers' behavior and to be managed by their peers using a peer-monitored token system targeted toward reducing disruption and increasing participation. Stern, Fowler, and Kohler (1988) had children without disabilities work in dyads in which one child served as a peer monitor and the other child earned points from his or her monitor for good behavior. Points were accumulated as part of a group contingency. When alternated on an every-other-day basis, the peer-monitor and point-earner roles were equally effective in substantially reducing disruptive and off-task behavior. Dougherty and colleagues

(1985) showed that peers can implement a token system to maintain reductions in previously high rates of negative interactions during recess. The results also suggest that classmates who serve as peer monitors may benefit significantly from their role. Undesirable rates of negative interactions immediately and substantially decreased among children appointed as monitors following their appointments. Furthermore, Dougherty and colleagues (1985) found that the improvements generalized within settings from days in which they monitored to days in which they did not monitor.

With regard to academics, Bentz and Shinn (1990) demonstrated that fourth-grade general education students can be trained to assess curriculum-based reading of second and third graders with the accuracy of trained adults. McCurdy and Shapiro (1992) studied progress monitoring of the oral reading rates of elementary-age students with learning disabilities. They found that students in the peer-monitoring conditions could collect reliable data on the number of correct words per minute. These studies illustrate that students can be trained as reliable data collectors, which can assist teachers in their evaluation of student progress in response to academic interventions.

Positive Peer Reporting

The PPR procedure involves asking peers to monitor and publicly acknowledge prosocial targeted behaviors (Ervin et al., 1996). Although the procedure was not called PPR, the concept of peer acknowledgement as a means of improving student behavior was initially described by Grieger, Kauffman, and Grieger (1976). Through the use of PPR, prosocial behaviors are supported and reinforced, which encourages students to engage in socially appropriate behaviors within their natural environment (Skinner, Neddenriep, Robinson, Ervin, & Jones, 2002). Typically, the teacher randomly selects a target student as "star of the week." Classmates are then told that they can earn rewards (e.g., tokens) if they observe and report that peer's positive behaviors (e.g., "Jill shared her cards at lunch"). A brief period of time is allotted in the day in which peers are given the opportunity to publicly report any specific positive behaviors they observed from the "star of

the week" student that day (Skinner et al., 2002).

With implementation of PPR in school settings, studies have demonstrated increases in positive peer interactions and in target students' initiation of social interactions and reductions in negative peer interactions of socially rejected children (Skinner et al., 2002; Jones, Young, & Friman, 2000). Ervin and colleagues (1996), for example, showed that a socially rejected girl's interactions and acceptance improved and negative social interactions were reduced when peers were rewarded for publicly reporting about the prosocial behaviors of the rejected girl. They also found that this intervention effectively influenced positive peer interactions and peer acceptance ratings. In another study, Bowers and colleagues (1999) found that through PPR the daily problem behaviors of a 15-year-old boy in residential care were reduced. In a group home setting, PPR resulted in substantial improvements in social interactions by previously isolated peers (Bowers et al., 2000).

Peer Modeling

Peer modeling is largely based on Bandura's (1977) social cognitive theory of observational learning through modeling. In general, a student's learning and motivation is strongly influenced by what his or her peers say and do. An advantage to the peer modeling strategy is that students can identify better with the demonstrated skills and learning strategies of a peer than with those of an adult (Schunk, 1998).

In this strategy, a task or distinctive behavioral feature is made explicit to the target student. This identified task is then successfully modeled by a peer and observed by the target student. Factors important when selecting peer models include developmental status and self-efficacy of the learner, model–observer similarity (e.g., gender, age), and model competence. Teachers and school psychologists should be aware that goal setting, vicarious consequences, and outcome expectations have also been found to influence peer modeling effectiveness (Schunk, 1987).

Peer modeling has been shown to be effective in the acquisition of academic skills. Schunk and Hanson (1985) investigated how children's self-efficacy and achievement were influenced by observing peer models learn an academic skill. The target students in this study had experienced difficulties learning subtraction with regrouping. Children who observed a same-sex peer demonstrate either rapid (mastery model) or gradual (coping model) attainment of subtraction skills experienced higher self-efficacy for learning and achievement than those in the teacher-model or no-model conditions. No significant differences due to type of peer-modeled behavior (mastery or coping) were found. Schunk, Hanson, and Cox (1987) examined how attributes of peer models influenced achievement behaviors of children who experienced difficulties learning mathematical skills. They had students observe either one or three same-sex peer models demonstrating mastery or coping behaviors while solving fractions. Children in the single-coping-model, multiple-coping-model, and multiple-mastery-model conditions demonstrated higher self-efficacy, skill, and training performance than children who observed a single-mastery model. Those children who observed coping (vs. mastery) models judged themselves more similar in competence to the models.

Group Contingencies

As classwide interventions, group contingencies allow peers to encourage appropriate behavior among their classmates. There are three different group contingency systems: independent, interdependent, and dependent. With an independent group contingency, everyone in the class is presented with the same target behavior and criterion, and those students meeting the criterion are reinforced (Alric, Bray, Kehle, Chafouleas, & Theodore, 2007; Skinner, Cashwell, & Dunn, 1996). For example, a class is given a spelling test, and only those students who score 85% or above are rewarded. In an interdependent group contingency system, the class receives access to the reinforcer contingent on the behavior of the entire group (Kelshaw-Levering, Sterling-Turner, Henry, & Skinner, 2000). For example, everyone in the class must get 85% or above on the spelling test for the class to receive the reinforcer. With a dependent group contingency, the group is provided access to the reinforcer

based on the behavior of one or a few students (Kelshaw-Levering et al., 2000). For example, the group receives the reinforcer if Sarah, Jay, and Sean score 85% or above on the spelling test.

Dependent group contingencies were used to increase the on-task behavior of general education students in third- and fourth-grade classrooms during math instruction. The mean levels of on-task behavior rose from 35% and 50% in the third- and fourth-grade classes, respectively, to above 80% for both classrooms during the intervention phases. In addition, social validity measures suggested that the procedure was feasible for classroom staff to implement, acceptable to students, and produced few, if any, adverse effects on student social standing (Heering & Wilder, 2006).

Alric and colleagues (2007) conducted a comparative investigation of independent, interdependent, and dependent group contingencies and found that all three strategies effectively increased reading fluency in grade 4 students. In the first condition, the independent group contingencies, students were told that they would work hard to obtain a set individual criterion of words read correctly per minute (WCPM) that would be individually reinforced. In contrast, the interdependent treatment condition encouraged students to work hard to achieve a group reward based on the WCPM class average relative to a preset criterion (everyone had to work in partnership to obtain the reward). In the third, dependent contingency, condition, the teacher announced that rewards would be provided on the basis of a selected student's WCPM performance (to encourage all the children to work their best and to help fellow confederates, the children were not told who would be selected). At the beginning of each of the 12 sessions, the teacher restated the contingency expectations to the students, and at the end of every lesson the reinforcers were distributed accordingly. They included game, drawing, and computer time, as well as selection of a small tangible item.

Cooperative Learning

Within cooperative learning groups, students work through academic assignments together in a structured format under the management of the classroom teacher. Johnson and Johnson (1994) describe five broad conditions that need to be met for cooperative learning to be successful. The first factor is *positive interdependence*. Students are held accountable for learning assigned material themselves and for ensuring that all members of the group also do so. For example, each group member has a specific responsibility to contribute to the joint task. Second, individuals are encouraged to assist their group members through *face-to-face interaction*. This can be done through sharing resources or giving feedback. The third important factor of cooperative learning is *individual accountability*. Students are held individually responsible for contributing their portion to the group's final outcome. The fourth essential element of cooperative learning is the appropriate use of *interpersonal and small-group skills*. Students must be taught this essential skill set in order to achieve mutual goals. The fifth feature is *group processing*. The purpose here is to clarify the contributions of the members to the collaborative efforts and to improve the effectiveness of the members to achieve the group's goals. Within cooperative learning, individual competitiveness is incompatible with success (Aronson & Patone, 1997).

Cooperative learning has strong empirical support. Johnson and Johnson (2000), in their extensive meta-analysis ($N = 164$ studies) of eight well-established cooperative strategies, found significant achievement gains across all eight methods. The following discussion expands on five of these strategies.

Student Teams–Achievement Divisions

In student teams–achievement divisions (STAD), students work in cooperative teams to learn new material presented by the teacher. Teams practice and study together, then take individual tests on which each score contributes to an overall team score. An individual's contribution to the team score is based on that person's improvement, not on an absolute test score (Slavin, 1990).

Team Games Tournaments

Throughout the week, group members help each other master new material. Students then compete in a three-person tournament with classmates of comparable ability from other teams to earn points for their original teams. Team games tournaments (TGT) use the same format as STAD, but mastery is demonstrated through competition in a class tournament (Aronson & Patone, 1997).

Jigsaw II

Jigsaw II is a commonly used adaptation of Aronson's (Aronson, Stephan, Sikes, Blaney, & Snapp, 1978) original Jigsaw method. This group–regroup activity extends and consolidates students' understanding of teacher-presented materials (Jigsaw Classroom, 2008). The class is split into groups, given a general topic, and then, within this general topic, individuals are given a subtopic. The students from different teams with the same subtopic meet in groups to read and identify the key points and become "experts." These experts then return to their original teams to teach what they have learned. All students are tested on a quiz that covers all topics, and the quiz scores are summed to form team scores. In the original Jigsaw, students received only individual grades based on their own test scores (Slavin, 1983).

Co-op, Co-op

Following teacher-presented material, heterogeneous teams select a topic. The topic is then divided into minitopics for each individual in the group to become an "expert" on. Each expert in the group prepares and presents his or her individual topic to the group. The group as a whole then prepares, presents, reflects, and evaluates their work together.

Numbered Heads Together

Within this question-asking strategy, heterogeneous groups of students are formed and then numbered 1–4. The groups each consist of one student of high ability, two students of average ability, and one student of low ability. A teacher-directed lesson is then presented, followed by questions that the group discusses as a whole, ensuring that every group member understands the content being covered and can answer the questions. Finally, the teacher randomly calls on specific numbered students to answer the questions.

Social Skills Training

As discussed earlier, social skills training with peers can involve observational, antecedent, and consequent approaches (e.g., group contingencies, contingent social reinforcement, peer modeling; Gresham, 1981). In peer-mediated social skills interventions teachers commonly train confederates to initiate, prompt, and reinforce positive social exchanges. Strain (1977) demonstrated that peer confederates can be coached to provide appropriate initiation (e.g., "Come on, let's all play tag"), leading to increased prosocial behaviors and interactions with generalization effects observed in later free-play settings. In their study of six preschool students with moderate mental handicaps, Strain and Shores (1977) illustrated how peers can augment both appropriate physical/gestural and verbal reciprocity. PMIs have been particularly effective in enhancing the social skills and interactions of students with autism (Bass & Mulick, 2007). Odom and Strain (1986) have developed a protocol whereby teachers specifically train peers to initiate prosocial interactions and play organizers (e.g., sharing, assistance requests, affection, compliment statements) and are then prompted to initiate these skills with target students around certain selected toys and activities. Another promising approach for children with autism is peer buddies, which increases social interaction by training peers to elicit appropriate social skills, such as asking for an object, getting someone's attention, or waiting their turn (English, Goldstein, Shafer, & Kaczmarek, 1997). In addition, the buddy skills script by Laushey and Heflin (2000) was designed for children with autism and involves three components: (1) stay with your buddy, (2) play with your buddy, and (3) talk with your buddy. Systematically structuring peer-mediated social networks in integrated high school settings has also been shown to improve the quantity and quality of social interactions among students with moderate and severe disabilities (Haring & Breen, 1992).

Special Considerations When Using PMIs in School Settings

A number of special considerations surrounding PMIs should be addressed before implementation. These special considerations include informed consent, time and resources required, the teacher's role, grouping or pairing of students, quality of peer training, and systematic monitoring of the intervention.

Informed Consent

Even though peer-mediated strategies intuitively seem to be a natural part of classroom instruction, it is important to address the areas of informed parental consent and voluntary participation in the initial stages of creating a program (Garcia-Vazquez & Ehly, 1995). Holding an informal information session with resource handouts and consent forms distributed to parents may be an efficient and effective way to avoid ethical controversy. This approach also provides parents with a forum to ask questions, discuss their concerns, and review literature related to potential advantages of PMIs for the students.

Time and Resources Required

When consulting with classroom teachers who are considering PMI strategies, it is important to acknowledge the initial time and resources that are potentially required. Providing background information on evidence-based approaches for target behaviors, procedures for peer selection, and training protocols will help reassure and guide teachers through this process. In advance, consultants can help prepare some of the materials needed (e.g., consent form, implementation/procedural checklists, monitoring/feedback logs) and resources (e.g., practical activity books, training videos) to ensure a successful setup. Although certain PMIs may initially demand additional time and material development, once integrated into the daily routine these interventions have proven to be well worth the effort (Maheady et al., 2001). Not surprisingly, high-quality professional development has been linked to better student outcomes and program sustainability (Baker et al., 2004). School psychologists can work closely with the classroom teacher to implement PMI programs and should be involved in the process of inservice training. Generally, PMI approaches do not require significant expenditure for equipment, material, and personnel. Many curriculum materials and classroom settings can be easily adapted to most methods (e.g., reciprocal paired reading and math problem solving). When considering the startup cost, it is important to note that in the long term, peer-mediated interventions may be more cost-effective than other methods (e.g., reducing class size; Levin et al., 1987).

The Teacher's Role

One potential drawback of having peers as the primary instructional agent in the classroom is that the role of the teacher sometimes is underestimated. Many parents express concerns that peer programs take away valuable teacher-directed instructional time, making it important to document and share the benefits of peer-mediated instruction (Maheady, 1998; Hoff & Robinson, 2002). In order to address these concerns, the teacher can use measures (e.g., curriculum-based assessment, computer-based systems, procedural/observational checklists) that are available in prepackaged programs such as PALS (Baker et al., 2004). Also, problems associated with PMIs, such as elevated classroom noise or small behavioral issues (e.g., students' complaints about partners, peers not working cooperatively, point inflation), often occur because of inadequate preplanning and teacher monitoring (Maheady et al., 2001).

Some teachers are apprehensive about adopting alternative instructional methodologies such as PMIs because they feel the strategies may compromise the breadth and pace of content coverage (Maheady, 1998). Although teacher-directed lessons may set a more rigorous pace, with instruction covering greater breadth of content, this does not necessarily mean that the students are mastering the material or learning more quickly (Maheady, 1998). This potential drawback regarding content coverage needs to be carefully considered in the preplanning stage. Paired and group activities should be well chosen, relevant to curriculum, and linked to student progress.

Grouping or Pairing of Students

Thoughtful recruitment, matching, and monitoring of students can prevent potentially negative peer interaction between students. If peer partners are poorly matched, forced, or not carefully monitored, there can be harmful outcomes, such as peer rejection or resentment (Sutherland & Synder, 2007). Understandably, students should not be coerced into these roles but instead given the choice to participate. Consideration of student characteristics (e.g., cognitive level, academic skills), student feedback, and opportunities for role reciprocity are essential parts of the planning process (Kunsch et al., 2007).

Quality of Peer Training

Poorly trained peers and insufficient contact time with peer partners can also create problems that undermine the benefits of PMI strategies (Fuchs et al., 2001). Peer training should involve explicit procedural instruction, guided practice, and feedback. More structured roles and explicit understanding of teacher expectations have been shown to lead to greater academic outcomes (Ginsburg-Block, Rohrbeck, Fantuzzo, & Lavigne, 2006; Cohen, Kulik, & Kulik, 1982). Once training is implemented, students need to meet at least three times a week to become fluent and comfortable with these procedures (Fuchs et al., 2001). A peer booster training session or designated feedback time can be implemented to deal with low motivation, procedural drift, or other problematic situations that might arise.

Systematic Monitoring of the Intervention

A commonly overlooked yet integral component of peer-mediated strategies is systematic monitoring. Once an intervention is in place, teachers need to circulate, supervise, carefully evaluate, and reward tutoring procedures, as well as achievement and behavioral performance outcomes (Topping & Ehly, 1998). Often procedures of error correction and reinforcement need adjustments (Greenwood, Terry, Arreaga-Mayer, & Finney, 1992). Collecting performance data will allow teachers to assess (1) whether or not learning objectives are actually being met, (2) the degree to which target students are responding to interventions, and (3) the need for program refinements. Individual instances of pupil failure to respond can be addressed subsequently through systematic analyses of treatment failures (Maheady et al., 2001).

Unfortunately, due to time constraints and new demands being placed on teachers daily, it is not uncommon for teachers to enthusiastically start PMIs and then leave them unmonitored, assuming they will run themselves. Continued support by the consultant during the monitoring and evaluation stage is essential to successful PMI implementation. In addition to monitoring student progress and treatment integrity, peer relationships should be assessed to ensure that there are no detrimental outcomes. Consistent feedback regarding students' performances as tutors and learners may reinforce their efforts and create program sustainability. Being able to share the academic and social–emotional benefits at the local level (i.e., with parents and teaching staff) can build program momentum and credibility.

Summary and Conclusions

Many methods have been developed that use peers as support agents for their classmates. These peer-mediated interventions encompass academic, behavioral, and social changes; they may involve dyads of students or groups; and the peer may reinforce a target behavior directly, indirectly, or via group contingencies. A plethora of studies exist documenting the utility of peer-mediated interventions across diverse populations and academic domains. Thus the studies we discussed herein are far from an exhaustive overview but rather are cited to highlight the versatility of peer-mediated intervention strategies available in the empirical literature.

Given the general consensus that peer-mediated approaches can have a powerful influence on both academic achievement (Kunsch et al., 2007; Stern et al., 1988) and social–emotional and behavioral outcomes (Cohen et al., 1982; Ginsburg-Block, Rohrbeck, & Fantuzzo, 2006; Johnson &

Johnson, 1989), school psychologists responsible for professional development, intervention, and consultation and monitoring will find it useful to be well versed in the potential advantages of PMIs discussed here.

Extensive research on the efficacy and the social validity of peer-mediated interventions suggests numerous benefits of peer-mediated interventions in the classroom. Favorable findings have been documented for a diverse range of techniques, including CWPT (Greenwood et al., 1989), RPT (Fantuzzo et al., 1990), PPR (Ervin et al., 1996), group contingencies (Skinner et al., 1996), peer monitoring (Henington & Skinner, 1998), and social skills training (Bass & Mulick, 2007). PMIs facilitate inclusion and acceptance of those with individual differences into the regular classroom (Utley, 2001). In this chapter a rationale was provided for the use of peer-mediated interventions, the salient features were described, and a number of advantages to using peer-mediated interventions were discussed, with a brief review of the existing literature. Readers interested in learning more about PMIs are encouraged to explore the vast literature on this topic, beginning with the references and resource links provided within this chapter.

References

Alric, J. M., Bray, M. A., Kehle, T. J., Chafouleas, S. M., & Theodore, L. A. (2007). A comparison of independent, interdependent, and dependent group contingencies with randomized reinforcers to increase reading fluency. *Canadian Journal of School Psychology*, 22(1), 81–93.

Anliker, J. A., Drake, L. T., & Pacholski, J. (1993). Impacts of a multi-layered nutrition program: Teenagers teaching children. *Journal of Nutritional Education*, 25, 140–143.

Aronson, E., & Patone, P. (1997). *The jigsaw classroom: Building cooperation in the classroom*. Menlo Park, CA: Longman.

Aronson, E., Stephan, C., Sikes, J., Blaney, N., & Snapp, M. (1978). *The jigsaw classroom*. Beverly Hills, CA.: Sage.

Baker, S., Gersten, R., Dimino, J. A., & Griffiths, R. (2004). The sustained use of research-based instructional practice: A case study of peer-assisted learning strategies in mathematics. *Remedial and Special Education*, 25(1), 5–24.

Bandura, A. (1977). *Social learning theory.* New York: General Learning Press.

Barbetta, P. M., Miller, A. D., & Peters, M. T. (1991). Tugmate: A cross-age tutoring program to teach sight vocabulary. *Education and Treatment of Children, 14,* 19–37.

Bass, J. D., & Mulick, J. M. (2007). Social play skill enhancement of children with autism using peers and siblings as therapists. *Psychology in the Schools, 44,* 727–735.

Bentz, J., & Shinn, M. R. (1990). Training general education pupils to monitor reading using curriculum-based measurement. *School Psychology Review, 19*(1), 23–32.

Block, M. E., Oberweiser, B., & Bain, M. (1995). Using classwide peer tutoring to facilitate inclusions with disabilities in regular physical education. *Physical Educator, 52*(1), 47–56.

Bowers, F. E., McGinnis, J. C., Ervin, R. A., & Friman, P. C. (1999). Merging research and practice: The example of positive peer reporting applied to social rejection. *Education and Treatment of Children, 22,* 218–226.

Bowers, F. E., Woods, D. W., Carlyon, W. D., & Friman, P. C. (2000). Using positive peer reporting to improve the social interactions and acceptance of socially isolated adolescents in residential care: A systematic replication. *Journal of Applied Behavior Analysis, 33*(2), 239–242.

Burks, M. (2004). Effects of classwide peer tutoring on the number of words spelled correctly by students with LD. *Intervention in School and Clinic, 39,* 301–304.

Carden-Smith, L. K., & Fowler, S. A. (1984). Positive peer pressure: The effects of peer monitoring on children's disruptive behavior. *Journal of Applied Behavior Analysis, 17*(2), 213–227.

Cochran, L., Feng, H., Cartledge, G., & Hamilton, S. (1993). The effects of cross-age tutoring on the academic achievement, social behaviors and self-perceptions of low achieving African-American males with behavioral disorders. *Behavioral Disorders, 18,* 292–302.

Cohen, P. A., Kulik, J. A., & Kulik, C. C. (1982). Education outcomes of tutoring: A meta-analysis of findings. *American Educational Research Journal, 19,* 237–248.

Cushing, L. S., & Kennedy, C. H. (1997). Academic effects on students without disabilities who serve as peer supports for students with disabilities in general education classrooms. *Journal of Applied Behavior Analysis, 30,* 139–152.

Delquadri, J. C., Greenwood, C. R., Whorton, D., Carta, J. J., & Hall, R. V. (1986). Classwide peer tutoring. *Exceptional Children, 52,* 535–542.

DeVries, R. (1997). Piaget's social theory. *Educational Researcher, 26,* 4–17.

Dougherty, B. S., Fowler, S. A., & Paine, S. C. (1985). The use of peer monitors to reduce negative interaction during recess. *Journal of Applied Behavior Analysis, 18,* 141–153.

DuPaul, G. J., Ervin, R. A., Hook, C. L., & McGoey, K. E. (1998). Peer tutoring for children with attention-deficit/hyperactivity disorder: Effects on classroom behavior and academic performance. *Journal of Applied Behavior Analysis, 31,* 579–592.

DuPaul, G. J., & Henningson, P. N. (1993). Peer tutoring effects on the classroom performance of children with attention deficit and hyperactivity disorder. *School Psychology Review, 22*(1), 134–143.

English, K., Goldstein, H., Shafer, K., & Kaczmarek, L. (1997). Promoting interactions among preschoolers with and without disabilities: Effects of a buddy skills training program. *Exceptional Children, 63,* 229–243.

Ervin, R. A., Miller, P. M., & Friman, P. C. (1996). Feed the hungry bee: Using positive peer reports to improve the social interactions and acceptance of a socially rejected girl in residential care. *Journal of Applied Behavior Analysis, 29*(2), 251–253.

Fantuzzo, J. W., King, J. A., & Heller, L. R. (1992). Effects of reciprocal peer tutoring on mathematics and school adjustment: A component analysis. *Journal of Educational Psychology, 84*(3), 331–339.

Fantuzzo, J. W., Polite, K., & Grayson, N. (1990). An evaluation of school-based reciprocal peer tutoring across elementary school settings. *Journal of School Psychology, 28,* 309–324.

Franca, V. M., Kerr, M. M., Reitz, A. L., & Lambert, D. (1990). Peer tutoring among behaviorally disordered students: Academic and social benefits to tutor and tutee. *Education and Treatment of Children, 3,* 109–128.

Fuchs, D., & Fuchs, L. S. (1998). Researchers and teachers working closely together to adapt instruction for diverse learners. *Learning Disabilities Research and Practice, 13,* 126–137.

Fuchs, D., Fuchs, L. S., & Burish, P. (2000). Peer-assisted learning strategies: An evidence-based practice to promote reading achievement. *Learning Disabilities Research and Practice, 15,* 85–91.

Fuchs, D., Fuchs, L. S., Mathes, P. G., & Simmons, D. C. (1997). Peer-assisted learning strategies: Making classrooms more responsive to diversity. *American Educational Research Journal, 34,* 174–206.

Fuchs, D., Fuchs, L. S., Phillips, N. B., Hamlett, C. L., & Karns, K. (1995). Acquisition and transfer effects of classwide peer-assisted learning strategies in mathematics for students with varying learning histories. *School Psychology Review, 24*, 604–620.

Fuchs, D., Fuchs, L. S., Thompson, A., Svenson, E., Yen, L., Otaiba, S. A., et al. (2001). Peer-assisted learning strategies in reading. *Remedial and Special Education, 22*(1), 15–21.

Garcia-Vazquez, E., & Ehly, S. W. (1995). Best practices in facilitating peer tutoring programs. In A. Thomas & J. Grimes (Eds.), *Best practices in school psychology: III* (pp. 403–411). Washington, DC: National Association of School Psychologists.

Giesecke, D., Cartledge, G., & Gardner, R. (1993). Low-achieving students as successful cross-age tutors. *Prevention School Failure, 37*, 34–43.

Gifford-Smith, M., Dodge, K. A., Dishion, T. J., & McCord, J. (2005). Peer influence in children and adolescents: Crossing the bridge from developmental to intervention science. *Journal of Abnormal Child Psychology, 33*, 255–265.

Ginsburg-Block, M. D., & Fantuzzo, J. W. (1997). Reciprocal peer tutoring: An analysis of "teacher" and "student" interactions as a function of training and experience. *School Psychology Quarterly, 12*, 134–149.

Ginsburg-Block, M. D., Rohrbeck, C. A., & Fantuzzo, J. W. (2006). A meta-analytic review of social, self-concept, and behavioral outcomes of peer-assisted learning. *Journal of Educational Psychology, 98*, 732–749.

Ginsburg-Block, M. D., Rohrbeck, C. A., Fantuzzo, J. W., & Lavigne, N.C. (2006). Peer-assisted learning strategies. In G. Bear & K. M. Minke (Eds.), *Children's needs: III. Development prevention, and intervention* (pp. 631–645). Washington, DC: National Association of School Psychologists.

Greenwood, C. R. (1991). Classwide peer tutoring: Longitudinal effects on the reading, language, and mathematics achievement of at-risk students. *Reading, Writing, and Learning Disabilities, 7*, 105–123.

Greenwood, C. R., Arreaga-Mayer, C., Utley, C. A., Gavin, K. M., & Terry, B. J. (2001). Classwide peer tutoring learning management system: Applications with elementary-level English language learners. *Remedial and Special Education, 22*(1), 34–47.

Greenwood, C. R., & Delquadri, J. C. (1995). Classwide peer tutoring and the prevention of school failure. *Preventing School Failure, 39*(4), 21–29.

Greenwood, C. R., Delquadri, J. C., & Hall, R. V. (1989). Longitudinal effects of classwide peer tutoring. *Journal of Educational Psychology, 81*, 371–382.

Greenwood, C. R., Horton, B. T., & Utley, C. A. (2002). Academic engagement: Current perspectives on research and practice. *School Psychology Review, 20*, 249–264.

Greenwood, C. R., Maheady, L., & Delquadri, J. C. (2002). Classwide peer tutoring programs. In M. Shinn, H. M. Walker, & G. Stoner (Eds.), *Interventions for academic and behavior problems: II. Preventive and remedial approaches* (pp. 611–649). Bethesda, MD: National Association of School Psychologists.

Greenwood, C. R., Terry, B., Arreaga-Mayer, C., & Finney, R. (1992). The classwide peer tutoring program: Implementation factors moderating student's achievement. *Journal of Applied Behavior Analysis, 25*, 101–116.

Gresham, F. M. (1981). Social skills training with handicapped children: A review. *Review of Educational Research, 51*, 139–176.

Gresham, F. M. (2006). Response to intervention. In G. G. Bear & K. M. Minke (Eds.), *Children's needs: III. Development, prevention, and intervention* (pp. 525–540). Washington, DC: National Association of School Psychologists.

Grieger, T., Kauffman, J. M., & Grieger, R. M. (1976). Effects of peer reporting on cooperative play and aggression of kindergarten children. *Journal of School Psychology, 14*, 307–313.

Haring, T. G., & Breen, C. G. (1992). A peer-mediated social network intervention to enhance the social integration of persons with moderate and severe disabilities. *Journal of Applied Behavior Analysis, 25*, 319–333.

Harper, G. F., Mallette, B., Maheady, L., Bentley, A., & Moore, J. (1995). Retention and treatment failure in classwide peer tutoring: Implications for further research. *Journal of Behavioral Education, 5*, 399–414.

Heering, P. W., & Wilder, D. A. (2006). The use of dependent group contingencies to increase on-task behavior in two general education classrooms. *Education and Treatment of Children, 29*(3), 459–468.

Henington, C., & Skinner, C. H. (1998). Peer monitoring. In K. J. Topping & S. W. Ehly (Eds.), *Peer-assisted learning* (pp. 237–253). Hillsdale, NJ: Erlbaum.

Heward, W. L. (1994). Three "low-tech" strategies for increasing the frequency of active student response during group instruction. In R. Gardner, D. M. Sainato, J. O. Cooper, T. E. Heron, W. L. Heward, J. Eshleman, et al. (Eds.), *Behavior analysis in education: Focus on measurably superior instruction* (pp. 283–320). Monterey, CA: Brooks/Cole.

Hoff, K. E., & Robinson, S. L. (2002). Best practices in peer-mediated interventions. In A. Thomas & J. Grimes (Eds.), *Best practices in school psychology* (4th ed., pp. 1555–1567). Bethesda, MD: National Association of School Psychologists.

Individuals with Disabilities Education Improvement Act of 2004 (IDEA 2004), Pub. L. No. 108-446, 118 Stat. 2647 (2004) (amending 20 U.S. C. §§ 1400 et seq.).

Jigsaw Classroom. (2008). Overview of the technique. Retrieved February 20, 2008, from *www.jigsaw.org/overview.htm*.

Johnson, D. W., & Johnson, R. T. (1986). Mainstreaming and cooperative learning strategies. *Exceptional Children*, 52(6), 552–561.

Johnson, D. W., & Johnson, R. T. (1989). *Cooperation and competition: Theory and research*. Edina, MN: Interaction Book.

Johnson, R. T., & Johnson, D. W. (1994). *An overview of cooperative learning*. Retrieved September 23, 2007, from *www.co-operation. org/pages/overviewpaper.html*.

Johnson, R. T., & Johnson, D. W. (2000). *Cooperative learning methods: A meta-analysis*. Retrieved September 15, 2007, from *www.co-operation.org/pages/cl-methods.html*.

Jones, K. M., Young, M. M., & Friman, P. C. (2000). Increasing peer praise of socially rejected delinquent youth: Effects on cooperation and acceptance. *School Psychology Quarterly*, 15, 30–39.

Kamps, D. M., Kravits, T., Lopez, A. G., Kemmerer, K., Potucek, J., & Harrell, L. G. (1998). What do peers think? Social validity of peer-mediated programs. *Education and Treatment of Children*, 21(2), 107–134.

Kelshaw-Levering, K., Sterling-Turner, H. E., Henry, J. R., & Skinner, C. H. (2000). Randomized interdependent group contingencies: Group reinforcement with a twist. *Psychology in the Schools*, 37(6), 523–533.

Klingner, J. K., & Vaughn, S. (1996). Reciprocal teaching of reading comprehension strategies for students with learning disabilities who use English as a second language. *Elementary School Journal*, 96, 275–293.

Klingner, J. K., & Vaughn, S. (1999). Promoting reading comprehension, content learning and English acquisition through collaborative strategic reading. *Reading Teacher*, 52, 738–747.

Kunsch, C. A., Jitendra, A. K., & Sood, S. (2007). The effects of peer-mediated instruction in mathematics for students with learning problems: A research synthesis. *Learning Disabilities Research and Practice*, 22, 1–12.

Laushey, K. M., & Heflin, L. J. (2000). Enhancing social skills of kindergarten children with autism through the training of multiple peers as tutors. *Journal of Autism and Developmental Disorders*, 30, 183–193.

Levin, H. M., Glass, G. V., & Meister, G. M. (1987). Cost-effectiveness of computer-assisted instruction. *Evaluation Review*, 11, 50–72.

Maheady, L. (1998). Advantages and disadvantages of peer-assisted learning strategies. In K. Topping & S. W. Ehly (Eds.), *Peer-assisted learning* (pp. 45–65). Mahwah, NJ: Erlbaum.

Maheady, L., Harper, G. F., & Mallette, B. (2001). Peer-mediated instruction and interventions and students with mild disabilities. *Remedial and Special Education*, 22, 4–14.

Maheady, L., Harper, G. F., Mallette, B., & Winstanley, N. (1991). Implementation requirements associated with the use of class-wide peer tutoring systems. *Education and Treatment of Children*, 14, 177–198.

Maheady, L., Harper, G. F., & Sacca, M. K. (1988). Peer-mediated instruction: Promising alternative for secondary learning disabled students. *Learning Disability Quarterly*, 11, 108–114.

Mathes, P. G., Howard, S. H., Allen, S., & Fuchs D. (1998). Peer-assisted learning strategies for first-grade readers: Responding to the need of diverse learners. *Reading Research Quarterly*, 33, 62–95.

McCurdy, B. L., & Shapiro, E. S. (1992). A comparison of teacher-, peer-, and self-monitoring with curriculum-based measurement in reading among students with learning disabilities. *Journal of Special Education*, 26(2), 162–180.

O'Connor, R. E., Fulmer, D., Harty, K. R., & Bell, K. M. (2005). Layers of reading intervention in kindergarten through third grade: Changes in teaching and student outcomes. *Journal of Learning Disabilities*, 38, 440–455.

Odom, S. L., & Strain, P. S. (1984). Classroom-based social skills instruction for severely handicapped preschool children. *Topics in Early Childhood Special Education*, 4, 97–116.

Odom, S. L., & Strain, P. S. (1986). A comparison of peer-initiation and teacher-antecedent interventions for promoting reciprocal social interaction of autistic preschoolers. *Journal of Applied Behavior Analysis*, 19, 207–219.

Palincsar, A. M., & Brown, A. L. (1984). Reciprocal teaching of comprehension-fostering and comprehension-monitoring activities. *Cognition and Instruction*, 1, 117–175.

Piaget, J. (1965). *The moral judgment of the child*. London: Free Press.

President's Commission on Excellence in Special Education. (2002). *A new era: Revitalizing special education for children and their families*. Washington, DC: U.S. Department of Education, Office of Special Education and Rehabilitative Services.

Rohrbeck, C. A., Ginsburg-Block, M., Fantuzzo, J. W., & Miller, T. R. (2003). Peer-assisted learning interventions with elementary school students: A meta-analysis review. *Journal of Educational Psychology*, 95, 240–257.

Rosenthal, S. (1994). Students as teachers: At-risk

high school students teach science to fourth-graders. *Thrust for Educational Leadership, 23*, 36–38.

Schneider, R. B., & Barone, D. (1997). Cross-age tutoring. *Childhood Education, 73*, 136–143.

Schunk, D. H. (1987). Peer models and children's behavioral change. *Review of Educational Research, 57*(2), 149–174.

Schunk, D. H. (1998). Peer modeling. In K. J. Topping & S. W. Ehly (Eds.), *Peer-assisted learning* (pp. 185–202). Hillsdale, NJ: Erlbaum.

Schunk, D. H., & Hanson, A. R. (1985). Peer models: Influence on children's self-efficacy and achievement. *Journal of Educational Psychology, 77*(3), 313–322.

Schunk, D. H., Hanson, A. R., & Cox, P. D. (1987). Peer-model attributes and children's achievement behaviors. *Journal of Educational Psychology, 79*(1), 54–61.

Skinner, C. H., Cashwell, C. S., & Dunn, M. S. (1996). Independent and interdependent group contingencies: Smoothing the rough waters. *Special Services in the Schools, 12*, 61–78.

Skinner, C. H., Neddenriep, C. E., Robinson, S. L., Ervin, R. A., & Jones, K. (2002). Altering educational environments through positive peer reporting: Prevention and remediation of social problems associated with behavior disorders. *Psychology in the Schools, 39*(2), 191–202.

Slavin, R. E. (1983). When does cooperative learning increase student achievement? *Psychological Bulletin, 94*(3), 429–445.

Slavin, R. E. (1990). *Cooperative learning: Theory, research, and practice.* Englewood Cliffs, NJ: Prentice Hall.

Spencer, V. G., Scruggs, T. E., & Mastropieri, M. A. (2003). Content area learning in middle school social studies classrooms and students with emotional or behavioral disorders: A comparison of strategies. *Behavioral Disorder, 28*, 77–93.

Stern, G. W., Fowler, S. A., & Kohler, F. W. (1988). A comparison of two intervention roles: Peer monitor and point earner. *Journal of Applied Behavior Analysis, 21*, 103–109.

Stokes, T. F., & Baer, D. M. (1977). An implicit technology of generalization. *Journal of Applied Behavior, 10*, 349–367.

Strain, P. S. (1977). Training and generalization effects of peer social initiations on withdrawn preschool children. *Journal of Abnormal Child Psychology, 5*, 445–455.

Strain, P. S., & Odom, S. L. (1986). Peer social initiatives: Effective interventions for social skill development of exceptional children. *Exceptional Children, 52*, 543–552.

Strain, P. S., & Shores, R. E. (1977). Effects of peer social initiations on behavior of withdrawn preschool children. *Journal of Applied Behavioral Analysis, 10*(2), 289–298.

Sutherland, S. K., & Snyder, A. (2007). Effects of reciprocal peer tutoring and self-graphing on reading fluency and classroom behavior of middle school students with emotional or behavioral disorders. *Journal of Emotional and Behavioral Disorders, 15*, 103–118.

Thurston, J. A. (1994). Art partners: A new focus on peer teaching. *School Arts, 94*, 41–42.

Topping, K. J., & Ehly, S. W. (1998). Introduction to peer-assisted learning. In K. J. Topping & S. W. Ehly (Eds.), *Peer-assisted learning* (pp. 1–24). Hillsdale, NJ: Erlbaum.

Utley, C. A. (2001). Introduction to the special series: Advances in peer-mediated instruction and interventions in the 21st century. *Remedial and Special Education, 22*, 2–3.

Vanderbilt Kennedy Center for Research on Human Development. (1998). *Peer-assisted learning strategies.* Retrieved January 25, 2008, from *kc.vanderbilt.edu/pals/.*

Webb, N., & Farivar, S. (1994). Promoting helping behavior in cooperative small groups in middle school mathematics. *American Educational Research Journal, 31*, 369–395.

Wheldall, K., & Colmar, S. (1990). Peer tutoring for low-progress readers using "pause, prompt, and praise." In H. C. Foot, M. J. Morgan, & R. H. Shute (Eds.), *Children helping children* (pp. 117–134). New York: Wiley.

Yarrow, F., & Topping, K. J. (2001). Collaborative writing: The effects of metacognitive prompting and structured peer interaction. *British Journal of Educational Psychology, 71*(2), 261–282.

Chapter 20

Self-Management Interventions

Kathryn E. Hoff
Kristin D. Sawka-Miller

Self-management represents a collection of skills that individuals can engage in to become more self-reliant. Self-management interventions can be implemented in a wide variety of settings, can be used to improve academic, social, emotional, or behavioral outcomes, and are effective for many diverse populations. Self-management interventions have multiple advantages in schools, including ease of implementation and adaptability. Further, teaching students to use self-management skills promotes strategies and self-control skills that can be used throughout the lifespan in many different situations. In this chapter, we define and review the benefits of using self-management interventions and describe four types of self-management interventions used in schools.

Self-Management Interventions

Self-management refers to actions purposefully taken by individuals to change or maintain their own behavior (Shapiro & Cole, 1994). For example, a student could be taught to engage in one action (such as self-monitoring—routinely monitoring and recording his or her behavior) with the goal of altering a target behavior (such as raising his or her hand in class before speaking).

Self-management strategies exist along an intervention continuum, with varying levels of adult and student control, to fit particular target behaviors and circumstances. At one end of the intervention continuum, all components of the behavior-change program are controlled by an external change agent (e.g., teacher or parent), such as a teacher who provides a verbal prompt telling a student what to do, records the occurrence of a target behavior, administers points for appropriate behavior, and provides feedback. A middle ground in the continuum might include a combination of teacher-directed components (e.g., identifying student goals and problem behaviors, developing interventions, and delivering consequences) coupled with student-managed components (e.g., observing and recording target behaviors, then graphing performance). At the opposite end of the self-management continuum lies an entirely self-managed program in which students direct the entire intervention themselves, such as setting goals, monitoring target behaviors, evaluating progress, and administering self-reinforcement.

When considering the implementation of a particular self-management intervention, the degree to which self-management strategies are used will vary based on the child's developmental level, target behaviors, and intervention complexity. Some students will be able to independently manage their behavior, and, in such circumstances, a self-management program can be used as a stand-alone procedure. Other situations (e.g., interventions with younger children) might involve self-management as a part of a multiple-component intervention. For example, a teacher using a classroom token economy could incorporate self-management components, such as having students set their own goals or graph their performances. There is no "one size fits all" approach to self-management implementation; one must carefully tailor the self-management strategy to the particular circumstances of each student.

In examining the self-management literature, several terms are used interchangeably, including *self-regulation*, *self-management*, *self-control*, and *self-determination*. The relevant literature also approaches self-management from various conceptual analyses and theoretical perspectives. Briefly, self-management strategies have been described from both contingency management and cognitive viewpoints (Shapiro & Cole, 1994). Contingency-based self-management strategies emphasize what the individual does after the target behavior occurs (e.g., recording whether or not a task was completed or evaluating a response), whereas cognitively based self-management interventions typically involve antecedent strategies, focusing on cognitive control (what the individual says, thinks, or does prior to engaging in the target behavior). Although there are differences in terminology and explanations for efficacy, both approaches to self-management share the same basic objectives. In both approaches, students are taught to monitor and evaluate their own behavior and make adjustments when needed, with the ultimate goal of performing the necessary steps of a desired sequence of coordinated behaviors without the need for supervision from others. Additional discussion of theoretical issues is beyond the scope of this chapter; thus readers are encouraged to explore additional sources to acquire a more in-depth theoretical understanding of self-management and associated procedures (e.g., Kanfer, 1977; Nelson & Hayes, 1981; Shapiro & Cole, 1994; Zimmerman & Schunk, 2001). Further definitions of several

specific self-management strategies are provided later in the chapter.

Self-management has proven effective across a wide variety of populations, settings, and behaviors. For example, self-management interventions have produced positive academic and social behavior changes for diverse populations of students, including students with autism (Ganz & Sigafoos, 2005), learning disabilities (Konrad, Fowler, Walker, Test, & Wood, 2007), emotional and behavioral disorders (Mooney, Ryan, Uhing, Reid, & Epstein, 2005), health-related concerns (Todd, Horner, & Sugai, 1999), visual impairments (Jindal-Snape, 2004), dually diagnosed speech and language impairments (Hughes et al., 2004), mild to severe cognitive impairments (Crawley, Lynch, & Vannest, 2006), and students with no identified disability (McDougall & Brady, 1998).

Self-management interventions can be used across the full age range of students, from preschool through high school. At the preschool level, a student might self-monitor a concrete skill such as greeting the teacher or carrying out a morning routine (e.g., brushing teeth and getting dressed), whereas a high school student might self-manage a more complex set of skills, such as completion of a long-term project. Interventions based on self-management are effective in a broad range of school environments, including general and special education classes, and even in less structured settings (e.g., physical education, cafeteria, hallways, playground; Shapiro & Cole, 1994). Self-management has the additional advantage of adaptability for use as an individual, targeted, or universal intervention (e.g., Mitchem, Young, West, and Benyo, 2007).

Self-management interventions are easy to implement, adaptable for individualized use, and easily taught, and they require minimal demands on teacher time and on curricular modifications (e.g., Dunlap, Dunlap, Koegel, & Koegel, 1991). Self-management programs are particularly attractive because they shift some responsibilities to the child for changing his or her behavior, they promote active involvement in the educational process, and they encourage skills that children use throughout their lifetimes. Self-management strategies permit teachers to spend more time on instruction and less time managing problem behaviors (Shapiro & Cole, 1994). Students can apply self-management strategies to monitor covert behaviors that are perceptible only to the individual, such as feelings of depression or positive thoughts (Stark et al., 2006). Finally, participants using self-management interventions can learn to generalize the skills they gain, apply them beyond the immediate training environment or intervention setting (e.g., Hoff & DuPaul, 1998), and maintain behavior changes after the intervention has been discontinued (e.g., Gureasko-Moore, DuPaul, & White, 2007).

In the sections that follow, we illustrate four commonly used school-based self-management interventions: self-monitoring, self-evaluation, self-instruction, and stress inoculation training. For each intervention, we describe the specific self-management strategy, provide research-based examples supporting its use, and discuss special considerations and/or applications. Please note that there is considerably more research in the area of self-monitoring and that its applications are more diverse than those of the other self-management interventions. Consequently, we focus more attention on the topic of self-monitoring. Following the descriptions of the four self-management interventions, we provide a case example of a self-evaluation intervention.

Self-Monitoring

Self-monitoring is the most frequently used self-management intervention. Self-monitoring is a straightforward intervention that involves two processes: self-observation and self-recording. Self-observation requires students to pay attention to a specific aspect of behavior and to discriminate whether the behavior being monitored has occurred. For example, a student who calls out an answer during teacher instruction may be taught to ask herself, "Did I raise my hand?" after she provides an answer in class. Alternately, a student who engages in high levels of off-task behavior may assess whether or not he was paying attention in response to a specific prompt (e.g., when a prerecorded tone sounds). Next, the student records whether the behavior being monitored has occurred (Nelson & Hayes, 1981), such as checking

"yes" or "no" on a self-monitoring form placed at his desk.

Common Applications in Schools

School-based applications of self-monitoring generally include (1) academic performance behaviors, such as academic productivity, work accuracy, and strategies used in task completion; (2) the process of self-regulated learning, such as outcome goals or strategic thinking (e.g., Zimmerman & Schunk, 2001); (3) attention or on-task behaviors; (4) problem behaviors, such as disruptive behaviors and internalizing difficulties; (5) social skills, such as initiating peer interactions, appropriate and inappropriate social responding, complimenting, and conversational abilities; and (6) skills to promote independence, such as homework completion, classroom preparation, and vocational, domestic, or organizational skills (Gureasko-Moore et al., 2007; Shapiro, Durnan, Post, & Levinson, 2002). Selected applications are highlighted next.

Self-Monitoring Attention

The majority of school-based self-monitoring research has focused on students monitoring attending behaviors, such as on-task behavior or academic engagement. For example, a student who displays frequent off-task behavior could assess and subsequently record whether or not he or she was on-task when a tone sounded. Additional examples that involve self-monitoring attention include a student monitoring whether or not he or she kept his or her eyes on the assigned work or the speaker, was working on the assigned activity, or followed a direction (e.g., started an activity when the teacher asked). Research demonstrates that self-monitoring attention is associated with decreased disruptive behavior (e.g., Lam, Cole, Shapiro, & Bambara, 1994) and increased on-task behavior (e.g., Reid, Trout, & Schartz, 2005). Collateral effects of self-monitoring of attention also are apparent. Specifically, self-monitoring of attention is associated with positive changes in academic performance, such as academic productivity and academic accuracy (e.g., Harris, Graham, Reid, McElroy, & Hamby, 1994; Maag, Reid, & DiGangi, 1993).

Self-Monitoring Academic Performance

Self-monitoring has been applied to three general areas of academic performance: (1) strategy use; (2) academic productivity; and (3) work accuracy (Shapiro et al., 2002). First students can self-monitor strategies they used for task completion by recording whether the steps in an academic task or operation were completed. For example, students can check off whether they completed each step of subtraction with regrouping problems on a self-instruction checklist (Dunlap & Dunlap, 1989) or monitor whether they followed a plan for completing a long-term project (Lenz, Ehren, & Smiley, 1991). Second, students can self-monitor academic productivity by recording the number of responses they completed, without regard to accuracy. Monitoring academic productivity (e.g., how many math problems were completed when a tone sounded; Maag et al., 1993) can lead to improvements in productivity, as well as improvements in academic accuracy and on-task behavior (Shimbukuro, Prater, Jenkins, & Edelen-Smith, 1999).

Third, self-monitoring work accuracy involves having students monitor the accuracy of their responses. Students typically compare their work with an answer key. Examples in the literature demonstrate improved accuracy for students who recorded the number of correct math problems completed (e.g., Lam et al., 1994) and counted the number of correctly written words (e.g., Harris, Friedlander, Saddler, Frizzelle, & Graham, 2005). One specific example of an interven-

tion for evaluating correct spelling words or math facts is the Cover, Copy, and Compare technique (Skinner, Turco, Beatty, & Rasavage, 1989). Readers are referred to Figure 20.1 for specific steps in this strategy.

A few studies have examined the differential effectiveness of having students self-monitor attention versus academic performance (e.g., counting the number of math problems completed or words spelled correctly). In general, researchers found both self-monitoring of attention and self-monitoring of performance strategies result in improvements in on-task behavior for students with learning disabilities (e.g., Harris et al., 1994; Reid & Harris, 1993) and ADHD or behavior disorders (e.g., Harris et al., 2005). Conclusions about academic performance are less clear. Reid and Harris (1993) found that students spelled more words correctly when they monitored their performances rather than attention; however, other researchers found that students did not make substantial academic gains when they monitored academic performance (Harris et al., 2005).

Self-Monitoring Internalizing Problems

Self-monitoring techniques are frequently included in treatments for internalizing disorders, such as depression or anxiety (e.g., Kaufman, Rohde, Seeley, Clarke, & Stice, 2005). Children might be taught to self-monitor covert behaviors (e.g., monitoring thoughts, feelings, or mood) or pleasant activities and events (Lewinsohn & Clarke,

---

1. Students are given a sheet of math problems with the problems and their answers listed in a column on the left-hand side of the paper
2. Students are instructed to look at the first problem and its answer
3. Students cover the answer with a piece of construction paper
4. Students write the problem and answer on the right-hand side of the original math problems
5. Students uncover the problem and evaluate if their answer was correct
6. If correct, students place a "+" mark next to the problem
7. If incorrect, students repeat the procedure until they respond correctly

Look	Cover	Copy	Compare

$$\begin{array}{r} 5 \\ + 3 \\ \hline 8 \end{array}$$

FIGURE 20.1. Cover, copy, compare. Reprinted from Shapiro and Cole (1994). Copyright 1994 by Guilford Press. Reprinted by permission.

1999). To implement self-monitoring, school psychologists might ask the child to keep a thought log or diary and record events as they occur. For example, in a school-based depression treatment program for adolescent girls, Stark and colleagues (2006) taught participants to monitor enjoyable activities, positive qualities, and successful coping strategies in a "Catch the Positive Diary" in order to teach girls to focus on more positive events. Research demonstrates that self-monitoring mood and/or pleasant activities (e.g., students assigning a pleasantness rating to their moods or self-reporting their pleasant activities) can improve mood quality and increase the number of pleasant activities in which the person engaged (e.g., Harmon, Nelson, & Hayes, 1980; Lewinsohn & Graf, 1973).

Self-Monitoring to Enhance Social Skills

Finally, self-monitoring has been used to enhance social skills. A series of studies by Hughes and colleagues demonstrated an increase in peer engagement and quality social interactions when students with cognitive impairments were taught to self-monitor peer initiations and appropriate social response (Hughes et al., 2002) or steps performed in a recreational activity with peers (Hughes et al., 2004). Other researchers have documented improved social performance when students monitored conversational abilities, the number of times they performed a social skill, or appropriate and inappropriate social responding (e.g., Moore, Cartledge, & Heckaman, 1995).

Considerations and Application Issues

When implementing a self-monitoring intervention, one needs to consider a number of things in developing, implementing, and monitoring progress. The following discussion highlights some of the more salient issues to consider when using self-monitoring interventions.

Reactivity

The act of self-monitoring can have a reactive effect on the target behavior, meaning that merely observing and recording one's own behavior can result in desired behav-

ior change (Kirby, Fowler, & Baer, 1991). Although reactivity may be an undesired source of variance in some cases (e.g., student reactivity to a measurement system when one is trying to get an accurate assessment of behavior), the reactive effects of self-monitoring are generally considered positive from an intervention perspective. The empirical literature documents a number of variables that influence the degree of reactivity during self-monitoring procedures, such as number of discrete target behaviors monitored, valence of the target behavior, obtrusiveness of self-monitoring procedures, length of monitoring interval, provision of external contingencies, adult surveillance, performance feedback, motivation, and expectations for change (Mace, Belfiore, & Hutchinson, 2001). Considerations for enhancing reactivity are incorporated throughout this section.

Selecting and Defining a Target Behavior

The initial step in implementing a self-monitoring intervention is selecting and defining a target behavior. The target behavior may consist of almost any response, provided that it is discrete, clearly defined, and understandable to the student (Shapiro et al., 2002). For example, if students are self-monitoring on-task behaviors in a classroom, the target behaviors should be defined using clear, specific, and observable terms (e.g., raising a hand to talk to the teacher, staying in one's seat, and working on the assignment) so that students can accurately discriminate whether or not the target behavior occurred. Further, the self-monitoring form could clearly list the definitions of the on-task behaviors expected of the student (Maag et al., 1993).

Student considerations are also important factors in selecting a target behavior. Self-management interventions are more effective when the targeted behaviors or the desired intervention outcomes are valuable to the student and when individuals are motivated to change the self-monitored response (Mace et al., 2001). In addition, the student should be able to perform the target behavior, at least to some degree, because self-monitoring does not teach the student *how* to perform a behavior. Finally, the type and number of target behaviors should be matched to the child's developmental level. For example, when working with young children or children with cognitive impairments, one might select a fewer number of observable target behaviors so that students learn to assess their behavior accurately. In contrast, a high school student could monitor several overt and covert target behaviors.

Selecting and Using Prompts to Self-Monitor

When monitoring behavior, students may need an additional prompt or cue to signal when to observe and then record the target behavior of interest. A typical audible prompt is a tape recorder that emits a prerecorded tone that prompts a student to record the target behavior of interest. For example, students record whether or not they were paying attention (e.g., Hallahan, Marshall, & Lloyd, 1981) or record how many math problems they have completed (Maag et al., 1993) when the tone sounds. Other audible methods of prompting include verbal reminders by the teacher to self-monitor (e.g., Crum, 2004). A visual cue is something a student sees that serves as a reminder. Examples include pictures that prompt self-monitoring, such as a picture of a hand on a self-monitoring form to signal hand raising (Brooks, Todd, Tofflemoyer, & Horner, 2003) or looking at a drawing of an individual engaging in the target behavior (e.g., Hughes et al., 2002). Finally, tactile cues are something the student feels. Examples include a teacher tapping a student on the shoulder when it is time to self-monitor (Maag, Rutherford, & DiGangi, 1992) and students wearing a small device that vibrates when it is time to self-monitor (Amato-Zech, Hoff, & Doepke, 2006).

One consideration in selecting the type of prompt depends on how self-monitoring is used in the classroom. For example, if all students in the class are participating in a self-monitoring intervention, a verbal prompt from the teacher may be the most effective. If the intervention is being implemented with an individual student, a tactile or auditory prompt (e.g., an MP3 player with a small earpiece) may be more appropriate. Practical considerations are the second factor in selecting the type of self-monitoring prompt. Although a salient prompt is associated with increased reactivity, one must weigh this benefit against the practical use in the classroom. Noticeable cues (e.g., wearing headphones or using audible cues that others can hear) may be perceived as stigmatizing or aversive to the target student participating in the intervention and can be distracting to other students in the classroom who are not directed to self-monitor. In these cases, a more discreet cue might be selected (e.g., the teacher pointing to a picture or tapping the student on the shoulder).

Using a Self-Monitoring Form

School psychologists should consider how students will record the target behavior of interest. The most common method is to use a paper-and-pencil recording form adapted to the specific behavior of interest and child's ability (see Figure 20.2 for an example of a self-monitoring sheet). Examples include students checking a "yes" or "no" box on a form taped to their desks, circling a happy or sad face on a form they keep in a folder, tallying the number of peer initiations on an index card, recording negative thoughts in a notebook, or using a checklist to check off steps in completing an assignment. Recording forms should be made accessible and easy to use so that students can record the behavior immediately after the behavior occurs. The recording form should be convenient and portable for use across multiple environments. Finally, the recording form should be sufficiently salient for students, but not so obtrusive that it is stigmatizing or distracting (Shapiro et al., 2002).

Self-Monitoring Schedule

School psychologists need to consider how often the student should self-monitor and the length of the self-monitoring interval. This decision depends on the nature of the target behavior, the current frequency of the behavior, and student characteristics. For example, if the student is engaging in a high-rate behavior, she or he might monitor her or his behavior more frequently. Students with attention difficulties or cognitive impairments or younger children will likely require a shorter self-monitoring interval. When initially implementing a self-monitoring intervention, one should allow frequent self-monitoring opportunities to increase profi-

When the first bell rings, I will indicate whether I have done the following:		
Morning Routine	Yes	No
Coat Hung Up on Hook		
Book Bag Emptied		
Completed Homework on Desk		
Pencil on Desk		
All Other Items Put away in Desk		

Morning Seatwork: When I hear the beep, I will place an "X" in the box if I am working.										
	1	2	3	4	5	6	7	8	9	10
Am I Working?										

Name: Date:			
Rating Period (Circle): Math Reading Science Social Studies English			
Behavior	My Rating	Teacher's Rating	Pointed Earned
Raised My Hand Before Talking	0 1 2 3 4 5		
Stayed in My Seat	0 1 2 3 4 5		
		Points Earned	

FIGURE 20.2. Examples of self-monitoring and self-evaluation forms.

ciency and shorter time intervals to increase accuracy. After students have some success, the self-monitoring interval can be extended to avoid interference with the academic environment (i.e., interrupting a task to monitor) and to enhance generalization and maintenance over time. Finally, it is helpful to keep the monitoring times random instead of on a fixed schedule so that students cannot anticipate when cues will occur (Maag et al., 1992, Shapiro et al., 2002).

Training

Initial training is critical to the ultimate success of the intervention; thus it is important to commit adequate up-front time to teaching teachers, parents, and students the self-management procedures. We suggest that the teacher or consultant provide a structured training session for students prior to the implementation of the intervention in which explicit training steps and intervention procedures are described (see, e.g., Young, West, Smith, & Morgan, 2000). A

training session might include (1) introducing the self-management strategy, describing the rationale and specific steps of intervention implementation; (2) modeling the procedure, using examples and nonexamples that are individualized to the student and situation; (3) role-playing self-management skills with praise and corrective feedback; and (4) providing performance feedback. Practice of self-management strategies in the training session should continue until students can use the particular set of self-management skills independently.

Self-Monitoring Accuracy

How important is it that a student monitors the target behavior accurately when using self-monitoring? Interestingly, some research demonstrates that the act of self-monitoring can produce behavior change despite inaccuracy of self-recording (e.g., Hallahan et al., 1981). In contrast, other researchers have found that giving adult feedback and rewards for accuracy resulted in increased treatment gains compared with self-monitoring in isolation (e.g., Freeman & Dexter-Mazza, 2004). Consequently, best practices indicate that working to increase accuracy of students' ratings might be required, at least initially.

Accuracy can be increased in several ways. One method is to have the child try to match his or her recordings of a target behavior with those made by an external observer, a procedure described in detail in the "Self-Evaluation Procedures" section of this chapter. Accuracy of self-monitoring also can be increased by thoroughly training participants, letting students know their accuracy will be evaluated, reducing the length of the self-monitoring interval, and reducing distractions or competing activities during self-monitoring. Finally, Shapiro and colleagues (2002) recommend that a minimum accuracy criterion be set prior to starting the self-monitoring intervention (e.g., 80% accuracy on three consecutive occasions) and suggest that accuracy be monitored periodically throughout the intervention.

Adult Monitoring

Despite the term *self-management*, many aspects of the intervention are overseen by adults to some degree. When self-monitoring interventions are used, the teacher's primary role shifts from direct intervention implementation to overseeing and supervising the intervention and monitoring progress to determine whether additional changes are necessary. Practical examples of such monitoring include walking around the room and monitoring accurate use of self-monitoring procedures, prompting the use of necessary self-management skills or responses, providing reinforcement for appropriate behavior, and ensuring that behavior is performed at a desirable level. Continued adult involvement in a supervisory role is almost always necessary to ensure the intervention's success.

Encouraging Generalization and Maintenance

The issue of generalization of treatment gains (i.e., students applying strategies they learn outside the particular intervention context) is another important consideration in implementation of any intervention. In their review of 16 studies on self-management interventions for students with behavior disorders, Nelson, Smith, Young, and Dodd (1991) concluded that the interventions produced moderate to large treatment effects but that positive gains related to self-management typically failed to generalize to other people, other times of the day, and/or other settings unless systematically programmed. Some methods to encourage generalization include gradually extending self-management periods (e.g., increasing the time from an average of every 10 minutes to an average of every 30 minutes) until the self-monitoring prompt is removed completely, covert use of self-monitoring (e.g., instructing students to self-monitor only when they "happen to think of it"), or a sequential introduction of self-management procedures in other settings (e.g., Peterson, Young, Salzberg, West, & Hill, 2006).

School psychologists can help maintain the continued use of self-management interventions by using procedures that are relatively easy for both the teacher and student to follow (Shapiro et al., 2002). Further, school psychologists can provide detailed instructions and steps to follow, prepare school staff for potential pitfalls and identify possible solutions specific to self-management interventions (e.g., responding to students when they monitor their behavior inaccurately), remain available for troubleshooting sessions, and implement treatment integrity checks.

Self-Evaluation Procedures

In self-monitoring interventions, the student is taught to answer the question, "What did I do?" by observing some aspect of his or her own behavior and providing an objective recording of that behavior. In self-evaluation interventions, an extension of self-monitoring, the student is also taught to ask the question, "How well did I do?" and to provide an appraisal of his or her performance against a self-determined standard (e.g., a personal goal for improvement), an externally determined standard (e.g., the teacher expectations for adequate performance), or, more often, both (Shapiro & Cole, 1994). A specific type of self-evaluation procedure that has most typically been used in the context of addressing concerns related to externalizing behavior problems is "matching."

The matching procedure generally involves the student evaluating some dimension of his or her own behavior (e.g., on a scale from 0 to 5) and someone else (e.g., a teacher, peer) also independently evaluating that student's behavior on the same scale (Rhode, Morgan, & Young, 1983). The student earns points based on how well the two ratings match; a perfect rating would earn bonus points, "close" ratings would earn points, and ratings that were widely discrepant would earn no points, regardless of how well the behavior was performed. The points earned for matching can then be traded for desirable items or activities. The matching strategy is predicated on the assumption that the student's skill at accurately self-assessing behavior is as important as the level of behavior in meeting success.

In their seminal study on self-evaluation, Rhode et al. (1983) devised a matching procedure specifically geared toward facilitating generalization and maintenance of treatment gains. An examination of their methodology gives insight into the proper use of a matching procedure in typical settings. Participants in Rhode et al.'s (1983) study were six elementary students with behavior disorders in a self-contained classroom. Following baseline assessment, the intervention consisted of four major phases:

• *Phase 1: Token reinforcement–systematic feedback.* Students were taught the resource room classroom expectations and were given two ratings by the teacher at the end of 15-minute intervals reflecting academic performance and behavior. Ratings were given on a 5-point scale (0 = totally unacceptable; 5 = excellent) and students earned points for their ratings to be turned in for rewards. The purpose of phase 1 was to teach expectations and provide more frequent feedback.

• *Phase 2: Matching student evaluation with teacher evaluation.* Following improvement in student behavior, students were instructed to rate themselves at the end of each 15-minute interval and to compare their ratings with the teacher's independent rating. A perfect match earned the number of points plus a bonus point; a match within one point earned the student the number of points they gave themselves; more than a point difference earned no points for that rating period.

As the level of behavior and accuracy of self-evaluation improved, the length of the rating period and the number of matching sessions were faded. The purpose of phase 2 was to teach students to accurately self-evaluate and to establish improvements in behavior in a restricted setting.

• *Phase 3: Generalization to another classroom.* The matching procedure was implemented in the students' general education classroom. The students and the general education teacher each rated the students' behavior at the end of 30-minute intervals. The ratings were recorded, and the students carried the ratings back to their special education classroom, where the special education teacher determined the number of points awarded for accuracy. The purpose of phase 3 was to extend the matching technique and the gains experienced in the self-contained setting to a general education classroom.

• *Phase 4: Fading of self-evaluation.* The matching and reward procedures were gradually eliminated in a series of steps. The time period for matching was extended to 60 minutes, the point exchanges became variable such that the student did not know in advance what days carried point exchanges, matches became random (i.e., a "surprise"), and, finally, the students eventually no longer wrote their ratings on paper.

Using this procedure, students increased their levels of appropriate behavior to 80% or better in the self-contained classroom, and these results were transferred to the general education classroom for all students. Further, gains were maintained in both settings for four students when all of the intervention components were faded. These findings suggest that this matching procedure can be an effective tool to facilitate treatment gains into novel settings and that some students can learn to completely self-manage their behavior in the absence of external prompts and rewards.

Several replications and variations of the general matching procedure described in Rhode et al. (1983) have demonstrated similar improvements in on-task and disruptive behavior by eliminating the token reinforcement–systematic feedback phase in the process (e.g., Smith, Young, Nelson, & West, 1992; Smith, Young, West, & Morgan, 1988; Peterson, Young, West, & Peterson, 1999), by utilizing peers (vs. teachers) in the matching student evaluation phase (Smith et al., 1992; Peterson et al., 2006), by targeting specific gains in academic quality and quantity (Smith et al., 1988), and by extending the number of programmed generalization settings to up to six general education classrooms (Peterson et al., 1999; Peterson et al., 2006). The self-evaluation procedure has been implemented effectively in self-contained classrooms (e.g., Smith et al., 1988) and general education settings (e.g., Hoff & DuPaul, 1998). Further, it has been utilized with students with behavior disorders (e.g., Peterson et al., 2006), learning disabilities (e.g., Smith et al., 1992), attention-deficit/hyperactivity disorder (e.g., Shapiro, DuPaul, & Bradley-Klug, 1998), and developmental disabilities (Harchik, Shermann, & Sheldon, 1992), as well as with children at risk for behavior disorders (e.g., Hoff & DuPaul, 1998).

In the effort to educate students in the least restrictive environment, the use of self-management matching procedures may be particularly useful to the general education teacher. However, despite the effectiveness of self-management interventions in general and self-evaluation matching procedures in particular, Mitchem and Young (2001) point out that the procedures are not widely used and that implementing a matching procedure with several students in a general education class may not meet the general educator's requirements for acceptability in terms of time and resources. For example, it would be difficult for one teacher to individually match with several students at the end of each class period. Mitchem and Young (2001) and Mitchem et al. (2001) therefore suggest a modified procedure from Rhode et al. (1983) for adopting the matching strategy on a classwide basis, utilizing peers as the evaluation agent and a dependent group contingency.

In one example of a classwide matching intervention, Mitchem et al. (2001) identified 10 students at risk for behavior disorders in three seventh-grade language arts classrooms. Following whole-class instruction of the classroom rules, every student in each class was assigned a partner, and partners were randomly assigned to one of two teams. At the end of specified intervals, all students rated their behavior and their partners' behavior with respect to classroom expecta-

tions on a 4-point scale, and students earned points for their ratings and bonus points for accurate matching. Each pair's total points were added to their team's points, and rewards were earned as a team. To support accuracy of ratings, students were told that each period one pair would be randomly selected to be observed by the teacher and that if each partner's ratings matched with the teacher's ratings (i.e., "mystery match"), the pair would earn additional bonus points. Following implementation of the classwide peer-assisted self-management program, the on-task behavior and appropriate use of social skills increased for the 10 targeted at-risk students, and overall levels of on-task behavior of the classes as a whole improved. Following systematic withdrawal of the intervention, most at-risk students and all classes maintained behavioral gains.

Self-Instruction

Self-instruction is an antecedent intervention designed to teach children to alter the thought processes that precede the behavior, with the expectation that thinking differently about a situation will produce different and improved outcomes (Shapiro & Cole, 1994). Self-instruction requires students to prompt themselves to perform particular behaviors and often involves teaching the student a verbal "script" that will help guide his or her verbal or nonverbal behavior (Shapiro & Cole, 1994). For example, Smith and Sugai (2000) taught a 13-year-old male with behavior disorders to self-monitor his reaction to peers' negative comments to prevent himself from engaging in a previous pattern of disruptive behavior. Specifically, the student was instructed to read a written prompt on his desk ("Did I keep my cool?"), to count to 10 with his eyes closed, and to return to work without comment. If he successfully completed this sequence, he circled "yes" on a self-management card; he circled "no" if he did not. In combination with self-monitoring for work completion and hand raising, as well as self-recruitment of adult attention, the self-management package was associated with improvements in work completion and on-task behavior and declines in the number of inappropriate verbalizations.

In an example of self-instruction targeting improvements in written expression, Reid and Lienemann (2006) taught three elementary students with ADHD and below-average writing achievement a script for planning and story-writing strategies. Planning was taught using the "POW" acronym (i.e., "Pick my ideas," "Organize my notes," "Write and say more"), and story writing was taught using the mnemonic "WWW, What = 2, How = 2" (i.e., "*Who* are the main characters? *Where* does the story take place? *When* does the story take place? *What* do the main characters want to do? *What* happens next? *How* does the story end? *How* do the main characters feel?"). Following implementation of the self-instruction strategies, students more than doubled the length of their stories and showed marked gains on measures of completeness and quality of their narratives. Comparable results have been obtained utilizing similar procedures for improving the completeness, accuracy, and neatness of creative writing homework assignments in middle school students with behavior disorders (Glomb & West, 1990), and large effects for self-instruction techniques targeting academic outcomes for students with behavior disorders have been found (Mooney et al., 2005).

Finally, self-instruction methods have been used as an effective strategy to recruit praise. Recruiting praise can enhance the reinforcing qualities of engaging in prosocial behavior in both academic and nonacademic situations (Sutherland, Copeland, & Wehby, 2001). Numerous studies have demonstrated that students with developmental disabilities (e.g., Craft, Alber, & Heward, 1998) and learning disabilities (e.g., Alber, Heward, & Hippler, 1999) can be taught to recruit teacher attention and that outcomes such as improved academic engagement and accuracy are associated with this practice (Alber et al., 1999). Based on their review of the literature, Sutherland et al. (2001, p. 48) offer the following five-step self-instruction procedure that could be taught in general or special education classrooms:

1. Discuss the rationale for recruiting teacher attention with the students.
2. Instruct students on when, how, and how often to ask for help.
3. Model the recruiting strategy using a "think-aloud" procedure.
   a. "OK, I've finished about half of my math problems and want to know how I'm doing."

b. "Now I will look for the teacher."
   c. "She's not busy. I'll raise my hand now."
4. The teacher and the students then role-play five different recruiting episodes.
5. The teacher asks the students to state the steps.

Although numerous studies support the use of self-instructional training, it is important to note that not all researchers have found positive outcomes. Based on their reviews, Shapiro and Cole (1994) note that strategies designed to increase the frequency of specific skills have generally been highly effective, provided the student has the prerequisite skills. However, when self-instructional strategies are taught to change more general work behaviors (e.g., "follow the rules," "check my work carefully"), results are more variable. Further, self-management techniques teaching general self-regulation (e.g., "stop, look, and listen") have generally been shown to be minimally effective when used with students with ADHD (e.g., Abikoff, 1985; Shapiro et al., 1998). Finally, it is important to note that cognitive-based self-management approaches such as self-instruction are typically used in conjunction with other interventions (i.e., a "package" approach), and Maag (1990) specifically suggests that these approaches may be best suited as generalization enhancers.

Stress Inoculation Training

Originally developed by Meichenbaum more than 30 years ago, stress inoculation training (SIT) is a cognitive approach designed to teach a person skills for adapting to stressful events (i.e., "inoculating" oneself to stress) in a way that is functional and productive (Meichenbaum, 2007). It generally involves teaching the individual to reconceptualize or reframe his or her problem (e.g., "I failed not because I'm stupid but because I didn't study correctly or enough"), to learn specific skills to respond to identified stressors (e.g., "I have the intelligence to do well in this class, and I have learned effective study skills"), and to implement those skills effectively. SIT is typically used as a supplement to other forms of intervention to manage anger or anxiety, and most research has been conducted with adults (Meichenbaum, 2007), although effective demonstrations with children and adolescents are becoming more common (Maag & Kotlash, 1994; Meichenbaum, 2007).

Dwivedi and Gupta (2000) implemented a group SIT program with eight 9th-graders identified as having significant anger management problems. The intervention consisted of eight 40-minute sessions across 10 weeks. Sessions involved teaching students to identify situations that triggered anger and specific skills related to relaxation, assertiveness, thought stopping, and problem solving. Prior to and after the training program, students completed "Lost-It Logs" in which they analyzed recent incidents of anger with respect to what went through their minds, what they did, and how they evaluated the quality of their responses. Following training, students reported feeling better about their behavioral responses to anger-inducing situations and reacted less aggressively in these situations. Interestingly, the intensity of the students' feelings about the situations did not change, suggesting that even though they still found the situations provocative, they felt less anger, were able to exercise more self-control, and felt happier about their responses.

Although SIT has been demonstrated to be a promising intervention in schools, Maag (1994) cautions that self-management strategies utilizing stress inoculation with children and adolescents often fail to address the nature of the student's problem and do not include adequate methods for systematically programming for generalization. Overall, results suggest that SIT can be effective but must be approached with caution. As with any intervention, the choice of self-management strategies should be based on a thorough assessment of the context in which the problem behaviors occur—including the hypothesized function of behavior and a determination of whether the problem is a performance deficit or skill deficit—and approached within the context of the problem-solving model with clear goals of maintenance and generalization of behavior.

Case Example of a Self-Evaluation Procedure

Mo is a third-grade student enrolled in a general education class who has been referred to the intervention team. The following example illustrates how each stage of the problem-solving model was used to select and evaluate a self-management intervention to address her needs.

Problem Identification

Mo's problem behavior was initially described by the teacher as "acting out." In operational terms, it was determined that specific problem behaviors included talking without raising her hand and getting out of her seat during instruction. The teacher collected baseline frequency counts of these behaviors for 3 days during math period, the time in which the problem most frequently occurred, and it was determined that Mo was on average engaging in these behaviors 30 times per class period.

Problem Analysis

Brief interviews with Mo and her teacher and a direct observation by the school psychologist revealed that a reliable consequence of Mo's acting-out behavior was laughter and comments from her classmates. Math, art, and music periods were identified as the most problematic times. Therefore, the team hypothesized that the function of Mo's problem behaviors was to gain access to peer attention. In order to teach Mo how to regulate her behavior and to provide a strategy that would allow her to gain peer attention in more appropriate ways, the school psychologist and teacher decided to use a self-management matching intervention.

Intervention Plan Implementation

The classroom expectations were reviewed with Mo, with specific emphasis on hand raising and remaining in one's seat. For 1 week a token economy was instituted such that at the end of math period each day the teacher provided Mo with two ratings on a 0- to 5-point scale (one for hand raising and one for remaining in her seat), as well as an explanation of her ratings. Based on these ratings, Mo could earn access to a variety of rewards, including time to play games with her classmates.

After Mo's behavior improved on the token system, she was provided with a self-management form and instructed to write down her own rating for her hand-raising and in-seat behavior at the end of each math period (see Figure 20.2 for an example rating form). Additionally, she was told that she would earn points based on how well her ratings matched her teacher's ratings. Perfect matches earned her a bonus point, a near match within one point earned her the number of points she gave herself, and no near-match earned her no points for that rating period. Mo was instructed that if she argued with the teacher's rating she would earn no points for that period.

Following the implementation of this self-management procedure, Mo's behavior improved in math, but she was still experiencing problems in art and music. To facilitate generalization of the gains in her math class, Mo was sent to these classes with a self-management form. Mo was instructed to rate herself at the end of each class period, and her teachers were asked to write down their ratings of Mo's behavior. Mo's general education teacher determined matches and points later in the day. To ensure integrity of implementation of procedures, on random occasions the school psychologist observed the process in the classroom and provided feedback to teachers as necessary.

Intervention Plan Evaluation

After 3 weeks using the self-management matching procedure, Mo's talk-outs and out-of-seat behavior declined to zero levels in all three of the targeted classes (see Figure 20.3). In addition, positive collateral effects, such as Mo being invited by her classmates to eat with them at lunch and to attend birthday parties outside of class, were observed, as well as improvements in completion of in-class math worksheets. The social validity of the self-management intervention was judged to be high; Mo's teachers reported liking the process (and using it with other students), and Mo similarly enjoyed the procedures.

At the 1-month follow-up, it was decided by the team that the intervention would continue but that fading procedures would be instituted. Mo would be instructed that she should continue to self-evaluate each period but that matches with teachers would become a "surprise." Specifically, at the end of each period, the teacher would pull a "Yes we match" or "no we don't" slip from a hat. The team scheduled a 2-week review to evaluate Mo's progress on the modified intervention.

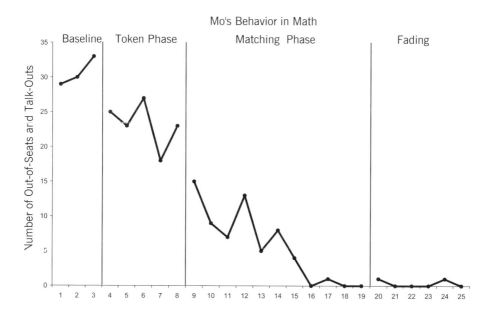

FIGURE 20.3. Sample data for contingency-based self-evaluation matching procedure.

Summary

The school psychologist can serve a primary role in developing, implementing, and evaluating a wide variety of self-management interventions. Results from empirical studies suggest that self-management strategies are efficacious across a wide range of behaviors, settings, and individuals. This is particularly important in light of current legislation that requires the use of evidence-based practices to address academic, social, and behavioral concerns. In addition, self-management interventions offer advantages over other strategies in their flexibility, potential for enhanced generalization effects, and high consumer satisfaction.

References

Abikoff, H. (1985). Efficacy of cognitive training interventions in hyperactive children: A critical review. *Clinical Psychology Review, 5,* 479–512.

Alber, S. R., Heward, W. L., & Hippler, B. J. (1999). Teaching middle school students with learning disabilities to recruit positive teacher attention. *Exceptional Children, 65,* 253–270.

Amato-Zech, N. A., Hoff, K. E., & Doepke, K. J. (2006). Increasing on-task behavior in the classroom: Extension of self-monitoring strategies. *Psychology in the Schools, 43,* 211–221.

Brooks, A., Todd, A. W., Tofflemoyer, S., & Horner, R. H. (2003). Use of functional assessment and a self-management system to increase academic engagement and work completion. *Journal of Positive Behavior Interventions, 5,* 144–152.

Craft, M. A., Alber, S. R., & Heward, W. L. (1998). Teaching elementary students with developmental disabilities to recruit teacher attention in a general education classroom: Effects on teacher praise and academic productivity. *Journal of Applied Behavior Analysis, 31,* 399–415.

Crawley, S. H., Lynch, P., & Vannest, K. (2006). The use of self-monitoring to reduce off-task behavior and cross-correlation examination of weekends and absences as an antecedent to off-task behavior. *Child and Family Behavior Therapy, 28,* 29–48.

Crum, C. F. (2004). Using a cognitive-behavior modification strategy to increase on-task behavior of a student with a behavior disorder. *Intervention in School and Clinic, 39,* 05–309.

Dunlap, L. K., & Dunlap, G. (1989). A self-monitoring package for teaching subtraction with regrouping to students with learning disabilities. *Journal of Applied Behavior Analysis, 22,* 309–314.

Dunlap, L. K., Dunlap, G., Koegel, L. K., & Koegel, R. L. (1991). Using self-monitoring to increase independence. *Teaching Exceptional Children, 23,* 17–22.

Dwivedi, K., & Gupta, A. (2000). "Keeping cool": Anger management through group work. *Support for Learning, 15,* 76–81.

Freeman, K. A., & Dexter-Mazza, E. T. (2004). Using self-monitoring with an adolescent with disruptive classroom behavior. *Behavior Modification, 28,* 402–419.

Ganz, J. B., & Sigafoos, J. (2005). Self-monitoring: Are young adults with MR and autism able to utilize cognitive strategies independently? *Education and Training in Developmental Disabilities, 40,* 24–33.

Glomb, N., & West, R. P. (1990). Teaching behaviorally disordered adolescents to use self-management skills for improving the completeness, accuracy, and neatness of creative writing homework assignments. *Behavioral Disorders, 15,* 233–242.

Gureasko-Moore, S., DuPaul, G. J., & White, G. P. (2007). Self-management of classroom preparedness and homework: Effects on school functioning of adolescents with attention-deficit/hyperactivity disorder. *School Psychology Review, 26,* 647–664.

Hallahan, D. P., Marshall, K. D., & Lloyd, J. W. (1981). Self-recording during group instruction: Effects on attention to task. *Learning Disabilities Quarterly, 4,* 407–413.

Harchik, A. E., Shermann, J. A., & Sheldon, J. B. (1992). The use of self-management procedures by people with developmental disabilities: A brief review. *Research in Developmental Disabilities, 13,* 211–217.

Harmon, T. M., Nelson, R. O., & Hayes, S. C. (1980). Self-monitoring of mood versus activity by depressed clients. *Journal of Consulting and Clinical Psychology, 48,* 30–38.

Harris, K. R., Friedlander, D. B., Saddler, B., Frizzelle, R., & Graham, S. (2005). Self-monitoring of attention versus self-monitoring of academic performance: Effects among students with ADHD in the general education classroom. *Journal of Special Education, 39,* 145–156.

Harris, K. R., Graham, S., Reid, R., McElroy, K., & Hamby, R. S. (1994). Self-monitoring of attention versus self-monitoring of performance: Replication and cross-task comparison studies. *Learning Disability Quarterly, 17,* 121–139.

Hoff, K. E., & DuPaul, G. J. (1998). Reducing disruptive behavior in general education settings: The use of self-management strategies. *School Psychology Review*, 27, 290–303.

Hughes, C., Copeland S. R., Agran, M., Wehmeyer, M. L., Rodi, M. S., & Pressley, J. A. (2002). Using self-monitoring to improve performance in general education high school classes. *Education and Training in Mental Retardation and Developmental Disabilities*, 37, 262–272.

Hughes, C. A., Fowler, S. E., Copeland, S. R., Agran, M., Wehmeyer, M. L., & Church-Pupke, P. P. (2004). Supporting high school students to engage in recreational activities with peers. *Behavior Modification*, 28, 3–27.

Jindal-Snape, D. (2004). Generalization and maintenance of social skills of children with visual impairments: Self-evaluation and the role of feedback. *Journal of Visual Impairment and Blindness*, 98, 470–483.

Kanfer, F. H. (1977). The many faces of self-control. In R. B. Stuart (Ed.), *Behavioral self-management: Strategies, techniques, and outcomes* (pp. 1–48). New York: Brunner/Mazel.

Kaufman, N. K., Rohde, P., Seeley, J. R., Clarke, G. N., & Stice, E. (2005). Potential mediators of cognitive-behavioral therapy for adolescents with comorbid major depression and conduct disorder. *Journal of Consulting and Clinical Psychology*, 73, 38–46.

Kirby, K. C., Fowler, S. A., & Baer, D. M. (1991). Reactivity in self-recording: Obtrusiveness of recording procedure and peer comments. *Journal of Applied Behavior Analysis*, 24, 487–498.

Konrad, M., Fowler, C. H., Walker, A. R., Test, D. W., & Wood, W. M. (2007). Effects of self-determination interventions on the academic skills of students with learning disabilities. *Learning Disability Quarterly*, 30, 89–113.

Lam, A. L., Cole, C. L., Shapiro, E. S., & Bambara, L. M. (1994). Relative effects of self-monitoring on task behavior, academic accuracy, and disruptive behavior in students with behavior disorders. *School Psychology Review*, 23, 44–58.

Lenz, B. K., Ehren, B. J., & Smiley, L. R. (1991). A goal attainment approach to improve completion of project-type assignments by adolescents with learning disabilities. *Learning Disabilities Research and Practice*, 6, 166–176.

Lewinsohn, P. M., & Clarke, G. N. (1999). Psychosocial treatments for adolescent depression. *Clinical Psychology Review*, 19, 329–342.

Lewinsohn, P. M., & Graf, M. (1973). Pleasant activities and depression. *Journal of Consulting and Clinical Psychology*, 41, 261–268.

Maag, J. W. (1990). Social skills training in schools. *Special Services in Schools*, 6, 1–19.

Maag, J. W. (1994). Promoting social skills training in classrooms: Issues for school counselors. *School Counselor*, 42, 100–113.

Maag, J. W., & Kotlash, J. (1994). Review of stress inoculation training with children and adolescents. *Behavior Modification*, 18, 443–469.

Maag, J. W., Reid, R., & DiGangi, S. A. (1993). Differential effects of self-monitoring attention, accuracy, and productivity. *Journal of Applied Behavior Analysis*, 26, 329–344.

Maag, J. W., Rutherford, R. B., & DiGangi, S. A. (1992). Effects of self-monitoring and contingent reinforcement on on-task behavior and academic productivity of learning-disabled students: A social validation study. *Psychology in the Schools*, 29, 157–172.

Mace, F. C., Belfiore, P. J., & Hutchinson, J. M. (2001). Operant theory and research on self-regulation. In B. J. Zimmerman & D. H. Schunk (Eds.). *Self-regulated learning and academic achievement: theoretical perspectives* (2nd ed., pp. 39–65). Mahwah, NJ: Erlbaum.

McDougall, D., & Brady, M. P. (1998). Initiating and fading self-management interventions to increase math fluency in general education classes. *Exceptional Children*, 64, 151–166.

Meichenbaum, D. (2007). Stress inoculation training: A preventative and treatment approach. In P. M. Lehrer, R. L. Woolfolk, & W. S. Sime (Eds.), *Principles and practice of stress management* (3rd ed., pp. 20–32). New York: Guilford Press.

Mitchem, D. J., & Young, K. R. (2001). Adapting self-management programs for classwide use: Acceptability, feasibility, and effectiveness. *Remedial and Special Education*, 22, 75–88.

Mitchem, K. J., Young, K. R., West, R. P., & Benyo, J. (2001). CWPASM: A classwide peer-assisted self-management program for general education classrooms. *Education and Treatment of Children*, 24, 111–140.

Mooney, P., Ryan, J. B., Uhing, B. M., Reid, R., & Epstein, M. H. (2005). A review of self-management interventions targeting academic outcomes for students with emotional and behavioral disorders. *Journal of Behavioral Education*, 14, 203–221.

Moore, R. J., Cartledge, G., & Heckaman, K. (1995). The effects of social skill instruction and self-monitoring on game-related behaviors of adolescents with emotional or behavioral disorders. *Behavioral Disorders*, 20, 253–266.

Nelson, R. O., & Hayes, S. C. (1981) Theoretical explanations for reactivity in self-monitoring. *Behavior Modification*, 5, 3–14.

Nelson, R. J., Smith, D. J., Young, R. K., & Dodd, J. M. (1991). A review of self-management outcome research conducted with students who exhibit behavioral disorders. *Behavioral Disorders, 16,* 169–179.

Peterson, L. D., Young, K. R., Salzberg, C. L., West, R. P., & Hill, M. (2006). Using self-management procedures to improve classroom social skills in multiple general education settings. *Education and Treatment of Children, 29,* 1–21.

Peterson, L. D., Young, K. R., West, R. P., & Peterson, M. H. (1999). Effects of student self-monitoring on generalization of student performance to regular classrooms. *Education and Treatment of Children, 22,* 357–372.

Reid, R., & Harris, K. R. (1993). Self-monitoring of attention versus self-monitoring of performance: Effects on attention and academic performance. *Exceptional Children, 60,* 29–40.

Reid, R., & Lienemann, T. O. (2006). Self-regulated strategy development for written expression with students with attention-deficit/hyperactivity disorder. *Exceptional Children, 73,* 53–68.

Reid, R., Trout, A. L., & Schartz, M. (2005). Self-regulation interventions for children with attention-deficit/hyperactivity disorder. *Exceptional Children, 71,* 361–377.

Rhode, G., Morgan, D. P., & Young, K. R. (1983). Generalization and maintenance of treatment gains of behaviorally handicapped students from resource rooms to regular classrooms using self-evaluation procedures. *Journal of Applied Behavior Analysis, 16,* 171–188.

Shapiro, E. S., & Cole, C. L. (1994). *Behavior change in the classroom: Self-management interventions.* New York: Guilford Press.

Shapiro, E. S., DuPaul, G. J., & Bradley-Klug, K. L. (1998). Self-management as a strategy to improve the classroom behavior of adolescents with ADHD. *Journal of Learning Disabilities, 31*(6), 545–555.

Shapiro, E. S., Durnan, S. L., Post, E. E., & Levinson, T. S. (2002). Self-monitoring procedures for children and adolescents. In M. R. Shinn, H. M. Walker, & G. Stoner (Eds.), *Interventions for academic and behavior problems: II. Preventive and remedial approaches* (pp. 433–454). Bethesda, MD: National Association of School Psychologists.

Shimbukuro, S. M., Prater, M. A., Jenkins, A., & Edelen-Smith, P. (1999). The effects of

self-monitoring of academic performance on students with learning disabilities and ADD/ADHD. *Education and Treatment of Children, 22,* 397–414.

Skinner, C. H., Turco, T., Beatty, K., & Rasavage, C. (1989). Cover, Copy, and Compare: A method for increasing multiplication performance. *School Psychology Review, 18,* 412–420.

Smith, B. W., & Sugai, G. (2000). A self-management functional assessment-based behavior support plan for a middle school student with EBD. *Journal of Positive Behavior Interventions, 2,* 208–217.

Smith, D. J., Young, R. K., Nelson, R. J., & West, R. P. (1992). The effect of a self-management matching procedure on the classroom and academic behavior of students with mild handicaps. *School Psychology Review, 21,* 59–73.

Smith, D. J., Young, R. K., West, R. P., & Morgan, D. P. (1988). Reducing the disruptive behavior of junior high school students: A classroom self-management procedure. *Behavioral Disorders, 13,* 231–239.

Stark, K. D., Hargrave, J., Sander, J., Custer, G., Schnoebelen, S., Simpson, J., et al. (2006). Treatment of childhood depression: The ACTION treatment program. In P. C. Kendall (Ed.), *Child and adolescent therapy: Cognitive-behavioral procedures* (3rd ed., pp. 169–216). New York: Guilford Press.

Sutherland, K. S., Copeland, S., & Wehby, J. H. (2001). Catch them while you can: Monitoring and increasing the use of effective praise. *Beyond Behavior, 11,* 46–49.

Todd, A. W., Horner, R. H., & Sugai, G. (1999). Self-monitoring and self-recruited praise: Effects on problem behavior, academic engagement, and work completion in a typical classroom. *Journal of Positive Behavior Interventions, 1,* 66–76.

Young, R. K., West, R. P., Smith, D. J., & Morgan, D. P. (2000). *Teaching self-management strategies to adolescents.* Longmont, CO: Sopris West.

Zimmerman, B. J., & Schunk, D. H. (Eds.). (2001). *Self-Regulated Learning and Academic achievement: Theoretical perspectives* (2nd ed.). Mahwah, NJ: Erlbaum.

Chapter 21

Interventions for Homework Problems

Donna Gilbertson
Rebecca Sonnek

Homework is a common instructional procedure used by teachers to improve academic achievement. Approximately 20% of the time that students are engaged in performing academic tasks is spent doing homework that influences the class grade (Cooper & Nye, 1994). Teachers opt to use homework as one method of increasing student engagement and time with academic tasks (Cooper, Robinson, & Patall, 2006). Results of empirical studies examining homework effects on achievement tests and class grades suggest that students who complete assigned homework academically outperform students who do not complete homework (Cooper, Lindsay, Nye, & Greathouse, 1998; Trautwein, 2007). Teachers, however, report that many students at risk for failure have difficulty completing homework assignments successfully (Rhoades & Kratochwill, 1998; Salend & Gajria, 1995; Weiner, Sheridan, & Jenson, 1998). Although special education students have the most significant homework problems, 30% of general education students also struggle with completing homework assignments (Polloway, Foley, & Epstein, 1992). Given the large portion of time spent on homework completion and the contribution of homework to academic grades, identification of effective strategies

for improving homework performance is an important concern for parents and teachers.

An emerging research base supports the use of classwide homework programs to increase homework completion (Bryan, Burstein, & Bryan, 2001; Keith & Keith, 2006; Miller & Kelley, 1994; Olympia, Sheridan, & Jenson, 1994). However, despite these positive findings, some students in a class may be unresponsive to classwide efforts. Homework problems may occur for several reasons, making it difficult to design a classwide homework program to address the needs of all students. Some students, for example, are able to do the work but have low motivation to do the homework (i.e., a performance deficit). Other students can do the work but need support organizing a consistent home–school routine in order to get the homework turned in on time (i.e., an organizational deficit). For some students, difficulties with homework accuracy and completion can result from academic skills deficits (Daly, Lentz, & Boyer, 1996; Daly, Witt, Martens, & Dool, 1997; Malloy, Gilbertson, & Maxfield, 2007). Individual differences in skill acquisition, efficiency, retention, and generalization to novel tasks are potential causes of academic deficits that might interfere with successful home-

353

work progress. Finally, some students lack basic tool skills, or prerequisite skills, that are needed to do complex tasks on homework assignments (Binder, 1996; Johnson & Layng, 1992). Common prerequisite skills for homework, for example, might include fluent reading with comprehension, math computation, and writing letters and words. Given the complexity of homework assignments, individual differences in the effectiveness of classwide programs are not surprising. To meet these individual differences, a more intensive homework intervention for an individual homework problem should be based on the reasons homework is not being turned in or completed accurately.

The purpose of this chapter is to discuss proven intervention strategies that address different types of homework problems. The first section provides an overview of research findings on strategies for five different types of homework problems. Specifically, we review interventions designed to address classwide homework problems, performance deficits, organizational deficits, academic skill deficits, and tool skill deficits. Following this section on proven intervention strategies, we describe a problem-solving approach to develop a hypothesis about the reason for a homework problem that would indicate what type of intervention is needed. Finally, the development of a progress monitoring system is discussed to determine whether the selected intervention is effectively resolving the problem.

Effective Homework Intervention Strategies for Common Problems

Classwide Homework Interventions

Ideally, a homework program provides effective support to all students in a classroom. When many students in a class are struggling with homework completion and accuracy, then a classwide intervention may be most appropriate. Results from several studies suggest that using a series of consistent steps when giving and receiving homework increases the likelihood of homework completion for most students (Hughes, Ruhl, Schumaker, & Deshler, 2002; Miller & Kelley, 1994; Olympia, Sheridan, & Jenson, 1994). An example of a classwide homework routine is presented in Table

21.1. As the table illustrates, an effective routine begins with a systematic presentation of homework instructions. Providing a student with sufficient knowledge about homework requirements enhances the likelihood that the student will be able to do the homework at home with little parental assistance. For example, explicit instruction on how to do the work, followed by modeling of accurate performance on several brief work examples, shows students how to complete the work (Ysseldyke & Elliott, 1999). Having students practice skills that are presented on the homework also promotes accuracy (Walberg, 1991). This brief practice session allows the teacher to directly observe whether or not the students understand the assigned work. This is important because many students report that they fail to do well on homework when assignments are not clearly presented and they do not understand what they are to do (Bryan & Nelson, 1994; Sawyer, Nelson, Jayanthi, Bursuck, & Epstein, 1996). Completing homework that is similar to work that the student has previously used in class likely decreases the need for parental assistance. Most parents want to be supportive, but in surveys of parents, most reported that they did not have adequate skills to assist their child (Christenson, Rounds, & Gorney, 1992), felt ill prepared to handle homework problems, and believed special training was needed to solve academic problems (Kay, Fitzgerald, Paradee, & Mellencamp, 1994).

Next, the routine should consist of steps to help students remember and keep track of homework assignments when working at home. Use of a homework planner is one effective strategy for increasing students' completion and return of homework. A homework planner is a weekly or monthly calendar that is used by the students to record homework assignments on a daily basis. Having the student bring the planner home each day also provides information about homework assignments to parents. Bryan and Sullivan-Burstein (1998) examined the effects of a homework planner and three other interventions (i.e., reinforcement for homework completion, graphing homework completion, and assigning "real-life" assignments) on student homework performance and teacher use of intervention over time. All four interventions effectively improved

TABLE 21.1. Example of Classwide Intervention Using a Homework Planner

Step	Student's role	Teacher's role	Parent's role
1	Pay attention to teacher's instructions during lesson on homework skill.	Tell students what to do on homework.	
2	Observe how to do the work and ask questions if unclear.	Model correct work.	
3	Practice a few work samples and ask for help.	Provide guided practice on a few work samples to gauge student accuracy	
4	Copy homework assignments and due dates in planner.	Write assignments on board in the same place daily.	
5	Prepare needed materials.	Write or tell students what to bring home.	
6	Show teacher the planner.	Check planner.	
7	Ask teacher about any unclear assignments.	Answer questions.	
8	Bring home the planner and show parent.		Check planner for homework.
9	Do homework, asking parent for help if needed.		Provide help if requested; make notes of difficult areas to teacher. Sign completed assignments.
10	Return to school, show teacher.	Review planner and check for parent's signature.	
11	Review graded work for errors and ask questions if needed.	Grade or have students grade work and reteach skill if more than 80% of the students do poorly.	Review graded work and provide positive feedback for correct homework.
Optional	Participate and support peers in your group.	Use peer cooperative groups.	

homework completion, but on a 2-year follow-up survey, teachers reported using only homework planners and graphing.

Setting up a homework-planner routine requires teacher, student, and parent participation. First, the teacher develops and uses a system to present homework assignments that students are to record in the planner. Useful information that teachers may provide about assignment requirements may include homework requirements for each subject and details such as what must be done to complete the homework assignment, the needed materials, the due date, an estimated time to complete daily tasks, and how the work will be evaluated. Next, the student completes the planner by recording all homework assignments and bringing it home. Teachers can quickly monitor student recording of accurate information in the planner and prompt students to bring their planners home while the students are packing to go home at the end of the school day. Finally, the parent sits down with the student to review the planner and monitor completion of homework requirements in the home setting (Epstein, Munk, Bursuck, Polloway, & Jayanthi, 1999). Providing space for the teacher and parent to write messages about homework successes and difficulties further enhances the school–home communication system.

To initiate a homework program, students are trained in the procedure, and an overview of the homework-planner procedures and homework policies (e.g., missed and late assignments, extra credit) should be sent home. Information can be given to parents on how to review information in the planner and completed homework on a daily basis to determine whether all homework is completed as required. After initiating a homework program, attention to completed homework is critical. Students are more apt to complete assignments and return quality homework when their homework is reviewed and evaluated in a timely manner (Walberg, 1991). Studies that examined the effects of students scoring their own work suggest that academic performance increases when students receive immediate feedback and that the procedure has the added benefit of decreasing grading time for the teacher (Trammel, Schloss, & Alper, 1994). Hundert and Bucher (1978), for example, evaluated the use and accuracy of a practical self-scoring procedure in two special education classrooms. In this study, teachers provided answers on an overhead while students graded their work. Assignments were graded with a different color pen than the pen color used to complete the assignment in order to track correction of work that occurred during grading. Immediately following the grading of papers, the teacher randomly selected one student's paper to check for accurate grading and gave the class bonus points for correct work and penalty points for errors. With this procedure in place, 83% of the students had accurately graded papers.

An interesting option for homework routines is to use a peer-managed routine (O'Melia & Rosenberg, 1994). For example, Olympia, Sheridan, Jenson, and Andrews (1994) evaluated the effectiveness of a group contingency procedure on homework completion and accuracy. Sixth-grade students were organized into cooperative learning teams and were trained to assume various roles, including coach, scorer, and manager. Each team earned rewards for exceeding a daily goal, and goals were based on the homework accuracy scores of all the team members. Homework completion improved for the majority of the students, but

accuracy results were mixed. The authors proposed that the lack of direct testing to determine whether the students had a skill deficit or a performance deficit might have contributed to the inconsistent accuracy results. In this study incentives were provided to prompt behavior for students who may have a performance deficit, but the students who lacked the ability to perform the skill were not given additional instructional components needed to successfully complete the assignments.

An effective classwide homework routine results in complete and accurate homework for most students in the class. However, there may be some students who still struggle with homework and need additional assistance with homework completion. For these students, the selection of homework support in addition to the classroom routine should address the reasons that homework is not being turned in or accurately completed.

Interventions for a Performance Deficit

When a student has the skills to complete homework but chooses not to do the work, the problem is considered a performance deficit. Motivational homework strategies can be useful to address such problems. Immediately grading homework provides most students with the motivation to do and return the homework at school. If this does not work for a student, the addition of an incentive program for homework accuracy may be warranted (Miller & Kelley, 1994). The intervention example in Table 21.2 presents an incentive procedure that can be added to a classwide homework-planner routine.

The use of goal setting may also enhance performance. A goal provides students with the expected level of performance that enables parents or teachers to immediately respond with praise when the goal is met or to provide specific feedback when the student is attempting to meet the goal. Trammel et al. (1994) showed that self-graphing with goals set by high school students enhanced homework completion. In this study, students set a goal for homework completion and recorded the number of daily homework assignments on a graph. Students reviewed graphs to determine when goals were met and to set new goals. No contingencies for meeting set goals were in place. Study-

TABLE 21.2. Example of Incentive Intervention for Performance Skill Deficits using a Homework Planner

Steps	Student's role	Teacher's role	Parent's role
Prepare	Set a goal. For example, three homework assignments are completed at 80% accuracy.	Work with student to ensure goal is reasonable.	Work with student to ensure goal is reasonable.
Prepare	Select rewards to earn for meeting the goal.		Develop a weekly or daily reward system with school psychologist support, if needed.
1	Follow steps for homework planner (Table 21.1)	Follow steps for homework planner.	Follow steps for homework planner.
2	Collect graded homework from teacher. Ask teacher to mark grades in homework planner.	Give back graded homework and record grade in planner. Optional: Provide a reward if goal met.	
3	Bring planner and graded homework home and show parent. Earn reward if goal is met. Problem solve with the parent on how to complete any missed steps.		Review planner for grades. Praise student efforts and reward if goal is met.
4	Ask the teacher and/or parent questions about any assignment that did not meet goal.	Answer questions and contact parent to problem solve if needed.	Answer questions and contact teacher to problem solve if needed.

ing middle-class families, Kahle and Kelley (1994) compared the effect on homework performance of a parent-training program focusing on homework issues either with or without a goal-setting procedure. To implement the goal-setting intervention, parents divided homework assignments into small, specific goals and provided daily and weekly rewards if the goals were attained. Parents also recorded homework accuracy and the amount of time from the student's starting to completing a homework assignment. Students' performances in both treatment groups (goal setting with parent training or parent training alone) was compared with students' performances in a monitoring-only condition. In this third condition, parents were instructed to monitor homework accuracy and duration but received no intervention training. Results showed that the goal-setting procedure significantly improved accuracy and answers correct per minute on homework assignments between pre- and posttreatment scores. The monitoring and parent-training-only groups had similar pre- and posttreatment scores.

Homework completion problems may also occur when other activities interfere with homework completion at home. For example, students who are allowed to spend homework time doing preferred activities such as watching TV or playing with friends may be less likely to complete their homework. Parents also commonly report problem behaviors such as whining, procrastinating, frequent off-task behaviors, and constant need for prompts as interfering with timely completion of the homework (Jayanthi, Sawyer, Nelson, Bursuck, & Epstein, 1995). A behavior contract is easy to create and often resolves this type of problem (Murphy, 1988). A behavior contract is an agreement between a student and parent by which the student agrees to meet a goal and the parent agrees to provide something preferred, such as a tangible reward or enjoyable activity, following goal attainment. Contracts require the parent, teacher, and student to select expected behaviors, rewards for successful goal obtainment, and a criterion for goal obtainment (Bowen, Jenson, & Clark, 2004). Written contracts are developed to explicitly tell the student the homework expectations that will result in predetermined positive rewards for student efforts and that can be earned within a fairly short time (Reavis et al., 1996). For example, a student may earn so many minutes of computer time or time to play with friends if he or she immediately starts homework on arriving home from school, stays on task, and completes homework accurately. Bonus incentives may also be added for unmotivated students. Figure 21.1 presents an example of a contract that may be used to improve homework completion.

Interventions for an Organizational Skill Deficit

Organizational skill support is required when a student has the skills to complete homework but struggles with organizing the many activities needed to complete and turn in homework. Students need to accurately record assignments, take needed materials home, take time to work, organize a work setting, complete the work, put homework away, and bring the work back to school (Bryan & Nelson, 1994; Epstein et al., 1999). Setting up a structured routine for completing homework in the home setting is an effective intervention option for students who need assistance in developing organizational skills in order to get homework completed and turned in on time. Several details should be considered when setting up the routine. First, the student and parents should organize a study area that is free of distractions, with appropriate lighting and materials needed to complete homework (e.g., paper, pens, dictionary). Next, a study time should be selected that can be consistently adhered

---

As part of the contract, the student agrees to follow these behaviors:

(Here select important homework behaviors that will increase completed and accurate homework the student agrees to do as part of the contract. A few examples follow.)

        Write down homework in planner.

        Bring home planner and materials needed to complete homework.

        Start homework at the set homework time _____ .

        Stay on task with no more than two parent reminders.

        Complete homework neatly and accurately.

As part of the contract, the parent agrees to follow these behaviors:

Review planner and write initials next to all completed homework in the planner.

Provide one of the following activities after the student meets the above agreement.

(Here select several activities (or reward) options that the parent is willing to provide, that are easy to provide, and that the student would like to earn. Daily activities that the student can select immediately after completing behavior in the contract may be negotiated—for example, computer time, time spent with friends or listening to music.)

    1. _____   2. _____   3 _____

    4. _____   5. _____   6. _____

As part of the contract, the teacher agrees to follow these behaviors:

Review student progress and praise student successes.

If needed, the teacher may provide a weekly bonus incentive. For example, the teacher can agree to provide an incentive after the student meets the above agreement for _ days.

Date: _____   Student signature: _____

Parent signature: _____   Teacher signature: _____

FIGURE 21.1. An example of a homework contract.

to each day and when a parent is present and available to help. Enough time should be allocated for completing daily homework assignments. Study time begins with the student and parent reviewing the homework planner to preview and discuss homework requirements. At the end of the study time, the student and parent review completed homework, and the parent provides support as needed. Homework is then placed in a designated location (e.g., a backpack) to get it ready to return to school the next day.

Interventions to increase organizational skills may also include strategies such as self-monitoring, goal setting, and home–school note procedures (Jurbergs, Palcic, & Kelley, 2007; Toney, Kelley, & Lanclos, 2003).

These procedures combined with steps for setting up a homework routine are included in the sample intervention script for an organizational deficit presented in Table 21.3.

Having students monitor their organizational behaviors when learning how to manage their own homework behaviors helps students become aware of the accuracy and effectiveness of these behaviors (Reid, 1996). Callahan, Rademacher, and Hildreth (1998) successfully implemented a self-monitoring homework program with middle school students who were enrolled in a program for at-risk youths. Students and their parents were first trained in skills related to setting up a homework study location and time, to monitoring student progress on homework

TABLE 21.3. Example of Intervention for Organizational Skill Deficits Using a Homework Planner

Steps	Student's role	Teacher's role	Parent's role
Prepare	Work with parent and teacher on a home routine for homework and time management plan.	Discuss with the parent the estimated time and support typically required.	Set aside a consistent place and time with the student to do the homework when you are available to monitor.
Prepare	Set a goal. For example, homework is completed at 80% accuracy, and 80% of the steps for homework planner in Table 21.1 were completed.	Work with student to ensure goals are attainable and reasonable.	Work with student to ensure goals are attainable and reasonable.
Prepare	Select rewards to earn for meeting the goal.		May develop a weekly reward system with school psychologist support.
1	Follow steps for homework planner (see Table 21.1).	Follow steps for homework planner.	Follow steps for homework planner.
2	Check off each step in the routine after completed.		
3	Show parent checked-off steps and homework.		Sign steps completed and mark any missed steps.
4	Graph steps completed and graded homework performance.	Give back graded homework and prompt the student to graph work if needed.	
5	Show the teacher the graph. Problem solve with the teacher on how to complete any missed steps.	Sign graph and mark if accurately graphed or write missed steps. Contact parent to problem solve if needed.	
6	Bring home to show parent the graph and earn reward if goal is met. Problem solve with the parent on how to complete any missed steps.	Increase goal if the first goal is successful for several weeks.	Review graph and teacher notes. Praise student efforts and provide reward if goal is met. Contact teacher to problem solve if needed.

completion, and to getting materials ready to take back to school. After training in organizational skills, parents and students were then trained to set goals and to monitor and record the student's use of these skills when completing the homework process. If parents and students agreed that an organizational skill was employed (e.g., the student brought home the materials to complete the homework assignment), the student earned a point. Accumulated points were later traded for a student-selected and parent-approved reward. Callahan et al. (1998) found that student completion of math homework was significantly higher after the self-management and parent-participation intervention was introduced than before intervention training. Further, teachers reported that more homework was completed on work assignments that were not included in the study and that this positively affected the student's academic performance. During follow-up interviews, both parents and students reported that the program was successful and that they were planning to continue the process.

While learning to independently use organizational skills, some students need additional monitoring of skill use from parents and teachers. To effectively monitor student compliance on homework routines, teachers and parents commonly stress the importance of an effective home–school communication system (Bursuck et al., 1999; Epstein et al., 1999). Establishing communication in the form of a home–school note can help the parent and teacher understand what specific homework steps were completed with and without problems (Jurbergs et al., 2007; Riley-Tillman, Chafouleas, & Briesch, 2007). Use of school–home notes has improved homework completion and accuracy (Blechman, Taylor, & Schrader, 1981; Strukoff, McLaughlin, & Bialozor, 1987). The purpose of a home–school note for homework problems is to provide more specific communication about student behaviors than the typical homework planner does. In addition to having students record homework assignments in a notebook, for example, teachers may record what assignments were successfully turned in and the obtained grade. Parents can also rate positive and negative homework behaviors and time for homework completion. The parent and/ or teacher can reward the student for posi-

tive homework behaviors or reteach steps that the student has difficulty completing.

Interventions for an Academic Skill Deficit

Strategies to help with skill deficits are required when a student has the appropriate basic skills yet is struggling to learn new tasks. Intervention studies using motivational or organizational strategies have reported inconsistent effects on children with learning disabilities or skill deficits (Bryan et al., 2001). Many of these students need some type of instructional support to do the work in the home setting, but different children need different types of support. The question at this point is what type of academic support will work best for each student. Unfortunately, there is a paucity of studies that provide proven interventions for this type of homework problem (Cooper et al., 2006; Jenson, Sheridan, Olympia, & Andrews, 1994). Few studies have investigated the effects of instructional support or learning strategies on homework performance and how parents can best support this process (Hoover-Dempsey et al., 2001). Perhaps the method of brief experimental analysis (BEA), described by Daly, Hofstadter, Martinez, and Andersen in Chapter 8, this volume, may be one of the most useful methods for selecting an effective intervention for a student. This method applies and assesses the effect of several treatment options on academic performance to select the intervention that is most likely to work for an individual child over time. Tables 21.4 (a math example) and 21.5 (a reading example) illustrate how the BEA process might be used to select an intervention that produces the most accurate and complete homework (Dunlap & Dunlap, 1989; Gajria, Jitendra, Sood, & Sacks, 2007; Malloy et al., 2007; Palincsar & Brown, 1984; Skinner, McLaughlin, & Logan, 1997; Vaughn, Klingner, & Bryant, 2001). These interventions offer parents instructional tools or learning strategies that may provide sufficient support for the student to do the work. Included in Table 21.5 is a series of learning strategies known to enhance students' comprehension of reading assignments, which is needed to understand and complete assignments given in class (Palincsar & Brown, 1984; Vaughn et al., 2001). Teachers first explicitly teach the

TABLE 21.4. Description of Examples of Interventions for Skill Deficits for Math Assignments

Cover, Copy, and Compare

The teacher provides a math worksheet and answer key to the student for homework. At home, the parent monitors as the student works one problem at a time on a homework assignment. After completing one problem, the student reviews the answer on an answer key provided by the teacher and changes any errors. The student works on 50% of the problems on the worksheet, using the answer key to check the accuracy of the work. The student continues to complete the remaining problems without checking the answer sheet to determine whether skill is learned and/or to earn a reward for accurate work.

Step-by-step cue cards

During class instruction, the teacher makes a step-by-step checklist that tells the student how to do a problem. A simple sentence for each step and an example of that step in a problem informs the student what to do. For homework, the student brings the checklist home and works on several more problems, using the checklist with parent support. When a student does not follow a step on a problem, the parent will point to the missed step and tell the student to redo the problem. The teacher may also provide an answer key to the parent. After receiving help, the student works on half of the remaining problems before asking the parent to check work using a red pen. After the parent helps correct work, the student completes the assignment.

Highlighted errors

The teacher provides a math worksheet and answer key to the student for homework. At home, the student independently completes 2–5 problems. The parent then reviews the work using an answer key and highlights any errors with a yellow highlighter marker. The student reviews error marks, asks questions, and continues working on the worksheet.

TABLE 21.5. Description of Examples of Interventions for Skill Deficits for Reading Assignments

Key words

On a reading homework assignment, the parent asks student to circle five words from the passage that the student cannot define. The parent then reads the passage out loud to the student (modeled), followed by the student reading the passage out loud to the parent. As the student reads, the parent listens and marks errors. When a word is missed, mispronounced, or not read within 3 seconds, the parent immediately reads the word correctly out loud to the student. The student repeats the word and continues to read. Following reading practice, the parent selects the first five words circled by the student. The parent can also select additional words, to meet a total of five words, from words that were marked as reading errors or that represent main concepts. These five words are written and presented to the student on index cards as the parent reads each word aloud and asks the student to repeat the word. Next, the parent defines each word, followed by the oral presentation of the word in a sentence. Following the key word definition, the student reads the passage and works on the homework assignment.

Strategic reading strategies

Prior to a reading assignment, the parent first asks the student to scan the reading and search for clues on what the reading is about, what the student already knows about the material, and what may be learned or asked about the reading. Second, the parent reviews questions that are to be completed for the homework assignment with the student to determine answers that will be there in the reading ("What happened in the story?"), that will be implied from material in the text that needs to be searched and thought about (e.g., "What are the strengths and weaknesses of the plan that the characters used in the story?"), or that will require the student to predict or infer something after reading the material (e.g., "What may happen if they used a different plan?"). Finally, the parent prompts the student to review the reading structure to help determine the purpose of the material (e.g., narrative, sequence, cause–effect, description, problem–solution, comparison, time–order).

During reading, the parent prompts the student to write down words that he or she does not understand and needs to know more about. After the student reads several paragraphs, the parent helps the student to look up words or discuss any parts in the reading that the student does not understand. Finally, the parent listens as the student rephrases the main idea(s) in each paragraph or section. If needed, the parent can prompt the student to reread the material to confirm the main idea.

After reading a section or all material, the parent can prompt the student to complete the work for homework based on the reading material.

skills and then have students practice using skills in cooperative groups to promote independent comprehension of academic reading. Parents may potentially be trained to prompt and monitor use of learning strategies on reading homework conducted at home. Each reading strategy listed in Table 21.5 has been demonstrated to be effective in several studies (Gajria et al., 2007). Several recent studies have also demonstrated promising results on gains in student reading fluency performance when parents delivered a reading intervention that they learned during a single training session (Gortmaker, Daly, McCurdy, Persampieri, & Hergenrader, 2007; Persampieri, Gortmaker, Daly, Sheridan, & McCurdy, 2006). Thus BEA can be employed to determine whether one or more strategies effectively enhance homework performance for an individual child on homework assignments. However, additional studies need to be conducted to evaluate the long-term effects of interventions recommended on the basis of this type of brief assessment on homework performance.

Perhaps the least intrusive approach is to shorten the amount of time needed to complete homework when students are required to work on a skill that is not yet fully acquired (Cooper et al., 1998). Studies examining the differences between the time a teacher estimates for homework completion and the time a student reports found that students were working longer than teachers estimated and were still turning in inaccurate work (Bryan et al., 2001). Moreover, previously identified reinforcers failed to enhance performance of higher complex skills when students were not yet fluent on prerequisite skills. Shorter homework assignments that provide many response opportunities are completed more often and more accurately than longer assignments (Cooper, 1989). Using shorter homework assignments can also be effective on tasks that can be independently performed by the student and easily monitored by the parent.

Interventions for a Tool Skill Deficit

A small group of students may lack basic tool skills that are prerequisite skills needed to perform complex skills (Binder, 1996; Johnson & Layng, 1992). Common prerequisite skills for homework include fluent reading with comprehension, knowledge of math facts, and ability to write letters and words. For example, a third-grade student who does not have the basic skills to read homework texts will not be able to effectively respond to questions about the text. When students lack the prerequisite skills to complete homework assignments, assigning more homework or more time to complete homework is not an effective solution (Cooper et al., 1998; Trautwein, 2007; Cooper et al., 2006). Instead, a logical approach would be to assign homework that focuses on increasing practice and fluency with basic math or reading skills that are the basis for more advanced skills taught in class (Binder, 1996). Providing practice time on basic skills at home would Practice at help maintain the time the student spends involved in the ongoing core curriculum content at school.

Table 21.6 lists examples of proven interventions that can be used to increase basic reading or math skills (Gortmaker et al., 2007; Sante, McLaughlin, & Weber, 2001). It is important to note that these types of interventions, though clearly of benefit to specific students, require extensive resources and modified materials. Most of the interventions listed require an adult or peer tutor to provide some sort of modeling, guided practice, or frequent feedback (Fishel & Ramirez, 2005; Gortmaker et al., 2007). Major advantages of these interventions is that they can be completed within 15 minutes and that they produce desired results. However, parents who are provided with intervention materials and training that includes role playing and feedback have children who show more consistent positive academic gains (Bryan et al., 2001).

A Process for Selecting Homework Interventions

Knowledgeable school personnel, including school psychologists, can be key facilitators in identifying homework problems and developing effective intervention plans for students (Olympia, Sheridan, Jenson, & Andrews, 1994; Rhoades & Kratochwill, 1998). The following sections describe an assessment process for identifying homework problems, assessing contributing environmental factors, and developing and evaluating appropriate intervention strategies.

TABLE 21.6. Description of Examples of Interventions for Tool Skill Deficits

Repeated readings to increase reading fluency

A 200- to 400-word passage is read repeatedly out loud four times by the student to the parent with feedback about the speed of reading. As the student reads the fourth time, the parent listens and marks errors (a missed or mispronounced word or a word not read within 3 seconds). Following the key word definition, the student reads the passage to the parent for 1 minute as the parent marks any errors. The number of words read correctly per minute is recorded.

Listening preview with positive practice/overcorrection to increase fluency and accuracy

The parent first reads a 200- to 400-word passage out loud to the student (modeled) followed by the student reading the passage out loud to the parent. As the student reads, the parent listens and marks errors. When a word is missed, mispronounced, or not read within 3 seconds, the parent immediately reads the word correctly out loud to the student. The student repeats the word five times and repeats the whole sentence once. Following the practice reading, the student reads the passage to the parent for 1 minute as the parent marks any errors. The number of words read correctly per minute is recorded.

Practice on math facts for single-digit math facts to increase accuracy and fluency

The teacher provides a folder to the student each week consisting of 6–10 single-digit-problem flash cards, four math worksheets consisting of problems from the flash cards, answer keys, and a graph. At home, the student and parent practice the flash cards five times. During practice, the parent gives the student 3 seconds to say the answer to a presented problem before telling the student the correct answer. Following flash card practice, the parent administers a 2-minute math worksheet to the student using a timer. After completing the timed worksheet, the parent grades the probe using a red marker and answer key. The work is scored as the number of digits correct, and this score is written on the graph. The parent can also determine whether the student had exceeded the previous best math probe score, and, if so, provide a preferred activity. The student returns graded probes, graph, and flash cards to the teacher at the end of the week.

Homework Problem Identification and Intervention Selection to Resolve the Problem

Conducting an assessment to identify the nature of the homework problem is the first step to solving homework problems. As noted earlier, homework assignments begin and end in the classroom. Thus a logical first step in the homework process is to assess the current process the teacher is using for selecting, assigning, and grading homework. The homework process or routine becomes a concern when many students within the classroom fail to turn in accurately completed homework. When homework problems are apparent with many students in the class, it would behoove the teacher to proceed with a classwide intervention. Once a classwide problem has been ruled out or resolved through an intervention, then individual children's problems are considered.

Table 21.7 presents options for assessing the effectiveness of a classwide homework program. An initial review of classwide homework grades may be useful in categorizing a homework problem as a classwide problem (e.g., less than 80% of the students are returning accurate homework) or an individual problem (e.g., 80% or more of the children are returning accurate homework). If a classwide problem is identified, the steps presented in Table 21.1 (Keith & Keith, 2006; Ysseldyke & Elliott, 1999) can be used as a checklist to help identify effective strategies missing in the current routine. When missing steps are identified, they could be added on a classwide basis to improve homework completion.

For students who are unresponsive to classwide homework intervention efforts, additional assessments may need to be conducted and more intensive homework interventions implemented. Several homework questionnaires, including the Homework Problem Checklist (HPC; Anesko, Schoiock, Ramirez, & Levine, 1987) and the Homework Performance Questionnaire (HPQ; Power, Dombrowski, Watkins, Mautone, & Eagle, 2007), can be administered to assess teacher and parent perceptions of the problem. These types of instruments are easy to administer and may provide useful information regarding potential areas of concern for individual students. For example, on the

HPC, parents rate the frequency of 20 possible problems that may occur when a student tries to complete his or her homework. The listed problems include procrastinating, getting frustrated or distracted, producing sloppy work, making lots of mistakes, needing constant support, refusing to do the work, or failing to bring the work home or to school. Similarly, on the HPQ, parents rate how much support is needed (parental supervision and teacher communication), how well the student is engaged (starting homework and on-task behaviors), and how competent the student is in regards to the homework assignments. The teacher rates the percentage of time (i.e., 0 = 0–39%; 1 = 40–69%; 2 = 70–79%; 3 = 80–89%; 4 = 90–100%) the student exhibited homework competency behaviors (e.g., ease of independent completion; quality, accuracy, and comprehension) and responsibility behaviors (e.g., ability to record assignments, to organize needed materials at home, to manage homework time, and to return completed homework on time). Homework behavior problems that are rated as occurring often or very often or appropriate homework behaviors that are rarely observed by teachers may be useful in selecting specific homework-related behaviors to target for intervention (Power, Karustis, & Habboushe, 2001).

In addition to information collected from rating scales, teacher and parent interviews may be conducted to identify specific events in the child's classroom or home setting that are related to the homework problem. Information from teacher interview questions presented in Table 21.8 can be used to assess the student's motivation and ability to do the work at home. Information about common homework assignments may also indicate needed tool skills or useful academic strategies or supports that may be used by the student when completing homework. This information can also be used to help select intervention ideas. For example, identifying effective strategies used by the teacher in the classroom may suggest that these strategies may be similarly effective on homework performance if applied by the parent in the home setting. Information from the parent interview questions presented in Table 21.8 can be used to ascertain whether parents and students may benefit from an organizational intervention. Comparing teacher and parent information may determine whether additional academic supports are required when the parent and student are struggling more than expected or if modification of the communication system is required when important information about the student's progress is not successfully communicated between home and school.

Finally, observing students working on homework assignments can provide information from which to derive a hypothesis about a student's ability to do the work required. For example, children who are struggling with homework assignments could participate in a brief assessment of the impact of powerful

---

TABLE 21.7. Classwide Assessment of Homework Progress

Step 1: Conduct a record review of homework completion and grades in grade book.

Key findings from record review:
- Determine whether the homework completion and homework accuracy is at 80% or more for 80% or more of the class to rule out a classwide problem.
- If many children are not performing as expected, a classwide problem is indicated suggesting a need for a classwide intervention.
- If a classwide problem is ruled out or has been resolved with intervention, assess grade book homework scores to identify at-risk students whose homework is not completed 80% or more of the time at 80% or more correct.

Step 2: For a classwide problem, observe or review current homework routine with the teacher. Table 21.1 may be used to check off use of effective routine steps.

Key findings from review of routine:
- Identify missed or inaccurately implemented effective routine steps that would enhance classwide homework performance.
- Observe students' participation with the routine. Student training on effective steps may be needed when many students are not correctly implementing steps.

TABLE 21.8. Teacher, Parent, School Psychologist, or Consultant Interview Assessment for At Risk Students

Step 1: Conducts a teacher interview to ask questions such as:
- What is the homework problem? (Completion, accuracy?)
- Is there a similar problem on classwork? If not, what works in class?
- What happens *before* you give homework? (Instructions? Guided practice?)
- How do you present the assignments?
- What happens *after* the homework is completed? (Graded? Earns rewards?)
- What is the estimated time to complete work?
- What type of parent support should be needed to complete work?
- How do you communicate with parents about assignments? (Homework Planner?)
- What have you tried to do about changing homework behavior?

Step 2: With teacher, school psychologist, or consultant reviews homework return and grades in the grade book to collect data on any at-risk students' homework performance prior to intervention (i.e., baseline).
  Key findings from the teacher interview:
- Identify effective in-class strategies that parents may also use at home.
- Identify any additional homework support already given to child, in addition to the effective classwide homework routine.
- Identify the type and frequency of feedback given to student and parent on homework completion and accuracy.
- Identify the number and typical type of homework assignments per night or week.

Step 3: Teacher or school psychologist conducts a parent interview to ask questions such as:
- What is the homework problem? (Completion, accuracy?)
- When is homework or work completed accurately?
- What is your current homework routine? (Place? Time of day?)
- What happens during homework? How does your child behave?
- What type of support is needed to complete work?
- What is the estimated time for completion?
- What happens *after* the homework is completed?
- How do you communicate with the teacher? How do you know what homework is assigned? Completed?
- What have you tried to do about changing homework behavior?

  Key findings from the parent interview:
- Identify effective strategies that result in the student's completing homework.
- Identify problem behaviors.
- Estimate amount of support and time needed.
- Identify strengths and weaknesses of current routine.
- Identify the effectiveness of the communication between parent and teacher.

incentives on performance (i.e., performance or skill deficit assessment). Procedures for this type of assessment are described in Table 21.9. These procedures are based on previous research suggesting the utility of this type of assessment in selecting an effective intervention for students who need additional academic supports (Duhon et al., 2004). During the first step of the school performance/skill deficit assessment in Table 21.9, the consultant provides students with a copy of a homework assignment that had been previously administered but had not been completed as expected. Students are told that they can earn a reward of their choice (e.g., earned free time with a peer, lunch with the teacher, small toys, edibles) by exceeding their previous homework score. Students are given the teacher's estimated amount of time needed to complete the assignment. Improved performance following the offer of a reward within an expected score range (e.g., 80–100% accuracy) may suggest that the student has the ability to do the work. A hypothesis about why a homework problem is occurring may be developed based on the outcome of this assessment. First, an assignment that is accurately completed during this type of assessment suggests that the student would benefit from an individual intervention for a motivational deficit. Alternatively, inaccurate work on this assessment suggests that the student has difficulty doing the work and needs support for a skill deficit.

TABLE 21.9. Student Ability Assessment

Step 1: Conduct a school skill/performance deficit assessment with the student.

Ask the student to do a homework assignment in a quiet setting. Before the student works on the assignment, tell the student that he or she will earn an incentive if 80% or more of the work is completed accurately. The incentive is provided if homework is completed within a teacher estimated time and accurate at 80% or more. If the goal is met, then this assessment result suggests a potential *performance deficit*. If the goal is not met, then this assessment result suggests a *skill deficit*.

Step 2: Conduct a curriculum-based assessment of basic skills for reading and math.

For reading, ask the student to read a grade-level reading probe out loud. Record the number of words read correctly. For math, ask the student to complete a sheet of grade-level single and double computation problems (addition, subtraction, multiplication and/or division). Probes are scored as number of digits correct. Scores are compared with local norms and/or instructional or low-risk benchmark scores cited in the literature.

For students who appear to be exhibiting a skill deficit, a second brief assessment of the student's academic basic skill level may be conducted to identify those students who struggle on homework due to low reading and math fluency scores. This assessment, as presented in step 2 of Table 21.9, involves ad-ministering curriculum-based measurement (CBM) assessments that have been used to identify students at risk for severe academic difficulties (Stecker, Fuchs, & Fuchs, 2005). Results from a CBM screening assessment can be used to determine those students who exhibit large differences from typical levels of performance or growth rates in reading or math (Good, Simmons, Kame'enui, Kaminski, & Wallin, 2002; Hintze, Christ, & Methe, 2006; Shinn, 2007; Silberglitt & Hintze, 2007). These students will likely continue to struggle without additional academic support.

The purpose of this assessment is to use information to develop a hypothesis about the reason for the homework problem and to select the type of intervention that is most likely to resolve the homework problem. Table 21.10 summarizes four hypotheses about the type of homework problem that may be developed based on the assessment data described in this section. As presented in this table, a review of a student's performance on homework, a skill/performance assessment, and a curriculum-based assessment of basic skills may be useful for identification of one of four types of homework problems: a classwide problem, an individual performance deficit, and individual academic skills deficit, or an individual tool skill deficit. Knowledge about the function of the homework problem allows the selection of

TABLE 21.10. Data-Based Decisions to Identify Homework Problem and to Select an Intervention that Addresses the Problem

	Types of Homework Problems			
Type of assessment	Classwide problem	Individual performance deficit	Individual academic skill deficit	Individual tool skill deficit
Low homework completion and accuracy	Many students show low homework performance (more than 20%)	Low performance and classmates are performing as expected (80% or more)	Low performance and classmates are performing as expected (80% or more)	Low performance and classmates are performing as expected (80% or more)
School skill/ performance deficit assessment		Meets goals	Does *not* meet goal	Does *not* meet goal
Curriculum-based assessment of basic skills for reading and math		Score falls within expected range for math and reading	Score falls within expected range for math and reading	Score falls *below* expected range for math and/or reading

instructional and environmental strategies that logically resolve the homework problems and facilitates successful homework completion.

Progress Monitoring of Intervention Effects

Once a selected intervention is being used, frequent monitoring and evaluation of student progress are needed to determine the effect of the intervention. Given individual differences in skill acquisition and efficiency, prerequisite skills, practice opportunities, and motivation (Daly et al., 1996; Daly et al., 1997; Malloy et al., 2007), selecting an intervention that does not match the student's needs may not provide the student with adequate support to do the work as expected (Margolis & McCabe, 2004). Progress monitoring allows a teacher to determine when students master a skill and when to modify the intervention if skill mastery is not accomplished. Moreover, evaluation systems that incorporate graphical results, including self-graphing of results, enhance students' progress (Fuchs & Fuchs, 1986).

The behavior to be monitored should be selected carefully. Although it is important to monitor homework completion and return, studies commonly find that an increase in homework completion is not always associated with an increase in homework accuracy. For example, providing incentives for homework accuracy is more effective in increasing academic achievement than providing incentives for homework completion (Miller & Kelley, 1994).

The purpose of homework assignments also influences the development of a progress monitoring system. Homework assignments may be designed to give students opportunities to practice skills taught in class, to master and retain skills, to extend skills to novel situations, and to study for tests. Monitoring student accuracy on these types of tasks (e.g., percent correct) may sufficiently determine successful acquisition and retention of a practiced skill or the ability to generalize skills to novel tasks. Alternatively, assessment of progress on a test may be needed to determine the success of studying activities conducted at home or retention of skills over time. When intervening with students with tool skill deficits, the goal is to obtain mastery on prerequisite skills. For these stu-

dents, CBM procedures can be administered daily or weekly to determine when a student has mastered oral reading or math facts (Daly et al., 1997). Once skills are mastered, the intervention for a tool skill deficit can be terminated, and the student's accuracy on homework assignments will continue to be monitored when given the normal homework requirements (Good et al., 2002; Deno & Mirkin, 1977).

Summary

Homework is an integral part of a student's academic success. It not only provides a student with the opportunities to practice new skills and expand on them but also teaches the student critical organizational skills that can be generalized to many life experiences. School psychologists have the tools to assess homework problems and to implement intervention support to the teacher, parent, and student that will help struggling students find success in the homework process.

References

Anesko, K. M., Schoiock, G., Ramirez, R., & Levine, F. M. (1987). The Homework Problem Checklist: Assessing children's homework difficulties. *Behavioral Assessment*, 9, 179–185.

Binder, C. (1996). Behavioral fluency: Evolution of a new paradigm. *Behavior Analyst*, 19, 163–197.

Blechman, E. A., Taylor, C. J., & Schrader, S. M. (1981). Family problem solving versus home notes as early intervention with high-risk children. *Journal of Consulting and Clinical Psychology*, 49, 919.

Bowen, J., Jenson, W. R., & Clark, E. (2004). *School-based interventions for students with behavior problems*. New York: Kluwer Academic/Plenum Publishers.

Bryan, T., Burstein, K., & Bryan, J. (2001). Students with learning disabilities: Homework problems and promising practices. *Educational Psychologist*, 36, 167–180.

Bryan, T., & Nelson, C. (1994). Doing homework: Perspectives of elementary and junior high school students. *Journal of Learning Disabilities*, 27, 488–499.

Bryan, T., & Sullivan-Burstein, K. (1998). Teacher-selected strategies for improving homework completion. *Remedial and Special Education*, 19, 263–275.

Bursuck, W. D., Harniss, M. K., Epstein, M. H., Polloway, E. A., Jayanthi, M., & Wissinger, L. H. (1999). Solving communication problems about homework: Recommendations of special education teachers. *Learning Disabilities Research and Practice, 14,* 129–140.

Callahan, K., Rademacher, J. A., & Hildreth, B. L. (1998). The effect of parent participation in strategies to improve the homework performance of students who are at risk. *Remedial and Special Education, 19,* 131–141.

Christenson, S. L., Rounds, T., & Gorney, D. (1992). Family factors and student achievement: An avenue to increase students' success. *School Psychology Quarterly, 7,* 178–206.

Cooper, H. (1989). *Homework.* White Plains, NY: Longman.

Cooper, H., Lindsay, J. J., Nye, B., & Greathouse, S. (1998). Relationships among attitudes about homework, amount of homework assigned and completed, and student achievement. *Journal of Educational Psychology, 90,* 70–83.

Cooper, H., & Nye, B. (1994). Homework for students with learning disabilities: Implications of research for policy and practice. *Journal of Learning Disabilities, 27,* 470–479.

Cooper, H., Robinson, J. C., & Patall, E. A. (2006). Does homework improve academic achievement? A synthesis of research. *Review of Educational Research, 76,* 1–62.

Daly, E. J., Lentz, F. E., & Boyer, J. (1996). The Instructional Hierarchy: A conceptual model for understanding the effective components of reading interventions. *School Psychology Quarterly, 11,* 369–386.

Daly, E. J., Witt, J. C., Martens, B. K., & Dool, E. J. (1997). A model for conducting functional analysis of academic performance. *School Psychology Review, 26,* 554–574.

Deno, S. L., & Mirkin, P. K. (1977). *Data-Based Program Modification: A manual.* Reston, VA: Council for Exceptional Children.

Duhon, G., Noell, G., Witt, J., Freeland, J., Dufrene, B., & Gilbertson, D. (2004). Identifying academic skill and performance deficits: An examination of brief and extended assessments. *School Psychology Review, 33,* 429–443.

Dunlap, L. K., & Dunlap, G. (1989). A self-monitoring package for teaching subtraction with regrouping to students with learning disabilities. *Journal of Applied Behavior Analysis, 22,* 309–314.

Epstein, M. H., Munk, D. D., Bursuck, W. D., Polloway, E. A., & Jayanthi, M. (1999). Strategies for improving home–school communication problems about homework for students with disabilities: Perceptions of general educators. *Journal of Special Education, 33*(3), 166–176.

Fishel, M., & Ramirez, L. (2005). Evidence-based parent involvement interventions with school-aged children. *School Psychology Quarterly, 20,* 371–402.

Fuchs, L. S., & Fuchs, D. (1986). Effects of systematic formative evaluation on student achievement: A meta-analysis. *Exceptional Children, 53,* 199–208.

Gajria, M., Jitendra, A. K., Sood, S., & Sacks, G. (2007). Improving comprehension of expository text in students with LD: A research synthesis. *Journal of Learning Disabilities, 40,* 210–225.

Good, R., Simmons, D., Kame'enui, E., Kaminski, R., & Wallin, J. (2002). *Summary of decision rules for intensive, strategic, and benchmark instructional recommendations in kindergarten through third grade* (Tech. Rep. No. 11). Eugene, OR: University of Oregon.

Gortmaker, V. J., Daly, E. J., McCurdy, M., Persampieri, M. J., & Hergenrader, M. (2007). Improving reading outcomes for children with learning disabilities: Using brief experimental analysis to develop parent-tutoring interventions. *Journal of Applied Behavior Analysis, 40,* 203–221.

Hintze, J. M., Christ, T. J., & Methe, S. A. (2006). Curriculum-based assessment. *Psychology in the Schools, 43,* 45–56.

Hoover-Dempsey, K. V., Battiato, A. C., Walker, J. M. T., Reed, R. P., DeJong, J. M. & Jones, K. P. (2001). Parental involvement in homework. *Educational Psychologist, 36,* 195–209.

Hughes, C., Ruhl, K., Schumaker, J., & Deshler, D. (2002). Effects of instruction in assignment completion strategy on the homework performance of students with learning disabilities in general education classes. *Learning Disabilities Research and Practice, 17,* 1–18.

Hundert, J., & Bucher, B. (1978). Pupils' self-scored arithmetic performance: A practical procedure for maintaining accuracy. *Journal of Applied Behavior Analysis, 11,* 304.

Jayanthi, M., Sawyer, V., Nelson, J. S., Bursuck, W. D., & Epstein, M. H. (1995). Recommendations for homework-communication problems: Generated by parents, classroom teachers, and special education teachers. *Remedial and Special Education, 16,* 212–226.

Jenson, W. R., Sheridan, S. M., Olympia, D., & Andrews, D. (1994). Homework and students with learning disabilities and behavior disorders: A practical, parent-based approach. *Journal of Learning Disabilities, 27,* 538–548.

Johnson, K. R., & Layng, T. J. (1992). Breaking the structuralist barrier: Literacy and numeracy with fluency. *American Psychologist, 47,* 1475–1490.

Jurbergs, N., Palcic, J., & Kelley, M. L. (2007).

School–home notes with and without response cost: Increasing attention and academic performance in low-income children with attention-deficit/hyperactivity disorder. *School Psychology Quarterly, 22,* 358–379.

Kahle, A. L., & Kelley, M. L. (1994). Children's homework problems: A comparison of goal setting and parent training. *Behavior Therapy, 25,* 275–290.

Kay, P. J., Fitzgerald, M., Paradee, C., & Mellencamp, A. (1994). Making homework work at home: The parent's perspective. *Journal of Learning Disabilities, 27,* 550–561.

Keith, T. Z., & Keith, P. B. (2006). Homework. In G. G. Bear & K. M. Minke (Eds.), *Children's needs: III. Development, prevention, and intervention* (pp. 615–629). Bethesda, MD: National Association of School Psychologists.

Malloy, K. J., Gilbertson, D., & Maxfield, J. (2007). Use of brief experimental analysis for selecting reading interventions for English-language learners. *School Psychology Review, 36,* 291–310.

Margolis, H., & McCabe, P. P. (2004). Resolving struggling readers' homework difficulties: A social cognitive perspective. *Reading Psychology, 25,* 225–260.

Miller, D. L., & Kelley, M. L. (1994). Interventions for improving homework performance: A critical review. *School Psychology Quarterly, 6,* 174–185.

Murphy, J. J. (1988). Contingency contracting in schools: A review. *Education and Treatment of Children, 11,* 257–269.

Olympia, D. E., Sheridan, S. M., Jenson, W., & Andrews, D. (1994). Using student-managed interventions to increase homework completion and accuracy. *Journal of Applied Behavior Analysis, 27,* 85–99.

Olympia, D. E., Sheridan, S. M., & Jenson, W. R. (1994). Homework: A means of home–school collaboration. *School Psychology Quarterly, 9,* 60–80.

O'Melia, M. C., & Rosenberg, M. S. (1994). Effects of cooperative homework teams on the acquisition of mathematics skills by secondary students with mild disabilities. *Exceptional Children, 60,* 538–548.

Palincsar, A. S., & Brown, A. L. (1984). The reciprocal teaching of comprehension-fostering and comprehension-monitoring activities. *Cognition and Instruction, 1,* 117–175.

Persampieri, M., Gortmaker, V., Daly, E. J., Sheridan, S. M., & McCurdy, M. (2006). Promoting parent use of empirically supported reading interventions: Two experimental investigations of child outcomes. *Behavioral Interventions, 21,* 31–57.

Polloway, E. A., Foley, R. M., & Epstein, M. H. (1992). A comparison of the homework problems of students with learning disabilities and nonhandicapped students. *Learning Disabilities Research and Practice, 7,* 203–209.

Power, T. J., Dombrowski, S. C., Watkins, M. W., Mautone, J. A., & Eagle, J. W. (2007). Assessing children's homework performance: Development of multi-dimensional, multi-informant rating scales. *Journal of School Psychology, 45,* 333–348.

Power, T. J., Karustis, J. L., & Habboushe, D. F. (2001). *Homework success for children with ADHD: A family–school intervention program.* New York: Guilford Press.

Reavis, K., Seeten, M. T., Jenson, W. R., Morgan, D., Andrews, D. J., & Fister, S. (1996). *Best practices: Behavioral and educational strategies for teachers.* Longmont, CO: Sopris West.

Reid, R. (1996). Research in self-monitoring with students with learning disabilities: The present, the prospects, the pitfalls. *Journal of Learning Disabilities, 29,* 317–331.

Rhoades, M. M., & Kratochwill, T. R. (1998). Parent training and consultation: An analysis of a homework intervention program. *School Psychology Quarterly, 13,* 241–264.

Riley-Tillman, T. C., Chafouleas, S. M., & Briesch, A. M. (2007). A school practitioner's guide to using daily behavior report cards to monitor student behavior. *Psychology in the Schools, 44,* 77–89.

Salend, S. J., & Gajria, M. (1995). Increasing the homework completion rates of students with mild disabilities. *Remedial and Special Education, 16,* 271–278.

Sante, A. D., McLaughlin, T. F., & Weber, K. P. (2001). The use and evaluation of a direct instruction flash card strategy on multiplication math facts mastery with two students with developmental disabilities and attention-deficit/hyperactivity disorder. *Journal of Precision Teaching and Celeration, 17,* 68–75.

Sawyer, V., Nelson, J. S., Jayanthi, M., Bursuck, W. D., & Epstein, M. H. (1996). The views of students with learning disabilities of their homework in general education classes: Student interviews. *Learning Disability Quarterly, 19,* 70–85.

Shinn, M. R. (2007). Identifying students at risk, monitoring performance, and determining eligibility within response to intervention: Research on educational need and benefit from academic intervention. *School Psychology Review, 36,* 601–617.

Silberglitt, B., & Hintze, J. M. (2007). How much growth can we expect? A conditional analysis of R-CBM growth rates by level of performance. *Exceptional Children, 74,* 71–84.

Skinner, C. H., McLaughlin, T. F., & Logan, P. (1997). Cover, Copy, and Compare: A self-managed academic intervention effective across skills, students, and settings. *Journal of Behavioral Education, 7*, 295–306.

Stecker, P., Fuchs, L. S., & Fuchs, D. (2005). Using curriculum-based measurement to improve student achievement: Review of research. *Psychology in the Schools, 42*, 795–819.

Strukoff, P. M., McLaughlin, T. F., & Bialozor, R. C. (1987). The effects of a daily report card system in increasing homework completion and accuracy in a special education setting. *Techniques, 3*, 19–26.

Toney, L. P., Kelley, M. L., & Lanclos, N. F. (2003). Self-parental monitoring of homework in adolescents: Comparative effects on parent's perceptions of homework behavior problems. *Child and Family Behavior Therapy, 25*, 35–51.

Trammel, D., Schloss, J., & Alper, S. (1994). Using self recording, evaluation, and graphing to increase completion of homework assignments. *Journal of Learning Disabilities, 27*, 75–81.

Trautwein, U. (2007). The homework–achievement relation reconsidered: Differentiating home-work time, frequency, and effort. *Learning and Instruction, 17*, 372–388.

Vaughn, S., Klingner, J. K., & Bryant, D. P. (2001). Collaborative strategic reading as a means to enhance peer-mediated instruction for reading comprehension and content-area learning. *Remedial and Special Education, 22*, 66–74.

Walberg, H. J. (1991). Productive teaching and instruction: Assessing the knowledge base. In H. C. Waxman & H. J. Walberg (Eds.), *Effective teaching: Current research* (pp. 470–478). Berkeley, CA: McCutchan.

Weiner, R. K., Sheridan, S. M., & Jenson, W. R. (1998). The effects of conjoint behavioral consultation and a structured homework program on math completion and accuracy in junior high students. *School Psychology Quarterly, 13*, 281–309.

Ysseldyke, J., & Elliott, J. (1999). Effective instructional practices: Implications for assessing educational environments. In C. R. Reynolds & T. B. Gutkin (Eds.), *The handbook of school psychology* (pp. 497–518). New York: Wiley.

Chapter 22

Teaching Functional Life Skills to Children with Developmental Disabilities

Acquisition, Generalization, and Maintenance

Ronnie Detrich
Thomas S. Higbee

A developmental disability is a disability that typically is present at birth, such as Down syndrome, but that may also become apparent later (e.g., autism). Developmental disabilities, which can involve cognitive and/or physical impairments, are chronic and present throughout the child's life. A defining characteristic of these students is the failure to acquire functional life skills in the same manner as typically developing children. In most instances these skills must be directly taught. For the purposes of this chapter, we discuss teaching methods for those students with cognitive impairments.

Functional life skills are defined as those skills that are important in the typical contexts in which a student interacts—such as home, school, work, and recreation—and that are likely to be valued and supported by the members of these communities. Examples of these skills include dressing independently, preparing meals for oneself and others, using public transportation to get to work, and maintaining friendships. The goal is for the student to perform these skills as independently as a typically developing student of the same age can (Reid et al., 1985). If the student is not independent, the strategy is to provide the support necessary for the student to be successful. Until the goal

of independence is accomplished, teaching should continue. Life skills are usually divided into domains that reflect the emphasis on skills that are important in different contexts. The domains usually include self-care (dressing), domestic (meal preparation), vocational (working), recreation/leisure, community (using public transportation), functional academics (using a calculator to determine price of items), communication (making wants and needs known to others), and social and self-management (setting an alarm to wake up in time for school or work).

The idea of independence is an important concept in educating students with disabilities. The more a student functions independently, the more competent he or she is perceived to be. For every task that a student with disabilities can perform independently, someone else does not have to assist or perform the task. As a consequence the student may be perceived as (and is) making meaningful contributions to the community by taking care of him- or herself. There are several approaches to assessing and determining which skills to teach that are beyond the scope of this chapter (see Chapter 3 in Snell & Brown, 2000, for a thorough review of assessment). Effective teaching is fundamental to creating independent students. It is necessary to have effective instructional methods so that students learn new skills in the most efficient manner possible.

Teaching

The purpose of this chapter is to describe effective teaching methods that offer the best opportunity for students to become independent. Before we describe specific teaching procedures, a brief discussion of general concepts that guide all instructional practices is warranted. There are three separate phases of effective teaching: (1) acquisition, (2) maintenance, and (3) generalization of the skill being taught. Acquisition describes the process of directly teaching the student until a skill is mastered. This phase receives the most attention in the discussion of instructional methods.

The two remaining phases of effective teaching, maintenance and generalization, are just as important as acquisition. When beginning instruction for a new skill, acquisition is the primary focus; however, maintenance and generalization should be planned for at the same time. Attending to these dimensions of instruction in the beginning will make them more likely to be achieved. Maintenance is the process of ensuring that once a skill is learned the performance remains durable over time, even though direct instruction may have decreased or been terminated.

Generalization occurs when a skill is performed in circumstances that are different from those of the original teaching situation such as with different persons, settings, or behaviors. It is important to develop effective methods to promote generalization, because it is unlikely that instruction during the acquisition phase will encompass all of the settings and environments in which the skill is relevant. Consider the following example. In the course of teaching a student to do laundry, it is necessary that he or she learn to operate a coin-operated washing machine. There are at least two different dimensions that are likely to require generalization across washing machine types (front loading vs. top loading and coins flat vs. coins on edge) if the student is to be able to successfully do laundry. It cannot be as-

sumed that a student will be able to operate a front-loading or coins-flat machine if she or he has been taught on only a top-loading, coins-on-edge machine. It will be necessary to actively promote generalization if the student is to successfully wash clothes regardless of the type of machine.

In the research literature, methods for promoting generalization have received greater attention than maintenance-enhancing strategies. This discrepancy does not reflect the relative importance of the two phases of learning. If behavior generalizes but does not maintain, then the acquisition and generalization of the skill have resulted in no lasting benefit for the student. Although a thorough review of generalization and maintenance strategies is beyond the scope of this chapter, Stokes and Osnes (1988) have provided a nice framework for considering the topic (see also Daly, Barnett, Kupzyk, Hofstadter, & Barkley, Chapter 29, this volume). They outline three principles of generalization: (1) take advantage of natural communities of reinforcement, (2) train diversely, (3) incorporate functional mediators. The principle of taking advantage of natural communities of reinforcement is based on the idea that the environmental contexts in which students live and work will naturally support adaptive behavior once it is established. For example, when a young child learns to speak, the natural community of reinforcement of family, teachers, and friends will respond to most efforts to communicate. When using this principle, special programming for generalization is not required. It is likely that many other functional life skills will maintain and generalize once they have been acquired because others in the student's life will reinforce these behaviors.

The second principle of generalization, training diversely, is based on the notion that teaching across a wide variety of contexts with a large group of teachers and using multiple stimuli is more likely to result in generalization than teaching in which the training situations are narrowly defined, in which instruction is limited to one person, and in which a small array of materials are used as instructional tools. The latter may result in more rapid acquisition but result in limited generalization. Consider the example of teaching a student to shop for items in a grocery store. If the shopping is restricted to one store and a small list of items, one would expect the student to learn where the items are relatively quickly; but if he or she is required to shop at a different store or for different items, he or she may well perform no better than before training. On the other hand, if shopping occurs across a wide variety of stores and across a wider variety of items, initial acquisition of shopping skills may be delayed, but, once mastered, the student will be much more likely to be effective in novel settings.

The final principle of promoting generalization, incorporating functional mediators, relies on the concept of stimulus control in which stimuli associated with training in one setting are likely to occasion relevant behavior in a second setting if they are present. An example would be tying a string around your finger to remind you to do something. The idea is that the string functions as functional mediator and will occasion the behavior in the relevant situation. The same logic applies to promoting generalization for students with developmental disabilities. When students are provided with functional mediators, it is possible for them to perform much more effectively across a variety of situations. In a job setting, it would be possible to arrange a picture task analysis to prompt the student through a job sequence. Similarly, when the student is on break, he or she can be given a list of conversation starters on a series of index cards so that he or she will be more likely to initiate an appropriate conversation to engage coworkers. Each time one of the conversation starters is used, it can be moved from one pocket to another so that the student does not become repetitious. Topics can be expanded and updated over time.

The Learning Trial

There are three components to effective instruction, which are referred to as the *learning trial*: (1) instruction, (2) response, and (3) feedback. The instruction sets the occasion for the student to make some type of response for which feedback will be given. The instructor is responsible for the first and last of these three elements, and how they are approached, in large part, determines the quality of the learning for the student.

The function of the instruction is to specify to the student that a response of a particular type is to occur (e.g., saying, touching, doing). Effective instruction increases the probability of correct responding by the student. Instructions can include both verbal direction from the teacher, such as "brush your teeth," and gestural and physical prompts that guide the student through tooth brushing. Visual presentation of instructional materials such as a toothbrush can also be part of the instruction. In the early phase of acquisition, it is likely that the instruction will involve multiple forms of presentation. As the student's learning increases, the instructor will reduce the components of the instruction until the least prompt necessary to occasion the desired response is in place, such as a picture schedule indicating what comes next. The ultimate goal of instruction is for the student to respond only to naturally occurring cues in the environment and for the teacher's presence to be irrelevant.

The instruction does not have to be identical in form but, rather, should be of the same functional class. A functional class is a set of behaviors that all result in the same consequence. For example, if the goal is to teach a student to respond to greetings, it would be appropriate for the instruction to vary across forms of greetings, such as "hello," "hi," "good morning," and so forth. Because all of these forms of greeting are likely to result in the same response from others, they are considered to be in the same functional class. Early in the training it is likely that the spoken greeting would be paired with a wave of the hand as well. In addition, the student might be verbally instructed as well as physically guided to wave. Over time, the types of instructions and the level of instructions are faded until the only instructions would be a wave on one occasion, a verbal greeting on another, and a combination of the wave and verbal greeting on a third. This approach in the acquisition phase may facilitate generalization as well. Stokes and Baer (1977) describe this method of training loosely as a generalization-promoting strategy.

The response component of the learning trial requires careful consideration before initiating teaching of a skill. The first consideration is what constitutes an acceptable response so that positive feedback can be provided. There is a delicate balance between narrowing the acceptable form of the response so that any variation is unacceptable and having such a broad definition that almost all forms are acceptable. In the example of teaching the greeting response just discussed, there are many acceptable ways to respond to a greeting, including waving, speaking, activating a touch talker (an assistive technology devise which provides programmed speech output when a symbol is touched), or nodding one's head. When determining the response in the learning trial, it is important to consider what forms of the behavior are likely to be reinforced by the student's family, friends, and coworkers. If response forms are selected that are not reinforced by individuals in the student's social environment, the behavior will not maintain or generalize.

The student's abilities are a second consideration in determining the response form. For example, when trying to teach a student with poor fine motor skills to independently dress him- or herself, one should select shoes with Velcro rather than with laces. Requiring a student to perform a task that he or she is physically incapable of or for which he or she has not been taught the prerequisite skills is likely to result in behavior and learning difficulties. The student is likely to engage in problem behavior to escape or avoid the instructional activity or to become emotionally distressed over poor performance. In either instance, student learning will suffer.

The final component of the learning trial is feedback. The primary function of feedback is to increase the probability of correct responses occurring and decrease the probability of errors on subsequent learning trials. Feedback for correct responses is positive reinforcement. It is most effective when delivered immediately following the correct response. Error correction procedures generally involve nonreinforcement for incorrect responses and some type of additional prompting for the correct response. Reinforcement and error correction procedures are described in greater detail in subsequent sections of this chapter.

Opportunities to Respond

Once the three components of the learning trial are well developed, then the teacher must turn attention to the number of opportunities to respond during an instructional period. High rates of opportunities to respond increase the learning rate for students, because there are more opportunities for reinforcement for correct responses and for the shaping of incorrect responses to correct ones. Conversely, low rates of opportunities to respond result in slower learning because feedback occurs at a lower rate. Responding without feedback does little to increase learning. Once a skill has been mastered, practice without feedback may contribute to maintenance of the skill.

Component and Composite Skills

Many of the functional skills that are important to teach are composed of sequences of other, more discrete skills. The broad sequence of skills is referred to as a *composite* skill, and the individual, discrete skills are *component* skills (Johnson & Layng, 1992). If a student is to learn how to make a peanut butter sandwich (composite skill), it will be necessary for the student to learn the component skills of twisting the lid off the jar of peanut butter, opening the bread bag, and spreading the peanut butter with a knife. Until each of these component skills is mastered, the student will not be able to independently make a peanut butter sandwich. These skills can all be taught in the context of making a sandwich, or they can be taught separately and then combined to teach the composite skill of making a peanut butter sandwich. There is no clear agreement within the field about which is the preferable instructional method. Instructional methods are described in greater detail in the sections that follow.

The Teaching Environment

The teaching environment can be conceptualized as a continuum, with community settings as one end point and analogue settings as the other end point and with a series of intermediate environments such as classrooms between the two end points (Cuvo & Davis, 2000). An analogue setting is one such as a classroom in which the teaching materials are approximations of what may be found in a community setting but are not the same. For example, a teacher might arrange a mock intersection in the classroom to teach students the fundamental skills of crossing a street before taking them out to streets in the community. Proponents of analogue settings make the case that there is more control over the instructional environment and that distraction from irrelevant stimuli is minimized, making instruction during the acquisition phase more efficient. It is also argued that more instructional trials are possible in analogue settings so that learning occurs more rapidly. The proponents of community-based training argue that the instruction is more naturalistic and has the advantage of requiring less planning for generalization as the skills are being taught in the relevant setting.

Several studies have examined the effects of community-based training relative to training in analogue settings, and no clear advantage to either community-based or analogue settings has been found (Cuvo & Klatt, 1992; Neef, Iwata, & Page, 1978; Neef, Lensbower, Hockersmith, DePalma, & Gray, 1990; Page, Iwata, & Neef, 1976). It should be noted that the lack of differences between the two training settings was obtained when the training was being conducted and supervised by very skilled researchers. It is not clear whether these same results would have been achieved if implemented in typical settings by the usual staff in these settings. One could make the argument that because there were no differences between training in the two settings, then training should occur in natural settings to minimize issues of programming for generalization. A counterargument is that training in analogue settings may be less expensive and more efficient as more training trials can be completed in an instructional day and less time is spent in transportation to the natural setting where the instruction can occur. Although the efficiency argument is compelling, it is recommended that training occur as much as possible in community-based settings to minimize some of the problems of promoting generalization.

A second reason to teach in community-based settings is that analogue settings do not contain many of the distracting events that are found in the community setting. It is better to teach with the distracting stimuli present from the beginning rather than introducing the distractions later in the training and having them disrupt performance.

Finally, teaching in the community setting is more desirable because students with disabilities are allowed access to the same activities, events, and experiences as peers without disabilities. There are many subtleties of a community-based setting that cannot be replicated in analogue training settings. There may be instances in which it is not feasible to teach in community settings, but the community should be the first option when developing a teaching program.

Basic Principles of Reinforcement

In the discussion of the learning trial, the third component is described as feedback. The feedback given to students for correct responding is positive reinforcement. Reinforcement is the behavioral process by which behavior is strengthened, or made more likely to occur in the future. Positive reinforcement is the behavioral procedure in which the probability that a behavior will occur is increased by virtue of adding or delivering something following that behavior. The positive reinforcer, the "something" added, can be either external to the behavior (e.g., providing a student with access to a preferred activity following correct completion of a self-care task) or the natural environmental product of the behavior itself (getting to go out of an open door following the behavior of turning the door handle and opening the door). Positive reinforcement is a critical component of behavioral teaching procedures.

In addition to being highly effective at producing behavior change, positive reinforcement has a number of desirable side effects. First, students tend to enjoy participating in teaching programs that employ positive reinforcement because their behavior is consistently acknowledged. They may also gain access to preferred objects, activities, or situations (positive reinforcers). A second benefit is that students tend to enjoy working with instructors who deliver positive reinforcement because the instructors come to take on the same value as the reinforcers they deliver. A third benefit of using positive reinforcement is the positive effect that adding reinforcement can have on the overall learning environment. In many cases, if enough positive reinforcement is delivered to students, a decrease in some problem behavior will occur. For instance, if students are receiving a high rate of positive reinforcement in the classroom (e.g., teacher praise and attention), this can reduce problem behaviors exhibited to gain attention.

It is important to remember that reinforcement is defined by its effects. A particular item or activity is a reinforcer only if it effectively increases the future probability of the behavior that it follows. Based on this functional definition of reinforcement, it follows that what is "reinforcing" to one person may not be reinforcing to another. Also, what is "reinforcing" to someone at one point in time might not be at another point. There are no "universal" reinforcers that will always work with all students. For example, although praise and acknowledgment from a teacher or parent might be a powerful reinforcer for many students, it might be completely irrelevant or even punishing to some. Thus it is important to identify a variety of reinforcers for individual students in order for positive-reinforcement-based teaching programs to be successful.

Using Positive Reinforcement Effectively (Dimensions)

The manner in which reinforcement is delivered can influence the effectiveness of positive reinforcement as a teaching procedure. How immediately the reinforcer is delivered following the targeted behavior, the magnitude of reinforcement delivered, and the schedule of reinforcer delivery can determine the success or failure of a positive-reinforcement-based intervention. With regards to immediacy, the general rule of thumb is that positive reinforcement is most effective when it is delivered immediately (within a few seconds) after the targeted behavior. As students are constantly "behaving," if reinforcement is delayed, the teacher may end up inadvertently reinforcing the wrong behavior. Consider a situation in which a teacher is working with a student to teach him or her to follow one-step directions. The teacher gives the instruction "raise your hand," with which the student complies by raising his or her hand. As the teacher turns around to get the preferred item that she or he was planning on delivering, the student begins to wave his or her hand in front of his or her face in self-stimulatory fashion. The teacher then delivers the item along with verbal praise. Even though the teacher intended to reinforce hand raising, it is more likely that she or he reinforced the student's behavior of waving his or her hand in front of his or her face. Thus it is important that tangible reinforcers be readily available so that they can be delivered immediately (within a few seconds) following the desired behavior.

The magnitude, or amount and quality, of reinforcers delivered can also influence the effectiveness of a positive-reinforcement-based teaching procedure. Generally speaking, higher quality and greater amounts of reinforcement will be more effective than lower quality and smaller amounts of reinforcement when teaching new behaviors. Once behaviors have been acquired, the magnitude of reinforcement can often be reduced as part of a behavioral maintenance program. Another guideline to follow is that the magnitude of reinforcement delivered should roughly correspond to the difficulty of the task the student is asked to perform. The more difficult the task, the higher the magnitude of reinforcement that should be delivered when the student correctly completes the task. For example, if sitting down at a desk when given an instruction to do so is an easy task, then periodic delivery of a brief praise or acknowledgement statement such as "thanks for sitting" might be a sufficient reinforcer. In contrast, if a student completes a 10-step hand-washing task for the first time without adult assistance (a difficult task for this student), then a higher quality reinforcer, such as access to a preferred magazine for a few minutes, should be delivered. For more information about how response effort, schedule of reinforcement, and delay in reinforcement can influence responding, see Horner and Day (1991).

Reinforcers can be delivered following every correct student response (a continuous schedule of reinforcement) or following some correct responses (an intermittent schedule). Continuous reinforcement is most effective when teaching new skills, whereas intermittent reinforcement promotes maintenance of skills once they are acquired. Thus, when teaching new behavior to students, the most effective approach would be to start with a continuous schedule and then gradually change to an intermittent schedule once the behavior has been acquired so that the behavior is more likely to be maintained (see Hagopian, Contrucci-Kuhn, Long, & Rush, 2005, for an example of how to fade from a continuous to an intermittent schedule).

Reinforcer Identification Procedures

Behavioral instructional programs provide learners with developmental disabilities with opportunities to practice and acquire important skills. The success or failure of these programs often depends on the quality of reinforcement that is provided for appropriate learner behavior. Identifying effective reinforcers can be the most challenging and important part of the intervention program. Over the past several years, a behavioral technology, called *stimulus preference assessment (SPA)*, has been developed that allows practitioners to identify potentially effective reinforcers for learners with autism and other disabilities. Modern SPA techniques involve systematically providing learners with opportunities to choose between potentially reinforcing items or activities and then measuring their choices. Although there are multiple strategies for conducting preference assessments that may be effective, only the most time-efficient method, the *multiple stimulus without replacement (MSWO)* method, is discussed here.

The MSWO method was first developed by DeLeon and Iwata (1996) and then later streamlined by Carr, Nicholson, and Higbee (2000). In an MSWO assessment, multiple (usually 5–8) items or activities are presented simultaneously in a row (often called a stimulus array) in front of the learner. An instruction to make a selection such as, "Choose the one you want the most," is given, and the student is then allowed to choose between the items or activities by touching or picking up one of them. After making a selection, the individual is allowed to consume or interact with the item or activity for a brief period of time. The selected item is not replaced in the stimulus array, and the remaining items are resequenced by taking the item from the far right of the array, moving it to the far left of the array, and then centering the items in front of the student. The individual is then allowed to make another selection. This process continues until all items have been selected or no

item is selected within a brief period of time (usually 5–10 seconds). Usually, this entire process is repeated three (Carr et al., 2000) to five (DeLeon & Iwata, 1996) times, although comparable results may be obtained in some cases by completing the selection process only once (Carr et al., 2000). A selection percentage is calculated for each item or activity by dividing the number of times an item or activity is selected by the number of times an item or activity was available for selection and multiplying by 100. Items are then ranked according to the selection percentage. It is important to note that selection percentages in the MSWO procedure are used only for ranking stimuli and do not indicate relative preference for each of the items. Researchers suggest that items ranked first in MSWO preference assessments are most likely to function as reinforcers (e.g., Carr et al., 2000; Higbee, Carr, & Harrison, 2000). Data obtained by Daly et al. (in press) and Higbee et al. (2000) also suggest, however, that items ranked second and third may function as reinforcers in many cases.

Carr et al. (2000) attempted to reduce the amount of time required to complete the MSWO assessment by reducing the number of stimulus arrays from five to three. They conducted these "brief" MSWO procedures with three learners with autism and then examined the reinforcing effectiveness of items or activities identified as being high, medium, and low preference by the brief MSWO by delivering these items or activities contingent on learner academic behavior. They found that the brief MSWO procedure accurately predicted reinforcer effectiveness, as contingent delivery of high-, medium-, and low-preference stimuli produced responding that corresponded to the degree of preference. In a secondary analysis, Carr et al. (2000) calculated correlation coefficients for the stimulus rankings produced by learner selections in the first stimulus array with the rankings produced by the combined results of the three arrays and found that the correlations were high, indicating that conducting an MSWO preference assessment with one stimulus array may be sufficient to accurately rank items and activities. The authors reported that the brief MSWO assessments could be completed in 10 minutes or less when three stimulus arrays were used. The time could be further decreased if only one

Student: _____   Assessed by: _____

Date: _____   Time: _____

Stimulus Items	Rank by Trial			Sum of 1, 2, and 3	Overall Rank (smallest sum is #1)
	1	2	3		

FIGURE 22.1. Brief MSWO Preference Assessment data sheet.

stimulus array was used. The brief MSWO assessment data sheet (Figure 22.1) can be used to record and analyze the data from the assessment. For specific guidelines and suggestions for using the brief MSWO procedure, see Higbee (2009).

Issues in Preference Assessments

Preferences have been shown to be relatively stable for some students and to fluctuate greatly for others (Carr et al., 2000). As such, a conservative approach would be to conduct preference assessments at least daily. It would be preferable to complete a preference assessment multiple times per day, such as before each teaching session or when the student's performance starts to deteriorate, if possible. To determine which items to include in the preference assessment, a good strategy is to watch what the student interacts with during "free play." Informal interviews with parents or other caregivers can also provide information about what to include in the assessment. It is important to include new items so that the student is exposed to them during the stimulus sampling procedure. It is also important to keep trying new items in a search for new potential reinforcers.

Researchers suggest that combining edibles and nonedibles in the same preference assessments may be problematic in some cases, as some students tend to select edible items before nonedible items even though the nonedible items may actually function as reinforcers (DeLeon, Iwata, & Roscoe, 1997). Thus, if a student appears to be selecting all of the edible items before the nonedible items, consider whether it may be best to conduct separate preference assessments for edibles and nonedibles.

The use of pictures or symbols instead of actual items or activities has also been investigated (e.g., presenting pairs or arrays of pictures of potential reinforcers and asking learners to choose which one they would most like to earn for working). Presenting potential reinforcers in a verbal forced-choice format (e.g., "Would you like to work for candy or music?") has also been evaluated. Results of research on the use of verbal or picture/symbol-based preference assessments have been mixed, with some studies showing positive effects (e.g., Graff & Gibson, 2003) and others not (e.g., Higbee, Carr, & Harrison, 1999). A critical variable appears to be whether or not access to the chosen item or activity is provided following a selection response. Preference assessments appear to be more accurate when access to the chosen item is provided following a selection response (Tessing, Napolitano, McAdam, DiCesare, & Axelrod, 2006). A second critical variable when considering the use of pictures or symbols in preference assessments is the participant's history of using pictures or symbols to gain access to items. This history appears to be necessary in order for symbols or pictures to be effective in preference assessments. In summary, when possible, it is best to use the actual items or activities in preference assessments. Pictures and symbols or verbal preference assessments should be used with caution until further research determines the conditions under which they can most effectively be used.

General Teaching Methods

The methods of instruction described in this section can be used alone or with other instructional methods to develop new skills for students with disabilities. They have been demonstrated to be effective across a wide range of skills. As all of the methods described here employ positive reinforcement, using the procedures previously described to identify potent reinforcers is of particular importance.

Shaping

Perhaps the most fundamental teaching procedure is shaping, which is defined as the differential reinforcement of successive approximations to a terminal behavior. In other words, reinforcement is initially provided for a behavior that "approximates," or is similar in some form to, the desired behavior. Once that behavior is reliably occurring, the criteria for reinforcement are changed, and the individual must now engage in a behavior that is a closer approximation to the final form of the desired behavior than the initially acceptable behavior. This process of gradually "raising the bar" for reinforcement continues until the desired terminal behavior is reached. For example, suppose a teacher wishes to begin toilet training with one of her students, but the student refuses to enter the bathroom. The teacher might begin by providing reinforcement (e.g., access to a preferred book) for sitting in a chair that is facing the bathroom but is 10 feet away from the door. Once this is occurring reliably, the teacher might move the chair 3 feet closer to the bathroom door, providing reinforcement when the student sits in the chair. The process would be continued as the chair is gradually moved closer and closer to the bathroom until it is placed in

the doorway and then ultimately inside the bathroom. The chair might then be removed and reinforcement provided when the student sits on the toilet with the lid down and his or her pants up, then with the lid up and pants up, then lid up with pants down, and so forth.

One of the principal advantages of shaping is that it encourages participation in the learning activity because the individual comes in contact with reinforcement early in the process and is frequently reinforced for making closer and closer approximations to the target behavior. It is important to remember, however, that the shaping process is not necessarily linear and that adjustments will often need to be made during the shaping process. For example, shaping steps may need to be made smaller or larger depending on how the student is performing. For a detailed description of shaping procedures see Pryor (1999, Ch. 2; "Shaping: Developing Super Performance Without Strain or Pain").

Prompting

Prompting is defined as adding some type of external cue to an instructional situation to increase the probability of a correct response occurring. Prompts fall into three categories: (1) verbal, including signed and written prompts; (2) physical, ranging from partial physical to full physical; and (3) gestural, including modeling. Typically, physical prompts are considered to be the most intrusive and verbal prompts the least intrusive. Often prompts are combined, such as gestural and verbal prompts, to occasion behavior. In any teaching procedure that is selected, some type of prompting of behavior will likely be required so that reinforcement can be delivered. If the student could already perform the skill, then no teaching would be necessary. Prompting is an efficient means of "getting behavior going." The other alternative is to wait for the behavior to occur and then reinforce when it does occur. In classic shaping procedures, this is the approach that is most often used.

There are two general procedures for prompting that can be incorporated when teaching either component skills or composite skills. One approach is a least-to-most prompting sequence. In this approach, the lowest level of prompt is implemented, and then increasingly intrusive prompts are implemented until the desired response occurs. Least-to-most prompting sequences are often used to increase compliance with instructions. An example of instructing a student to throw some trash away is described in the sequence below:

1. Specific verbal direction to throw trash away. Student does not comply.

2. Verbal direction is repeated, and a gestural prompt of pointing toward the garbage is added. Still no compliance by student.

3. Verbal direction with gestural prompt is repeated, along with partial physical prompt of pulling student's chair back from the table. Still no response from the student.

4. Verbal direction with gestural prompt is repeated, and a more intrusive physical prompt of slightly tugging on the student's shirt is added. No response from student.

5. Verbal direction with gestural prompt is repeated, and a full physical prompt of lifting the student from the chair and guiding him or her to the garbage can is added. At this point, student complies.

Depending on where the student is in the teaching sequence, reinforcement can be added at any point of the sequence as compliance occurs. Often reinforcement is reserved for those occasions in which compliance occurs at the first step.

The other approach is to move from most-to-least prompts in which the highest level of prompt necessary to occasion behavior is implemented and then faded to less intrusive forms of prompts. This sequence is often used to teach a wide variety of self-care skills for students with developmental disabilities. An example of this procedure follows. The skill being taught is applying toothpaste to a toothbrush. The student has no ability with respect to this skill, so full physical prompts and visual prompts are used.

1. Instructor models the skill by placing an appropriate amount of toothpaste on a toothbrush while student observes. Using full physical guidance, the student is prompted to squeeze an appropriate amount onto his or her toothbrush. This level of prompting is continued until the student reliably applies an appropriate amount of toothpaste that matches the amount on the model toothbrush prepared by the instructor.

2. The next step in the prompting sequence is a partial physical prompt, in addition to the visual model of the toothbrush. In this sequence the student applies the toothpaste with the instructor's hands very close to the student's, shadowing the student's movements so that if another partial prompt is required it can occur at the moment the student is performing the task. When an appropriate amount has been dispensed, the instructor guides the student to put the toothbrush down.

3. The next step is to fade from the partial physical prompt to simply providing the model toothbrush with the appropriate amount of toothpaste on it. The student is verbally directed to put toothpaste on the toothbrush. Once the student is reliably performing this step, then the prompt is again faded.

4. The next step in the sequence is to eliminate the visual model of the toothbrush and place a toothbrush and toothpaste in front of the student, instructing the student to put toothpaste on it. When the student is consistently performing this step, the prompt is again faded.

5. In this step, as the toothbrush and toothpaste are placed in front of the student, the instructor gives the indirect verbal prompt, "What do you do next?" When the student is consistent at this level, the indirect verbal prompt is faded.

6. The last step in this prompting sequence is to place the toothbrush and toothpaste in front of the student and wait for the student to respond. The student will have mastered this component of the toothbrushing task when the toothpaste is applied to criterion level across a specified number of trials.

When using the most-to-least method of prompting, reinforcement is provided if the student responds correctly to the instructional prompt.

With the most-to-least method, it is likely that the student will make response errors or fail to respond on some occasion. On these occasions, some type of error correction is required. In many instances the appropriate error correction is to use the next most intrusive prompt in the sequence to occasion correct responding. This error correction prompt may be the prompt used previously for correct responding before fading to a less intrusive prompt. Reinforcement should not be provided if correct responding occurs with the error correction. Once the error correction has produced the correct response, then the instructor should move on to the next trial so that reinforcement is once again available when correct responding occurs.

Regardless of which prompting method is used, it is necessary to remove all external prompts before the student can be considered to be independent. Toward that end, when a teaching plan is initially developed, prompt fading should be a component of the plan. The prompt fading plan should include clear specification of the criteria for changing the prompt level, the next prompt in the fading plan, and criteria for returning to a previous prompt level if performance deteriorates. Typically, the criteria for fading to the next prompt are specified as number of consecutive correct trials over a specified time period.

Ultimately, the prompting plan and prompt fading plan have to be individualized with a specific student and skill in mind. There is no universal sequence of prompts that can always be followed. There are several considerations when selecting the prompting method, the specific sequence of prompts, and the fading plan. In terms of selecting a prompting procedure, the most-to-least sequence is most commonly used to teach self-care skills. The specific sequence of prompts depends on the skill being taught and characteristics of the student. If a student is uncomfortable being touched, it may be unwise to include physical prompts. Similarly, if the student has limited vision or hearing, visual and auditory prompts will be ineffective. The characteristics of the student may limit the types of prompts that can be used, but they are not limits to effective instruction. For a more comprehensive discussion of prompting, please see Snell and Brown (2000, Ch. 4). In Figure 22.2 there is an instruction data sheet that allows the instructor to define the current instructional prompt, as well as the correction prompt. This form allows for quick analysis of the effectiveness of the teaching plan.

Task Analysis

Many of the functional skills that we want to teach involve a complex sequence of steps. A task analysis is not a teaching method but rather a method for organizing how to sequence the instructional process. In the preceding section, we used applying toothpaste to a toothbrush to demonstrate how to use a most-to-least prompting sequence. Applying toothpaste is a component skill of the larger skill of toothbrushing and is of little value if the student cannot perform the remaining steps in the sequence.

There are several methods for developing a task analysis, with various levels of effort required of the instructor to generate the list of component steps (Bailey & Wolery, 1984; Horner & Keilitz, 1975; Moyer & Dardig, 1978; Wilson, Reid, Phillips, & Burgio, 1984). Perhaps the simplest method is for the instructor to perform the task and to note each discrete form of behavior that occurs (Moyer & Dardig, 1978). It is wise to perform the task several times to ensure that as many of the steps as possible are identified. It is likely that the some of the steps will have to be broken down into more discrete steps for the purposes of instruction. It is important to note the steps in as small units as possible. Following is an example of a task analysis for toothbrushing:

1. Pick up toothbrush by the handle with dominant hand.
2. Turn on cold water with other hand.
3. Holding toothbrush, place bristles of toothbrush under the water.
4. Turn off water.
5. Put toothbrush down.
6. Pick up tube of toothpaste.
7. Take cap off toothpaste.
8. Pick up toothbrush.
9. Hold toothbrush in one hand and toothpaste in other.
10. Apply appropriate amount of toothpaste onto the bristles of the brush.
11. Put toothbrush down.
12. Put cap back on toothpaste.
13. Pick up toothbrush.
14. Bring toothbrush to mouth and brush front outside surface of teeth.
15. Brush back outside surface of teeth on left side.

Instructions

1. In the section labeled *Task*, write in sequence the steps of the task analysis.
2. Next to each step, under column labeled *P*, list the type of teaching prompt that is currently being used, such as partial physical prompt. This is the level of prompting at which reinforcement is provided if the student responds correctly.
3. In the column labeled *C*, list the type of prompt that is to be used if the student does not respond correctly when the teaching prompt is used. If the teaching prompt is a partial physical prompt, then the correction prompt may be a full physical prompt.
4. The numbers across the top correspond to the number of teaching trials that have been conducted. They are noted by the date above each number. There may be more than one teaching trial per day. Each time a correct response occurs, mark a (+) in the correct column and row. Each time an incorrect response occurs, mark (−).
5. Depending on the instruction procedure being used, data can be calculated as percent correct per teaching trial or percent correct for each step in the sequence. To calculate percent correct per teaching trial, count the number of steps that were scored correct and divide by the number of steps. To score percent correct for each step, count the number scored correct across the teaching trials for each step and divide by the number of trials that were conducted. On the data sheet it is possible to score 10 trials.

Data Sheet

	Date											
	Initial											
TASK	*P*	*C*	*1*	*2*	*3*	*4*	*5*	*6*	*7*	*8*	*9*	*10*

FIGURE 22.2. Teaching Data sheet.

16. Brush back outside surface of teeth on right side.
17. Position toothbrush to brush inside surface of the teeth.
18. Brush front inside surface.
19. Brush back inside surface on left side.
20. Brush back inside surface on right side.
21. Put toothbrush down.
22. Turn on cold water.
23. Fill cup with water.
24. Turn off water.
25. Bring cup to mouth.
26. Take water into the mouth and rinse.
27. Spit water into the sink.
28. Pick up towel.
29. Wipe mouth.
30. Replace towel.
31. Place toothbrush and toothpaste in proper location.

As can be seen in this example, there are many discrete steps. In some instances the sequence is important, and in other instances the sequence is not. For example, placing the cap back on the toothpaste could be one of the last steps in the sequence, and filling the rinse cup could occur right after wetting the toothbrush. It is also likely that some of the steps will have to be reduced to even more discrete steps for the purposes of teaching. Teaching a student to rinse may require teaching the student to gargle and swish the water around in the mouth rather than swallowing it.

As a means of increasing the maintenance and generalization of the toothbrushing, picture prompts can be used in which the student is taught to follow the picture sequence when brushing his or her teeth. The picture sequence functions as the task analysis and can be used concurrently with other types of prompts to increase the probability of the student's completing each step. Time delay can also be incorporated into the teaching sequence with the picture prompts. Once a picture is presented, the instructor waits for a specified length of time before providing another prompt. The goal is for the student to become independent of adult prompts, with the picture prompts functioning as a common salient stimulus to facilitate toothbrushing in any setting in which it is required. The picture prompts can remain in place indefinitely and be used in the same

way that many of us use appointment books to manage our behavior.

Establishing Behavioral Chains

One method for teaching the skills identified in a task analysis is to consider them as a chain of behaviors, with each step in the sequence occasioning the next step. In the preceding task analysis of toothbrushing, there is a defined sequence of component skills that compose the composite skill of toothbrushing. Behavioral chains can be taught as forward chains in which the sequence of skills is taught from the first to the last component. The alternative is to teach in a backward chain, in which the last component skill in the sequence is taught first and then the next to last and so on until the entire sequence is taught. Both forward and backward chaining have been used to teach a variety of functional life skills. There is no compelling evidence to favor one method over the other (Bellamy, Horner, & Inman, 1979).

The primary advantage of backward chaining is that the student performs the last response in the chain first and immediately receives reinforcement for completing the sequence. For instance, when teaching shoe tying, the instructor would perform all of the steps except pulling the laces tight. The student is required to pull the laces tight as the last response in the chain. Once the laces are tightened, the student is praised for tying her shoes and allowed to go outside to play. Once the student has mastered pulling the laces tight, then pulling a loop through the lace and pulling the laces tight will be taught. Because the student has already mastered tightening the laces, getting to this step will function as a reinforcer for pulling the loop through the laces, and tightening the laces is reinforced by praise and going outside to play.

The primary advantage of forward chaining is that the task is taught in the sequence in which it typically occurs, and it may be that the student can perform some of the steps without explicit training. In forward chaining, it is possible to provide social reinforcement for each step correctly performed so that the student receives high rates of reinforcement during each instructional trial.

After completing a task analysis, a decision must be made about which chaining method to use. One step at a time can be systematically taught while the instructor guides the student through the rest of the sequence. This method can be used with either backward or forward chaining procedures. A total task approach is utilized only with the forward chaining method. In this approach, systematic teaching is used for each step of the sequence, and all steps are taught during each instructional session. Typically, total task approaches are used when the sequence is relatively short. The advantage is that each time teaching occurs, all steps are taught, which may result in getting to independence more quickly. However, more effort is required from the student when longer sequences of component steps are taught. This may result in increased resistance from the student toward instruction. Teaching one component at a time may reduce the overall effort required of the student during an instructional session.

When using chaining to teach a skill, it is likely that prompting will be incorporated into the instructional plan. Prompting facilitates the student's mastering of each step of the sequence and ultimately his or her being able to perform the entire skill independently. It is likely that various prompt levels will be necessary for different steps within the total task presentation sequence. One of the disadvantages of the total task presentation is that the instructor must keep in mind the appropriate prompt level and sequence for each component step in the chain. Teaching only one component step at a time may be easier for the instructor to implement, because it is necessary to remember only one prompt during an instructional session.

Instructional Methods

In this section we describe specific methods for instruction that have been used to teach a wide variety of skills across all of the domains of functional life skills.

Discrete Trial Teaching

Discrete trial teaching (DTT) is an effective, research-based technique for teaching students new skills (see Remington et al., 2007, as a recent example of the positive outcomes produced by DTT). Although it has received a significant amount of attention recently as an intervention strategy for students with autism, it has also been shown to be effective with students with other types of disabilities (e.g., cerebral palsy, communication delays, cognitive delays; Downs, Downs, Johansen, & Fossum, 2007). The basic logic of DTT involves presenting students with repeated opportunities to practice specific skills and to receive feedback and reinforcement from an instructor based on their performances. These opportunities to practice skills and receive feedback and reinforcement are called "discrete trials." The basic structure of each discrete trial is as follows: (1) the teacher obtains the student's attention, (2) the teacher presents an instruction, (3) the teacher waits for the student to respond to the direction and provides additional assistance in the form of prompts if necessary, and (4) the teacher provides a consequence based on how the student responds (reinforcement for correct responses, corrective feedback for incorrect responses).

It is important to gain the student's attention before delivering an instruction, both to increase the probability that the student will respond correctly and to allow the instructor to differentiate between errors made because the student was not paying attention or because he or she does not know how to perform the correct response. Eye contact, either with the instructor or with the instructional materials, has commonly been used as a means of determining whether a student is attending and is ready to receive an instruction. Whereas some students may readily give eye contact, others may need prompting to do so. Various strategies, including saying the student's name, giving a light touch to the cheek, or giving an attending instruction such as "look," have been used to gain eye contact (see Higbee, 2009, for a detailed discussion of methods of teaching attending skills).

Once the student is paying attention, the next step in DTT is to provide the student with an instruction and an opportunity to respond. When teaching new skills to students, instructions need to be simplified to promote correct responding (e.g., "brush teeth" instead of "Can you please come over here and brush your teeth?"). Once the student is consistently responding correctly to the instruction, it can be made more complex and naturalistic. It is important to avoid repeating instructions in DTT. Each instruction is presented only once, and a consequence must be provided before the student is given another opportunity to respond. This teaches students that it is important to pay attention to the first instruction rather than waiting for it to be repeated. As a general rule, students should be allowed up to 5 seconds to respond to the instruction.

The student can give one of three responses to an instruction: correct, incorrect, or no response (which is also incorrect). Following a correct response, the instructor should provide praise, as well as additional reinforcement based on the needs of the student. Incorrect or nonresponses can be given a variety of different consequences depending on the individual student. One approach is to provide brief verbal feedback using a neutral phrase such as "try again." Another approach is to avoid saying anything, break eye contact for a few seconds, and then represent the next instructional trial. Error correction procedures in which the student is prompted to make the correct response can also be added to either approach. Recent research by Worsdell and colleagues (2005) suggests that error correction procedures in which the student is prompted to repeat the correct response several times in succession may be more effective than repeating the correct response once.

Although DTT has often been used in relatively sterile, highly structured instructional environments in which distractions are minimized for the student, such an environment is not a requirement of this approach. DTT can be used to teach a variety of skills in educational, vocational, leisure, and home environments. Strategies to promote generalization of skills learned through structured DTT teaching include: practicing the skill in multiple locations, including the contextually appropriate location for using the skill (e.g., after learning to identify coins in a DTT preparation, practice selecting the appropriate coins for use in a vending machine); practicing the skill with multiple instructors; and using multiple examples during teaching (e.g., when teaching an individual to recognize restroom signs, use several different restroom signs as examples, including text signs and symbol signs).

One important strategy for promoting maintenance of skills learned during DTT is called *interspersal*. Interspersal involves mixing trials of skills that have been mastered with trials of new skills. It has the dual purpose of keeping the student in contact with reinforcement by providing him or her with opportunities to respond to skills he or she has mastered while simultaneously providing additional practice on the mastered skill to promote maintenance. Research on interspersal has shown that once a skill has been mastered, fewer trials are required to maintain it at acceptable levels of performance (Neef, Iwata, & Page, 1977, 1980).

Incidental Teaching

Incidental teaching is often characterized as child-led instruction (Hart & Risley, 1975; Koegel, Koegel, & Surratt, 1992) and has also been described as naturalistic teaching (Laski, Charlop, & Schreibman, 1988). Instruction is embedded into naturally occurring routines and interactions with adults, such as mealtimes and play periods. The instruction is considered to be child-led because the instruction occurs during an activity in which the child is showing interest and is already participating. Because of the child's interest in the activity, it is possible that the child's motivation is very high, so some of the problems of reinforcer identification are minimized. For example, if a child picks up a car during play, many goals can be taught using the car as the stimulus for teaching. The adult can briefly block play until the child names the color of the car, identifies whether it is large or small relative to another toy, or identifies the shape of the wheels. Similarly, if the goal is to learn to tie shoes, then each time the student goes outside, he must change into outside shoes and practice tying the laces. The reinforcer is going outside. The chaining and prompting methods described earlier can be incorporated into the teaching to ensure efficient learning.

The term *incidental teaching* can be a bit misleading in that it can be interpreted as a laissez-faire approach in which adults just wait around for the child to show an interest in an activity or routine. Effective incidental teaching encourages a high level of engagement by setting up the environment with interesting materials for the student. Different activities and routines can be arranged to teach specific skills. The activities and materials that are available to the student are selected with the instructional goals in mind and are routinely changed to facilitate generalization of the skill across different stimuli. For example, if the goal is to teach a child to ask for help, the environment can be set up in several ways to increase the motivation to ask for help. Preferred materials can be placed out of reach; tasks that require the assistance of a second person, such as moving something heavy, can be assigned; preferred items can be placed inside a jar with the lid on so tightly that the student cannot open it without assistance; and doors and cabinets can be locked so that it will be necessary for the student to ask for help to gain access. All of these efforts can be seen as increasing the motivation for the student to gain access to preferred activities for which only effective means is to ask for help.

One of the demands on the instructor using incidental teaching is to identify relevant "teachable moments." The task of the instructor is twofold. First, the instructor must provide the appropriate level of prompting and coaching to ensure student success at the task. This requires the instructor to be aware of where the student is in the instructional process on all of the skills that are being taught and to be able to provide the current teaching prompt and error correction if necessary. The second task for the instructor is to briefly obstruct access to preferred activities and routines until the correct performance has been demonstrated. If the obstruction lasts too long or the response requirement is too great, the student is likely to engage in problem behavior associated with the loss of reinforcement.

Although incidental teaching may minimize motivational issues, one of the challenges that instructors face with incidental teaching is ensuring that a sufficient number of learning trials occurs so that a skill can be learned as quickly as possible. One approach is to use analogue instructional methods such as discrete trial training to facilitate initial acquisition of the skill and then use incidental teaching methods to facilitate maintenance and generalization.

Incidental teaching effectively promotes generalization because many of the stimuli used during instruction are encountered across settings and contexts (Hart & Risley, 1980; McGee, Krantz, & McClannahan, 1985). The nature of incidental teaching minimizes the need for planning for generalization. Regardless of the teaching method selected for initial acquisition, at some point the teaching must move to the natural environment, and the methods of incidental teaching will become relevant.

Video Modeling

Video modeling is an instructional technique that is being used more commonly with individuals with autism and other developmental disabilities. In video modeling interventions, footage is created that depicts one or more individuals engaging effectively in a sequence of behaviors (the video model). The learner views the videotape or DVD and is given the opportunity to imitate the behavioral sequence. Video modeling procedures have been used to successfully teach learners with autism and related disabilities a variety of skills, including perspective taking (e.g., Charlop-Christy & Daneshvar, 2003), language (e.g., Charlop & Milstein, 1989), daily living skills (e.g., Charlop-Christy, Le, & Freeman, 2000), play (e.g., D'Ateno, Mangiapanello, & Taylor, 2003), and academic skills (Kinney, Vedora, & Stromer, 2003). Researchers have shown that participants rapidly acquire the target skills and demonstrate skill maintenance over long periods of time (e.g., Charlop & Milstein, 1989).

Technological advances have made video modeling more accessible by decreasing the cost and level of expertise necessary for creating video models (e.g., Charlop-Christy et al., 2000). All that is now required is a digital video camera and a computer with a DVD burner and basic video editing software (often included in software packages shipped with new computers). Of course, sufficient time, patience, and motivation to learn how to use the camera and video editing software are also required.

In addition to cost- and time-effectiveness, there may be several potential advantages to using video models to teach students with disabilities. One potential advantage is the systematic repetition and consistency of instruction that can be provided by having the learner view the same video model numerous times (Charlop & Milstein, 1989; Taylor, Levin, & Jasper, 1999) in contrast to using *in vivo* modeling, which can include small behavioral variations in the performance of the live models each time the target behavior is modeled for the learner. Video models can conveniently employ strategies that help promote generalization, such as programming multiple exemplars, incorporating common stimuli, and training using natural contingencies and environments by arranging these instructional features in the creation of the video model (e.g., Charlop & Milstein, 1989). Finally, videotaping may also facilitate the use of a variety of models that might not be available for repeated live modeling trials, such as typical peers (Nikopoulos & Keenan, 2003), siblings (Taylor et al., 1999), and the learner him- or herself (Wert & Neisworth, 2003).

Evaluating Progress

Inherent in effective instruction is the systematic evaluation of student progress. Ongoing measurement helps practitioners optimize their effectiveness and ensures that teaching programs are not terminated prematurely because subtle improvements in student performance are not readily apparent nor continued indefinitely when the student is clearly not making sufficient progress.

As the range of skills falling under the heading of "functional life skills" is quite broad, no one data collection system would be universally appropriate. Critical features of high-quality data collection systems allow the practitioner to track the accuracy of student performance and his or her level of independence (e.g., prompt levels). As important as it is to collect data on student behavior, it is useful only to the extent that it is analyzed and used to inform practice. Accurate data collection is a means to an end and not an end unto itself. Graphical data displays, particularly line graphs, can help practitioners to make sense of their data and make appropriate data-based decisions. Whether graphs are created using computer software

or handwritten is relatively unimportant, so long as the data are accurately represented in a way that allows the practitioner to evaluate the level (in general, how high or low the data are), trend (the general slope up or down in the data), and variability (the "bounce" or range of scores) in the data. See Daly et al., Chapter 29, this volume, for a more detailed discussion of evaluating outcomes, including summarizing data.

Conclusion

In this chapter we have tried to highlight the fact that effective instruction for students with disabilities requires consistent and systematic instruction that takes advantage of one or more of the methods described. The constant across all methods is that reinforcement has to be consistently provided for approximations to correct responses if learning is to progress. There are many variants to the methods that we have described in this chapter. They reflect that, ultimately, instructional methods have to be adapted to the individual student and the circumstances in which the student is being instructed. Effective instruction involves continuous evaluation and revision until the student is making measurable progress toward the greatest level of independence possible. If there is no progress, then there has been no teaching.

References

Bailey, D. B., & Wolery, M. (1984). *Teaching infants and preschoolers with handicaps*. Columbus, OH: Merrill.

Bellamy, G. T., Horner, R. H., & Inman, D. P. (1979). *Vocational habilitation of severely retarded adults: A direct service technology*. Baltimore: University Park Press.

Carr, J., Nicholson, A., & Higbee, T. (2000). Evaluation of a brief multiple-stimulus preference assessment in a naturalistic context. *Journal of Applied Behavior Analysis, 33*, 353–357.

Charlop, M. H., & Milstein, J. P. (1989). Teaching autistic children conversational speech using video modeling. *Journal of Applied Behavior Analysis, 22*, 275–285.

Charlop-Christy, M. H., & Daneshvar, S. (2003). Using video modeling to teach perspective taking to children with autism. *Journal of Positive Behavior Interventions, 5*, 12–21.

Charlop-Christy, M. H., Le, L., & Freeman, K. A. (2000). A comparison of video modeling with in vivo modeling for teaching children with autism. *Journal of Autism and Developmental Disorders, 30,* 537–552.

Cuvo, A. J., & Davis, P. K. (2000). Behavioral acquisition by persons with developmental disabilities. In J. Austin & J. E. Carr (Eds.), *Handbook of applied behavior analysis* (pp. 39–60). Reno, NV: Context Press.

Cuvo, A. J., & Klatt, K. P. (1992). Effects of community-based, videotape, and flash card instruction of community-referenced sight words on students with mental retardation. *Journal of Applied Behavior Analysis, 25*(2), 499–512.

D'Ateno, P., Mangiapanello, K., & Taylor, B. A. (2003). Using video modeling to teach complex play sequences to a preschooler with autism. *Journal of Positive Behavior Interventions, 5,* 5–11.

Daly, E. J., III, Wells, J. N., Swanger-Gagne, M., Carr, J. E., Kunz, G. M., & Taylor, A. M. (in press). Evaluation of the multiple-stimulus without replacement stimulus preference assessment method using activities as stimulus events. *Journal of Applied Behavior Analysis.*

DeLeon, I., & Iwata, B. (1996). Evaluation of a multiple-stimulus presentation format for assessing reinforcer preferences. *Journal of Applied Behavior Analysis, 29,* 519–533.

DeLeon, I., Iwata, B., & Roscoe, E. (1997). Displacement of leisure reinforcers by food during preference assessments. *Journal of Applied Behavior Analysis, 30,* 475–484.

Downs, A., Downs, R. C., Johansen, M., & Fossum, M. (2007). Using discrete trial teaching within a public preschool program to facilitate skill development in students with developmental disabilities. *Education and Treatment of Children, 30,* 1–27.

Graff, R., & Gibson, L. (2003). Using pictures to assess reinforcers in individuals with developmental disabilities. *Behavior Modification, 27,* 470–483.

Hagopian, L. P., Contrucci-Kuhn, S. A., Long, E. S., & Rush, K. S. (2005). Schedule thinning following communication training: Using competing stimuli to enhance tolerance to decrements in reinforcer density. *Journal of Applied Behavior Analysis, 38,* 177–193.

Hart, B., & Risley, T. R. (1975). Incidental teaching of language in the preschool. *Journal of Applied Behavior Analysis, 8,* 411–420.

Hart, B., & Risley, T. R. (1980). In vivo language intervention: Unanticipated general effects. *Journal of Applied Behavior Analysis, 13*(3), 407–432.

Higbee, T. S., Carr, J., & Harrison, C. (1999). The effects of pictorial versus tangible stimuli in stimulus preference assessments. *Research in Developmental Disabilities, 20,* 63–72.

Higbee, T. S., Carr, J., & Harrison, C. (2000). Further evaluation of the multiple-stimulus preference assessment. *Research in Developmental Disabilities, 21,* 61–73.

Higbee, T. S. (2009). Reinforcer identification strategies and teaching learner readiness skills. In R. A. Rehfeldt & Y. Barnes-Holmes (Eds.), *Derived relational responding: Applications for learners with autism and other developmental disabilities.* Oakland, CA: New Harbinger Publications.

Horner, R. D., & Keilitz, I. (1975). Training mentally retarded adolescents to brush their teeth. *Journal of Applied Behavior Analysis, 8*(3), 301–309.

Horner, R. H., & Day, H. M. (1991). The effects of response efficiency on functionally equivalent competing behaviors. *Journal of Applied Behavior Analysis, 24,* 719–732.

Johnson, K. R., & Layng, T. V. (1992). Breaking the structuralist barrier: Literacy and numeracy with fluency. *American Psychologist, 47*(11), 1475–1490.

Kinney, E. M., Vedora, J., & Stromer, R. (2003). Computer-presented video models to teach generative spelling to a child with an autism spectrum disorder. *Journal of Positive Behavioral Interventions, 5,* 22–29.

Koegel, R. L., Koegel, L. K., & Surratt, A. (1992). Language intervention and disruptive behavior in preschool children with autism. *Journal of Autism and Developmental Disorders, 22*(2), 141–153.

Laski, K. E., Charlop, M. H., & Schreibman, L. (1988). Training parents to use the natural language paradigm to increase their autistic children's speech. *Journal of Applied Behavior Analysis, 21*(4), 391–400.

McGee, G. G., Krantz, P. J., & McClannahan, L. E. (1985). The facilitative effects of incidental teaching on preposition use by autistic children. *Journal of Applied Behavior Analysis, 18*(1), 17–31.

Moyer, J. R., & Dardig, J. C. (1978). Practical task analysis for special educators. *Teaching Exceptional Children, 11*(1), 16–18.

Neef, N. A., Iwata, B. A., & Page, T. J. (1977). The effects of known-item interspersal on acquisition and retention of spelling and sight-reading words. *Journal of Applied Behavior Analysis, 10*(4), 738.

Neef, N. A., Iwata, B. A., & Page, T. J. (1978). Public transportation training: In vivo versus classroom instruction. *Journal of Applied Behavior Analysis, 11*(3), 331–344.

Neef, N. A., Iwata, B. A., & Page, T. J. (1980). The effects of interspersal training versus high-density reinforcement on spelling acquisition and retention. *Journal of Applied Behavior Analysis, 13*(1), 153–158.

Neef, N. A., Lensbower, J., Hockersmith, I., De-Palma, V., & Gray, K. (1990). In vivo versus simulation training: An interactional analysis of range and type of training exemplars. *Journal of Applied Behavior Analysis, 23*(4), 447–458.

Nikopoulos, C. K., & Keenan, M. (2003). Promoting social initiations in children with autism using video modeling. *Behavioral Interventions, 18*, 87–108.

Page, T. J., Iwata, B. A., & Neef, N. A. (1976). Teaching pedestrian skills to retarded persons: Generalization from the classroom to the natural environment. *Journal of Applied Behavior Analysis, 9*(4), 433–444.

Pryor, K. (1999). *Don't shoot the dog! The new art of teaching and training.* New York: Bantam Books/Random House.

Reid, D. H., Parsons, M. B., McCarn, J. E., Green, C. W., Phillips, J. F., & Schepis, M. M. (1985). Providing a more appropriate education for severely handicapped persons: Increasing and validating functional classroom tasks. *Journal of Applied Behavior Analysis, 18*(4), 289–301.

Remington, B., Hastings, R. P., Kovshoff, H., Espinosa, F. D., Jahr, E., Brown, T., et al. (2007). Early intensive behavioral intervention: Outcomes for children with autism and their parents after two years. *American Journal on Mental Retardation, 112*, 418–438.

Snell, M. E., & Brown, F. (2000). *Instruction of students with severe disabilities* (5th ed.). Upper Saddle River, NJ: Merrill.

Stokes, T. F., & Baer, D. M. (1977). An implicit technology of generalization. *Journal of Applied Behavior Analysis, 10*(2), 349–367.

Stokes, T. F., & Osnes, P. G. (1988). The developing applied technology of generalization and maintenance. In G. Dunlap, R. H. Horner, & R. L. Koegel (Eds.), *Generalization and maintenance: Life-style changes in applied settings* (pp. 5–19). Baltimore: Brookes.

Taylor, B., Levin, L., & Jasper, S. (1999). Increasing play-related statements in children with autism toward their siblings: Effects of video modeling. *Journal of Developmental and Physical Disabilities, 11*, 253–264.

Tessing, J., Napolitano, D., McAdam, D., DiCesare, A., & Axelrod, S. (2006). The effects of providing access to stimuli following choice making during vocal preference assessments. *Journal of Applied Behavior Analysis, 39*, 501–506.

Wert, B. Y., & Neisworth, J. T. (2003). Effects of video self-modeling on spontaneous requesting in children with autism. *Journal of Positive Behavioral Interventions, 5*, 30–34.

Wilson, P. G., Reid, D. H., Phillips, J. F., & Burgio, L. D. (1984). Normalization of institutional mealtimes for profoundly retarded persons: Effects and noneffects of teaching family-style dining. *Journal of Applied Behavior Analysis, 17*(2), 189–201.

Worsdell, A., Iwata, B. A., Dozier, C. L., Johnson, A. D., Neidert, P. L., & Thomason, J. L. (2005). Analysis of response repetition as an error-correction strategy during sight-word reading. *Journal of Applied Behavior Analysis, 38*, 511–527.

Chapter 23

Parents and School Psychologists as Child Behavior Problem-Solving Partners

Helpful Concepts and Applications

Patrick C. Friman
Jennifer L. Volz
Kimberly A. Haugen

Healthy socialized and optimally educated behavior is the primary goal of childhood. For the first 2 or 3 years of life, parents, with the periodic aid of child medical providers, are the persons primarily responsible for helping children achieve this goal. After age 3 (the age at which many children enter preschool), however, educational professionals (e.g., teachers) are increasingly involved in the process, and, by age 6, children often spend as much (or more) waking time with teachers as they do with parents. Although the primary task for teachers is the delivery of formal education, over the past few decades they have been increasingly recruited to train socialized behavior. The specialized knowledge needed to effectively satisfy the corresponding increase in teacher tasks (e.g., conducting behavior management programs, collaborating with parents to solve school behavior problems) has dramatically increased the need for involving school psychologists in the educational process. And, because many of the child problems teachers must now address at school are significantly influenced by what happens at home, there is an increased need for partnerships between parents and teachers.

The professional most frequently called on to broker these partnerships is the school psychologist. Accordingly, over the past 20 years, the curriculum used to train school psychologists has been steadily expanding its conventional dimensions (e.g., psychoeducational assessment, teacher consultation, classroom behavior management) to include training in an array of diverse subjects, including clinical applications across the diagnostic spectrum, health psychology, behavioral medicine, telemedicine, and parent training. The purpose of this chapter is to contribute to the latter, expanding subject area, parent training. The specific intent is to provide school psychologists with information that will enhance their ability to help parents solve their children's school-relevant behavior problems. The chapter has two primary dimensions. The first is obvious—the chapter provides examples of concepts and applications that significantly contribute to understanding the development and management of child behaviors exhibited at home and school. The second is more subtle—the chapter describes those concepts and applications in mostly non-technical, user-friendly language, the kind of language that is much more likely to reflect how parents speak in their everyday capacity as parents than the technical language that dominates most literature in psychology. If the descriptions seem simple from a technical perspective, then we have achieved our goal. If the descriptions seem to bypass or, worse, violate some technical aspect of highly operationalized concepts, that is one of the costs of employing user-friendly language. That is, some precision may be sacrificed for the sake of understandability and scope.

For example, the field of behavior analysis has precisely operationalized the concept of positive reinforcement: It involves a functional relation between a behavior and its consequences that leads to an increase in the probability of the behavior. The word *positive* does not refer to a quality of experience (e.g., pleasant) generated by the consequences; it refers to delivery (i.e., something is added), as contrasted with the word *negative*, as in negative reinforcement, which refers to withdrawal or escape from consequences (i.e., something is subtracted). These are subtle, sophisticated, and largely nonintuitive distinctions that even many professional psychologists do not fully understand. Here we refer to consequences as pleasant and preferred or unpleasant and nonpreferred, and we bypass the technical coverage of the concept of reinforcement altogether. There appears to be no reason to attempt to educate parents about the technical nuances of a behavioral concept that even experts in the field often misunderstand, especially when the primary goal of the discussion is to persuade parents to appreciate how significantly the consequences of behavior (intended and unintended) contribute to child learning. More generally, our intent is to describe important concepts and applications in ways that are similar to how we would describe them to parents.

Of the numerous concepts relevant to our task, we have selected the following for discussion: doing (vs. saying), child learning, creating motivational consequences through limits, rule-governed behavior, child development, and behavioral function. Of the numerous relevant applications, we have selected two types of behavioral assessment, Typical Day and functional, and four types of interventions: time-in/-out, task-based

grounding, the classroom pass program, and home–school notes.

Emphasis on Doing

The distinction between knowing how to do something and knowing how to say it (or to specify verbally what is to be done) is an important one for school psychologists to communicate to parents. The distinction has been drawn in many ways and fields (e.g., cognitive knowing vs. behavioral knowing, knowing a rule vs. behaving consistently with the rule, declarative vs. procedural knowledge, information capacity vs. procedural capacity, theory vs. practice). There are at least three reasons why the distinction is important in programs for child behavior problems: (1) knowing how to say does not entail knowing how to do; (2) adult attempts to change child behavior typically emphasize saying much more than doing; (3) the combination of 1 and 2 is an important source of child behavior problems.

For example, during toilet training, it is routine to ask a 2- or 3-year-old child if he or she has to go to the bathroom. Accurately answering the question can be difficult for such young children. First, the child must determine whether the question refers merely to a change in location (i.e., just going into the bathroom) or to an act of elimination. If the child believes the question involves elimination, he or she must examine bodily sensations to determine whether elimination is imminent. If it is, the child has to decide whether it is in his or her best interests to say so. Children in the early stages of toilet training are typically wearing toileting garments that absorb moisture and retain warmth when an accident occurs, and most children would typically rather eliminate in the garment than stop what they are doing, go into the bathroom, take off their clothes and the garment, sit on the toilet, and attempt to eliminate there.

Thus the difficulty occasioned by the question "Do you have to go to the bathroom?" is potentially problematic in at least four ways. First, the question places emphasis on an answer about toileting and not on a toileting action. In other words, it calls for children to say, not to do. Second, the developmental limitations of 2- and 3-year-old children, coupled with children's natural tendency to protect their own comfort, dramatically decrease the chances of an affirmative answer, even when elimination is imminent. Third, nonaffirmative answers in such situations (e.g., child says "no" and has an accident shortly thereafter) set the occasion for punishment (or at least unpleasant parent–child interactions) because such answers make it seem as if the child has been dishonest, stubborn, or stupid. Fourth, unpleasant interactions during or following toileting episodes can lead to unpleasant associations, toileting resistance, and delayed attainment of toileting skills.

A focus on doing instead of saying at the beginning of parent–child interactions involving toileting can avoid these problems and expedite training. For example, when timing (i.e., time elapsed since last act of elimination) or child responses (e.g., shifting weight from foot to foot) suggest that elimination is imminent, rather than making an inquiry about toileting urge, parents could instead issue a toileting instruction requiring that their child attempt to eliminate in the toilet, guide them as they do so, and praise performance and any success achieved. This method removes the focus on saying and places it on forms of doing that are central to toileting.

Focus on doing more than saying is important for other reasons. For example, in many domains of child life, children's ability to say what they should do is learned before their ability to do it. For example, children can easily say they should share their toys but not have the slightest inclination to do so because they lack the social and emotional skills that are essential to proficient sharing. Unfortunately for many children, the mere fact that children can say they should share indicates to their parents that they actually know how. When these children do not share, their parents, often assuming the children "should know better," are more inclined to attribute the absence of sharing to a deficit in character or personality rather than skill.

That a disparity between saying and doing exists and that differential emphasis is more productively placed on doing should be no surprise to adults. Revealing examples are legion. For example, all golfers know they should keep their heads down during the golf swing, but many (most) routinely lift their heads up. As a sample of other examples, lovers say they should look before they leap, readers say a book should not be judged by its cover, and fools say they should not rush in. Yet lovers often leap, readers frequently judge by the cover, and fools often rush in, all because their knowledge involves a facility for saying far more than it does a capacity for doing what has been said. The importance of doing over saying also suffuses the marketplace. As an example, the January 2001 issue of issue of *Wired Magazine* included a symposium on marketing in the new millennium in which David Kelley, a prominent participant, said, "If you listen to the customers, they can't tell you anything. You have to *watch* the customer to really learn something. That's how you get at what they think and feel" (Pearlman, 2001, p. 181). We believe Kelley's assertion is also relevant for school psychologists and parents working with children.

Child Learning

Although it is possible to teach children effectively without actually knowing how they learn, knowledge of learning principles facilitates the process. Thus a significant way the school psychologist can assist parents attempting to solve child behavior problems is to teach them how children derive meaning from the flow of events that compose their day-to-day lives, why they exhibit appropriate or inappropriate behavior, or, more generally, how they learn. A century of research on learning shows that child learning largely results from the emergence of functional relations between what children do, what happens before they do it, and changes in experience produced by what they do. A simple, straightforward way to express this is that children learn from repetition followed by changes in experience.

In general terms, there are four classes of experience that produce learning, two that make behavior more likely and two that make behavior less likely. The two that make behavior more likely are (1) pleasant or preferred experiences and (2) avoidance of, or escape from, unpleasant or nonpreferred experiences. The two that make behavior less likely are (1) unpleasant or nonpreferred experiences and (2) loss, cessation, or reduction of pleasant or preferred experiences. In other words, when behavior produces desired outcomes, it becomes more likely, and when it produces undesired outcomes, it becomes less likely. Although this point seems obvious, what constitutes a desirable outcome may not be obvious at all. For example, negative or critical adult attention can be a preferred outcome for some children (for more on this point, see the section on behavioral function). An important corollary is that the number of repetitions necessary for children to learn (e.g., to change their behavior, make meaningful "connections") is determined by the amount of the experiential change that follows what they do. The more change occurs, the fewer repetitions are necessary to learn a meaningful relationship between a behavior and the changes in experience it produces.

For example, behavior that produces first-degree burns or worse is behavior that has produced an enormous and highly unpleasant change in experience. Very young children who initially encounter fire are typically unaware of its dangers but are enthralled with its beauty, and, if unsupervised, they will often try to touch it. If successful, an immediate, large, and highly unpleasant experience occurs (i.e., being burned), and a major life lesson is learned (i.e., do not touch an open flame). The change in experience is so great and so unpleasant that the learning is typically immediate and permanent. This is not to say that children who have been burned by touching an open flame will not be burned again, but it is unlikely that they will be burned in that particular way.

If the temperature of fire were lower, however—if it were much closer to skin temperature for example—the lesson would be learned much more slowly, would require many more repetitions, and probably would also require some supplemental aversive (e.g., disciplinary) consequences administered by a parent or teacher. That is, when behavior produces large changes in experience, fewer repetitions are necessary for learning-based changes (i.e., an increase or a decrease in frequency of behavior) to occur, but when behavior produces only small changes in experience, many more repetitions are needed to produce a comparable amount of learning.

Corroborative routine household examples are abundant. For example, giving an instruction, repeating the instruction, reminding the child that the instruction has not been followed, warning the child that it would be in his or her best interest to follow the instruction, and threatening the child with punishment if the instruction is not followed is a very common sequence of tactics that parents employ to get their children to do or not do things that are important to the parent (e.g., hanging up coats). A common complaint is that children often ignore most of what is said in the sequence. They do so because experience-changing consequences for ignoring the parent typically do not occur (i.e., there is no penalty); therefore, there is no learning-based reason for the child to comply. Quite the contrary, the learning dynamics in the sequence typically reward noncompliance. Children are always learning, and each time a parent repeats an instruction, the prior instruction (the one repeated) and the interval between it and the repetition of it compose a learning trial in which an instruction was given and then ignored, deferred, or refused by the child and no parent-mediated consequence was provided. The absence of a parent-mediated consequence means that a pleasant or preferred outcome was produced for the child; specifically, the child ignored the parent's instruction and continued engaging in an activity that was apparently preferable to the activity that the parent requested. In simple terms, the child got away with it. This sequence of events produces learning, but not of the sort that the parent intends. The tendency to ignore the parent becomes even more firmly imbedded in the child's repertoire. Furthermore, as indicated, warnings or threats are usually part of the parental tactics, and when the child does not heed the warning and the parent does not make good on the threat, the child also learns to ignore parental warnings and threats.

Another example is the converse of the first, and it can also lead to children ignoring parental instructions. Specifically, when children do follow parental instructions the first time they are given but the parent responds minimally or not at all, no pleasant or preferred experiential change is produced by the compliance. In fact, being ignored or responded to minimally after following an instruction may produce unpleasant or nonpreferred experience (e.g., the child feels that his or her good behavior was ignored) and thus lead to a decreased likelihood of future compliance. Collectively, the tendency to ignore the parent, established by frequent parental repetitions, warnings, and threats with no consequential follow-up, is made even more likely when the child complies with the parent and still receives no follow-up. More generally, the learning of inappropriate behavior (e.g., ignoring the parent) is often accompanied by learning trials in which appropriate alternatives (e.g., compliance) are not followed by the type (pleasant, preferred) or the amount of experiential contrast necessary to increase the likelihood of appropriate alternative behavior. In conclusion, many child behavior problems result from a confluence of learning trials in which inappropriate behavior receives more of an experiential payoff for the child than its appropriate alternatives.

Making matters even worse is the devolution in parent teaching tactics that can result from these problematic teaching and learning sequences. Many parents, frustrated by the extent to which their instructions and rules are ignored, resort to highly punitive consequences, especially yelling and sometimes even spanking. These consequences produce large amounts of experiential change and thus readily instigate learning, but their potential benefits are outweighed by several potential risks. For example, children quickly become accustomed (i.e., habituate) to yelling and spanking, so more is gradually needed, an escalatory process that can lead to abusive child treatment in extreme cases. Additionally, frequent use of punishing tactics often creates so much distress for the child, parent, and family that the quality of the family environment is diminished as a result. The effects of highly punitive tactics on child behavior are also reductive, and so they are less likely to teach new skills than they are to increase avoidance and escape. Punishing tactics can also cause unwanted side effects (e.g., fear, retaliation) that can further worsen the parent–child relationship. Finally, punishing behavior does not teach children appropriate alternatives to inappropriate behavior. For additional information on learning, consult a technical text on learning (e.g., Catania, 1997), behavior modification (e.g., Miltenberger, 2007), or applied behavior analysis (e.g., Cooper, Heron, & Heward, 2007).

Creating Motivational Consequences through Limits

One of the central themes of the preceding section is that children are motivated by the pleasant, preferred experiences that shape their behavior. Not only is it possible to create pleasant and preferred experiences to motivate children, but it can also be done with activities and commodities that are freely available; nothing new need be purchased or constructed. Motivational experiences can be created merely by placing limits on existing activities. A large body of basic and applied research shows that placing limits on activities establishes pleasant, preferred (i.e., reinforcing) properties in the activities that are limited (e.g., Timberlake & Farmer-Dougan, 1991). This line of scientific investigation is called the *response deprivation approach* to learning. Descriptions of the approach say that forced or programmed reductions of any activity that result in its rate or duration falling below its typical level establishes reinforcing properties in the activity. Thus the activity can be used as a learning-based consequence for behaviors that parents would like to see more of (e.g., homework, chores, compliance, being nice).

A persuasive selling point of response deprivation learning is that so many routine activities can yield motivational consequences. One good example involves staying up after bedtime. The key to turning bedtime into an effective consequence to be used for motivation is to establish and enforce a relatively early time for bed. For example, if parents establish an 8 P.M. bedtime but actually believe a 9 P.M. bedtime would be acceptable for their child, they have created an hour that could be used as a reward. Most children want to extend their bedtime even if it is already unreasonably late (Friman, 2005a). Therefore, when bedtime is early, a large amount of time (after the time set) that children would be motivated to obtain (e.g., by doing homework or chores) is created. Furthermore, the time (e.g., 1 hour) can be divided up into portions (e.g., four 15-minute portions), and each can be used as its own independent reward.

As indicated, the process works for any activity, not just bedtime. Placing limits on any child activity increases the value of that activity for the child. This effect is similar to the "scarcity creates demand" principle in economics. When working with parents who are puzzled by how difficult it is to motivate their children or who are reluctant to buy new items or to create new privileges in an attempt to increase motivation, another option is merely to place limits on their children's routine recreational activities and to allow the child to earn relaxation of those limits through compliance with parental rules and requests. Our standard suggestion is for parents to freely permit small amounts of regular recreational activity (e.g., 30 minutes of television, computer gaming, telephoning, text messaging) and require that increased amounts be earned through child behaviors requested by parents.

Rule-Governed Behavior

One of the more complicated concepts in behavioral psychology is rule-governed behavior. Definitive descriptions range from contingency-specifying stimuli (Skinner, 1969) to derived relational responding (Hayes, Barnes-Holmes, & Roche, 2001). We forgo a technical account of rule-governed behavior and merely describe it as behavior that is strongly influenced by the semantic properties (i.e., meanings) of language. The emphasis on semantics here is important because the behavior of nonhuman animals can be strongly influenced by words, but not through their semantic properties or meanings; rather, the influence of words on nonhuman animals is merely the result of direct associations.

For example, most dogs can easily be taught to sit in response to the word *sit*, but the dog's sitting response is the direct result of an association between the spoken word "sit" and the rewards it receives for doing so. The dog does not actually know what the word means; any word could be substituted for the word *sit*. For example, dogs can be trained to lie down in response to the word *sit*, to roll over when told to lie down, or to respond in other ways that are obviously unrelated to the actual meaning of commands that are used in their training. This type of contrarian dog training can be humorous because it so clearly shows that dogs do not really know the meaning of words. Children, on the other hand, learn the meaning of words such as *sit* very early in their lives and learn to respond to them appropriately in all of their forms (spoken, written, or illustrated). In other words, humans derive meanings from words and those meanings influence behavior. In lower animals, words influence behavior only through direct associations and not at all through derived meanings. When the meanings of words influence behavior, it is referred to as rule governed.

There are many benefits of rule-governed behavior, the foremost one of which is its efficiency. For example, when teaching children to look both ways before crossing the street, parents begin with one street and teach the rule ("look both ways"). Very early in the training, sometimes at the first or second street, parents add the word *always* into the command ("always look both ways"), and the ultimate outcome is that children learn to look both ways before they cross any street anywhere, anytime. That is, they learn to apply the rule to streets on which they have had no direct training, a very efficient outcome of direct training. Lower animals cannot be trained with the same efficiency. The rule would have to be trained for every street encountered, because the animal's behavior would not generalize to untrained streets as the children's behavior does; lower animals cannot learn to derive meaning from an abstract word such as *always*.

Another advantage is that rule-governed behavior can neutralize or lessen the effect of direct experiences on child performance. This effect is beneficial when direct experience is unpleasant (but not harmful) and interferes with child performance. For example, children often want to quit an activity when it becomes physically difficult. But children's desire to quit can be overridden by thinking or saying a rule related to continued performance (e.g., "when the going gets tough, the tough get going," "I think I can, I think I can, I know I can"). Once again, lower animals are not capable of this type of responding because they are not capable of responding to the meaning of the rules. Unfortunately, the neutralizing effect of rule-governed behavior on direct experience can also result in disadvantages. The effect is especially problematic when rules inhibit a performance the continuation of which is needed to produce beneficial outcomes. For example, arithmetic and math can be difficult for some children, and some children derive a rule that they are just not good at math. Subsequently, regardless of how often they have pleasant experiences in math-related situations (e.g., sitting next to a desirable peer, doing well on a math test, having a fun and effective math teacher), they resolve to avoid math. More generally, an instance or two of failure can induce some children to decide that they are not smart (talented, good, athletic, etc.) enough for success, and they simply stop trying for success. Following the decision (i.e., formation of a rule), the experience of occasional or even frequent success can be overridden by the pessimistic notion derived from the first failure. In other words, pessimistic rules about ability can be derived from just a few instances of failure, and those rules can neutralize the experience of success in future activity and ultimately severely limit the extent to which a child is even willing to try.

Cognitive-behavioral therapy, perhaps the dominant form of clinical psychology in North America, includes multiple methods for determining when rules are adversely influencing the quality of clients' lives and for modifying those rules (e.g., Hersen, 2005; also see Bushman & Gimpel Peacock, Chapter 25, this volume). School psychologists with some specialized training in cognitive-behavioral therapy can help children whose performances are influenced by self-defeating rules and can coach parents on how to augment that help at home.

Child Development

Child development is another conceptual area in which some knowledge could enhance parent's effectiveness as they partner with school psychologists to solve their children's behavior problems. This subject, like child learning, is very broad, and here we merely discuss one major dimension of child development: children's developing ability to understand and make use of concepts. The most authoritative person studying and writing on that subject was Jean Piaget. He spent his entire career studying the incremental nature of cognitive abilities (cf. Flavell, 1963). Among Piaget's many discoveries was the relatively slow development of children's ability to competently understand and use concepts. Concepts are semantic tools that categorize phenomena according to at least one quality or dimension (e.g., color, size, length). Competent use of concepts requires a developmental process that Piaget referred

to as conservation. Conservation involves the capacity *to conserve* a quality of an object or event and meaningfully apply that quality to another object or event. Conservation involving objects or events that physically resemble each other emerges early in a child's life, but conservation involving objects or events that are physically dissimilar emerges much later (averaging between 5 and 7 years) and does not fully develop until the teen years.

Piaget (and many other researchers) conducted numerous studies that reveal young children's limited capacity to conserve. For example, when asked to hold a pound of lead and a pound of feathers and then asked to choose which weighs more, young children are likely to choose the lead. When faced with two containers with identical volume capacities but different forms (e.g., one tall and thin the other short and wide) and asked to choose which holds more water, young children are likely to choose the taller container. When shown two similar apples, one cut into fourths and one cut into eighths, and asked which they prefer, young children are likely to pick the one cut into eighths ("because there is more apple"). When shown five quarters in a bunch and five quarters in a row and asked to choose which grouping has more quarters, young children are likely to choose the row.

That children are slow to develop conservation is an important message for school psychologists to communicate to parents, because parents use so much language to teach their children about appropriate behavior; the success of that teaching is heavily dependent on the children's capacity to understand that language (e.g., Blum, Williams, Friman, & Christophersen, 1995; Friman & Blum, 2003). No two episodes of behavior are completely alike, and thus, to learn conduct-relevant relations between different episodes, children must be able to conserve aspects of the episodes that are formally or functionally similar. Parents can easily discern similarities between differing episodes (e.g., "he is doing it again!"), and when they speak to their children about the episodes, their language likely reflects the similarities that they see. But the children may have difficulty seeing the similarity due to their limited capacity to conserve (contrasted with the parents' very well-developed capacity to conserve). For example, the onset of a disciplinary event often includes a parental attempt to forcefully assert similarities between a current and a previous behavioral episode (e.g., "Isn't that the same thing I warned you about yesterday?"). There are at least two conservation-based assumptions implicit in parental language of this kind: (1) the child should have been able to see conduct-relevant sameness in the two behavioral episodes; and (2) the child can currently see the sameness because the parent has pointed it out verbally. When conservation is weakly developed, however, as it is among most young children, both assumptions are likely to be incorrect. If children have a difficult time seeing quantitative sameness between five quarters in a row and five quarters in a bunch, it seems safe to say that they would also have difficulty seeing conduct-relevant sameness between something they have just done and something they did hours or even days ago. Furthermore, the test situations with quarters are simple and uniform, with the exception of the differing arrangement of the quarters. Behavioral episodes are often very complex and differ in many ways, including time frames, persons present, and physical locations. Additionally, when conducting tests of conservation capacities in the laboratory, investigators exhibit calmness, acceptance, and perhaps even gentleness. As much as possible, investigators avoid any hints of disappointment, judgment, or implied punishment. Most children respond in kind (by cooperating, trying their best, etc.). But in the prototypical disciplinary event, parents exhibit disappointment, judgment, and sometimes anger, and the possibility of punishment is always implicit and often very explicit. Many (probably most) children respond emotionally (by crying, yelling, denying, etc.), and high levels of emotional arousal can substantially diminish cognitive functioning. That is, while in an intensely emotional interaction with a parent, children's levels of cognitive functioning are much lower than their chronological age. Thus even children who routinely exhibit a developed capacity to conserve in routine situations may be unable to do so in disciplinary situations.

Behavioral Function

Behavior always has a function, although it is not always obvious. The word *function, however, is a complex one, and when speaking with parents, the word purpose* may be a better substitute—but here we stick with *function.* The four general classes of function that have received the most scientific attention are (1) tangible outcomes (e.g., access to video game or cell phone); (2) social outcomes (e.g., attention); (3) avoidance or escape (e.g., noncompletion of homework or chores); and (4) automatic, nonsocially mediated outcomes (e.g., relief provided by scratching an itch; Iwata, Dorsey, Slifer, Bauman, & Richman, 1994).

The primary reason for assessing the function of behavior is that knowledge of function can be used to design interventions that teach children (more) appropriate ways of satisfying the function. For example, a boy who goes into his brother's room to play with his brother's toys can be taught to ask first or can be supplied with similar toys of his own. A girl who engages in inappropriate attention seeking can be taught more appropriate methods for recruiting attention. A girl who avoids homework may be offered assistance and small breaks. A boy who is soothed by thumb sucking can be taught more appropriate methods for self-soothing. There are myriad other examples.

When the function of behavior is not obvious, it is often necessary for the school psychologist and parent to work together to determine plausible possibilities. A methodology for making the determination is discussed in the section of this chapter focused on assessments. To illustrate the kind of clinically relevant findings that can result, consider the following example. An 11-year-old sixth-grade boy was referred to a school psychologist for assessment of violent outbursts and fighting at school. A review of social and academic history revealed that his family was intact, that his relations with his parents were good, and that, although he had occasional quarrels with his three younger siblings, his relations with them were also good. The boy was largely nondescript. He was average in all areas of his school and family life. His intelligence, grades, athletic skills, musical aptitude, speaking skills, and even appearance (e.g., height, weight) were all average. He had friends in school but not close ones. Even his teacher had a difficult time describing him other than in terms of the referral problems, which involved frequent fights with classmates and even with older children from higher grade levels. In terms of those problems, he truly did stand out, and the function of his behavior is revealed in that phrase. One month prior to the referral, the boy had been accosted by an older, larger boy who had a reputation for being a bully. The encounter took place in an enclosed coatroom, and during it the older boy attempted to take the younger boy's lunch. The younger boy lost his temper (his description was that he "blacked out") and fought back wildly, bloodying the older boy's mouth and nose and persuading him to back away. The commotion drew the attention of the teacher, and the younger boy began to struggle with her. He was restrained and taken to the principal's office. When he emerged from the coatroom restrained and when he returned to class, he was no longer nondescript. Although his classmates were not interviewed, the teacher reported that they all viewed him in an entirely different way—with a mixture of fear, respect, and concern. And, almost immediately, the referral behaviors began to appear. The frequent outbursts, arguments, and fights always resulted in some sort of discipline, ranging from detention to out-of-school suspension, and yet their frequency remained unabated. School staff speculated about problems at home, but, as indicated, the social history revealed nothing of significance. School staff also speculated about psychopathology, but his assessments yielded elevations only in areas topographically related to the target behaviors (e.g., yelling, fighting, anger); there was support for neither internalizing conditions such as anxiety or depression nor for externalizing problems such as attention-deficit/hyperactivity disorder (ADHD), oppositional defiant disorder (ODD), or conduct disorder (CD). As indicated, prior to the fight in the coatroom, he had not stood out in any particular way, including those ways that would have been suggestive of an underlying psychological condition.

Direct observations and functional assessments suggested that the target behaviors had a social function. That is, the behaviors produced an abundance of attentional outcomes across teachers and students, not all of which were negative. An interview with the boy indicated that he had begun to think of himself as tough and fearsome, and that opinion appeared to be shared by most classmates. The teacher and principal reported that the older boy he had fought with in the coatroom was now afraid of him, and direct observations indicated that the older boy avoided him on the playground. The overall outcome of the original fight and those that ensued appeared to be a substantial enlargement of the boy's reputation in the class and at the school. Whereas formerly he was nondescript to the point of being a social cipher, he had become the subject of frequent conversations among students and teachers alike. The consequences administered for his fighting did not function as deterrents; rather, they appeared to enhance his new reputation and thus served as pleasant, preferred outcomes (i.e., the type that strengthen rather than weaken behavior).

Based on the attentional-outcomes hypothesis, a new intervention that supplied social attention in multiple other, more appropriate ways was implemented. For example, the boy was selected for the lead role in a school play about George Washington. His teacher significantly increased the number of times she called on him in class (and prepared him for answers in advance if the question was going to be difficult). Some of his drawings were pinned to the school bulletin board (formerly reserved for only the most skilled members of the class). He was selected to bring the attendance slips to the office after the first hour. Multiple other changes occurred. Privately, the school psychologist coached the boy about earning attention appropriately and explained that his new social advantages would be reduced or lost if he exhibited the target behaviors. The school psychologist also worked with the boy's parents and established a home-based response system for appropriate and inappropriate school behavior. Additionally, the psychologist explained the attentional-outcomes hypothesis and recommended that his parents design ways for him to earn increased attention at home. For example, his positive school reports were taped to the refrigerator. For each positive daily report, he earned 15 minutes of special time with the parent of his choice. The parents also began to solicit his input during family conversations (e.g., dinner) more often (historically he had been easy to overlook). The ultimate outcome resulted in a dramatic decrease in the target behaviors at school, with a corresponding increase in his social status at home and at school.

This case example is just one of many that illustrate some of the benefits of determining the function of problematic school behavior. Six published examples from our clinic alone include cases involving classroom disruption (Ervin, DuPaul, Kern, & Friman, 1998), school aggression coupled with social phobia (Friman & Lucas, 1996), school disruption and simple phobia (Jones & Friman, 1999), habitual self-injury and anxiety (Swearer, Jones, & Friman, 1997), aggression and self-injury (Field, Nash, Handwerk, & Friman, 2004) and ADHD–ODD (Hoff, Ervin, & Friman, 2005). More generally, data demonstrating the value of assessing function to better understand and treat child behavior problems are rapidly forming one of the largest bodies of empirical evidence in the broad field of behavioral psychology (e.g., Hanley, Iwata, & McCord, 2003; Neef, 1994). In sum, helping parents determine the function of the child's problematic behavior can significantly augment the problem-solving process.

Assessments

There are myriad methods for assessing child behavior problems, and there is a continuum of the degree to which parents are involved in the process among them. Here we describe two methods of assessment; one requires full involvement of parents, and the other is optimal when parents are involved but can be conducted without them. When parents are involved, it is important to establish a partnership whose purpose is the identification of child behavior problems and their causal circumstances. Great care should be taken to avoid explicit or implicit judgments about the quality of home life or parenting. Although assessment can be reactive and generate behavior change even prior to intervention, that is not the goal. The goal is maximal procurement of clinically relevant information that can inform diagnosis and treatment of problems. The first method is the Typical Day Interview (TDI), and it is used entirely with parents. When done well, it is nonthreatening, technically simple, and jargon free, and yet it produces an abundance of information relevant to child behavior problems. Its purpose to obtain a full picture of a child's day with special emphasis

on the points of potential conflict between parental expectations and child desires (e.g., bedtime, morning routine). The second method is functional assessment, and it can be conducted with any combination of child, parent, and teacher. Although it is moderately more technical than the TDI, the type of information it yields pertains directly to behavioral function (as described earlier) and thus is directly pertinent to treatment.

Typical Day Interview (TDI)

The TDI involves a discussion between psychologist and parent during which the psychologist asks for a description of events that typically occur in the daily life of the child. The purpose of the TDI is to investigate the potential points of conflict between child and parent during a typical day, especially in terms of child preferences, desires, and practices on the one hand and parental requests, requirements, and rules, as well as methods used for teaching and enforcement, on the other. The interview should highlight all points of potential conflict between child and parental preferences (e.g., early vs. late bedtime). We recommend beginning the interview with bedtime and proceeding from there around the clock and back to bedtime. Special emphasis should be placed on points in the day at which child and parent interests and desires are likely to conflict. At bedtime, for example, children usually prefer to stay up later, whereas parents want them to go to bed. Queries should focus on what the parental expectation actually is, how motivated the parent is to see it met, the extent to which it has been communicated clearly to the child, what (if any) enforcement procedures are used, what (if any) rewards are used, and the level of child compliance and resistance. So the following set of questions could be used to assess bedtime:

1. "What bedtime have you set?"
2. "What is the bedtime routine?"
3. "How much resistance does your child exhibit?"
4. "What type of resistance does your child exhibit (e.g., passive, active, stalling, requesting, begging, pleading, bargaining)?"
5. "How do you respond to the resistance?"

6. "What is the rule about reading in bed?"
7. "What is the lighting arrangement in the room?"
8. "Does your child stay in bed for the night?"

Although this list is reasonably thorough, several other queries could be added depending on the behaviors of concern. The next logical daily event is the morning routine, and queries about it should pertain to topics similar to the preceding (e.g., wake-up time, resistance, responses). At points at which independence is a developmental issue, related queries should be made (e.g., "What percentage of the morning routine is independent?"). The interview should also address how the child spends free time, what the homework arrangements are, conduct at the dinner table, household rules and expectations, chores, behavior in public, and discipline. All aspects of a child's typical day can yield clinically relevant information, so, in theory, no aspect is too small to query. The ultimate yield of a TDI is a picture of a child's day, complete with reasonably evident and often very obvious areas that could productively be targeted for intervention (e.g., amount and timing of homework, disciplinary practices, amount of sleep). Another indirect outcome of the TDI is information potentially pertinent to questions about the function of problematic behavior. However, there are more direct ways to address these questions, the most informative and widely used of which is functional assessment.

Functional Assessment

As stated in the section on behavioral function, the directly relevant research has focused on four general types of functions of behavior. The primary purpose of a functional assessment is to determine the function (what a child gets out of exhibiting a particular behavior) of behavior. Functional assessment specifically focuses on the A-B-C's: Antecedent (what comes before the behavior), Behavior (description of what the child does), and Consequence (the changes in experience produced by behavior). The ultimate reason for a functional assessment is to identify the variables that maintain problem behavior so that they can be used in

applications designed to modify it. Parents and teachers are obvious resources for information used in the functional assessment of child behavior. Jones and Wickstrom (Chapter 12, this volume) describe functional assessment procedures in detail. Here we focus on their use with parents.

The first step in a functional assessment is identify behaviors whose function is to be determined. Although any behavior can be the object of a functional assessment, typically the behaviors selected are problematic at home and/or school, and the order in which they are arranged for assessment is established by the seriousness of the problems. Thus it is important to ask the child's parents and teachers which behaviors they find the most problematic and why. Subsequently, each behavior should be defined in clear, observable, and quantifiable terms. Some examples of good operational definitions include: number of words read per minute, number of instances of physical aggression toward others (hitting, kicking, biting, or spitting), latency of following directions, duration of time out of seat (buttocks not touching seat), percentage of homework assignments completed on time and turned in, and so forth.

After a target behavior has been selected, the method of its measurement needs to be determined. Functional assessment is an umbrella category that includes a number of indirect and direct assessment methods. Some examples include surveys, self-reports, interviews, observation, scatterplots, A-B-C records, frequency counts, and functional/experimental analyses. Due to space limitations, we discuss only two: the functional interview and direct observation.

The functional interview is a versatile and informative method for home and school, and it is the most logical step to follow if problem behavior has been identified on a TDI. The information obtained from the TDI can be used to inform the functional interview and to generate more questions related to the target behavior. Multiple informants should be considered when conducting a functional interview, and, as indicated earlier, parents and teachers are prime candidates, but the child him- or herself is also a very good source of functional information. Wording and questions will differ depending on the informant. Following is a sample of questions that are commonly posed to parents and teachers in a functional interview.

1. "When did you first notice this behavior?"
2. "Could you describe the behavior?"
3. "When is the behavior most likely to occur?"
4. "Where is the behavior most likely to occur? "
5. "Who is the child usually with when the behavior occurs?"
6. "When is the behavior least likely to occur?"
7. "What usually happens right before the behavior? "
8. "What do you usually do when the behavior occurs? "
9. "What do others usually do when the behavior occurs?"

Another type of functional assessment involves in-school and/or in-home direct observation and/or data collection. Many different observation methods are available; partial-interval recording, whole-interval recording, duration measurement, latency measurement, event recording, and rate are notable examples. Partial-interval recording is often used for high-frequency behaviors. This entails observing the child for a period of time (typically no more than 30 minutes) and noting (typically on a sheet designed for data collection) whether the target behavior occurred within specified time increments (e.g., 10 seconds). The observer should also plan to take data during a time suggested by a parent and/or teacher as a time that the behavior is most likely to occur.

The school psychologist should select a simple and efficient method of data collection and train the observer accordingly. For example, a parent could be asked to complete a log indicating the date, time, and description of the behavior, what occurred before the behavior, and what happened after the behavior (including how the parent reacted to the behavior). This form of data collection is intended to identify patterns that may not be noticeable without the aid of data taken over extended time periods.

The type of functional assessment conducted will depend on the complexity and severity of the behavior to be assessed, how much time is available, what level of training is necessary, and what resources are at hand. The school psychologist may wish to begin with more indirect measures, such as interviews and surveys, as these are the least effortful and intrusive and to use other methods only if it becomes clear that additional information is needed to develop an effective intervention. For a much more comprehensive description of functional assessment, consult any current text on behavior modification (e.g., Miltenberger, 2007) or applied behavior analysis (e.g., Cooper et al., 2007).

Applications

Time-Out and Time-In

Time-Out

Of all treatment applications derived from behavioral science, time-out (TO) is most frequently used by parents in the United States (for additional information, see Shriver & Allen, Chapter 24, this volume, on parent training). TO is an abbreviation for time-out from positive reinforcement, a procedure first tested with laboratory animals in the 1950s (e.g., Ferster, 1958) and subsequently widely used for treatment of child misbehavior, the successes of which have been reported regularly since the early 1960s (e.g., Wolf, Risley, & Mees, 1964). The laboratory version typically involved limiting an animal's access to motivating activities such as eating or drinking. The child version involved limiting a child's access to preferred experiences, especially social interaction and all forms of entertainment. In both versions, TO regularly produced substantial reductions in the behaviors for which it was used as a consequence. Numerous replications of this effect, coupled with the fact that TO proved to be much more socially acceptable than corporal punishment, resulted in widespread dissemination of TO as a child disciplinary tactic. At present, a professional or popular book on child management techniques that does not include a section on TO would be hard to find (Friman & Blum, 2003; Friman, 2005b; Friman & Finney, 2003).

The virtual ubiquity of TO makes it unnecessary for school psychologists to inform parents about its availability; parents are as aware of TO as psychologists. But establishing optimal utility for TO will almost always require professional input. In fact, a common parental complaint is that TO was tried and did not work. The implicit assumption is that what was done in the name of TO closely resembles the procedure developed in the laboratory long ago. Unfortunately, close resemblance is the rare exception rather than the rule. Animals exposed to TO in the laboratory had no possibility of getting the experimenters to provide preferred experiences during the TO period. In colloquial terms, nothing preferred was happening for the animal, and for a specified period of time, there was nothing that the animal could do about it. The laboratory experience for the animal, however, differs substantively from the typical experience children have in TO in homes (and schools) across the country.

For example, the majority of parents and teachers using TO have not been specifically trained to do so, and thus they have not been trained to ignore a child's attempts to control the situation. Thus children in TO often have substantial capacity to change their situation through inappropriate behavior. For example, simply calling out, crying out, or coming out of TO (without permission) often successfully recruits the attention of parents (and teachers) and thereby neutralizes the desired aversive effects of TO. Other types of inappropriate behaviors (e.g., profanity, disrobing) also typically engage parental attention. The attention thus engaged is usually negative but, because it is delivered when the child is in TO, it results in a temporary escape (the instant attention is delivered, TO functionally ends), which is more likely to increase rather than decrease the inappropriate behavior. In other words, negative attention is something, and for children in TO, something is usually better than nothing. Therefore, the school psychologist should train parents to minimize the attention directed to obnoxious behavior that children exhibit in TO. All verbal contact should cease until the child is informed TO is over, and physical contact should be confined to the amount needed to seat children in TO and sustain their presence there. For more information on TO, refer to multiple publications that specifically address it (e.g., Friman & Blum, 2003; Friman, 2005b; Friman & Finney, 2003) and to Shriver and Allen (Chapter 24, this volume).

Time-In

As indicated in the section on child learning, learning results from the changes in experience produced by behavior; the fundamental basis for the effectiveness of TO is that children's lives outside of TO are fun and enjoyable, or at least mildly pleasant. In other words, children must experience pleasant situations, the removal from which generates unpleasant, nonpreferred experience. If nothing pleasant or preferred was occurring prior to a TO, the TO itself may not make much difference to the child, and thus there is little likelihood that much would be learned. Conversely, if engagement, fun, and/or affection were abundant prior to a TO, the TO would cause a very unpleasant change in the child's life, and reduction in behavior that led to the TO is much more likely. Therefore, prior to using TO, it is necessary to establish a high degree or level of what has come to be called time-in (TI). For early scientific evidence of this point, see Solnick, Rincover, and Peterson (1977). From a more colloquial perspective, if hockey players did not like playing hockey, the penalty box (a form of hockey TO) would mean little to them. Heuristically, TI can be thought of as the functional opposite of TO. TO is a procedure that minimizes preferred experience and is used in response to inappropriate child behavior. TI is a procedure that maximizes preferred experience (e.g., physical affection, parental participation in child activities) and is used in response to appropriate child behavior.

In conclusion, TO is a widely used disciplinary tactic but one that is often used ineffectively. Nonetheless, for children between 2 and 7 years of age (we discuss methods for older children in the next subsection), it can be the primary method used for discipline and can produce good results when used in strategically and tactically sound ways. Helping parents achieve strategic and tactical effectiveness with TO can be an important goal for the school psychologist. A critical component of this assistance involves helping parents eliminate sources of social stimulation (e.g., warnings, criticisms, expressions of parental anger) that often occur while children are in TO. Perhaps an even more important component is helping parents to see that to be effective, any form of discipline—TO as well as others that we describe—must involve unpleasant or nonpreferred experience that stands out starkly from what was happening before the discipline was imposed. Yelling or spanking can serve this purpose, but we have already discussed the problems associated with their use. TO is much more subtle, but it can produce good results if three conditions are met: (1) sources of social stimulation are eliminated during the TO (as discussed); (2) the child's inappropriate attempts to terminate TO are ignored outright; and (3) the child's life was generally interesting and fun before TO was imposed.

Task-Based Grounding

Although TO is a very effective first line of defense against child behavior problems in young children, its effectiveness declines as children grow older, which leads parents to seek other methods for managing their older children's behavior problems. The most frequently used alternative involves extended withdrawal of privileges and freedoms, the colloquial term for which is "grounding." Virtually by definition, the procedure is time-based, and its most common form consists of restricting the privileges to which the child is allowed access for a specific period of time (e.g., day, week, month). For example, parents might ground their children by restricting them to the house for a week (except for school) following inappropriate behavior. Unfortunately, time-based grounding has an inherent limitation that violates some primary principles of learning. Specifically, the release criteria merely involve the passage of time and not the performance of appropriate behavior. Thus there is no clear incentive for prosocial performance during the time-based restriction. If prosocial behavior does not lead to termination of grounding (i.e., an escape-based incentive for performing prosocial behavior is established), then coercive behavior (e.g., defiance, pouting, and/or aggressive behaviors) often emerges. It is as if grounded children try to make parents so uncomfortable that they are compelled to end the grounding prematurely—an outcome that is pleasant and preferred and that could inadvertently strengthen coercive behavior in the formerly grounded child.

An alternative to time-based grounding that is more consistent with the principles of learning combines the customary elements of grounding (e.g., restriction of privileges) with performance-based release criteria. This alternative approach, called task-based grounding (TBG), has been developed for older children (i.e., ages 7–16). The advantage of TBG over time-based grounding is that the children determine the length of the restriction by their behavior. To start the procedure, parents create a list of jobs that are not essential to the running of the house—jobs that if left undone for an extended period of time would produce minimal inconvenience for the household. Some examples include cleaning the garage floor, washing windows (every large window would be one job), cleaning car windows, cleaning grout, washing baseboards, or seasonal outdoor tasks such as weeding (unless being outdoors is a highly preferred activity). There are numerous other examples. These jobs should then be described on note cards and arranged in a deck. When children misbehave, they should be given cards and told that until the jobs written on them are completed, they will be grounded. Being grounded means restriction from all recreational activities that are not part of an organized educational program (e.g., soccer team). While at home, grounded children are not allowed access to electronics for any form of recreation or entertainment (e.g., no TV). In essence, they are allowed to do only their assigned jobs and their homework. Violating the rules or exhibiting additional misbehavior should lead to room-based TO and/or additional job cards. Parents are instructed not to nag, remind, or lecture; rather, they are instructed to let the TBG condition motivate the children to do the jobs and gain their freedom. The number of jobs is determined by the parental view of the gravity of the offense. For example, bickering in the car after an unheeded instruction to stop might lead to one job for each bickerer. Major violations of curfew or sneaking out of the house would lead to many jobs. A final point is that jobs are not complete until the parent is completely satisfied.

The ubiquity of time-based grounding contrasts sharply with a paucity of research on the effectiveness of its use. In fact, a literature search yielded no published research directly evaluating it or even research that directly evaluated withdrawal of privileges as an intervention for the behavior problems of typically developing children.

There was, however, a relatively recent published description of TBG (Eaves, Sheperis, Blanchard, Baylot, & Doggett, 2005), as well as an evaluation showing that TBG reduced high-rate behavior problems to near-zero levels in a group of children ages 8–15 who were exhibiting behavior problems (Richards, 2003).

The Classroom Pass Program

A recent development in treatment for bedtime problems is the bedtime pass program. In single-subject studies (e.g., Friman et al., 1999) and in a randomized clinical trial (Moore, Friman, Fruzetti, & MacAleese, 2007), the pass program reduced the high-rate bedtime behavior problems of virtually all participants to zero or near-zero levels. The program involves supplying children with a pass after they have gotten in bed and then allowing them to use it for one penalty-free trip out of bed or one summons of a parent to their bed for the satisfaction of one request (e.g., drink, hug, bathroom visit). Once the pass has been used, the children are required to surrender it and to stay in bed for the rest of the night. A routine artifact of the pass program is that children often do not use their passes; it is as if they were saving them until they really needed to leave their rooms. This artifact has led to a modification of the bedtime program— children earn incentives for unused passes. Conceptual analysis suggests that the pass program works largely because it allows children an exercisable escape option in an aversive situation, which, in turn, provides them with a sense of control while in that situation. The incentive adds another function-based dimension to the program.

Although it is possible that school psychologists may be asked to consult with parents on child bedtime problems (fatigue is a significant contributor to daytime behavior and school problems), that is not the reason the pass program is discussed here. The reason is that the pass program can be extended to other circumstances that are unpleasant but that cannot (or should not) be avoided. For example, some schoolchildren find that being in class is highly aversive (e.g., children with school phobia or severe attentional problems). For these children, avoidance of, or escape from, school or class produces experientially preferred outcomes such as relief, which, in turn, decreases the likelihood that children will go to school or class or remain once they are there. A classroom-based pass program is one intervention that school psychologists could use to help children go to and stay in class. Similar to the bedtime pass program, before class the children are given a pass that they can use for a penalty-free trip out of class for a set period of time (e.g., 15 minutes). Possession of the classroom pass appears to reduce the unpleasant experience of being in class for children in the program (perhaps by giving them a sense of control over their situation). If the children use the pass, they have to surrender it when they return to class. Unused passes are exchanged for incentives that can be provided at home, school, or both. In severe cases, children can be given more than one pass.

Although there are no published studies on the utility of the classroom-based pass system—it was only recently derived from the bedtime pass program—results from our clinical applications of it are often successful. Furthermore, its strict derivation from the highly effective bedtime pass program, coupled with its consistency with the principles of learning, suggests that it would survive empirical evaluation. Thus, as with TBG, the classroom pass is offered not only as an optional application for some child behavior problems but also as a potentially productive line of school psychology research.

Home–School Notes

The home–school note is an intervention that does precisely what the name implies. It facilitates two-way communication between the home and school settings. The benefits of this type of partnership are difficult to overstate. Central to the theme of this chapter is the fact that parents and teachers have the most contact with children throughout the day and thus shape critical facets of children's lives. Consequently, collaborative work between the home and school settings has increasingly become an objective in educational reform efforts. Teachers and parents routinely correspond as needs arise, though, when using the home–school note, communication occurs on a consistent basis and targets specific areas of children's behavior. In addition, it requires few resources and little time to implement, which is important considering the increasing expectations on classroom teachers paired with parents' demanding work schedules and time constraints.

The design of the home–school note is not technically complex, and neither is its use. The first step is to identify the areas of concern. Once the target behaviors are identified, a scale for rating those behaviors must be devised, and it must be consistent with the target child's developmental level. Examples of scale indices include images (e.g., smiley face, star, thumbs-up), colors (e.g., green, yellow, red), a checklist (e.g., "yes/no," "good/needs improvement"), or numeric ranges (e.g., 1–10, with identifiers for each rating). Then the frequency of the ratings, rewards, and delivery of information pertaining to the target behaviors must be determined. Next, rewards have to be identified, and the criteria for earning rewards must be explicit. Finally, all involved parties need to agree on individual responsibilities.

There are myriad forms of the home–school note, some examples of which include: tablets with handwritten comments, templates that are placed in a binder and completed daily, small pieces of construction paper with notes for each period of the school day, and Post-it notes that provide an indication of whether the child met the criteria for the day. At a minimum, the note should include the date, target behaviors for the intervention, progress in the targeted areas, designation of whether the child met the criteria necessary to earn a reward, the reward that was issued (at home and/or at school), and signatures of the people who were involved. Regardless of the form, the sophistication of the system should parallel the intensity of children's needs and be minimally invasive. For additional information, a large body of literature describes how to use the home–school note (e.g., Kelly, 1990).

Home–school notes are helpful in addressing a wide variety of developmental, academic, and behavioral concerns (e.g., Jurbergs, Palcic, & Kelley, 2007). As an example, for children who have special needs and require intensive support in the school setting, the note could address eating habits and progress on individualized goals related to communication and motor skills. Both parents and teachers could communicate through the note to ensure continuity of care and progress on educational objectives. As another example, for children who have learning disabilities, the note could target work accuracy, work completion, homework submission, and strategies to practice at home. A reading teacher would include specific interventions to complete at home, allowing parents to supplement children's academic development. Home–school notes can also address such problems as aggression, talking out of turn, problematic peer interactions, poor organization, and many other school problems.

Some potential problems are associated with the implementation of the home–school note, despite the relative ease of its use. For example, sometimes the note is implemented inconsistently (e.g., teachers or parents forget, children lose it) and is thus prematurely thought to be ineffective. Similarly, sometimes the rewards that are promised to children for positive notes are delivered inconsistently or not at all, resulting in significant decreases in motivation. Another potential problem involves parent and teacher expectations that are too high and reward criteria that are too difficult to meet. For example, if a third-grade boy leaves his seat without permission an average of three times each hour, or approximately 20 times in a school day, it is unreasonable to expect him to remain seated for the entire day in the 1st week of a treatment program using a home–school note. Targets for success and criteria for rewards should reflect a gradual progress toward full-day performance.

School psychologists can help parents and teachers avoid these problems by incorporating information from the various sections of this chapter (e.g., learning, development, behavioral function) into the design of home–school note programs. School psychologists can also help by conducting classroom observations, setting reasonable reward criteria, designing the actual note, providing copies, consulting with parents and teachers regularly to ensure that the intervention is being implemented as agreed on, conducting functional assessments to ensure that the rewards are in fact an incentive to the child, and offering assistance throughout the entire process of intervention design and implementation.

Concluding Remarks

Optimally assisting parents in the school-based behavior problem-solving process involves a broad range of critical components, ranging from interpersonal skill to technical proficiency. Here we have emphasized a limited set of these components, but ones we believe are among the most important. The most subtle of these may also be the most crucial. The relevant communication taking place between school psychologists, teachers, and parents must be easily understood by all parties. Psychologists of every stripe, including school psychologists, have a tendency to discuss familiar subjects with unfamiliar words, phrases, and concepts (e.g., positive and negative reinforcement) or familiar words, phrases, and concepts in unfamiliar ways (e.g., "response to intervention" used as the name for a procedure rather than a description of an outcome). Although this tendency does not typically deter effective communication between professionals, it can thwart effective communication between school and home.

In this chapter, we emphasized the importance of readily understood communication and attempted to demonstrate ways to discuss highly technical concepts in broadly and easily understandable ways. For example, we provided a small sample of concepts that could be useful to anyone working with children, whether he or she is a parent, a professional, or both. Learning, development, motivation, the role of rules, and the function of behavior are concepts that are important but not just in the school context; they are central to a child's life in general. It seems safe to say that it is not possible for parents to know too much about these subjects, and providing parents with information on them significantly augments the partnership between parents and school psychologists.

Another component involves participation in the assessment process, and, although only two examples of the countless assessment methods were discussed—TDI and functional assessments—they both depend on parent participation and yield information that is directly relevant to treatment applications, the final critical component covered in the chapter. Although treatments can be conducted solely by school personnel, child behavior problems often occur both at home and at school; or, if they occur only at school, they can be influenced positively and negatively by events that happen at home. Thus, four of the applications that we covered directly involve the parents: TI, TO, TBG, and the home–school note. TO and grounding are the most frequently used disciplinary methods in this country, and in our coverage of them, we supplied information that could substantially improve their effectiveness. The home–school note is the most frequently used method for linking events happening at school to events at home. Finally, the classroom pass program is implemented only at school; however, if incentives are available for unused passes, they can involve home-based privileges and thus involve parents as partners in the program. As indicated, there are many other concepts, assessment methods, and applications that we could have included. Those actually chosen are broadly relevant and applicable to the most frequently occurring child behavior problems and thus provide a solid foundation for the partnership between parents and school psychologists as they seek to optimize healthy child education and socialization.

References

Blum, N., Williams, G., Friman, P. C., & Christophersen, E. R. (1995). Disciplining young children: The role of verbal instructions and reason. *Pediatrics, 96,* 336–341.

Catania, C. (1997). *Learning.* Upper Saddle River, NJ: Prentice Hall.

Cooper, J. O., Heron, T. E., & Heward, W. L. (2007). *Applied behavior analysis* (2nd ed.). Upper Saddle River, NJ: Prentice Hall.

Eaves, S. H., Sheperis, C. J., Blanchard, T., Baylot, L., & Doggett, A. (2005). Teaching time out and job card grounding procedures to parents: A primer for family counselors. *Family Journal, 13,* 252–258.

Ervin, R. A., DuPaul, G. J., Kern, L., & Friman, P. C. (1998). Classroom-based functional assessment: A proactive approach to intervention selection for adolescents diagnosed with attention-deficit/hyperactivity disorder. *Journal of Applied Behavior Analysis, 31,* 65–78.

Ferster, C. (1958). Control of behavior in chimpanzees and pigeons by time out from positive reinforcement. *Psychological Monographs, 72*(8, Whole No. 461).

Field, C., Nash, H., Handwerk, M. L., & Friman, P. C. (2004). Using functional assessment and experimental functional analysis to individualize treatment within a residential care setting for out of home adolescents. *Clinical Case Studies, 3*, 25–36.

Flavell, J. H. (1963). *The developmental psychology of Jean Piaget*. New York: Van Nostrand.

Friman, P. C. (2005a). *Good night, we love you we will miss you, now go to bed and go to sleep: Managing sleep problems in young children*. Boys Town, NE: Boys Town Press.

Friman, P. C. (2005b). Time out. In S. Lee (Ed.), *Encyclopedia of school psychology* (pp. 568–570). Thousand Oaks, CA: Sage.

Friman, P. C., & Blum, N. J. (2003). Primary care behavioral pediatrics. In M. Hersen & W. Sledge (Eds.), *Encyclopedia of psychotherapy* (pp. 379–399). New York: Academic Press.

Friman, P. C., & Finney, J. W. (2003). Time out (and time in). In W. O'Donohue, J. E. Fisher, & S. C. Hayes (Eds.), *Cognitive behavior therapy: Applying empirically supported techniques in your practice* (pp. 429–435). New York: Wiley.

Friman, P. C., Hoff, K. E., Schnoes, C., Freeman, K., Woods, D., & Blum, N. (1999). The bedtime pass: An approach to bedtime crying and leaving the room. *Archives of Pediatrics and Adolescent Medicine, 153*, 1027–1029.

Friman, P. C., & Lucas, C. (1996). Social phobia obscured by disruptive behavior disorder: A case study. *Clinical Child Psychology and Psychiatry, 1*, 401–409.

Hanley, G. P., Iwata, B., & McCord, B. E. (2003). Functional analysis of problem behavior: A review. *Journal of Applied Behavior Analysis, 36*, 147–186.

Hayes, S. C., Barnes-Holmes, D., & Roche, B. (2001). *Relational frame theory: A post Skinnerian account of language and cognition*. New York: Plenum.

Hersen, M. (Ed.). (2005). *Encyclopedia of behavior modification and cognitive behavior therapy*. Thousand Oaks, CA: Sage.

Hoff, K. E., Ervin, R. A., & Friman, P. C. (2005). Refining functional behavioral assessment: Analyzing the separate and combined effects of hypothesized controlling variables during ongoing classroom routines. *School Psychology Review, 34*, 45–57.

Iwata, B., Dorsey, M. F., Slifer, K. J., Bauman, K. E., & Richman, G. S. (1994). Toward a functional analysis of self-injury. *Journal of Applied Behavior Analysis, 27*, 197–209.

Jones, K. M., & Friman, P. C. (1999). Behavior assessment and treatment of insect phobia: A preliminary case study. *Journal of Applied Behavior Analysis, 32*, 95–98.

Jurbergs, N., Palcic, J., & Kelley, M. L. (2007). School–home notes with and without response cost: Increasing attention and academic performance in low-income children with attention-deficit/hyperactivity disorder. *School Psychology Quarterly, 22*, 358–379.

Kelly, M. L. (1990). *School–home notes: Promoting children's classroom success*. New York: Guilford Press.

Miltenberger, R. G. (2007). *Behavior modification: Principles and procedures* (4th ed.). Belmont, CA: Wadsworth/Thomson Learning.

Moore, B., Friman, P. C., Fruzetti, A. E., & MacAleese, K. (2007). Brief report: Evaluating the bedtime pass program for child resistance to bedtime: A randomized controlled trial. *Journal of Pediatric Psychology, 32*, 283–287.

Neef, N. (Ed.). (1994). Functional analysis approaches to behavioral assessment and treatment [Special issue]. *Journal of Applied Behavior Analysis, 27*, (2).

Pearlman, C. (2001). A conversation about the good, the bad, and the ugly. *Wired Magazine, 9*, 168–169; 176–183.

Richards, D. F. (2003). Evaluation of task-based grounding as a parent-implemented disciplinary procedure. *Dissertation Abstracts International: Section B. The Physical Sciences and Engineering, 63* (10-B), 4885.

Skinner, B. F. (1969). *Contingencies of reinforcement: A theoretical analysis*. Englewood Cliffs, NJ: Prentice Hall.

Solnick, J. V., Rincover, A., & Peterson, C. R. (1977). Some determinants of the reinforcing and punishing effects of time-out. *Journal of Applied Behavior Analysis, 10*, 415–424.

Swearer, S. M., Jones, K. M., & Friman, P. C. (1997). Relax and try this instead: Abbreviated habit-reversal for maladaptive oral self-biting. *Journal of Applied Behavior Analysis, 30*, 697–700.

Timberlake, W., & Farmer-Dougan, V. A. (1991). Reinforcement in applied settings: Figuring out ahead of time what will work. *Psychological Bulletin, 110*, 379–391.

Wolf, M., Risley, T., & Mees, H. (1964). Application of operant conditioning procedures to the behavior problems of an autistic child. *Behavior Research and Therapy, 1*, 305–312.

Chapter 24

Parent Training

Working with Families to Develop and Implement Interventions

Mark D. Shriver
Keith D. Allen

Parent training is a model of service delivery in which parents are directly taught specific skills to improve child functioning (Shriver, 1997). Parent training may be used to treat a multitude of different child problems (e.g., Briesmeister & Schaefer, 1998), but it has received the most empirical support in the treatment of oppositional, noncompliant, and aggressive behaviors in young children (Brestan & Eyberg, 1998). As a model of service delivery in the treatment of antisocial behaviors in young children, parent training has substantial empirical support going back over 40 years (Dangel & Polster, 1984; Patterson, 1976; Reid, Patterson, & Snyder, 2002; Shriver & Allen, 2008). Parent training is also a key component in prevention programs targeting children at risk for poor outcomes, such as school failure (e.g., Conduct Problems Prevention Research Group, 1992, 2004; Kumpfer & Alvarado, 2003).

Parent training is most likely to be implemented in clinical settings; however, parent training is also an important service that may be provided by school psychologists in a school setting. For example, federal educational legislation, as described by the Individuals with Disabilities Education Improvement Act (IDEIA; 2004) has identified parent training as a related service, one that involves counseling and training for parents to help them acquire the necessary information and skills to support the implementation of their child's individual education plan (IDEIA, 2004, Sec. 300.34, 8). In addition, in light of the evidence that parent training can reduce child risk for poor outcomes at school (e.g., Conduct Problems Prevention Research Group, 1992, 2004), it can be argued that parent training is a psychological service that should be available to all parents in support of their child's education.

So what is meant by "parent training"? It can mean, in part, parent education. For example, the first two components of the IDEIA (2004) definition of parent training refer to the *educational* aspect; namely, assisting parents in understanding the special needs of their child and providing parents with information about child development. This educational aspect of parent training may occur when a school psychologist meets with individual parents to discuss evaluation findings regarding the learning and development of their child. It may also occur when a school psychologist conducts an informational parent meeting or parent support group to discuss typical child development or learning processes. These types of parent education activities may be described as Tier

1 interventions, as they are primarily implemented for purposes of prevention.

Perhaps more important than the parent education component in parent training is the effort to help parents actually acquire the skills they need to help their children change and grow. Indeed, parent training has been defined as "the active, targeted teaching of specific parenting skills with the goal of positively affecting child behavior" (Shriver & Allen, 2008, p. 4). Consistent with this definition, IDEIA also states that parent training involves "helping parents to *acquire the necessary skills* that will allow them to support the implementation of their child's [educational plan]" (italics added). Parent training defined as such may be described as a Tier 2 or 3 intervention, as parent training is conducted to implement interventions to improve child outcomes at home and/or school.

Interestingly, hundreds of programs that have been developed to assist in the training of parents, and it seems as though new parenting programs are being introduced and promoted all the time. Some parent training programs make rather extraordinary claims about their successes; offer vivid testimonials and anecdotes; aggressively pursue dissemination through self-published materials, workshops, and advertising; and offer certification through specialized training. Faced with many choices and an abundance of supporting evidence, many school psychologists may be left with uncertainties and confusion about which parent training program to choose. Fortunately, there is an extensive base of research on the efficacy of parent training.

The purpose of this chapter is, in part, to provide school psychologists with information about parent training programs with strong evidentiary support. In addition, we provide information on how school psychologists might implement parent training in a school setting based on current evidence. Much of the best evidence supporting parent training comes from nonschool settings. However, the content, instructional methods, and conceptual foundations of current empirically supported parent training programs are so similar that school psychologists can translate that evidence to their school setting with confidence that they are delivering an evidence-based practice.

Empirically Supported Parent Training Programs

Evidence-based practice explicitly encourages the identification of the "best available research" (American Psychological Association, 2005). Toward that end, the identification of "empirically supported" interventions is a movement that has spread in the past decade or so across most, if not all, of the social science and medical disciplines (e.g., Chambless & Hollon, 1998; Kratochwill & Stoiber, 2000; No Child Left Behind, 2002; Sackett, Straus, Richardson, Rosenberg, & Haynes, 2000). There are at least four common criteria for defining empirically supported interventions in psychology: First, the intervention must demonstrate significant effects in two or more randomized control group treatment designs or in three or more well-controlled single-n (interrupted time series) designs. Second, the treatment must have a manual or detailed treatment protocol for dissemination. Third, research on the intervention must have been conducted by two or more independent experimenters or experimenter teams. Fourth, it is typically assumed, if not outright stated, that the research must be published in a peer-reviewed forum.

To date, four parent training programs are consistently identified as meeting scientific criteria for identification as empirically supported programs (Brestan & Eyberg, 1998; Chambless & Hollon, 1998; Kumpfer, 1999). These parent training programs are: Living with Children (LWC; Patterson, 1976; Patterson, Reid, Jones, & Conger, 1975); Incredible Years (IY; Webster-Stratton, 1992), Helping the Noncompliant Child (HNC; McMahon & Forehand, 2003) and Parent–Child Interaction Therapy (PCIT; Hembree-Kigin & McNeil, 1995).

A multitude of other parent training programs are available that do not meet criteria as empirically supported programs. Some of these programs have little to no empirical research support for producing positive parent and/or child behavior change (e.g., Dembo, Sweitzer, & Lauritzen, 1985), whereas others have some research support, but not yet enough to meet the criteria of "empirically supported" as described earlier (Barkley, 1997; Burke, Herron, & Schuchmann, 2004; Kazdin, 2005; Sanders, 1999). Any time lines are drawn regarding which program may be included in a particular category, there will be disagreement or controversy. It is expected that with continuing research regarding parent training programs, and particularly research regarding parent training in schools, additional programs will be listed as "empirically supported" particularly for application in schools (e.g., Carlson & Christenson, 2005). In addition, as the criteria for what constitutes "empirically supported" become more consistent across professional disciplines, there is likely to be more agreement about which programs meet that standard.

Although each of the empirically supported parent training programs listed previously has unique features, there are also important commonalities between the programs. Commonalities can be identified in the specific skills that parents are taught, how parent training is conducted, and the conceptual and scientific foundation of each program. Understanding these commonalities can make the translation from research to an evidence-based practice much easier because they suggest which core components are most important to maintain even when modifications may be required because of unique demands imposed by setting or client. In this section, we review these core components and their common conceptual foundations.

Summary Description of the Programs

All of the empirically supported parent training programs target young children (typically between 3 and 10 years of age) who are exhibiting problems with noncompliance, tantrums, aggression, oppositional behavior, hyperactivity, and/or antisocial behavior. Three of the programs (LWC, HNC, PCIT) target individual children and families. Only Incredible Years is a group-based parent training program. HNC has developed a group-based parent training program similar to the individually based parent training program, but this particular group-based program has not yet undergone empirical scrutiny (McMahon & Forehand, 2003; Shriver & Allen, 2008). All of the parent training programs were developed in the context of an outpatient clinical service model. Parent training sessions are offered weekly, ranging from 1 to 2 hours each session and from 8 to 14 weeks.

What Is Taught (Program Content)

Parents are taught to implement behavior intervention strategies to both increase desired behavior and decrease problem behavior. All of the programs teach parents how to identify, monitor, and reinforce desired behavior. Reinforcement procedures may include differential social attention and/or token reward systems. For example, parents are typically taught to attend to their children and to "catch them being good" with praise and physical touch while trying to ignore minor inappropriate behavior. The programs also teach parents how to establish rules and give commands so that children are more likely to comply. Finally, parents are typically taught at least one effective discipline procedure, such as time-out (sitting alone for a short time, restricted from contact with preferred people or activities) or response cost (e.g., loss of points and/or privileges) as a result of misbehavior.

How Parents Are Trained (Instructional Method)

A behavioral-skills-training model is used across all the programs to teach parents behavior intervention strategies. A behavioral-skills-training model includes four steps: (1) instruction, (2) modeling, (3) practice, and (4) feedback (Miltenberger, 2001). Instruction means providing parents with information about what they are going to be expected to do. Instruction is best delivered in simple, sequential steps, using language and examples that parents may best understand. For example, a parent might be told, "You are going to learn how to describe or narrate your child's play." The instruction should be followed immediately by a model of the desired behavior.

Modeling provides a demonstration for the parents of what they have been instructed to do and even what they should not do. Modeling may involve having parents watch a video demonstrating parent–child interactions, observing the parent trainer working with the parent or two parents working together (i.e., one parent pretends to be the child), or, perhaps best, observing the parent trainer demonstrating a particular skill directly with the child. For example, the trainer might now say, "Let me show you how to describe or narrate your child's play" (trainer says, "Johnny, I see you have built a big tower with red and blue blocks and you are still stacking them higher and higher … "). The model should be followed immediately by an opportunity to practice.

Practice refers to the parent immediately trying to imitate the skill he or she just saw demonstrated. For example, the parent trainer might say, "OK, now let me see you try it; it's OK if your descriptions sound just like mine" (parent drops to the floor and says, "Yes, I see Johnny building a big tower with red and blue blocks. Is that a house?"). Practice can sometimes involve role-playing implementation of the skill, with the parent trainer taking the role of the child. Practice can also refer to actual implementation of the skill with a child under the supervision of the parent trainer. Finally, practice can include implementing parenting skills outside the training sessions (i.e., homework). However, the best practice is always practice that is followed immediately by feedback.

Feedback is two-pronged. First, and most important, the parent trainer provides immediate reinforcing feedback for accurate or near accurate (i.e., shaping) demonstration of parent skills during parent training sessions. For example, the trainer might say, "Wow! You did such a nice job of describing their play. You used descriptors like *big*, *red*, and *blue*, and you described actions you saw, such as building. That was terrific!" Trainers can also provide important feedback in response to parents' adherence to homework recommendations.

Second, the parent trainer will often need to provide corrective feedback (including additional instruction and modeling as needed) for errors during rehearsal or in response to identified problems with adherence to homework recommendations. For example, the trainer might say:

> "Asking Johnny if he is building a house is a question. We want to stick with descriptions rather than questions [corrective feedback]."
> "You can turn your questions into descriptions [instruction] … by simply saying 'that looks like a house' [modeling]."
> "You try it [practice]."

The more opportunities parents have to observe modeling, to practice, and to receive feedback on skills, the more likely it is that they will learn these skills.

Scientific Foundation

The common scientific and conceptual thread tying these programs together is behavior analysis. The programs all rely on behavioral technology derived from research in applied behavior analysis. The common techniques used across programs, such as differential attention, token systems, rules and commands, and punishment procedures (response cost and time-out), all have solid empirical support. In addition, there is strong empirical support in the experimental analysis of behavior for the principles of behavior that underlie these techniques; namely, reinforcement, stimulus control, extinction, and punishment. (For those interested in further reading on these topics, one can find reviews of the basic principles with numerous illustrations from parent training [Shriver & Allen, 2008] or with examples from the empirical literature [Miltenberger, 2001]). Having a firm understanding of basic behavioral principles and behavioral technology (including behavioral skills training) can be an important element in providing effective parent training.

Implications of Empirically Supported Parent Training for School Psychologists

The applicability of empirically supported parent training programs may not be readily apparent for school psychologists, as most of the programs are individually based and developed within an outpatient clinical service model. School psychologists will likely have more opportunities for group-based parent training in schools. These programs do provide guidance, however, regarding the components of parent training that will likely be most successful regardless of setting. Understanding that parent training largely involves teaching parents behavior intervention strategies using behavioral skills instruction provides school psychologists with some direction on what parent training in schools should, at a minimum, include.

There are some good examples of group-based parent training programs that can be used in schools. Of the empirically supported programs, Incredible Years is the only group-based program. HNC has a group program derived from the individually based parenting program. Common Sense parenting is a parent training program that does not yet meet criteria to be labeled "empirically supported" but has promising research support (Burke et al., 2004). Likewise, Barkley's defiant children parenting training program and Kazdin's parent management training are other group-based parent training programs that have promising research support (Barkley, 1997; Kazdin, 2005). All of these programs contain the same common elements described earlier in that they all teach parents behavioral strategies, use behavioral skills instruction, and are generally grounded in behavioral theory. These programs and their corresponding manuals can help guide the school psychologist in leading a parent training group.

An Example of a Parent Training Group

Table 24.1 provides an example of one way in which school-based group parent training sessions might be organized. The topical focus of this particular parent training group is child noncompliance. The content of the sessions is derived from the content typically taught in the empirically supported parent training programs for child noncompliance. In the following example, behavioral skills training that includes instruction, modeling, practice, and feedback is incorporated in almost every session. Parents are provided specific homework assignments in most sessions, and data are collected during and between sessions to monitor progress.

In the first session, the parent trainer has three main goals: (1) to establish group boundaries and rapport, (2) to develop commitment to the group through effective rationale, and (3) to teach the first skill—data collection. Defining boundaries and establishing rapport occurs through introductions, reviewing rules for the group, and allowing participants to talk about themselves and their children, as well as their own concerns, strengths, and goals. Second, the trainer must provide an effective rationale for training parents (instead of the child) to effect child behavior change. For example, parents can be helped to see that they are the

logical choice to implement treatment because they have the greatest amount of contact with the child and the greatest amount of control over the home environment, in which most of the daily life learning experiences occur. The manuals for the empirically supported parent training programs provide helpful guidance for trainers on how to present a rationale for the role of parents in child behavior change. Finally, parents are taught to operationally define the problem behavior (e.g., noncompliance) and target behavior (e.g., compliance), and data collection begins during role plays. For example, one parent might give instructions to another parent (role playing a child), who intersperses episodes of compliance with noncompliance while the parent codes the frequency of each. Parents are then given homework to collect data on their children's behaviors during the next week.

In the second session, the parent trainer continues to build rapport, usually through review and problem solving related to homework completion. Behavioral skills training of differential attention is then introduced. Differential attention refers to providing children with positive adult attention (e.g., social praise, positive touch, descriptions of behavior, reflecting child language) contingent on appropriate child behavior and withdrawing adult attention contingent on negative or inappropriate child behavior. The skill is described and modeled by the trainer, then practiced by the parents with each other or with their children during the session. Videotapes may be used for modeling. Practice of the skill may take place during a short-duration (i.e., 5-minute) structured-play situation in which the parent and child are interacting. As parents practice with each other or with their children, the parent trainer provides feedback focused on shaping effective differential attention skills. This typically involves the trainer providing labeled praise to parents for positive skills (e.g., "Nice job praising Sally for sharing her blocks with you"), as well as corrective feedback for mistakes observed (e.g., "Oops, that was a question. Try to phrase as a statement instead"). The emphasis for the parent trainer centers on providing more praise than corrective feedback to the parent. Handouts summarizing the parenting skills may be provided. For example, a typical handout on

TABLE 24.1. Session Outline for Group-Based Parent Training to Improve Child Compliance

Session 1
(all sessions 1½ hours)

Introductions
Preview session
Review goals
Review rules
Gather information from parents about children, concerns, strengths, goals
Define compliance and noncompliance
Present theory of child behavior change
Discuss importance of monitoring behavior and data collection
Model and practice data collection with parents and children
Homework: Have parents collect data on compliance

Session 2

Review goals of group, preview session, parent questions from preceding week
Review data
Present and discuss differential attention
Model differential attention with parent (videotapes may be helpful)
Have parents practice with each other while trainer provides feedback
Have parents practice with their children while trainer provides feedback
Homework: Practice providing differential attention at home as part of a play interaction with child

Session 3

Review preceding week, preview session, parent questions
Review differential attention home practices and problem-solve parent concerns
Introduce effective commands
Model and practice
Practice with children
Homework: Practice effective commands at home

Session 4

Review, preview, parent questions
Practice effective commands with differential attention
Introduce and discuss token reward programs
Homework: Negotiate reward list with children and continue effective commands and differential attention

Session 5

Review, preview, parent questions
Review reward lists
Discuss criteria for earning tokens, exchanging rewards
Have parents practice with their children during play activity
Homework: Implement token reward program for targeted behavior

Session 6

Review, preview, questions
Review implementation of token reward program and problem-solve difficulties
Present use of time-out as consequence for noncompliance
Model time-out with parents
Role-play with children with trainer feedback
Homework: Implement time-out at home and monitor

Session 7

Review, preview, questions
Discuss time-out implementation successes and problems
Introduce response cost as a consequence
Model and practice with parents with trainer feedback
Practice with children
Homework: Implement response cost and monitor

Session 8

Review, preview, questions
Review implementation of response cost and discuss success and problems
Discuss generalization of skills to other problems

attending to children (from the McMahon and Forehand, 2003, program, "Helping the Noncompliant Child") includes reminders to parents that during practice, they should (1) follow rather than lead, (2) describe their child's behavior, (3) describe enthusiastically, (4) describe only OK behavior, (5) avoid asking questions. Another handout describes how to use rewards, such as labeled praise and physical attention, during practice at home. Homework involves requesting parents to practice the skill at home and to collect data on the frequency of practice.

In Session 3, the group begins with a review of the homework implementation data, as well as problems (and problem solving) and successes in implementing differential attention. The trainer provides some additional behavioral skills training related to generalizing differential attention to everyday situations (e.g., in the grocery store, in the car, while getting dinner ready), but then the focus shifts to behavioral skills training in giving effective commands. An effective command (sometimes called an "alpha" command) refers to a command statement that has been demonstrated in research to increase the probability of child compliance (e.g., Matheson & Shriver, 2005). The trainer provides a description of the characteristics of effective (e.g., one instruction, clear voice, "do" command, simple language) and ineffective (e.g., vague, phrased as question, chained with multiple demands) commands and typically includes handouts. In addition, parents are taught to establish clearly defined "house rules," or daily expectations. The parent trainer should model effective commands but may find that modeling ineffective commands can help parents learn to discriminate between the two. Parents should, of course, practice effective commands in role plays with each other or in practice with their child, but they may also find that demonstrating ineffective commands for other parents to "catch" may be both fun and effective. Finally, the trainer assigns homework to parents to practice using effective commands at home. For example, a parent may practice providing effective commands during a prescribed time period or activity each day and monitor the child's response. Or the parent may be given homework to provide a certain number of

effective commands per day (e.g., 2–10) and to monitor the child's response.

In Session 4, following homework review and problem solving, the trainer provides behavioral skills training related to using effective commands and differential attention together. In this way, parents begin learning to attend to good behavior in general but to compliant behavior in particular. At this point, parents often want specific guidance about recommended discipline for noncompliance; however, consistent with the approach of the empirically supported programs, the emphasis remains on increasing reinforcement for compliance and ignoring noncompliance. Indeed, in the final portion of this session, to further strengthen the reinforcement for compliance, a token reward program is introduced and discussed. Some parents will object to the use of tangible rewards for basic compliance, and the trainer will need to have a well-developed rationale to support this component of parent training. Although it is certainly true that "we all work for rewards," it may prove more effective to remind parents that rewards are like many medical interventions (e.g., casts), which are cumbersome and disruptive but are tolerated because they are effective and temporary (see Shriver & Allen, 2008). The assigned homework then involves asking parents to work with their child to negotiate a list of acceptable rewards that can be earned for increasing compliance.

In session 5, the reward lists are reviewed to assess practicality (e.g., can they be delivered frequently?) and potential effectiveness (e.g., do they appear to be reinforcing for the child?). Actual tokens to be earned for compliance (e.g., poker chips, tickets, tallies on a sheet, stickers, happy faces) are developed for each child, and the criteria for daily exchange of tokens for rewards are discussed. For example, a child might earn a marble, placed in a jar, for each instance of compliance, thereby enabling the child to trade the marbles for more TV time, for a later bedtime, for an extra snack, or for a quarter. The trainer will need to help parents decide how much each reward costs and how often tokens can be exchanged each day. This will vary depending on how often commands are given (determined from the command-based homework data in Session 3) and the child's current level of compliance (determined from the compliance-based homework data collected after Session 1). Of course, the trainer may model token and attention delivery contingent on compliant behavior, but it may be more effective by Session 5 to have parents model and give feedback to each other. Parents are then asked to implement the token reward system during the coming weeks, with data collection focused on tracking the number of tokens and rewards earned daily. These data will provide some indication of parents' treatment integrity, as well as child compliance.

In Session 6, data from token reward system implementation are reviewed, and parents themselves are recruited to help problem-solve any difficulties with implementation and follow-through. Time-out for noncompliance is then introduced, and behavioral skills training ensues. Note that there is no evidence that parents must understand why time-out works in order to implement it effectively. Still, each of the empirically supported programs takes steps to help parents see that removing a child from a reinforcing environment (e.g., one with praise, tokens, and attention) to a less reinforcing environment (e.g., sitting alone and being ignored) can be an effective discipline and that past failures of time-out are often tied to not enough of the former and too little of the latter (Shriver & Allen, 1996). Of course, modeling and role playing with feedback can be extremely important in overcoming common pitfalls such as scolding, threatening, and warning a child who is crying in time-out or who is negotiating an early release. It can be both entertaining and effective to have a parent role-play a child in time-out (based perhaps on his or her experiences with his or her own child) and exhibit the sorts of behaviors that might occur (e.g., falling to the floor, begging for release, claiming he or she is not loved, claiming potty needs, saying "I hate you"). The trainer can help parents problem-solve how to ignore these behaviors or to deal with more difficult escape attempts by children who will not stay put. Recommended homework includes implementing time-out at home and collecting data on frequency and durations of time-outs daily. However, it is equally important that parents continue to track performance

on the token reward system to ensure that the child still finds the "time-in" environment reinforcing.

In Session 7, the trainer should expect numerous questions about challenges and difficulties experienced by parents who implemented time-out. The trainer must resist spending too much time on any one parent's problems, and there may be times a parent requires a referral for more intensive individualized services to solve unique problems. Of course, a common obstacle to successful implementation of time-out is enforcement of the procedure. Some children will not stay put. Although isolation in another room (e.g., bedroom) can be an effective backup for some parents, in many cases it may not, either because the room has too many potential reinforcers or because the available rooms are not safe (e.g., bathroom). In these cases, response cost can be an effective alternative, and it is introduced here as a punitive consequence for noncompliance. Response cost involves the removal of tokens or privileges contingent on noncompliance. Response cost could be used as an alternative to time-out or as an enforcement of time-out. For example, as an alternative to time-out, a child who refuses to put on his or her shoes might lose two tokens, earning one back if he or she now complies. However, as enforcement, a child who refuses to put on his shoes might be sent to time-out and lose two tokens only if he or she refuses to stay in his or her assigned area. Not all parents would require the response-cost component, but all would benefit from understanding how it would work and contribute to enforcement and learning. Recommended homework consists of implementing a response-cost strategy (if necessary) and continuing to collect data on token rewards and time-out implementation.

In Session 8, the final session, the trainer spends some time reviewing and problem solving the implementation of response-cost system. However, the majority of this session targets the generalization of the parenting skills to address problems outside the home (e.g., at school, at the store, visiting relatives, at church) and problems other than noncompliance (e.g., physical aggression, bedtime problems, schoolwork completion). Parents are allowed some latitude in developing solutions to their own and others' unique problems. Here, the trainer serves as a moderator, keeping the parents focused on using the skills derived from empirically supported programs and taught in the preceding sessions. Parents are encouraged to contact the trainer by phone with any questions or to address other concerns.

Developing and Implementing Parent Training Groups in Schools

In this section we outline some essential considerations for school psychologists interested in conducting group-based parent training in schools. These considerations are described in the subsections on practical considerations and group leadership considerations. These are issues that must be thought about prior to developing and conducting a parent training group.

Practical Considerations

Like all interventions, successful parent training requires planning. It is important that the school psychologist give careful consideration to the needs of the school and community, to the resources available in the school, and, of course, to the school psychologist's own time, interest, and expertise needed for training a group of parents.

Needs Assessment

The first step in developing a parent training group is to determine whether the need for such a group exists within the particular school community served by the school psychologist, and, if so, what the needs of the parents in the school community are. The first part of this needs assessment may seem relatively straightforward, as school psychologists can usually make a strong case that parents would benefit from training. However, this needs assessment is largely about determining whether other school professionals and the parents themselves see a need for parent training. The school psychologist will want to talk with teachers in the school, the principal, the school counselor, and/or the family liaison to assess their perceptions of parents' needs in the community. The

school psychologist may also address the Parent–Teacher Organization or other parent groups within the community to assess their perceptions of need for parent training in the community. The school psychologist may want to send out a brief survey to ask whether parents would be interested in parent training and asking them to check off topics or to list topics on which they would be interested in receiving training and for which they would actually attend sessions. The survey might also inquire about best times for groups to meet and whether child care will be required.

As described in the example earlier, parent training often focuses on issues of child noncompliance, but parent training may also address myriad other child problems (Briesmeister & Schaefer, 1998; Shriver & Allen, 2008). If parents in a group are seeking solutions to vastly different problems, then it can be difficult for the parent trainer to address all participants' needs effectively. Thus, when establishing a parent training group, it will be important that the parents in the group are there to address the same problem behaviors. Parents seeking solutions to similar problems will be in a better position to provide support to each other and may be able to provide other parents with ideas for intervention and implementation. Parent training groups can be developed to address academic issues (i.e., skill deficits, performance deficits, homework and study skills), strategies for addressing behavioral characteristics of children with attention-deficit/hyperactivity disorder (ADHD) or high-functioning autism or Asperger disorder, sleep hygiene issues, or managing adolescent behavior problems. For anyone just starting to conduct parent training, we recommend starting with parent training to address child noncompliance, as that is the topic with most research support and available information (i.e., manuals).

Size of Group

Given that parent training involves the active teaching of skills, including frequent feedback from the trainer, the size of the group must be limited. A parent trainer would be hard-pressed to engage in behavioral skills training with a group of parents numbering

12 or more. Indeed, group training is usually most effective with groups of 8–12 individuals (Corey & Corey, 2006). Although the number of children who benefit by having trained parents may vary considerably depending on the numbers of single parents or couples in the group or number of children in one home, for purposes of group management and training, it is probably best to limit group size to 8–12 parents. If there is a greater need, the school psychologist will need to make a decision as to whether to ask someone (e.g., another school psychologist, a school counselor, teacher) to help him or her provide training or consider organizing two parent training groups or perhaps put some parents on a waiting list.

Time of Day

Because of work schedules and other commitments, parents are often not available to meet during the school day. Typically, parent training groups take place in the late afternoon or early evening. The groups will most commonly meet about 90 minutes per week and may meet for anywhere from 6 to 10 weeks. An alternative to early evening may be early morning, particularly if there are before-school programs for the children to attend. The school psychologist will need to plan a time that works best for the parents based on the needs assessment described earlier. In addition, some school psychologists may need to work out arrangements with their school administration regarding hours of availability. For example, if the school psychologist works late one evening a week, perhaps he or she will be able to arrange coming in later one day a week.

Child Care

Certainly one determinant of attendance for many parents will center on the availability of child care. Many parents will have one or more children who require care during the parent training group and would find it more convenient to bring their children with them rather than securing their own child care every week. In fact, many may consider this an absolute necessity and will not attend otherwise. However, there are other reasons to make child care available. Although the trainer may plan to have children involved with training from time to time (e.g., for role playing and practice with parents), it is likely that their continuous attendance would be distracting and possibly disruptive. In addition, some children will be too young to assist with practice. One alternative is to invite some children to participate in some of the parent training activities but also plan for the children to be engaged for part of the time with other children in child-oriented activities in another room. This type of arrangement would require child-care staff. If child care will not or cannot be provided and children will not be welcomed during the parent training group, then this needs to be made clear to parents up front; this is not recommended, however.

Space, Equipment, Materials, and Personnel

Because meeting space can, at times, be limited, the school psychologist will need to discuss with the principal, appropriate administrative professionals, and teachers which rooms are available for a parent training group. Likewise, projectors, DVD players, and monitors, although not necessary, may be helpful for some components of the parent training. In particular, if videos from the Incredible Years program are used, then a monitor and DVD player are certainly needed. Space for child care and materials for activities for the children may be needed and personnel for child care may need to be identified. Chairs for parents to sit on will be needed. Handouts and other materials for parents will need to be developed. Perhaps an assistant to help with the parent training will be needed. All of these issues require planning and oftentimes permission from school administration prior to proceeding.

School Budget and/or Parent Pay

Child care, materials, and videos usually come at a price. Training for implementation of parent training programs, such as the Incredible Years, also may cost schools. The school psychologist and school administration will need to decide up front how much they are willing to budget for parent training. At a minimum, the school administration will need to provide space, chairs, and a small budget for copying materials and handouts. If more is desired to increase and improve parent involvement in the groups (e.g., child care) or to improve training procedures (e.g., video examples), then the school administration will have to make a commitment to these needs. In addition, some school districts or communities may have parents who are capable of paying a fee for the parent training program. If so, then decisions about the appropriate amount will need to be made, as well as decisions about whether to implement a sliding scale for income and whether to provide "scholarships" for parents who cannot pay. Sometimes local grants may be available from foundations, community agencies, or corporations to underwrite the costs associated with parent training. The school psychologist may want to talk with the principal about these possibilities.

Evaluating Outcomes

It is best to consider how outcomes will be evaluated prior to starting a parent training group because evaluation requires planning. At a minimum, the school psychologist will want to obtain a measure of satisfaction with the parent training group at the end of the process. McMahon and Forehand (2003) provide a very nice example of a parent satisfaction questionnaire in the appendix of their manual.

Consideration should also be given to administering a pre- and posttest of expected knowledge to be gained from the parent training group. Patterson's LWC (1976) provides some nice examples of quiz questions with answer keys for everything from social reinforcement to time-out. Of course, in practice, the pre- and posttest measures selected should address the primary needs and goals for the group that were developed based on the original needs assessment.

A satisfaction measure and a measure of acquired knowledge will provide information as to whether the groups functioned well as an educational enterprise. However, these measures will not provide information as to whether actual changes in parent and child behavior occurred. Evaluation of behavior change can include measures of parent adherence to recommendations and/

or adherence to homework assignments, as well as data collected on target child behaviors. These data collection procedures will require that each week the school psychologist consider what specific changes are expected in parent and child behavior and how these changes will be measured through homework assignments or other means (e.g., a weekly phone call assessing parent adherence to recommendations). For example, parents might be asked to simply track the frequency of child noncompliance for 1–2 weeks prior to training and then track for another 1–2 weeks after training has concluded. In addition, parents might be asked, during treatment, to simply record whether they remembered to practice providing differential attention during structured play interactions at home. The appendix of the Parent–Child Interaction Therapy manual (Hembree-Kigin & McNeil, 1995) provides a nice sample of just such a self-monitoring form.

Assessing Time and Effort for the School Psychologist

Parent training can be an extremely rewarding experience as parents are observed making positive changes and acquiring new parenting skills and children achieve positive outcomes. Parent training can help remediate child problem behaviors at home and school, can help prevent problems from developing, and can assist with improving relationships between parents and schools. Parent training, however, even in a group context, requires a substantial amount of time, planning, and effort. In addition, the parent training group may need to occur at a time that can interfere with the school psychologist's personal time and activities. Administrative support of parent training may be questionable in some schools or districts. The school psychologist may realize that she or he requires additional training or supervised experience in developing and implementing behavior interventions, collaborating with parents, and/or running groups. In addition, it is highly recommended that school psychologists receive training (didactic and supervised experiences) in conducting parent training and implementing behavioral interventions prior to implementing parent training. It is important that the school psychologist carefully conduct a personal cost–benefit analysis of developing and conducting a parent training group prior to proceeding.

Group Leadership Considerations

At the initial group meeting, the leader must recognize and establish up front that the parent training group is a "psychoeducational" group, not a support or therapy group (Corey & Corey, 2006). A psychoeducational group is primarily conducted for the purpose of imparting information and/or teaching skills. Therapy or support groups are conducted for the purpose of addressing members' personal psychological or behavioral health needs. Parent training groups are not appropriate venues for parents to discuss marital discord or individual mental health problems (e.g., depression, substance abuse, anxiety). These are topics that may arise in discussing the difficulty of managing child problems, but they should be addressed in the context of managing the child problems. If parents do have individual and personal difficulties that interfere with their ability to participate effectively in the group and/or to address child problems, then the school psychologist should refer these parents to another provider for treatment.

Although therapy or support services are not the purpose of a parent training group, member support will likely become an active component of the group. This is often a natural outgrowth of a group of individuals coming together to address common personal goals. They will discuss with each other their own difficulties and successes with their individual children. This type of support is a benefit of group-based parent training. The parent trainer's responsibility will be to manage these supportive interactions so that they do not interfere with teaching the skills to parents. It is important that the parent trainer establish early in the first session with parents the goals and rules of the group. Rules may include that only one person at a time is allowed to talk, that the group leader decides when to change topics or activities, and that criticism of other parents in the group is not allowed. Parents may need to be taught how to use supportive and reinforcing statements with one another. In addition, parents may need to be taught early how to provide constructive critical feedback to one another during group discussion.

Group Dynamics

Parents bring their own unique learning histories, culture, and personalities to the parent training situation and interaction with the parent trainer. Likewise, the parent trainer also brings his or her own unique learning history, culture, and personality to the parent training interaction, as well. This mix of individual variables must be managed by the parent trainer to facilitate learning and to prevent distractions from learning. Establishing rules and expectations early in the group (see the preceding example) may assist in effectively managing these personalities.

In addition to different personality characteristics, parents may come to the parent training group with different parenting skill needs. Those who arrive with many of the skills necessary to achieve the goals of the group may require only some minor instruction and feedback. Those with few positive parenting skills may require substantial behavioral skills training to achieve the goals of the group. The parent trainer will need to consider whether parents with very limited skills require referral to another provider for individualized parent training.

Similarly, some parents will have children with more severe behavior problems (e.g., more frequent, intense, longer duration) than those of children of other parents in the parent training group. These children may require more intensive intervention, and the parents will need more intensive training and supervision. These are also parents who will likely require referral to another provider for individualized parent training.

Whereas the science of parent training may lie in the content of what is taught (behavioral principles and strategies) and the methods used to teach (i.e., behavioral skills training), the art of parent training may lie in the dynamics of the process. That is, the development of a positive relationship between the parent trainer and parents and between the parents themselves may significantly enhance parents' learning of and adherence to recommended strategies. Establishing an effective dynamic can involve a wide variety of clinical skills that include the effective use of rationales, metaphors, humor, disclosure, rapport, and collaboration, as well as careful attention to cultural issues. Webster-Stratton and Herbert (1994) provide an excellent resource on developing effective group process in which they describe a variety of strategies for building rapport. These clinical skills are also discussed in more detail specific to parent training in Shriver and Allen (2008). Other general texts on running groups often incorporate information on effectively managing group dynamics (Corey & Corey, 2006; Delucia-Waack, Gerrity, Kalodner, & Riva, 2004). Finally, the manuals for the empirically supported parent training programs provide advice on how to present information to parents regarding child behavior change and how to engender greater parental adherence.

Summary and Conclusions

Parents can be effective partners with school professionals in facilitating the success of their children in the classroom. Parent training can be an important role for school psychologists working with students in special education, as well as general education, contexts to assist with remediating and/or preventing child problems at home and school and developing collaborative home–school partnerships. Although most parent training programs with empirical support were developed for individual families in a clinical context, this does not mean that parent training is not effective in a school setting, but rather that adaptations regarding how parent training is delivered will likely need to be considered in order for parent training to be effective in a school setting. Review of the literature and the manuals that accompany empirically supported parent training programs provide direct guidance for school psychologists in what and how to train parents.

When we consider parent training as part of the role of a school psychologist, it appears that group-based parent training is probably the most efficient and efficacious model for parent training in terms of time, effort, and impact on a larger number of children and families. Conducting group-based parent training requires knowledge of research to inform parenting skills and child interventions, managing group dynamics, using effective clinical skills, and applying data-based decision making. Although continued research on the efficacy and effectiveness of parent training groups in schools is sorely needed, the empirical support for parent training as a service delivery model and treatment is certainly sufficient to incorporate these skills as part of typical school psychology graduate training and practice.

References

American Psychological Association. (2005). Policy statement on evidence-based practice in psychology. Available at *www2.apa.org/practice/ebpstatement.pdf*.

Barkley, R. A. (1997). *Defiant children: A clinician's manual for assessment and parent training* (2nd ed.). New York: Guilford Press.

Brestan, E. V., & Eyberg, S. M. (1998). Effective psychosocial treatments of conduct disordered children and adolescents: 29 years, 82 studies, and 5272 kids. *Journal of Clinical Child Psychology, 27*, 180–189.

Briesmeister, J. M., & Schaefer, C. E. (1998). *Handbook of parenting training: Parents as cotherapists for children's behavior problems* (2nd ed.). New York: Wiley.

Burke, R., Herron, R., & Schuchmann, L. (2004). *Common sense parenting: Learn at home workbook and DVD*. Boys Town, NE: Boys Town Press.

Carlson, C., & Christenson, S. L. (Guest Eds.). (2005). Evidence-based parent and family interventions in school psychology [Special issue]. *School Psychology Quarterly, 20*, 345–351.

Chambless, D. L., & Hollon, S. D. (1998). Defining empirically supported therapies. *Journal of Consulting and Clinical Psychology, 66*(1), 7–18.

Conduct Problems Prevention Research Group. (1992). A developmental and clinical model for the prevention of conduct disorder: The FAST Track Program. *Development and Psychopathology, 4*, 509–527.

Conduct Problems Prevention Research Group. (2004). The effects of the Fast Track program on serious problem outcomes at the end of elementary school. *Journal of Clinical Child and Adolescent Psychology, 33*, 650–661.

Corey, M. S., & Corey, G. (2006). Groups: Process and practice (7th ed.). Belmont, CA: Thomson Learning.

Dangel, R. F., & Polster, R. A. (Eds.). (1984).

Parent training: Foundations of research and practice. New York: Guilford Press.

Delucia-Waack, J. L., Gerrity, D. A., Kalodner, C. R., & Riva, M. T. (Eds.). (2004). *Handbook of group counseling and psychotherapy.* Thousand Oaks, CA: Sage.

Dembo, M. H., Sweitzer, M., & Lauritzen, P. (1985). An evaluation of group parent education: Behavioral, PET, and Adlerian programs. *Review of Educational Research, 55,* 155–200.

Hembree-Kigin, T. L., & McNeil, C. B. (1995). *Parent–Child Interaction Therapy.* New York: Plenum Press.

Individuals with Disabilities Education Improvement of 2004, Pub. L. No. 108-446, §302, 118 Stat. 2803.

Kazdin, A. E. (2005). *Parent management training: Treatment for oppositional, aggressive, and antisocial behavior in children and adolescents.* New York: Oxford University Press.

Kratochwill, T. R., & Stoiber, K. C. (2000). Empirically supported interventions and school psychology: Conceptual and practical issues: Part 2. *School Psychology Quarterly, 15,* 233–253.

Kumpfer, K. L. (1999). Strengthening America's families: Exemplary parenting and family strategies for delinquency prevention. Retrieved December 12, 2007, from *www.strengtheningfamilies.org.*

Kumpfer, K. L., & Alvarado, R. (2003). Family-strengthening approaches for the prevention of youth problem behaviors. *American Psychologist, 58*(6/7), 457–465.

Matheson, A., & Shriver, M. D. (2005). Training teachers to give effective commands: Effects on student compliance and academic behaviors. *School Psychology Review, 34,* 202–219.

McMahon, R. J., & Forehand, R. L. (2003). *Helping the noncompliant child: Family based treatment for oppositional behavior* (2nd ed.). New York: Guilford Press.

Miltenberger, R. G. (2001). *Behavior modification: Principles and procedures* (2nd ed.). Belmont, CA: Wadsworth/Thomson Learning.

No Child Left Behind Act of 2001, Pub. L. No. 107-110 (2002).

Patterson, G. R. (1976). *Living with children: New methods for parents and teachers* (Rev. ed.). Champaign, IL: Research Press.

Patterson, G. R., Reid, J. B., Jones, R. R., & Conger, R. E. (1975). *A social learning approach to family intervention: Families with aggressive children* (Vol. 1). Eugene, OR: Castalia.

Reid, J. B., Patterson, G. R., & Snyder, J. (2002). *Antisocial behavior in children and adolescents: A developmental analysis and model for intervention.* Washington, DC: American Psychological Association.

Sackett, D. L., Straus, S. E., Richardson, W. S., Rosenberg, W., & Haynes, R. B. (2000). *Evidence-based medicine: How to practice and teach EBM* (2nd ed.). New York: Churchill Livingstone.

Sanders, M. R. (1999). Triple P-Positive Parenting Program: Toward an empirically validated multilevel parenting and family support strategy for the prevention of behavior and emotional problems in children. *Clinical Child and Family Psychology Review, 2*(2), 71–90.

Shriver, M. D. (1997). Teaching parenting skills. In T. S. Watson & F. Gresham (Eds.), *Child behavior therapy: Ecological considerations in assessment, treatment, and evaluation* (pp. 165–182). New York: Plenum Press.

Shriver, M. D., & Allen, K. D. (1996). The time-out grid: A guide to effective discipline. *School Psychology Quarterly, 11,* 67–75.

Shriver, M. D., & Allen, K. D. (2008). *Working with parents of noncompliant children: A guide to evidence-based parent training for practitioners and students.* Washington, DC: American Psychological Association.

Webster-Stratton, C. (1992). *The Incredible Years: A trouble-shooting guide for parents of children aged 3–8.* Toronto, Ontario, Canada: Umbrella Press.

Webster-Stratton, C., & Herbert, M. (1994). *Troubled families—problem children: Working with parents: A collaborative process.* New York: Wiley.

Chapter 25

Problem-Solving Skills Training

Theory and Practice in the School Setting

Bryan Bushman
Gretchen Gimpel Peacock

Nine-year-old Michael seemed unable to contain himself any longer. During small-group-circle time, he fidgeted and made a clumsy attempt to unobtrusively scoot closer to the girl seated on his right. Michael's teacher could see what was coming. Before she could intercede, Michael shouted a loud "oink" in the girl's ear and grinned expectantly as his classmate recoiled. After being mildly pushed away by the girl, Michael, now looking more disappointed and angry, began to push back. As the teacher quickly approached, Michael engaged several other students in a pushing and name-calling match that seemed to quickly engulf the classroom. ... After sitting in time-out for several minutes, Michael looked dumbfounded and teary-eyed as the teacher asked why, yet again, he was unable to keep to himself during group activities.

This chapter presents theory, research, and a practical treatment approach to helping students like Michael who have difficulty demonstrating appropriate behavior. Such students often demonstrate maladaptive, impulsive, or aggressive behaviors during interactions with fellow students, teachers, or family members. They do not seem to think through or learn from the consequences of their actions, frustrating parents, teachers, and peers. Because these behaviors are typically impairing for the child and problematic for important others in a child's life (e.g., teachers, parents), many students who exhibit such behaviors will be referred for services in the school context. In this chapter we describe a treatment method commonly referred to as problem-solving skills training (PSST; e.g., Kazdin, 2003; Kendall & Braswell, 1985). PSST is a cognitive-behavioral intervention that is aimed at helping children stop and think through potential solutions before they respond. Students are taught specific problem-solving steps that can be applied to a variety of social situations and are provided with opportunities to practice these steps in session, as well as outside of session, in "real" social situations. PSST can be an appropriate treatment method for students who demonstrate a variety of problem behaviors (e.g., aggression, defiance, impulsivity) related to problem solving in social contexts.

We begin this chapter with an overview of some of the empirical literature and theory related to children who frequently engage in aggressive, defiant, and impulsive social behavior. Specifically, we first provide a brief review of the literature regarding the proposed cognitive differences between such children and their same-age peers. Here the term *cognitive differences* implies a difference in the cognitive strategies a student uses to solve problems; it does not imply a global cognitive deficiency or developmental delay. To help put these differences within a conceptual framework, we provide an overview of a social-information-processing model. We then provide a general overview of the PSST treatment methods and techniques, followed by a review of some of the empirical support for PSST and similar cognitive-behavioral interventions. We conclude the chapter with a session-by-session overview of an abbreviated PSST program with specifics on how to implement this treatment in the school context.

Several caveats are important to mention before continuing. First, this chapter focuses primarily on the theoretical and practical aspects of working directly with students using a PSST model. It does not provide information on other evidenced-based treatment options, such as parent training or classroom-based behavior management programs, that focus on how to enact behavioral contingencies, which are clearly an important treatment component when working with children with externalizing behavior problems. Readers are encouraged to review other chapters in this volume to familiarize themselves with treatment methods that may be used in conjunction with PSST. For example, Shriver and Allen (Chapter 24, this volume) provide an overview of behavioral parent training, which is often used in combination with PSST, and Kern, Benson, and Clemens (Chapter 27, this volume) provide an overview of behavioral interventions for children with challenging problem behaviors. The intervention presented in this chapter is also geared toward children who have the developmental capacity (e.g., understanding of language) to utilize more advanced cognitive methods; thus it will be less applicable to very young children or to those who have significant developmental delays (see Friman, Volz, & Haugen, Chapter 23, this volume for a discussion of children's understanding of language in the context of behavioral interventions). Finally, although the theory and practices presented in this chapter may have some applicability to children with pervasive developmental disorders,

such as Asperger disorder, these students will likely require more intensive treatment (Coie, 1990; Spivack, Platt, & Shure, 1976).

Research, Theory, and Practical Implications of Problem-Solving Deficits Underlying Aggressive and Impulsive Behaviors

Research and Theory of Problem-Solving Deficits

Several researchers have suggested that students who consistently demonstrate defiant, impulsive, and aggressive behavior frequently demonstrate social skill problems (Crick & Dodge, 1994; Dodge, 1993; Gifford-Smith & Rabiner, 2004; Walker, Colvin, & Ramsey, 1995). In addition, these children often differ from their peers across a number of cognitive factors that underlie effective problem solving, such as attentional control, cognitive flexibility, planning, and self-monitoring (Lochman, Powell, Whidby, & FitzGerald, 2006; Webster-Stratton & Lindsay, 1999). Rather than that these phenomena (e.g., social skill problems, cognitive deficits) simply co-occur, it has been suggested that these cognitive problem-solving deficits may contribute to the expression of problematic social behaviors (Webster-Stratton & Lindsay, 1999) and can result in an ongoing reactive pattern of aggression, defiance, and impulsivity (Giancola, Moss, & Martin, 1996). As a result, students are at increased risk for long-term peer rejection and further deterioration of social behavior (Loeber & Farrington, 2000).

Crick and Dodge's (1994) social-information-processing model adequately captures many of the findings of the literature and fits nicely with the fundamental tenets of the intervention method described in this chapter. Their model delineates several steps, as outlined here, that students typically use when processing interpersonal material and reacting to their environment:

1. *Encoding:* A student encodes cues related to social interactions. These cues can be either external (e.g., what is said by others) or internal (e.g., the amount of emotional arousal the youth is experiencing at that time).
2. *Interpretation:* The student interprets the cues and either clarifies a goal for the

interaction or attempts to regulate the arousal being experienced.

3. *Response generation:* The student constructs various responses to either regulate arousal or achieve the desired goal.

4. *Response decision:* A response decision is made based on an evaluation of what the child perceives to be positive outcomes.

At each stage of this process, the child uses a memory store of learned social interactions and schema (i.e., organized mental constructs). It is assumed that a fair amount of overlap exists between stages and that the stages interact with one another, resulting in substantial feedback between stages.

Although all children follow this process, it is hypothesized that many children with behavior problems differ from their "normal" peers in several ways (Crick & Dodge, 1994). First, students with behavior problems may have a deficit in *encoding* information from their environment (Step 1). Specifically, students who are aggressive selectively attend to any cues of hostility in the environment. For example, a student is walking down the hall at school and three of his peers say "hello," while another student bumps into him. The student may focus selectively on the potentially "hostile" action of being bumped. Next, these students are hypothesized to have what is referred to as a *hostile attributional bias*, or faulty mental representation. In Step 2 of Crick and Dodge's (1994) model (i.e., interpretation), these students perceive either neutral or unknown stimuli from the environment as being hostile, whereas other children do not necessarily perceive the same stimuli as being threatening. Due to the perception of threat, they are more likely to believe that retaliation is warranted. Using our preceding example, students without this hostile attributional bias may interpret being bumped into in the hall as just an accident, something that commonly occurs when the halls are busy. However, a student with a hostile attribution bias may interpret being bumped into as a purposeful act meant to be harmful. A third difference, according to Crick and Dodge (1994), is that such children do not have access to as many socially acceptable ways of responding (Step 3, response generation and memory store), a tendency that is referred to as *response access.* In

other words, after one or two well-rehearsed prosocial responses are generated, only aggressive or impulsive ways of responding are recalled by the student. Thus the student's response to being bumped may be to retaliate with physical aggression. Finally, when determining how to respond, it is theorized that these children often give an inappropriate amount of consideration and approval to aggressive or impulsive actions in their *response evaluation* (Step 4). In our example, the student may think that using physical aggression in response to being bumped in the hall will make it less likely that he will be bumped again and may believe this behavior will increase his social status with other children. Of course, it is possible to understand the same student's behavior as a function of reinforcement—for example, classmates move out of the student's way the next time they see him in the hall. Nevertheless, cognitive theorists such as Crick and Dodge assume that a lack of cognitive skill underlies (or at the very least contributes to) persistent problematic behaviors—especially in light of the cognitive skill deficits referenced earlier. It is important to be clear, though, that these cognitive processes and attributions may not be causal factors in the expression of the inappropriate social behaviors. Children with these hypothesized deficits may selectively respond to environmental stimuli and, via this selective responding, learn inappropriate behaviors.

Practical Implications: Identifying Students for Treatment

Theories such as Crick and Dodge's provide direction regarding which students may benefit the most from treatments such as PSST (although it is important to note that additional empirical research is needed to support these theory-based suggestions). In line with this theory, an appropriate candidate for the problem-solving treatment described in this chapter would be a student who has difficulty *interpreting* social cues, *generating* multiple prosocial solutions to problems, and *evaluating* which solutions will lead to effective outcomes. The child's general level of emotional arousal should also be kept in mind. Dodge and colleagues have observed that a high level of emotional arousal negatively influences a child's interpretation of social cues, as well as accessibility and selection of response options (Dodge, 1980; Dodge & Coie, 1987; Dodge, Prince, Bachorowski, & Newman, 1990). Consequently, a child who is greatly upset yet who may normally possess adequate problem-solving skills may react in a way similar to a child who possesses problem-solving deficits.

Practically speaking, when deciding which students to target for intervention, students might first be nominated by their teachers as demonstrating difficulties with peer social interactions (e.g., see the discussion by McIntosh, Reinke, & Herman in Chapter 9, this volume, on screening methods; also see Martens & Ardoin, Chapter 10, this volume, for additional information on assessment of disruptive behaviors). School psychologists can then more fully evaluate which students would benefit from PSST by using behavioral checklists and behavioral observations during time periods in which social skill problems typically occur (e.g., recess). It is important to note that the hypothesized cognitive constructs discussed previously are not directly observable but instead are inferred based on observable behavior in interaction with events occurring before and after it. Therefore, it is of utmost importance to note patterns of interaction between behavior and environmental events. During observations, specific attention to the following can be important: (1) behaviorally operationalizing (i.e., defining in specific, behavioral terms) the maladaptive behavior(s) in question; (2) noting antecedent social interactions that occur before the behavior; and (3) noting consequential social responses to determine whether the maladaptive behavior plays an instrumental or functional role in obtaining a desired outcome (e.g., attention, access to a desired object). As with all behavior observations, the practitioner may also wish to monitor the frequency and duration of the maladaptive behavior as a way of determining the student's baseline of functioning.

Noting antecedent triggers and consequential outcomes are both important because they relate specifically to intervention. Having a list of antecedent social situations will help the practitioner decide which social situations need to be role played during the intervention sessions, as the student may be unaware of or unwilling to divulge the types of social situations he or she finds difficult.

The practitioner may also want to note the child's level of emotional arousal (e.g., frustration, anger), as the child may need to be taught how to employ relaxation strategies before he or she can effectively implement problem-solving skills. It is also important to determine what consequence the maladaptive behavior has on the child's social environment to determine whether the child engages in reactive or instrumental social behavior. If the child engages in reactive behavior, the child may have cognitive problem-solving deficits, and an intervention such as PSST may be appropriate. In contrast, if the student engages in instrumental behavior (i.e., behavior intended to gain some desired outcome), it will be more important for the practitioner to work with the teacher and, potentially, parents to alter behavioral contingencies so that there is less of a "payoff" for maladaptive behavior. Of course, for many students, such a simple dichotomy does not exist, and both components will be necessary for treatment. Interviews with the student's teachers and, ideally, parents are important supplements to the information obtained through observation.

Overview of PSST

Many of the PSST treatments utilized by researchers and clinicians are based loosely on Kendall and Braswell's cognitive-behavioral therapy for impulsive children program (Kendall & Braswell, 1985), although others have also developed and evaluated similar programs (e.g., Kazdin, 2003; Webster-Stratton & Reid, 2003). Kendall and Braswell (1985) identify five treatment principles used with varying emphasis in each session of their PSST program: (1) teaching the student the problem-solving steps, (2) using self-instructional training as much as possible, (3) applying behavioral contingencies for demonstrating the steps both in session and out of session, (4) using modeling techniques, and (5) practicing responses through role-playing exercises. Each of these is described next; later in the chapter we provide a detailed overview of a PSST treatment program that incorporates these principles.

Treatment begins by teaching students the basic skills of problem-solving using a step-by-step method. Kendall and Braswell (1985) use the following steps: (1) "What am I sup-posed to do?" (2) "What are all the possibili-ties?" (3) "Relax," (4) "I think this is the one … ", and (5) "How did I do?" (p. 120). With other PSST programs, the exact wording of the steps may vary somewhat; however, they are very similar. For example, Kazdin's (2003) steps as worded in self-statements are: (1) "What am I supposed to do?" (2) "I have to look at all the possibilities"; (3) "I'd better concentrate and focus in"; (4) "I need to make a choice"; and (5) "I did a good job" or "Oh, I made a mistake" (p. 246). In both models, children are instructed to evaluate the solutions generated in the second step during the third step.

Self-instructional approaches are used throughout treatment to assist youths in integrating the problem-solving steps into their own language and level of understand-ing. For instance, in one of the first treat-ment sessions, the student is taught to ver-balize the problem-solving steps in his or her own words. Ideas are also solicited from the student regarding basic rules that he or she can use to determine whether a solution is appropriate (e.g., "Is it fair to others?" "Is it dangerous?"). Of course, the therapist pro-vides some general rules; however, the stu-dent is to be an active participant in generat-ing rules to determine whether solutions are effective.

The use of behavioral contingencies is also an important aspect of treatment. The prac-titioner uses tokens (e.g., poker chips) dur-ing sessions that the child can exchange for rewards. Initially, the child is able to earn tokens simply for engaging in treatment, for remembering concepts, for completing homework assignments ("experiments"), and for demonstrating the problem-solving steps. Eventually, however, it is impor-tant for the practitioner to implement a response-cost program, as data suggest that many children (especially those with symptoms of attention-deficit/hyperactivity disorder) often do not demonstrate improve-ment if a reward system is used in isolation (e.g., Acker & O'Leary, 1987; Pfiffner & O'Leary, 1987). The child can lose tokens in the session for (1) forgetting to use one or more of the problem-solving steps or (2) going "too fast" during task completion. The practitioner provides the child with a matter-of-fact explanation for the token

being removed and uses clinical judgment regarding the timing and frequency of token removal so as not to provoke an adversarial relationship. When developing a reinforce-ment system, it is important to involve the student's teacher(s) and/or parent(s) when at all possible so that students can exchange to-kens for out-of-session rewards that parents and teachers control. In addition, parents and teachers can provide reinforcement to the child for practicing the problem-solving steps outside of session. It should be made clear to parents and teachers that their role is to provide praise when the child is behav-ing appropriately and/or when it seems likely that the child has used the problem-solving steps, not to punish or "nag" the child into using the problem-solving steps.

The practitioner and, as much as possible, the student's parents and teachers model the problem-solving steps by stating out loud the use of the steps. Obviously, this requires the child's parents and teachers to be informed regarding the steps. When the practitioner models the steps in the session, he or she starts with a "mastery" model by doing the steps perfectly. Eventually the practitioner uses a "coping" model once the student has become accustomed to using the steps. The practitioner intentionally makes mistakes, catches him- or herself, and makes coping statements to correct the "error" (e.g., "This is stupid. I give up. No, wait … [deep breath] It's OK. I'll catch myself next time"). The modeling of this skill is important because it is hypothesized that many children who exhibit aggressive and disruptive behaviors may have difficulties in effectively cop-ing with errors. Near the end of treatment, the child ideally views him- or herself on a videotape using the steps (i.e., the child is a self-model) and is asked to generate feedback about his or her use of the steps.

Role plays are often used conjointly with modeling during treatment. Initially, the problem-solving steps are practiced in ses-sion using games (e.g., checkers), during which the practitioner models the problem-solving steps and the child is expected to practice applying the problem-solving steps. After these initial exercises, role plays that mirror real-life social situations that the child may encounter are used to practice the application of the problem-solving steps. Near the end of treatment, the practitioner solicits situations that have caused problems for the student in the past from his or her teachers or parents, and the practitioner and student role-play these situations. During all role plays it is important that the clinician help the child generate at least three or four potential solutions to problems. Doing this may be more difficult with cognitive tasks in which only one or two solutions present themselves (e.g., checkers); however, as the practitioner moves with the student into actual social situations, generating multiple alternative solutions becomes more of a priority. If students become stuck or attempt to escape generating further solutions with an "I don't know" answer, it can often be helpful to suggest outrageous or silly solutions to problems. For example, if a child generates only one or two solutions to being bullied, the practitioner can suggest that the student curl up in a ball and meow like a cat. This strategy can help demonstrate the brainstorming element entailed in problem solving: All ideas need to be considered. It is important that the child's ultimate solution be respected (e.g., the child may still think it is worth it to hit another student); otherwise, an adversarial relationship may be created between the child and the therapist and the child may not feel comfortable expressing his or her true thoughts. As long as the practitioner has helped the child think through all potential consequences of solutions and the child has demonstrated an ability to do this on his or her own, the main objectives of treatment have been met. As Kendall and Braswell (1985) stated, treatment involves helping the child "learn *how* to think, not *what* to think" (p. 204).

Obviously, it is possible that a student will generate a solution that the practitioner cannot ignore or even consider as a potential solution (e.g., suggestions of seriously harming oneself or others). Consequently, it is always recommended that the therapist review with the child the limits of confidentiality before treatment begins. For instance, the child needs to be told that if he or she is thinking of seriously of hurting him- or herself or someone else, the practitioner will have to tell the child's parents and others. During the session, if the child mentions a plan that includes harming him- or herself or others (e.g., "I could stab my sister with a knife"), the therapist should stop the session and discuss the likely outcomes with the child. The practitioner should also query about the child's access to such methods (e.g., "Where are the knives in your house?") and past instances in which the child may have acted out such behaviors (e.g., "Have you ever tried to hurt someone with a knife before?"). If the practitioner determines that the likelihood of danger is real, the child can be reminded at the end of the session about the limits of confidentiality. He or she should be told directly that his or her parents (and potentially others) will need to be immediately informed "so that everyone stays safe."

Empirical Support for PSST

Several investigators have formulated specific cognitive-behavioral treatments to teach students problem-solving skills (e.g., Kazdin, 2003; Kendall & Braswell, 1985). For the purposes of the current discussion, these treatments are referred to under the broad category of PSST. A handful of studies have compared PSST or similar interventions with alternative treatment methods or no-treatment controls. In two randomized controlled trials, Kazdin and colleagues compared PSST with relationship-based therapy (Kazdin, Bass, Siegel, & Thomas, 1989; Kazdin, Esveldt-Dawson, French, & Unis, 1987a). In both studies, children who received the PSST treatment demonstrated greater reductions in problem behaviors at home and at school and showed an increase in prosocial behaviors at posttreatment and at a 1-year follow-up compared with children in the relationship-based therapy treatment. Other researchers have also found positive effects for treatments similar to PSST. For instance, Arbuthnot and Gordon (1986) found that adolescents enrolled in a program similar to PSST demonstrated increased moral reasoning and more improvement than those in a no-treatment control group on several behavioral indexes, including a decrease in the number of behavioral referrals to the principal's office, a decrease in the number of court or police contacts, and an increase in grades (in English and humanities classes). However, there were no significant differences between groups on teacher ratings of behavior problems. Lochman, Burch, Curry, and Lampron (1984) compared an anger-coping treatment (a cognitive-behavioral treatment similar to PSST), goal setting (GS) alone, anger coping plus GS, and no treatment. Compared with children in the GS-only condition, children in the anger coping plus GS conditions demonstrated decreases in aggressive behaviors in the classroom and at home. Children in the anger coping group showed a significant decrease in parent-reported aggressive behavior compared with those in the GS-only group. However, no significant differences between groups were noted in the number of alternatives generated on a problem-solving measure and in social acceptance scores based on ratings of peers and teachers.

Other researchers have concluded that, although students exposed to PSST or similar cognitive-behavioral social-problem-solving treatments may demonstrate improved assertiveness and prosocial coping compared with controls, results are not maintained over time, and teacher, parent, and peer perceptions of the child are more difficult to change (Kolko, Loar, & Sturnick, 1990; Prinz, Blechman, & Dumas, 1994). Maintenance of results over time is a particular area of concern. Two meta-analyses on social skills interventions (including cognitive-behavioral therapy [CBT] programs similar to PSST) noted initial positive results but with a decline in positive effects at follow-up (Beelmann, Pfingsten, & Losel, 1994; Losel & Beelmann, 2003). Despite such limitations, many recent reviews of the literature have concluded that relationship or play therapy techniques do not improve social skills outcomes as effectively as cognitive-behavioral treatments such as PSST (Borduin et al., 1995; Eyberg, Nelson, & Boggs, 2008; Kazdin & Weisz, 1998). Therefore, although PSST has limitations, it currently seems to have more empirical support than other traditional forms of individual psychotherapy.

Combining PSST with behavioral methods focused on altering environmental contingencies seems to be a logical way to improve overall outcomes and increase generalization of treatment effects (Gross, Fogg, & Webster-Stratton, 2003). However, only a few studies have used both behavioral methods and PSST to determine whether a combined approach is more beneficial than a single-treatment-modality approach (Dishion & Andrews, 1995; Kazdin, Esveldt-Dawson, French, &

Unis, 1987b; Kazdin, Siegel, & Bass, 1992; Webster-Stratton & Hammond, 1997). In examining these studies, a few conclusions are evident. First, studies that have compared PSST plus parent training (PT) with PSST indicate that PSST in isolation has only a mild to moderate effect on oppositional behaviors (Kazdin et al., 1992; Webster-Stratton & Hammond, 1997). For instance, Webster-Stratton and Hammond (1997) found that mothers' scores on the Child Behavior Checklist (CBCL) demonstrated a moderate effect size change at the completion of therapy for the PSST-only group (0.57), whereas a much larger effect size change was obtained for children enrolled in both PT and PSST (1.20). Results such as these indicate that the child has a much greater likelihood of exhibiting fewer oppositional behaviors at posttreatment when PT is included in the treatment plan. Second, children in a PT-only treatment, as opposed to those in a PT-plus-PSST treatment, demonstrated nearly no change in social skills or problem-solving ability (Dishion & Andrews, 1995). Third, some data suggest that treatment outcomes are greater immediately posttreatment and at follow-up when both child and parent are involved in treatment (i.e., a combination of PT plus PSST rather than either one alone; Kazdin et al., 1992; Webster-Stratton & Hammond, 1997). In addition to evaluating the additive effects of PT plus PSST, Webster-Stratton, Reid, and Hammond (2004) looked at the addition of teacher training on classroom management and promoting positive relationships and social skills to PT, PSST, and PT plus PSST. Although all treatment groups demonstrated some gains in prosocial behaviors and declines in problem behaviors relative to a wait-list control group, different domains of functioning were affected differently by the treatments (e.g., child social competence improved only for those children involved in PSST; improvements on teacher measures were noted in all groups except the PT-only group). Given these findings, school personnel should consider using PSST as part of a broader treatment package for children demonstrating problematic behaviors in social contexts. And, of course, school personnel should monitor any intervention they implement to ensure that it is having the intended effect on a child's behavior.

Implementing a PSST Treatment

In this section we present an abbreviated and modified version of Kendall and Braswell's (1985) PSST treatment. Kendall and Braswell (1985) utilized approximately 12 sessions in their PSST program; however, the treatment described here is delivered in 6 sessions. Although this is a significant departure from the length of treatment advocated by the original authors, there is some empirical support for this abbreviated form of treatment when behavioral contingencies in the form of parent training are first employed (Bushman, 2007). Furthermore, 6 sessions is a more practical goal than 12 sessions for most school-based professionals. Of course, some aspects of treatment may need to be lengthened or shortened for individual students as the practitioner's clinical judgment indicates (see "Final Thoughts and Clinical Considerations" section for additional ideas related to this issue). In the outline of each session, example dialogues between students and practitioners are presented as a sample of how therapy may be conducted. The dialogues are included to illustrate the process and are not scripts that should be used verbatim by practitioners.

When using a PSST treatment within the school setting, it will most likely be used as a Tier 3 intervention (see Ervin, Gimpel Peacock, & Merrell, Chapter 1, and Hawkins, Barnett, Morrison, & Musti-Rao, Chapter 2, this volume) as it is typically delivered in a one-on-one format. However, school psychologists may be able to adapt some of the treatment components to present the basic problem-solving steps as a Tier 2 intervention to small groups of students who have been identified as being at risk for increases in social-behavioral problems. As noted earlier, school psychologists who implement PSST should work through the problem-solving model before implementing a PSST treatment with a student to ensure that the identified problem is one of a social-behavioral nature and that there is reason to suspect that the child's lack of social-problem-solving skills is contributing to the problem.

Introduction to Problem-Solving Steps (Session 1)

The objectives of the first session are to introduce the child to the problem-solving steps and to establish a positive alliance with the child. As noted earlier, problem-solving steps can vary slightly from one PSST program to another. The steps provided in Table 25.1 are those used in the empirical evaluation of this abbreviated PSST treatment (Bushman, 2007) and were modified slightly from Kendall and Braswell's (1985) steps. They include:

1. What is the problem?
   This step is designed to help students provide a clear definition of the problem to be solved.
2. Look at all the possibilities.
   At this step, students are instructed to brainstorm as many solutions as possible to the identified problem.
3. Focus in and relax.
   Students are instructed to relax so that they can take time to think through each of the solutions rather than immediately reacting to the identified problem.
4. What happens next?
   At this stage, students evaluate the solutions they have generated.
5. Pick a solution. How did I do?
   Using evaluations of each solution to the identified problem, students pick one solution to implement and then evaluate the consequences (positive and negative) of the implementation of this final solution.

In addition to introducing the problem-solving steps in the first session, session rules, including the use of tokens, are introduced to the child. It is important that the practitioner have permission from the student's parent(s) or teacher(s) regarding the use of tokens and the associated reinforcers (e.g., candy, stickers, bouncy balls, small cars). It can be helpful to start the session with a preapproved list of potential privileges from the student's parent(s) and/or teacher(s). The practitioner first explains to the student how he or she can earn tokens in session, as well as for completing the out-of-session "experiments." The list of privileges and the associated token "costs" are finalized in session and shared later with the student's parents and teachers. Practitioners can also work with teachers and parents on out-of-session rewards children can earn.

An example dialogue regarding the use of tokens follows:

PRACTITIONER: I'm going to give a copy of this list to your parent(s) [or teacher] so they can see what you are working toward and how many chips you need to earn something. We're also going to keep one copy here to remind us. At the end of every session, I will write down how many chips you earned. You can earn chips in session and by remembering to complete the "experiments" I will give you at the end of each session. Do you know what an experiment is?

STUDENT: Is it like what scientists do?

PRACTITIONER: Yeah. They do things that are new to see what will happen. I want you to do the same thing. At the end of each session, I will give you an example of something new to try. This will be your experiment for the week. For example, I may ask you to talk with your parents about the steps you will learn today. That would be an example of an experiment. As long as you try it, I will give you five chips at the beginning of the next session. Remember, things don't have to work out perfectly when you do the experiment to get the tokens; you only have to try. Of course, there are also some ways you can lose chips. Let's list them on this piece of paper together. They are:

1. Going too fast. It is important to take your time and be careful. If you go too fast, you lose one chip. Don't worry. I will warn you first if I think you are going too fast.
2. Forgetting a step. If you don't say a step or forget to say a step you will lose a chip. Are there any other rules we should come up with about how to either earn chips or lose chips?

Following this discussion, the practitioner and student brainstorm any additional rules or guidelines the student wishes to add, with the practitioner keeping in mind that such a list should not be too lengthy or too difficult for a student to achieve or remember.

To help illustrate the concept of "going too fast," which is still not well defined for the child, the practitioner and the child play two games of checkers; one is played at the regular pace, and one is played in which each person has only 2 seconds to make a move. The practitioner discusses with the child the difficulties of making good moves in the fast game of checkers and draws a parallel between this and thinking through decisions in other situations. This discussion can easily lead to an introduction of the problem-solving steps. The practitioner can spend some time with the child defining "problem solving" and generating examples of situations in which the student might have used problem-solving methods in the past. The practitioner then engages the child in a dialogue about the specific problem-solving steps covered in the PSST program:

PRACTITIONER I have a handout that you can keep that will help us remember the problem-solving steps. (*Uses Table 25.1 to make a handout for the student with the problem-solving steps.*) The first step is, "What is the problem?" One of the first ways we know if we have a problem is if we have a feeling like anger, fear or sadness. What was the problem in the situation you just mentioned? [*Spends time defining problems with the student until he believes the student understands the general concept.*] The second thing we say is, "Look at all the possibilities." Why is that important?

STUDENT: So you don't miss something?

PRACTITIONER: Right. We want to think of many different ways to solve problems; not just one or two. A good problem solver can think of as many as four to five different solutions to a problem. Next, we tell ourselves to "focus in and relax." It is important to just think about the problem and not anything else. Sometimes it helps to take three to four deep breaths to help focus in. Let's practice.

(*The practitioner coaches the student in the deep-breathing routine, emphasizing the importance of breathing slowly and evenly. While the student breathes, the practitioner may model coping statements, such as "I can calm down" or "I can solve this problem." The practitioner emphasizes that the student must breathe deeply several times before continuing.*)

TABLE 25.1. The Problem-Solving Steps

Step	Cognitive skills being developed
1. What is the problem?	Problem definition
2. Look at all the possibilities.	Solution generation
3. Focus in and relax.	Focusing attention/arousal regulation
4. What happens next?	Solution evaluation
5. Pick a solution. How did I do?	Behavioral enactment/self-reinforcement

Note. Adapted from Kendall and Braswell (1985, p. 120). Copyright 1985 by The Guilford Press. Adapted by permission.

PRACTITIONER: The fourth step is to think of each solution you came up with and ask "what will happen next?" if you do it. Like if I tried to trip some boy in the hall who I thought was making fun of me, what might happen next?

STUDENT: He would fall down.

PRACTITIONER: Yes ... and then what?

STUDENT: My friends and I would laugh.

PRACTITIONER: OK ... and then what?

STUDENT: I don't know. ... (*The practitioner allows the pause to linger, silently communicating the need for the student's active participation.*) He might pick a fight with me.

PRACTITIONER: Good job thinking through what happens next. We could also think of other things that might happen, like him telling the teacher. Either one may not be what you want. So this step reminds us to think ahead not just to what will happen right after you do your solution, but what will happen over the whole day or longer. The last step reminds us to pick a solution and ask ourselves how we did. If we chose a good solution, we need to tell ourselves that we did a good job. What are some ways you could tell yourself you did a good job? (*The practitioner and the student brainstorm positive self-statements. It may be helpful to write some of these down in a place where the student can see them.*) If our solution did not work out, we don't need to get mad at ourselves. Do you know what I mean when I say 'get mad at ourselves'? How do people do this?

STUDENT: Is that like saying, "I suck at this"?

PRACTITIONER: Yeah. I have a list here of good things people can say to help themselves when they make a mistake [see Figure 25.1]. Let's read them together and circle some that you would like to use. ...

This example dialogue emphasizes the type of interaction that must occur when the therapist is "teaching" the child to use the steps. Notice how, in this example, the practitioner

"It's no big deal."

"I can do better next time."

"People make mistakes."

"It's not that bad. I will still be OK."

"Things will get better."

"I can calm myself down."

"I just need to try again."

"I can do it."

"Relax. These things happen."

"I can handle making a mistake."

"As long as I learn from my mistakes, everything will be OK."

"I learned a good lesson here. I should remember it for next time."

"Just because I made a mistake doesn't mean I have to get angry or sad."

What are some other coping thoughts you can think of?

_____

_____

_____

_____

FIGURE 25.1. Coping statements: Things to say to yourself when you make a mistake.

is not flustered by the consequences the student initially generates. Instead a friendly, gentle style of questioning is used to keep the child engaged in treatment.

After the introduction to the token economy and the problem-solving steps, the practitioner and child again play checkers—this time attempting to use the problem-solving steps prior to each move. The practitioner should use the response-cost system sparingly during this initial session (no more than twice) and should model coping statements for the student when things do not go the practitioner's way (e.g., "You jumped me again! This is kind of frustrating. Wait [breathes]. It is okay. It is just a game"). The student is given the "experiment" of writing down at least one time when using the problem-solving steps may have been helpful. If possible, following this session, parents and teachers are also informed of the problem-solving steps and encouraged to model these steps for the child, as well as to reinforce the child if he or she uses the steps. Parents can be encouraged to model the steps by speaking them out loud as they consider how to solve problems. For example, a parent might engage in a self-dialogue such as the following:

"Let's see ... what is for dinner? [Step 1] ... I could go to the store and pick something up, we could go with leftovers, or make something new. [Step 2] ... Let's see ... what would be best? (*pause and breathe deeply*) [Step 3] ... If I go to the store I may spend money that we don't have, I'm tired of leftovers, and spaghetti might be good." [Step 4] ... That worked out. [*or* Well, that didn't work out, but it is OK. I know better for next time.]" [Step 5]

Teachers (and parents) can be encouraged to use existing reward programs they have in place to reward the child when they observe him or her following the problem-solving steps.

Application of Problem-Solving Steps (Session 2)

After the problem-solving steps have been introduced, the focus turns to helping the student apply the steps. The "experiment" for the week is always reviewed at the beginning of the sessions. Even if the student forgets to do the experiment, the practitioner spends time reviewing similar material. For instance, if the experiment was to think of one situation in which the student could have used the problem-solving steps, the practitioner can spend 5 minutes brainstorming with the student one such situation. As long as the child actively participates, he or she can receive at least partial credit and associated reinforcers. Next, the student is asked to list the problem-solving steps in his or her own words. For instance, the practitioner might say, "Now I'd like us to think about putting these steps or statements into your own words. Let's first draw a picture that looks like a stop sign. Let's make it nice and big so we can write some words in it." The practitioner and the student create a stop sign using crayons and paper, with the practitioner introducing the task by saying, "Great. Now we can use this as a cheat sheet. The first step is, 'Find out what I'm supposed to do.' What's the way you might say the same thing?" This process is continued with each step. The practitioner and child can then play another in-session game to help illustrate the use of the problem-solving skills. For example, a game Kendall and Braswell (1985) suggest is "cat and mouse," which also makes use of the checkers and board. In this game, four black checkers (the cats) and 1 red checker (the mouse) are used. The "cats" try to catch the "mouse" in a game similar to checkers; however, the cats can move only forward (though the mouse can move in both directions), and the pieces do not jump each other. The game starts with the mouse in the center of the board and the cats at one end of the board. The game is "won" when either the mouse successfully evades the cats or the cats surround the mouse by occupying all squares around the mouse. As this game is being played, the practitioner and child each talk through the problem-solving steps. Initially this is done out loud, but as the child is able to demonstrate mastery of the steps, this moves to whispered speech. The practitioner may introduce whispered speech by saying, "These steps can help you with all kinds of problems, but you probably don't want others hearing you using them. So what we're going to do now [*practitioner starts whispering*] is to practice whispering the steps while we take turns." The practitioner can also discuss with the student a signal that can be helpful for others (e.g., parents, teachers, the practitioner) to use to remind the child to use the problem-solving steps. For example, the person may make a stop signal with a hand or say "slow it down." During this session the practitioner should also make sure to use the token system set up during the first session. The experiment given after this session is for the child to use the problem-solving steps in at least one situation. Following the session, parents and teachers are informed of the agreed-on signal and, ideally, agree to reward the student if he or she responds to the signal by slowing down (the child may not be able to use all the steps by this phase of the program). In addition, parents and teachers are asked to think of and provide the practitioner with specific social situations in which the child reacted impulsively, aggressively, or disruptively so that these can be used in later sessions to facilitate skill generalization in "real-life" social situations.

Using Skills in Social Situations (Sessions 3 and 4)

Once the student becomes adept at applying the problem-solving steps to game situations in session, the practitioner can begin to assist the student in applying the steps to social situations. After reviewing homework, the practitioner asks the student which of the steps are easiest for him or her and which are the hardest to use. This information helps the practitioner emphasize those steps that the child perceives (and the practitioner has observed) as being the most difficult to use. Next, the practitioner and child can play checkers again; the child continues to use the problem-solving steps, but the practitioner purposely misses a step or goes too fast. The student's job is to catch the practitioner doing this. In terms of applying steps to social situations, the practitioner can start with a list of social situations and ask the child to respond using the problem-solving steps. Nine potential scenarios are presented in Figure 25.2 ("Typical Problems Some Kids Have"). Practitioners are also encouraged to create their own scenarios for use in this exercise. Each scenario can be cut into strips and chosen out of a hat, with the practitioner and student taking turns applying the steps to different scenarios. It may be helpful to first talk about what may hap-

You promised your mom you would start your homework, but some friends come by and want you to go to the movies with them just as you are getting started.

You are playing checkers, and you think the other person might be cheating.

You're playing basketball with some other kids at school, but they never pass you the ball.

Your mom promised to pick you up after school, but she isn't there when school ends. You feel yourself starting to get worried.

You say the wrong answer in class and the person behind you laughs. You feel angry.

You want cereal in the morning. When you go downstairs for breakfast, you find that your sister ate all the cereal.

You trip at recess, and someone makes fun of you.

You are taking a test in school, and your friend starts talking to you.

Other kids say "no" when you ask them nicely to let you join in a game they are playing.

FIGURE 25.2. Typical problems some kids have. Some situations adapted from Kendall and Braswell (1985).

pen if someone does not using the problem-solving steps so that the student can draw a comparison between using and not using the steps. It is important for the practitioner to go first, modeling how to apply the steps in social situations:

PRACTITIONER: First, I must figure out the problem. (*reading from the strip of paper*) "You promised your mom you would start your homework, but some friends come by and want you to go to the movies with them just as you are getting started." My problem is that I want to hang out with my friends but I made a promise to my mom. How would something like that make you feel?

STUDENT: I would probably feel angry.

PRACTITIONER: How would you know you were feeling angry?

STUDENT: I start to yell.

PRACTITIONER: I sometimes do that, but many times I feel my muscles get tense. That is one of the first ways I know that I am feeling angry. (*May go on to explain what "tense" muscles feel like.*) Second, I need to think of different ways to solve this problem. Any ideas?

STUDENT: Nope.

PRACTITIONER: What if I invited all my friends over for party where all we do is do homework? (mildly teasing the student to get him engaged)

STUDENT: No. (*laughing*) ... You could go anyway and tell your mom you'll do it later.

PRACTITIONER: OK, that is one idea. Let's put that down as a solution. (*Writes it down.*) I could also tell my friends that I can't go. ... (*Writes idea down.*) I need to think of at least three different things. ... I guess I could also tell them that I need to work first but I will catch up with them later. (*Writes last solution down.*) OK, that is three. Let's concentrate on these and focus in. (*Practices deep breathing with the student.*) OK, now let's play "What's next?" What will happen next if I do my first solution, "go anyway ... do it later"?

STUDENT: Mom would probably get mad.

PRACTITIONER: What would happen next?

STUDENT: We would get into a fight.

PRACTITIONER: Doesn't sound too good. What about the next solution?

The practitioner continues to look with the student at the possible consequence of each choice. It may be helpful to adopt a "pros and cons" approach with some solutions. This allows the practitioner to acknowledge the short-term advantages of some maladaptive solutions while increasing the likelihood that the student will be willing to examine the solution's disadvantages. Remember, if the student insists on a choice the practitioner thinks is negative, it is not the practitioner's job to talk the student out of his or her decision. The primary job of the practitioner is to (1) help the student think systematically about problems and (2) assist the student in thinking through the advantages and dis-

advantages of each decision. This communicates respect for the student's autonomy, while reducing unnecessary power struggles. This process is repeated throughout the third session until the student demonstrates some ability to generate multiple solutions and can generate pros and cons related to these solutions. Notice in the example how the practitioner also processed with the student how the situation made the student feel while discussing the first step. This form of affective education can often be integrated into the problem definition skill, as the student's initial emotional reaction is often the first cue to the student that a problem exists. Consequently, it is important for the practitioner to process with the student how the situation would make him or her feel, as many children may not be able to label their feelings. Some of the scenarios in Figure 25.2 provide the child with such a label (e.g., angry, embarrassed), but others do not provide a feeling, leaving it to the student to identify a feeling with the practitioner's help. The experiment for the third session is the same as in the previous session—to have the child use the problem-solving steps in at least one situation. The therapist should continue to work with the child's parents and teachers to obtain examples of situations in which the child had negative or impulsive reactions to social situations and can begin to incorporate these "real" situations in session.

The fourth session has the same goal as the previous session but adds to a student's understanding of how to evaluate potential solutions. After reviewing the student's take-home experiment, the practitioner and the student once again take turns pulling social situations out of a hat. However, this time the practitioner challenges the student to "catch" the practitioner when he or she intentionally misses a step. The student is rewarded with an extra token each time he or she is able to catch the practitioner in an error. This addition may be helpful given that the practitioner should now be using the response-cost system more frequently with the student. The practitioner also discusses using the problem-solving steps covertly rather than in a whispered manner. The practitioner and student may want to come up with signal they can use in session (e.g., student strokes his or her chin) to indicate that the steps are being used covertly.

Once the student demonstrates some ability to generate multiple solutions and pros and cons of these solutions, the practitioner teaches the child a more systematic way of knowing whether a solution will lead to a positive outcome. Webster-Stratton (1992) proposed that the student be trained to ask him- or herself the following questions when determining whether a solution is appropriate: (1) "Does the solution cause me or others to feel bad later?" (2) "Is the consequence fair?" and (3) "Is the consequence dangerous?" (p. 104). Therapy shifts to having the child evaluate solutions based on his or her answers to these (or similar) questions, not just in terms of what will likely happen if a given solution is implemented. Ideally, the practitioner solicits ideas from the student about how he or she will know whether a solution is positive or negative, with the aforementioned questions being a rough guide. This might be difficult for some children; however, the practitioner should attempt to have the student assist in generating a list of questions used for solution evaluation, because it will likely invest the student more in the process.

Throughout the time the student is learning to apply the problem-solving steps, the student's parents and teachers should be encouraged to praise the student when he or she is seen to be using the problem-solving steps or slowing down when prompted to do so. This praise can be incorporated into a home or a classroom behavioral plan if such a plan exists. For homework, the student is again asked to use the problem-solving steps in at least one social situation over the course of the week. The student is also told that he or she will no longer be rewarded for simply responding to the teacher's or parent's use of the "slow down" signal but instead will need to independently begin to engage in the problem-solving steps. However, it should be noted that if the student has difficulty spontaneously slowing him- or herself down, the signal may continue to be used before it is faded completely.

Self-Critique (Session 5)

After the student has become proficient at applying the problem-solving steps in session, the student is videotaped engaging in a role play and using the problem-solving skills.

The scenes used for the role plays should either be solicited from the child or should be based on information provided by parents and/or teachers. The student is told that he or she will get to be both an "actor" and a "director" during the session. The practitioner has several "scripts" that will need to be acted out using the problem-solving steps. The student gets to act as him- or herself and gets to direct the therapist, who plays a significant other in the scene. Initially, the therapist helps the student work through the problem-solving steps, but eventually the therapist provides little to no direction regarding the steps during the scene; however, after the role play, the practitioner and the student watch the video together, with the student critiquing his or her use of the steps. If the student presents as being defensive, the therapist may choose to first model a situation from his or her life in which he or she "could have thought through things better" (using clinical judgment regarding what is appropriate to reveal). Because this is a new experience for the student, the exercise may initially include a great deal of coaching:

PRACTITIONER: First, let's look at our list of scenes. Here is one. "While going out to recess, you trip, and another classmate, Johnny (*real classmate's name*), starts to laugh and call you names. How do you feel?

STUDENT: Embarrassed.

PRACTITIONER: I can understand that. How do you know when you are feeling embarrassed? (*Practitioner and student spend time identifying bodily cues for embarrassment and act out such cues for the camera.*) Do you want me to be Johnny or you?

STUDENT: You can be Johnny.

PRACTITIONER: OK, you be the director. I'm Johnny. What was Johnny doing before you tripped?

STUDENT: He was talking with his friends. So, you are over there (*points to the side of the room*) talking.

PRACTITIONER: OK, you come out to recess and trip. Remember to use the steps. This is your first try, so it doesn't have to be perfect.

STUDENT: OK. Action. (*Pretends to trip.*)

PRACTITIONER: Hey, look at (*child's name*)! Good move!

STUDENT: (*to the practitioner*) What do I do now?

PRACTITIONER: What is the first step?

STUDENT: What is the problem? (*Holds up one finger.*)

PRACTITIONER: Yep. ... What is the problem?

STUDENT: Johnny and his friends are laughing at me.

PRACTITIONER: OK, that's the problem, and you know you have a problem because of how you feel, so you could have said, "I feel embarrassed because I tripped." What's next?

STUDENT: What can I do about my problem? (*Note: The practitioner should substitute the child's way of saying the steps at this point in treatment.*)

PRACTITIONER: Yeah, we can act that out by stroking our chin. (*Does this with the student.*) What are some solutions?

STUDENT: Well, I can punch Johnny. (*Laughs.*)

PRACTITIONER: Yep that is one solution, but we want to think of more. What are some other solutions? (*The practitioner and student spend time coming up with multiple solutions.*) Now let's act out what will happen if you do each solution. What will happen if you hit Johnny?

STUDENT: The teacher will see me, and I will get detention again.

PRACTITIONER: All right, let's act it out. I don't want you to really punch—just pretend. Do you want me to be the teacher or still be Johnny?

STUDENT: You can be the teacher. ... (*The practitioner and student continue to act out each solution's potential outcome.*)

PRACTITIONER: OK, so let's now focus in and relax. How do we do that? (*The student begins to breathe deeply and the practitioner joins him.*) That was great. Which solution do you want to choose?

STUDENT: I think I will just ignore Johnny

because if I tell the teacher (*one of the other solutions*), all the other kids will make fun of me.

PRACTITIONER: OK, sounds like a good plan. Let's do the entire scene over again, but this time we only do the solution you want to do: ignoring Johnny. Remember to act out "embarrassed" at the beginning of the scene. You say "action" when you want to start. (*The role play begins with the practitioner reminding the student to use the covert steps.*) Nice job. Lets look at the tape and see how you did, but for the next scene you tell me how to use the steps.

As the tape is reviewed, the practitioner should pause the tape after each solution is acted out and evaluate with the student the solution based on the evaluation questions introduced in the previous session or by examining pros and cons. The practitioner should also brainstorm with the student either some positive self-statements (if the solution is socially effective) or some coping statements (if the solution is socially problematic) for the student to use.

If a video camera is not available, or if the student is reluctant to be videotaped, the role play can still occur. However, instead of the student watching and critiquing the video, the student will need to be prompted to critique his or her performance following the role play without the advantage of seeing the replay. The student's experiment for the week includes using the problem-solving steps in at least one situation that has been a problem for him or her in the past. Therefore, a good amount of time should be spent at the end of the session devising several options for the student to choose from and problem-solving any potential difficulties that may arise. It is important to communicate to the student's parent(s) or teacher(s) the student's goal for the week so they can supervise and motivate the student to complete the task and reward him or her for doing so.

Treatment Consolidation (Session 6)

In the final session, the student and practitioner continue to role-play scenarios, with particular emphasis placed on skill components the student has found to be difficult. Also during this session, the student is engaged in a role play in which he or she is asked to "teach" the problem-solving steps to someone else. During this role play, the practitioner can play the role of a child who does not know the steps. At the final session the practitioner can also discuss the progress he or she has seen in the student's ability to engage in appropriate social interactions through application of the problem-solving steps. Parents and teachers should be encouraged to continue to praise the student for using the problem-solving steps and to provide prompts to the student to use the steps if needed. Because many students have difficulty remembering to use the steps over time, scheduling follow-up sessions (over an increasing interval length between sessions) is generally recommended.

Final Thoughts and Other Clinical Considerations

In this chapter we have presented a practical approach to working with children who react impulsively, disruptively, and/or aggressively in social situations. The PSST approach primarily emphasizes a method of thinking that students can systematically use to solve interpersonal problems and conflict; however, skills other than those presented in this program may also need to be integrated into treatment. As mentioned previously, some children may have a limited ability to identify their own or another's feelings. If this is the case, skills related to affect identification may need to first be taught (for a helpful resource, see Merrell, 2008). Some children may need to first learn specific ways to relax before they can engage in problem solving. Although deep breathing is mentioned in Step 3, many students, especially those who have a history of responding reactively, will require greater time and practice before mastering this skill. For instance, the student can first be taught to identify when he or she is feeling upset as a cue that relaxation strategies are necessary. Consequently, a therapist may decide that Steps 2 (solution generation) and 3 (relaxation) need to be reversed before a student can engage in problem solving. In addition, many students may need more immediate feedback so they

can generalize the skills they are learning. For these children in particular, having a parent and/or teacher involved in the treatment plan is crucial to success. Finally, like most cognitive-behavioral treatments, this form of therapy assumes that the child is, at least partially, invested in changing. This may not be the case for all children, particularly those who perceive that they are being "forced" into treatment or who do not perceive that there are negative consequences of their socially inappropriate behaviors. In these situations, the practitioner may need to spend several sessions forming a relationship with the student and may also need to consider implementing a classroom and/or home behavior management system to ensure that the student is not being reinforced for inappropriate behaviors. As noted earlier, the PSST approach appears to produce the most changes when it is combined with a behavioral approach (e.g., parent training and/or a classroom behavioral intervention). Thus in most situations we advocate using the PSST method as part of a broader treatment plan for youth who lack social problem-solving skills and as a result engage in inappropriate social behaviors. As problem-solving change agents, school psychologists are in an excellent position to determine when PSST may be a useful part of an intervention package.

References

Acker, M. M., & O'Leary, S. G. (1987). Effects of reprimands and praise on appropriate behavior in the classroom. *Journal of Abnormal Child Psychology, 15*, 549–557.

Arbuthnot, J., & Gordon, D. A. (1986). Behavioral and cognitive effects of a moral reasoning development intervention for high-risk behavior-disordered adolescents. *Journal of Consulting and Clinical Psychology, 54*, 208–216.

Beelmann, A., Pfingsten, U., & Losel, F. (1994). Effects of training social competence in children: A meta-analysis of recent evaluation studies. *Journal of Abnormal Child Psychology, 5*, 265–275.

Borduin, C. M., Mann, B. J., Cone, L. T., Henggeler, S. W., Fucci, B. R., Blaske, D. M., et al. (1995). Multisystemic treatment of serious juvenile offenders: Long-term prevention of criminality and violence. *Journal of Consulting and Clinical Psychology, 63*, 569–578.

Bushman, B. B. (2007). *Does teaching problem-solving skills matter? An evaluation of problem-solving skills training for the treatment of social and behavioral problems in children.* Unpublished doctoral dissertation, Utah State University, Logan.

Coie, J. D. (1990). Toward a theory of peer rejection. In S. R. Asher & J. D. Coie (Eds.), *Peer rejection in childhood* (pp. 365–398). Cambridge, UK: Cambridge University Press.

Crick, N. R., & Dodge, K. A. (1994). A review and reformulation of social information processing mechanisms in children's social adjustment. *Psychological Bulletin, 115,* 74–101.

Dishion, T. J., & Andrews, D. W. (1995). Preventing escalation in problem behaviors with high-risk young adolescents: Immediate and 1-year outcomes. *Journal of Consulting and Clinical Psychology, 63,* 538–548.

Dodge, K. A. (1980). Social cognition and children's aggressive behavior. *Child Development, 51,* 162–170.

Dodge, K. A. (1993). Social-cognitive mechanisms in the development of conduct disorder and depression. *Annual Review of Psychology, 44,* 8–22.

Dodge, K. A., & Coie, J. D. (1987). Social information processing factors in reactive and proactive aggression in children's peer groups. *Journal of Personality and Social Psychology, 53,* 1146–1158.

Dodge, K. A., Prince, J. N., Bachorowski, J., & Newman, J. P. (1990). Hostile attributional biases in severely aggressive adolescents. *Journal of Abnormal Psychology, 99,* 385–392.

Eyberg, S. M., Nelson, M. M., & Boggs, S. R. (2008). Evidence-based psychosocial treatments for children and adolescents with disruptive behavior. *Journal of Clinical Child and Adolescent Psychology, 37,* 215–237.

Giancola, P. R., Moss, H. B., & Martin, C. S. (1996). Executive cognitive functioning predicts reactive aggression in boys at high risk for substance abuse: A prospective study. *Alcoholism: Clinical and Experimental Research, 20*(4), 740–744.

Gifford-Smith, M. L., & Rabiner, D. L. (2004). Social information processing and children's social competence: A review of the literature. In J. Kupersmidt & K. A. Dodge (Eds.), *Children's peer relations: From development to intervention to policy* (pp. 61–79). Washington, DC: American Psychological Association.

Gross, D., Fogg, L., & Webster-Stratton, C. (2003). Parent training of toddlers in day care in low-income urban communities. *Journal of Consulting and Clinical Psychology, 71,* 261–278.

Kazdin, A. E. (2003). Problem-solving skills training and parent management training for conduct disorder. In A. E. Kazdin & J. R. Weisz (Eds.), *Evidence-based psychotherapies for children and adolescents* (pp. 241–262). New York: Guilford Press.

Kazdin, A. E., Bass, D., Siegel, T. C., & Thomas, C. (1989). Cognitive-behavioral therapy and relationship therapy in the treatment of children referred for antisocial behavior. *Journal of Consulting and Clinical Psychology, 57,* 522–535.

Kazdin, A. E., Esveldt-Dawson, K., French, N. H., & Unis, A. S. (1987a). Problem-solving skills training and relationship therapy in the treatment of antisocial child behavior. *Journal of Consulting and Clinical Psychology, 55,* 76–85.

Kazdin, A. E., Esveldt-Dawson, K., French, N. H., & Unis, A. S. (1987b). Effects of parent management training and problem-solving skills training combined in the treatment of antisocial child behavior. *Journal of the American Academy of Child and Adolescent Psychiatry, 26,* 416–424.

Kazdin, A. E., Siegel, T. C., & Bass, D. (1992). Cognitive problem-solving skills training and parent management training in the treatment of antisocial behavior in children. *Journal of Consulting and Clinical Psychology, 60,* 733–747.

Kazdin, A. E., & Weisz, J. R. (1998). Identifying and developing empirically supported child and adolescent treatments. *Journal of Consulting and Clinical Psychology, 66,* 19–36.

Kendall, P. C., & Braswell, L. (1985). *Cognitive-behavioral therapy for impulsive children.* New York: Guilford Press.

Kolko, D. J., Loar, L. L., & Sturnick, D. (1990). Inpatient social-cognitive skills training groups with conduct-disordered and attention-deficit-disordered children. *Journal of Child Psychology and Psychiatry, 31,* 737–748.

Lochman, J. E., Burch, P. R., Curry, J. F., & Lampron, L. B. (1984). Treatment and generalization effects of cognitive-behavioral and goal-setting interventions with aggressive boys. *Journal of Consulting and Clinical Psychology, 52,* 915–916.

Lochman, J. E., Powell, N. R., Whidby, J. M., & FitzGerald, D. P. (2006). Aggressive children: Cognitive-behavioral assessment and treatment. In P.C. Kendall (Ed.), *Child and adolescent therapy: Cognitive-behavioral procedures* (3rd ed., pp. 33–81). New York: Guilford Press.

Loeber, R., & Farrington, D. P. (2000). Young children who commit crime: Epidemiology, developmental origins, risk factors, early interventions, and policy implications. *Developmental Psychopathology, 12,* 737–762.

Losel, F., & Beelmann, A. (2003). Effects of child skills training in preventing antisocial behavior: A systematic review of randomized evaluations. *Annals of the American Academy of Political and Social Science, 587,* 84–109.

Merrell, K. W. (2008). *Helping students overcome depression and anxiety: A practical guide* (2nd ed.). New York: Guilford Press.

Pfiffner, L. J., & O'Leary, S. G. (1987). The efficacy of all-positive management as a function of prior use of negative consequences. *Journal of Applied Behavior Analysis, 20,* 265–271.

Prinz, R. J., Blechman, E. A., & Dumas, J. E. (1994). An evaluation of peer coping-skills training for childhood aggression. *Journal of Clinical Child Psychology, 23,* 193–203.

Spivak, G., Platt, J. J., & Shure, M. B. (1976). *The problem solving approach to adjustment.* San Francisco: Jossey-Bass.

Walker, H. M., Colvin, G., & Ramsey, E. (1995). *Antisocial behavior in school: Strategies and best practices.* Pacific Grove, CA: Brooks/Cole.

Webster-Stratton, C. (1992). *The incredible years: A trouble-shooting guide for parents of children age 3 to 8.* Toronto, Ontario, Canada: Umbrella Press.

Webster-Stratton, C., & Hammond, M. (1997). Treating children with early-onset conduct problems: A comparison of child and parent training interventions. *Journal of Consulting and Clinical Psychology, 65,* 93–109.

Webster-Stratton, C., & Lindsay, D. W. (1999). Social competence and early-onset conduct problems: Issues in assessment. *Journal of Child Clinical Psychology, 28,* 25–43.

Webster-Stratton, C., & Reid, M. J. (2003). The Incredible Years parents, teachers, and children training series: A multifaceted treatment approach for young children with conduct problems. In A. E. Kazdin & J. R. Weisz (Eds.), *Evidence-based psychotherapies for children and adolescents* (pp. 224–240). New York: Guilford Press.

Webster-Stratton, C., Reid, M. J., & Hammond, M. (2004). Treating children with early-onset conduct problems: Intervention outcomes for parent, child, and teacher training. *Journal of Child Clinical and Adolescent Psychology, 33,* 105–124.

Chapter 26

Cognitive-Behavioral Interventions for Depression and Anxiety

Susan M. Swearer
Jami E. Givens
Lynae J. Frerichs

Collectively, anxiety and depressive disorders are the most common mental health conditions that affect school-age youths. However, despite the prevalence of internalizing disorders, most youths are referred for treatment for externalizing problems (Kazdin & Weisz, 2003). The stark reality is that many anxiety and depressive disorders remain undiagnosed, or worse, misdiagnosed. Depressive disorders in youths have been called the "hidden epidemic," as these youth are often overlooked in the classroom because they are typically the quiet, withdrawn students who are not creating any problems. Consider this example from the Child and Adolescent Therapy Clinic at the University of Nebraska–Lincoln: an elementary school-age boy was referred due to psychosocial difficulties related to his attention-deficit/hyperactivity disorder (ADHD) disorder; however, his parents were concerned about his sad affect. Parents reported a family history of major depressive disorder on both paternal and maternal sides. This young man presented as quite depressed: He never smiled, his hair covered his eyes, he rarely maintained eye contact, he had quit most of his activities (anhedonia), and his speech was replete with negative self-statements. During a school consultation session, the teacher

remarked, "I had no idea that John was depressed. He's such a nice, quiet young man and he never causes any problems." Although John's parents (given their family history of depression) were aware of his internalizing problems, not all children are so fortunate. John ended up receiving cognitive-behavioral treatment and medication management for his depression, which was the primary disorder affecting his functioning. As a result of successful combination treatment, his school and social functioning drastically improved. The purposes of this chapter are to provide a brief overview of childhood depression and anxiety, to present empirically based treatment protocols, and to describe cognitive-behavioral treatment strategies for these disorders in school-age youths.

The Role of the School Psychologist in Prevention and Intervention for Depression and Anxiety

Effective treatment must be preceded by accurate assessment. School psychologists serve an important problem-solving function in assessing students who may experience depressive and/or anxiety disorders. School psychologists trained in multidisciplinary service delivery models can work with these students and their caregivers to determine an appropriate course of treatment. There are three levels of services across which school psychologists can develop mental health programming in schools (Merrell, Ervin, & Gimpel Peacock, 2006). The first level, *primary prevention*, could include teaching students how to express feelings of anxiety, irritability, and/or sadness. The next level, *secondary prevention*, could include helping counselors and teachers identify students whose caregivers suffer from internalizing problems and/ or who live under multiple stressful conditions and then working with these students in small groups. The third level, *tertiary prevention*, includes providing treatment for students experiencing depressive and/or anxiety disorders. In treating depression and anxiety in youths, we would add a fourth component, *sustainability*, in which school psychologists can coordinate with community mental health practitioners and can help facilitate home–school–community connections (Cowan & Swearer, 2004). In the sections to follow, we briefly review the prevalence and diagnostic criteria for depression and anxiety in school-age youths. In order to be an effective problem solver, knowing the prevalence and diagnostic criteria for depression and anxiety is the first step. Accurate assessment is the next step (see Miller, Chapter 11, this volume). Finally, identifying effective treatments emanates from accurate knowledge of the disorders, assessment, and accurate diagnosis.

Depression in School-Age Youths

One of the most common psychological disorders in childhood and adolescence is depression. Prevalence of depression ranges from less than 1% to 2% in children and from 1 to 7% in adolescents (see Avenevoli, Knight, Kessler, & Merikangas, 2008). Three major categories of unipolar depression can be diagnosed with the text revision of the fourth edition of the *Diagnostic and Statistical Manual of Mental Disorders* (DSM-IV-TR; American Psychiatric Association, 2000), including major depressive disorder (MDD), dysthymic disorder (DD), and depressive disorder not otherwise specified (DDNOS). The affect of a youth with depression can be characterized as sad, depressed, irritable,

angry, or a combination of these emotions (American Psychiatric Association, 2000; Friedberg & McClure, 2002). Youths with depression typically exhibit a negative cognitive style, characterized by negative perceptions of themselves, the world, and their future (Beck, Rush, Shaw, & Emery, 1979). These children and adolescents often discount positive events and focus on their negative experiences (Beck et al., 1979; Compton et al., 2004; Friedberg & McClure, 2002). Additionally, youths with depression may exhibit problems in their interpersonal relationships and experience anhedonia or a decreased interest and involvement in pleasant events. They may experience distorted thinking and poor problem solving and self-assertion skills (Compton et al., 2004; Friedberg & McClure, 2002), as well as loss of appetite, insomnia, psychomotor agitation, fatigue, and suicidal ideation (American Psychiatric Association, 2000).

Anxiety Disorders in School-Age Youths

Anxiety disorders represent the most common psychiatric disorder diagnosed in children and adolescents (Anderson, 1994; Beidel, 1991; Costello & Angold, 1995). Although generalized anxiety disorder (formally overanxious disorder), separation anxiety disorder, and specific phobia are the most prevalent of anxiety disorders, estimated prevalence rates of any anxiety disorder have been reported to range between 5.8 and 17.7% (Silverman & Kurtines, 2001). Anxiety is an adaptive emotional response to a perceived physical or emotional threat. However, anxiety becomes nonadaptive when it is produced by a situation or object that is not actually a threat to the individual (Grills-Taquechel & Ollendick, 2007). Anxiety disorders are characterized by anxious responding that is excessive in intensity, frequency, and/or duration and that includes a combination of physiological, emotional, behavioral, and cognitive symptoms that interfere with daily functioning. Youths with anxiety may experience somatic symptoms as a result of their distress, appearing uneasy and uncomfortable. Behaviorally, youths who are anxious often avoid situations or circumstances that they view as threatening (e.g., school, social situations). Cognitively, youths with anxiety may elaborate on negative information and make catastrophic predictions and expectations about their coping abilities (e.g., "I can't do it"; "I'm bound to fail"; Friedberg & McClure, 2002).

DSM-IV-TR delineates nine diagnostic categories of anxiety disorders that can be diagnosed in children and adolescents. For complete diagnostic criteria for each of the nine anxiety disorders, see DSM-IV-TR (American Psychiatric Association, 2000). *Generalized anxiety disorder* (GAD) involves excessive and uncontrollable anxiety about a number of events or activities. Children and adolescents diagnosed with GAD often have excessive worry about general life concerns, including their past, present, and future (American Psychiatric Association, 2000). *Separation anxiety disorder* (SAD) is characterized by anxiety related to separation from a major attachment figure (American Psychiatric Association, 2000). *Social phobia* (also called social anxiety disorder) is persistent fear of social or performance situations in which embarrassment may occur. *Specific phobia* is defined as persistent fear of objects or situations that evoke an immediate anxious response, often in the form of a panic attack (American Psychiatric Association, 2000). *Panic disorder* (PD) is diagnosed when youths experience recurrent, unforeseen panic attacks (American Psychiatric Association, 2000) and subsequently fear the physical sensation of having a panic attack (Albano, Chorpita, & Barlow, 1996). *Agoraphobia* can accompany PD and is characterized by anxiety about being in a situation in which escape is difficult or embarrassing (American Psychiatric Association, 2000). *Obsessive–compulsive disorder* (OCD) is an anxiety disorder characterized by recurrent, time-consuming, and impairing obsessions and/or compulsions (American Psychiatric Association, 2000). OCD is distinguished from normal childhood rituals or behaviors by the excessive distress that is seen when the ritual or behavior is prevented or interrupted (Albano et al., 1996). *Posttraumatic stress disorder* (PTSD) occurs after an individual has experienced or witnessed or was confronted with an actual or perceived threat of death or serious injury. Those diagnosed with PTSD reexperience the traumatic event, avoid associations with the event, and have increased levels of arousal (American Psychiatric Association, 2000). *Acute stress disorder* occurs within one month of exposure to an extreme traumatic stressor (American Psychiatric Association, 2000) and has been characterized as a precursor to PTSD (Meiser-Stedman, Yule, Smith, Glucksman, & Dalgleish, 2005).

Comorbidity of Depression and Anxiety

Comorbidity occurs when two (or more) disorders are present. Both depression and anxiety are likely to co-occur with each other, as well as with other psychological disorders. Unfortunately, youths with comorbid disorders are more severely impaired (Lewinsohn, Rohde, & Seeley, 1998) and suffer from more negative long-term consequences (Harrington, Fudge, Rutter, Pickles, & Hill, 1991) than those with a single disorder.

It is estimated that depression has one of the highest rates of comorbidity with other psychiatric disorders, including anxiety and behavioral disorders (Schroeder & Gordon, 2002). It is likely that most youths with depression will experience an additional psychological disorder, with estimates being that up to three-quarters of youths with depression meet the criteria for additional diagnoses (Mitchell, McCauley, Burke, & Moss, 1988; Nottelmann & Jensen, 1995).

Anxiety disorders co-occur most often with other anxiety disorders (Kendall, 1994); however, they also co-occur with other internalizing disorders (e.g., depressive disorders) and externalizing disorders (e.g., attention-deficit/hyperactivity disorder, oppositional defiant disorder, conduct disorder, substance abuse; Kendall, 1994; Silverman & Kurtines, 1996) as well. Studies have found comorbid anxiety and internalizing disorders in 24–79% of children and adolescents in a clinic sample (Last, Strauss, & Francis, 1987) and 18.7% in a community sample (Lewinsohn, Zinbarg, Seeley, Lewinsohn, & Sack, 1997). Kendall (1994) noted higher rates of comorbid internalizing disorders (e.g., depressive disorders, 32%; simple phobias, 60%) in children with anxiety compared with externalizing disorders (attention-deficit/hyperactivity disorder, 15%; oppositional defiant disorder, 13%; and conduct disorder, 2%).

Comorbidity and Treatment of Depression and Anxiety

Comorbidity can significantly complicate treatment efforts. For example, choosing which diagnosis should be the primary focus of treatment (Curry & Murphy, 1995) can be difficult when more than one disorder is present. Curry and Murphy (1995) suggest three considerations when treating comorbid disorders. The first is the relationship between the disorders. For example, if one disorder is seen as a cause of the second, treatment should focus on the first disorder. A second consideration is specificity of treatment. If a specific, well-validated treatment exists for the primary disorder, focus should be given to that disorder (e.g., exposure and response prevention for the treatment of OCD). Similarly, specific components of manualized treatments can be extracted or combined for more comprehensive treatment. Third, the overall level of functioning should be considered regarding the nature of the disorders. For example, in the case of John, his depressive symptoms were far more impairing than his ADHD symptoms. Treating his depression then allowed his parents and teachers to focus on helping him manage his ADHD symptoms (i.e., disorganization, poor homework completion).

Because depressive and anxiety disorders often co-occur in school-age youths, programs that target the treatment of both disorders can be helpful for school psychologists (i.e., Merrell, 2008). With accurate knowledge about the depressive and anxiety disorders that can occur among school-age youths, accurate assessment of the symptoms of these disorders (see Miller, Chapter 11, this volume) and effective strategies for treating symptoms of anxiety and depression, school psychologists can prevent, reduce, intervene early, and treat these disorders. School psychologists are proponents of data-driven problem solving (Merrell et al., 2006) and use their knowledge of assessment and intervention to treat youths experiencing anxiety and/or depression. In addition to recommending the book *Helping Students Overcome Depression and Anxiety* (Merrell, 2008), in the next section of this chapter we review cognitive-behavioral interventions for treating depression and anxiety in school-age youths.

Empirical Support for the Treatment of Depression

The Treatment for Adolescents with Depression Study (TADS) is considered the most sophisticated of all internalizing clinical trials (Weisz, McCarty, & Valeri, 2006). The TADS participants included 439 youths age 12–17 years diagnosed with MDD from 13 clinical sites (see Treatment for Adolescents with Depression Study Team [TADS], 2005, for demographic and clinical information). TADS was a randomized controlled trial intended to evaluate the short-term (0–12 weeks) and long-term (0–36 weeks) effects of treatments through medication (i.e., fluoxetine), cognitive-behavioral therapy (CBT), and the combination of fluoxetine and CBT. Children in these treatment groups were compared with those in a pill placebo group. The TADS treatment groups were generally tolerable and acceptable, as 80% of the adolescents completed 12 weeks of their given treatment group (Emslie et al., 2006).

Results from the TADS study after 12 weeks of treatment (Treatment for Adolescents with Depression Study Team [TADS], 2004) demonstrated that the combination treatment of fluoxetine and CBT resulted in a greater decrease in depressive symptoms when compared with the placebo group, as well as either active treatment group. The fluoxetine-alone group was superior to the placebo and CBT-alone groups, whereas CBT alone proved no better than placebo. The authors reported several reasons for the low response rate to CBT alone, including treating participants who were more impaired than those in previous CBT treatment studies (who responded positively to CBT treatment).

Other TADS studies have expanded on initially published TADS findings. Emslie et al. (2006) found that the combination treatment had a better safety profile than fluoxetine alone. Specifically, suicidal ideation improved with all treatment groups; however, it showed the greatest improvement with combination treatment. Moreover, as depression improved, participants' reported physical symptoms (e.g., sleep problems, headaches, stomach pain) decreased. Curry et al. (2006) found that younger, less impaired adolescents responded better to acute (12 weeks) treatment than adolescents who were older, more impaired, or diagnosed with a comorbid disorder. Also, adolescents who expected treatment to result in symptom improvement showed a significantly greater improvement in depressive symptoms than those with lower treatment expectations.

Although it may seem counterintuitive that CBT treatment at 12 weeks is only as beneficial as placebo, those findings should be interpreted with caution. In weighing the risks and benefits of treatment for depression, it is important to look at the long-term outcomes. In their long-term study, the Treatment for Adolescents with Depression Study Team (TADS, 2007) found that the CBT treatment group caught up to fluoxetine treatment at the halfway point (Week 18) and caught up to combination treatment at the end of treatment (Week 36). Additionally, suicidal ideation was found to continue in adolescents receiving fluoxetine-alone treatment, perhaps lending itself to the notion that CBT protects against suicidal tendencies. In sum, in both the short and long term, the combination of CBT and fluoxetine seems to be superior to either CBT or fluoxetine alone. For a complete discussion of pharmacological treatment for depression, see DuPaul, Weyandt, and Booster, Chapter 28, this volume.

Treatment Protocols for Depression in School-Age Youths

Several cognitive-behavioral treatment protocols have been developed for treating children and adolescents with depression. Based on the cognitive-behavioral model, these treatments focus on the connection between thoughts, feelings, and behaviors. Youths are encouraged to develop specific strategies to change their beliefs and consequently improve their moods and behavior. Comprehensive manual-driven interventions may be especially relevant in schools, as they provide treatment packages useful for school psychologists. Three school-based treatment programs that have empirical support for their effectiveness were chosen to review in this chapter. The ACTION program (Stark et al., 2008; Stark, Schnoebelen, et al., 2007; Stark, Simpson, Schnoebelen, et al., 2007; Stark, Simpson, Yancy, & Molnar, 2007), the Coping with Depression Course (Lewinsohn, Clarke, Hops, & Andrews, 1990), and

Interpersonal Psychotherapy for Depressed Adolescents (Mufson, Moreau, Weissman, & Klerman, 1993) are described in the next section. Additionally, many of the specific techniques used in these programs are described in detail later in this chapter.

ACTION

The ACTION treatment program is a small-group CBT intervention for depressed girls, ages 9–13 years, conducted in the school setting. This manualized treatment follows a structured therapist's manual and workbook for both the girls and their parents (Stark et al., 2008; Stark, Schnoebelen, et al., 2007; Stark, Simpson, et al., 2007; Stark, Simpson, Yaney, & Molnar, 2007). The earlier version of this program, Taking Action (Stark & Kendall, 1996), is designed for both boys and girls.

The ACTION treatment program is based on a self-control model in which girls are taught coping skills using cognitive-behavioral components during 20 sessions over 11 weeks (Stark et al., 2008). The program consists of four components: (1) affective education, (2) coping skills training, (3) problem-solving training, and (4) cognitive restructuring. A session agenda is followed to provide the participants with a sense of security and knowledge of the session structure. Each session begins with a rapport-building activity; the therapist asks the girls to evaluate their progress toward their goals; the effectiveness of using coping skills is demonstrated; and a fun activity is experienced. ACTION workbooks and homework are used to reinforce the therapeutic components. The treatment program can be adapted for use with individuals, but Stark et al. (2008) notes that preliminary investigations have found some of the treatment effectiveness to be related to the group format.

In addition to the student treatment sessions, parent training is included to teach parents how to support their child's new skill acquisition and to teach parents the same skills their children are being taught. The parent training also focuses on behavior management and communication skills and helps parents reduce conflict and assist their children in identifying and changing their negative thoughts (Stark, Sander, Hargrave, et al., 2006). Furthermore, teacher consultation is included in the ACTION program, in which the therapist and teacher collaboratively help the girls use their coping skills in the classroom. Preliminary outcome results suggest that 70% of participating girls no longer experienced depressive symptomatology after participating in the ACTION program (Stark, Sander, Hauser, et al., 2006).

Adolescent Coping with Depression Course

Developed by Lewinsohn and colleagues (1990), the Adolescent Coping with Depression Course (CWD-A) combines cognitive, behavioral, and social skills to address symptoms of depression and facilitate improvement. This treatment is based on the assumption that youths with depression do not receive positive reinforcement and that their behavior in turn contributes to a loss of social support (Lewinsohn et al., 1990). The CWD-A program teaches adolescents coping and problem-solving skills (Rohde, Lewinsohn, Clarke, Hops, & Seeley, 2005). The program consists of sixteen 2-hour sessions over the course of 8 weeks. Seven components are taught, including assertiveness, relaxation, cognitive restructuring, mood monitoring, pleasant event planning, communication, and conflict resolution. A parent component is also integrated into the program (Lewinsohn et al., 1990; Rohde et al., 2005).

Lewinsohn et al. (1990) evaluated the effectiveness of the CWD-A program among 59 adolescents, ages 14–18 years. Placed into three groups—(1) adolescent only, (2) adolescent plus parent, and (3) control group— the depression scores of the participants in the two active treatment groups showed significant improvement that was maintained 2 years after treatment compared with the control group. Kahn, Kehle, Jenson, and Clark (1990) examined the impact of the CWD-A program among 68 middle school students who were randomly assigned to four groups: (1) CWD-A, (2) relaxation treatment (i.e., basic and progressive relaxation skills), (3) self-modeling treatment (i.e., observations of self-enacting desired behaviors), or (4) control group. All active treatments were more effective than the control condition in reducing depressive symptoms.

Interpersonal Psychotherapy for Depressed Adolescents

Interpersonal Psychotherapy for Depressed Adolescents (IPT-A), developed by Mufson and colleagues (1993), is a brief therapy developed to decrease depressive symptoms and enhance interpersonal functioning. The program focuses on damaged interpersonal relationships, specifically family relationships. This program was developed to treat nonpsychotic adolescents suffering from depression and is not designed to treat adolescents in crisis, those who are suicidal or homicidal, individuals who have bipolar disorder, those with cognitive delays, or those abusing substances (Mufson et al., 1993; Young & Mufson, 2008). IPT-A is a three-phase program with four sessions in each phase. During the initial phase, interpersonal problems related to the client's depression are identified. The problems are clarified during the middle phase, followed by the selection, development, and implementation of the treatment plan. The therapist continues to monitor the adolescent's depression and may consider referral for medication if depressive symptoms increase or do not show improvement. During this phase, several techniques are implemented, including linking the adolescent's depression to his or her interpersonal functioning, analyzing the impact of the adolescent's communication during interpersonal events, role playing, and practicing at home (Mufson et al., 1993; Young & Mufson, 2008). During the termination phase, the adolescent's progress is reviewed, and areas of further need are identified. The client is prepared for termination and for future problems related to his or her depression or a comorbid diagnosis (Young & Mufson, 2008).

IPT-A has been shown to be an efficacious treatment for depression. In a community setting, Mufson et al. (2004) found that IPT-A was more beneficial than treatment as usual (supportive, individual counseling). In a study of 12- to 18-year-old outpatients following IPT-A treatment, none met the diagnostic criteria for depression, and they were all functioning more adaptively at home and school (Mufson et al., 1994). Mufson, Weissman, Moreau, and Garfinkel (1999) compared IPT-A with clinical monitoring for 12 weeks. Those in the IPT-A group showed significant improvement over the clinical monitoring group in depressive symptoms and overall functioning. IPT-A has shown a higher depression recovery rate (82%) compared with CBT (52%) in a study of Puerto Rican adolescents (Rosselló & Bernal, 1999).

Empirical Support for the Treatment of Anxiety Disorders

Fewer controlled trial studies have focused on the treatment of anxiety in children and adolescents compared with those designed to study the treatment of depression in youths. However, evidence supports the use of CBT in treating childhood and adolescent anxiety disorders. In the most recently released clinical trial for anxiety disorders in youths, Walkup et al. (2008) conducted a randomized controlled trial for children diagnosed with moderate to severe anxiety disorders, called the Child–Adolescent Anxiety Multimodal Study (CAMS). Participants included 488 children ages 7–17 years. Their primary diagnoses included SAD, GAD, and/or social phobia. The study consisted of two phases. Phase 1 was a short-term 12-week treatment comparing three treatment groups— CBT, sertraline, and the combination of CBT and sertraline—with a placebo group. (For a complete discussion of pharmacological treatment for anxiety, see DuPaul et al., Chapter 28, this volume.) The second phase extended Phase 1 for 6 months for those participants who responded to Phase 1. CBT included fourteen 60-minute sessions based on the Coping Cat program developed by Kendall (1992). The medication group included eight sessions in which the participants rated their anxiety symptoms, treatment response, and adverse effects. The results of the study indicate that combination treatment was the most effective treatment in reducing anxious symptomatology; however, all three treatments (i.e., combination, CBT alone, and sertraline alone) were superior to the placebo. Three treatment programs that target the most commonly diagnosed anxiety disorders in children and adolescents are the Coping Cat program (Kendall & Hedtke, 2006); John March's OCD treatment protocol (March & Mulle, 1998); and Anne Marie Albano's treatment protocol for social

anxiety (Albano & DiBartolo, 2007). These programs are reviewed in the next section, and many of the specific techniques are described in detail later in the chapter.

Treatment Protocols for Anxiety in School-Age Youths

Coping Cat Program

Kendall and colleagues were pioneers in their development of a manualized treatment for anxiety in children and adolescents, Coping Cat (Kendall, 1992). Kendall and colleagues based their program on the assumption that youths with anxiety view the world as threatening. They developed a flexible application of CBT that includes emphasis on adherence to the theoretical underpinnings of CBT, knowledge of child development and psychopathology, and training in effective CBT treatment components (Albano & Kendall, 2002).

Coping Cat (Kendall, 1992; Kendall & Hedtke, 2006) is a cognitive-behavioral treatment program that helps children and adolescents 7–13 years old to recognize and cope with their anxious feelings. The treatment program involves 14–18 sessions through a 12- to 16-week period. Each session is intended to last 60 minutes. The focus of treatment includes learning (in the first 6 to 8 sessions) and practicing (in the second 8 sessions) new skills to manage anxiety. The Coping Cat program includes five principles of CBT: (1) recognition of anxious feelings and somatic anxious reactions, (2) identification of unrealistic or negative expectations, (3) development of a plan to cope with anxiety in a given situation, (4) exposure, (5) performance evaluation and reinforcement. The treatment program comprises two phases, including skill development (e.g., relaxation strategies, cognitive restructuring) and graded exposure. The protocol teaches youths to increase their coping skills and to reconceptualize feared situations. The therapist and client build the youth's repertoire of coping skills, including relaxation training, imagery, identifying and restructuring maladaptive cognitions, self-talk, problem solving, and reinforcement. Skill generalization and relapse prevention are incorporated through homework assignments. Parents are included throughout the course of the treatment, as they help with weekly updates, exposures, and coaching depending on the treatment plan and parental ability.

The Coping Cat treatment has proved efficacious for treating anxiety in children and adolescents and is transferable to a family or group format and across cultures (Albano & Kendall, 2002). Modifications can also be made to the treatment manual, depending on diagnosis (see Grover, Hughes, Bergman, & Kingery, 2006, for specific recommendations) and culture (Barrett, Dadds, & Rapee, 1996). To study the efficacy of the Coping Cat program, Kendall (1994) assigned 47 participants, ages 8–13 years, to either a treatment or control group. Following the treatment, 64% of the treatment group no longer met criteria for an anxiety disorder; compared with 5% of the control group.

The CAT project (Kendall, Hudson, & Webb, 2002) is a similar program to the Coping Cat program but is designed specifically for adolescents 14–17 years. This program also outlines 16 sessions. These manualized treatments (Coping Cat and the CAT project), available from Workbook Publishing, offer individual workbooks, as well as therapist manuals for individual, group, and family treatment. Video and DVD guides are also offered to assist with treatment.

Treatment for OCD

CBT for OCD uses both cognitive and behavioral strategies to alter behaviors and reduce distressing thoughts and feelings. March and Mulle (1998) developed a step-by-step guide for OCD treatment that includes four stages: (1) psychoeducation, (2) cognitive training, (3) OCD mapping, and (4) exposure and response prevention. A self-monitoring technique using a fear thermometer is used during exposure and response preventions to gauge the client's level of anxiety during the exposure. The treatment protocol takes place over 12–20 sessions (plus booster sessions). March and Mulle (1998) provide specific information for the therapist to follow during the course of treatment, including goal setting, previous session review, presentation of new material, assistance with session practice, homework, and rules for self-monitoring. Parents are included in Sessions 1, 7, 12, and 19. The authors encourage midweek phone calls to clients between

sessions to check at-home exposure and response prevention practice.

Treatment for Social Anxiety

Albano and DiBartolo (2007) developed a therapist guide for treating adolescents, ages 13–18 years, diagnosed with social anxiety. Based on CBT techniques, groups of five to seven youths learn how to cope in social situations. The treatment protocol is set up in a series of two stages, skill building and exposures. Skill building sessions include cognitive restructuring, problem solving, social skills, and assertiveness training. The group members systematically complete exposure exercises involving feared or avoided social situations. Parents of the group members are included during selected sessions, as deemed therapeutically necessary. They are educated about the goals of treatment and are included to improve adolescent and parent communication, as well as to learn ways to provide increased support to their child. The therapist manual outlines each session and provides sample dialogues, role-playing activities, and homework. Albano and DiBartolo (2007) also provide tips for treatment for children ages 8–12 and in the context of individual therapy.

Treatment of Depression and Anxiety in School-Age Youths

The treatment protocols discussed previously for depression and anxiety contain specific behavioral and cognitive strategies, emphasizing the acquisition of these cognitive and behavioral skills to manage depressive and anxious symptoms. CBT is based on the assumption that the symptoms are caused or maintained by deficits in all four domains of the cognitive model: (1) cognitions, (2) mood, (3) behavior, and (4) environmental factors (Reinecke & Ginsburg, 2008).

CBT for depressive disorders challenges and reconstructs the depressogenic cognitions of the child or adolescent ("I am helpless"; "I am unlovable") and increases engagement in pleasant events (Beck, 1995; Compton et al., 2004). The most common cognitive components in CBT interventions for depression include problem solving, self-monitoring, affective education, and cognitive restructuring. Common behavioral components include activity scheduling, relaxation training, behavioral rehearsal and experiments, reinforcement, and modeling (Maag & Swearer, 2005; Maag, Swearer, & Toland, 2009). The extant research has found that behavioral treatment is a necessary precursor for effective cognitive treatment (Stark, Sander, Hargrave, et al., 2006; Stark, Swearer, Kurowski, Sommer, & Bowen, 1996). This temporal sequence between behavioral and cognitive techniques helps children and adolescents elevate their moods before they are taught and helps them benefit from cognitive restructuring.

The mechanism of treatment for anxiety disorders involves reversing the tendency to avoid threatening situations (Rapee, Wignall, Hudson, & Schniering, 2000). CBT for anxiety disorders promotes habituation to or extinction of fears (Compton et al., 2004) through exposure and other techniques (e.g., thought exercises, rewards, praise, and differential reinforcement; Chorpita, 2007). Chorpita identified five components common to CBT for anxiety: (1) psychoeducation, (2) somatic symptom management, (3) cognitive restructuring, (4) exposure, and (5) relapse prevention. The most common behavioral components include exposure, modeling, relaxation training, systematic desensitization, extinction, contingency management, reinforcement, and rewards. Other common cognitive components for anxiety are self-monitoring and cognitive restructuring. The CBT techniques commonly used in treating both depression and anxiety are described in more detail.

Behavioral Strategies

Activity Scheduling

Children and adolescents diagnosed with depression tend to withdraw from other people and social situations and do not engage in pleasurable activities as they did prior to the onset of their depression (Stark, 1990). Therefore, activity scheduling is initiated at the beginning of treatment to increase the youth's social interactions and reduce his or her withdrawal behaviors (Friedberg & McClure, 2002). Activity scheduling involves intentional planning of pleasurable or goal-oriented activities, as well as psychoeduca-

tion about the connection between mood and behavior (Stark, 1990). The therapist provides the client and parent with a rationale for the importance of engaging the child or adolescent in pleasurable activities. Together, the therapist and client generate a list of activities the client finds pleasurable (Reinecke & Ginsburg, 2008; Stark, 1990). Initially, it may be difficult for a depressed youth to generate pleasurable activities. The therapist may need to ask about the activities he or she found pleasurable prior to his or her depression. For example, a child may have previously loved to play outside. The role of the therapist is also to ensure that the parent or guardian can facilitate the child's identified activities. The therapist may also need to help the child or adolescent create gradual steps before he or she is able to participate in a pleasurable activity (Friedberg & McClure, 2002). For example, consider a child who had previously participated in ballet but no longer finds her ballet classes enjoyable. In creating steps to participating in ballet again, the first step may be to call the ballet teacher and sign up for classes, followed by the girl's attending her first class, and so on.

Depending on the severity of the client's depression, activity scheduling may need to become very detailed (Stark, 1990). Eventually, the client is instructed to self-monitor his or her engagement in pleasurable activities by rating his or her mood before and after engaging in a pleasant activity (see Figure 26.1 for an example). This self-monitoring technique will help the youth with depression make the connection between his or her mood and behavior and identify changes in mood as being associated with the activities they complete (Stark, 1990).

A youth with depression may also predict that he or she will not enjoy an identified activity, and, through self-monitoring and behavioral experiments, he or she will become aware of a tendency to make negative predictions and be able to test the reality of those predictions (Friedberg & McClure, 2002). Consider the following example:

THERAPIST: How much do you think you will enjoy playing checkers with me in session?

ROB: Not that much, maybe a 3.

Monday	Tuesday	Wednesday	Thursday	Friday	Saturday	Sunday
Mood before: 4

Shot hoops after school

Mood after: 6 | Mood before: 3

Helped Dad in the garage

Mood after: 5 | Mood before: 5

Family game night (cards)

Mood after: 7 | Mood before: 6

Played video game with Steve

Mood after: 7 | Mood before: 7

Camping trip

Mood after: 8 | Mood before: 7

Fishing and hiking

Mood after: 9 | Mood before: 8

Leaving trip

Mood after: 6

Talked to friend on the phone

Mood after: 7 |

FIGURE 26.1. Sample pleasant events schedule with mood ratings (1 = low; 10 = high).

THERAPIST: What thoughts are going through your mind about playing checkers?

ROB: I stink at games. The only way I win is if I get lucky or if the other person messes up.

THERAPIST: How do those thoughts make you feel?

ROB: Frustrated.

THERAPIST: So, Rob, you are predicting that you won't have much fun playing checkers and said you are thinking "I stink at games," which is making you feel frustrated. What if we tested your prediction about checkers and play for a little bit? (*Plays checkers with Rob.*) Rob, I noticed you're smiling and that you laughed a couple of times during our game. How much fun did you have playing checkers?

ROB: I guess more than I thought, probably a 6.

THERAPIST: A 6 is more fun than you thought you would have playing the game, which was a 3.

ROB: Yeah, I guess it was.

Relaxation

Relaxation techniques are useful for youths with both depression and anxiety. Relaxation training helps youths cope with aversive levels of physical arousal (Stark et al., 1996). Relaxation training can help a youth learn to notice the tension in his or her body and recognize it as a symptom of his or her disorder (Weissman, Fendrich, Warner, & Wickramaratne, 2002). Relaxation techniques should be taught and practiced in ses-

sion (Beck, 1995). Therapists use progressive muscle relaxation to help the client achieve a relaxed state by instructing the child or adolescent to tense each muscle and subsequently relax it. Relaxation strategies can be presented in a graduated form, especially for younger children who may have more difficulty tensing and relaxing their muscles (Friedberg & McClure, 2002; Weissman et al., 2002; Wright, Basco, & Thase, 2006). A therapist should keep his or her relaxation script developmentally appropriate, using a metaphor or analogy to help younger children understand relaxation techniques (Chorpita, 2007). For example, instead of instructing a child to tense specific muscles, the therapist can ask him or her to pretend that he or she is squeezing lemons with his or her hands or squishing a bug with his or her foot. For a detailed relaxation script, see Wright et al. (2006).

Systematic Desensitization (Graded Exposure)

Systematic desensitization decreases fears and anxiety through counterconditioning. Relaxation is used to inhibit anxiety as the youth is gradually presented (using an exposure hierarchy described here) with fear-invoking situations (Friedberg & McClure, 2002; Wright et al., 2006). In creating exposure hierarchies, also called a fear ladder, the first objective is to establish a list of feared items with the child or adolescent. The stimuli at each step should be specifically described and then ranked according to the child's or adolescent's fear, using subjective units of distress (SUDS; Masters, Burish, Hollon, & Rimm, 1987) ratings (e.g.,

1–100; 1–10; Friedberg & McClure, 2002; Wright et al., 2006). The child or adolescent should be familiar with his or her rating system (e.g., fear thermometer) and practice ranking nontargeted stimuli in session prior to ranking the targeted stimuli (Chorpita, 2007). Graduated levels of fear should be created within the same concern or domain (e.g., only social phobia stimuli). A new fear ladder can be used to target other problem areas if needed. In setting up a fear ladder, at least 10 items should be identified by the youth (see Figure 26.2 for an example). The therapist can use a note card to write down each identified stimulus on one side and the fear rating on the other side. Then, each fear is hierarchically arranged, from the least to the most anxiety provoking. If less than 10 stimuli are identified, it may be helpful to look for variations within the same feared stimuli (Chorpita, 2007). For example, giving a speech in front of one person, giving a speech in front of a few people, and giving a speech in front of the whole class are graduated variations within the same fear of public speaking.

Ask someone to come over to play video games.	10
Call another student on the phone.	10
Talk to another kid for at least 5 minutes during lunch.	9
Introduce myself to someone new in the cafeteria.	8
Eat lunch in the cafeteria.	7
Tell three kids about a video game I am playing.	6
Ask another kid what they did over the weekend.	5
Ask another kid if I can borrow a pencil.	5
Say "hi" to the kid who sits behind me in math class.	4
Say "hi" to my teacher.	3

FIGURE 26.2. Sample fear ladder.

Behavioral Rehearsal/Experiments

Behavioral experiments are used to alter a child's or adolescent's behavior in order to change his or her thinking by testing the validity of negative cognitions (Stark et al., 1996). For example, an experiment can be designed to directly test the validity of a negative prediction that a child or adolescent makes about his or her ability to perform a task or about the outcome of an event (Beck, 1995). During behavioral assignments (such as asking a friend to come over to play or filling out a job application), the therapist provides the youth with feedback about his or her behavioral experiment. The therapist points out information that is inconsistent with the youth's schema (Stark, 1990). Prior to assigning a behavioral plan outside of session, the therapist should role-play with the youth to ensure that he or she is able to carry out the activity. It is also necessary to provide feedback, look for roadblocks, and provide coaching. The youth should guide the role play by making predictions as to which response he or she expects and then role playing various scenarios (i.e., best case, worst case, and most likely; Wright et al., 2006). Behavioral experiments for youths diagnosed with anxiety disorders are also known as exposures.

Exposure

Exposure procedures have received the most empirical support (e.g., Foa, Rothbaum, & Furr, 2003) and are the key therapeutic components in youth anxiety interventions (Silverman & Kurtines, 2001). For example, Chorpita and Southam-Gerow (2006) found exposure to be effective at reducing anxiety in more than 35 controlled studies. Exposure-based interventions for youths with anxiety include real (in vivo) or imagined (in vitro) exposure to feared stimuli in order to assuage the anxiety the child or adolescent pairs with the stimuli (Chorpita, 2007; Compton et al., 2004). Exposure to the feared stimuli is completed within a hierarchy of feared stimuli, so that the client is first exposed to less anxiety-provoking stimuli, followed by increasingly anxiety provoking stimuli (Chorpita, 2007; Compton et al., 2004). Imagined exposure exercises introduce the youth to the feared stimuli as the therapist describes a scene while the youth listens and imagines the details of the scene. This is helpful for situations that are not easily performed *in vivo* (Chorpita, 2007).

Exposure and response prevention plays a key role in March and Mulle's (1998) protocol for OCD treatment. Exposure to a feared stimulus creates an aversive physiological state; however, with repeated exposures to the feared stimulus, the body eventually returns to homeostasis. Thus after exposures the client realizes the feared stimuli can be faced and overcome (Wright et al., 2006). Response prevention entails not engaging in the ritual or compulsion during the *in vitro* or *in vivo* exposure (March & Mulle, 1998).

Contingency Management, Reinforcement, and Rewards

A child's behavior may be shaped through contingency management, reinforcement, and rewards. Through contingency management, focus is on the consequences of the behavior, using reinforcement, shaping, and extinction (Kendall, Chu, Pimentel, & Choudhury, 2000). Caregivers and teachers provide the youth with positive reinforcement for desirable behaviors while ignoring undesirable behaviors (Farris & Jouriles, 1993; Friedberg & McClure, 2002). Parents provide a link between a child's ability to acquire skills during therapy and generalize them to the natural environment (Stark et al., 1996). Developing and reinforcing small steps or identifying targeted time periods for the desired behaviors to occur may be necessary in order to gradually shape desired behavior. Contingencies can be developed using if–then strategies. For example, Julie, who is diagnosed with social phobia, avoids going to school. An if–then contingency for her could be, "If Julie is on time to school today, she can choose what the family has for supper."

For youths diagnosed with anxiety disorders, parents and other family members often unintentionally reinforce the child's avoidance behaviors or participation in a ritual to reduce anxiety. Family anxiety management sessions should be implemented by the therapist in order to increase treatment effectiveness (Barrett, Rapee, Dadds, & Ryan, 1996) and create a team to overcome anxiety (March & Mulle, 1998). For example,

consider an adolescent diagnosed with OCD who engages in reassurance seeking related to his or her germ obsession. When his or her parents answer such questions as "Is this clean?" they are unintentionally reinforcing the adolescent's fear of germs. During parent sessions, parents learn to ignore these behaviors (i.e., extinction) and reinforce habituation and more desired behaviors (e.g., the youth's touching an object he or she fears is contaminated).

Modeling

Modeling is based on the social learning theory of Bandura (1986) and is used in treating youths with depression and anxiety. The therapist or adult models alternative, adaptive thoughts for the child or adolescent by verbalizing his or her thoughts about problems or situations. When coping thoughts and problem-solving skills are modeled, the youth with depression learns more adaptive ways of thinking (Stark, 1990). Modeling can be done in this observational or vicarious manner or through video. When using modeling for youths with anxiety, the therapist helps the youth learn an adaptive approach to a feared stimulus (Weissman, Antinoro, & Chu, 2008). For example, in working with Lydia who has a phobia of dogs, the therapist and Lydia, first watch a video of someone playing with a dog. The person on the video is modeling appropriate coping, and the therapist can also verbalize coping statements aloud as a way to model for Lydia. Next, modeling and exposure are combined (Chorpita, 2007), and a dog is brought into session. The therapist pets the dog while verbalizing appropriate coping statements for Lydia.

Cognitive Strategies

Problem Solving

Direct instruction and practice in problem solving helps youths who lack the skills to effectively solve problems (Beck, 1995). Teaching youths to problem-solve helps them expand their thinking, gives them another coping strategy, and can empower them to help themselves (Stark, 1990). Problem solving is broken into multiple components (Kendall et al., 2000; Stark et al., 1996), with the objective of teaching youths how to think, *not* what to think, about problems and stressful situations they encounter (Reinecke & Ginsburg, 2008). Games are especially helpful in teaching the problem-solving model (e.g., Jenga, checkers), as they provide a concrete way to teach problem solving in session. Games teach the relevance of using the problem-solving strategy and provide immediate feedback through the natural consequences of the game (e.g., Jenga blocks falling). Once the problem-solving steps have been learned, the therapist guides the youth through hypothetical problem-solving situations and then through the youth's own problems (Stark et al., 1996). The following is an example from Kendall et al. (2000) of how problem solving is broken into multiple components (also see Bushman & Gimpel Peacock, Chapter 25, this volume): (1) What is the problem? (2) What are my options? (3) What will happen if I do those things? (4) Which solution will work best? and (5) How did it work?

Affective Education

Through affective education, a client learns to recognize his or her emotions and the accompanying physical features. For example, in the ACTION treatment program for depressed adolescent girls, the girls are instructed to recognize their emotions by using the "three B's": body, brain, and behavior. They are taught to pay attention to what their bodies are doing, what they are thinking, and how they are acting (Stark et al., 2008). Affective education is first based in the abstract. The therapist refers to the emotions of others to distance both pleasant and unpleasant emotions from the youth. Then several activities are implemented to help the youth learn to recognize and label his or her emotions. The child or adolescent learns to identify emotions through pictures, magazines, books, and other activities. Role-playing emotions and their physical expressions using emotional charades is a useful activity for affective education (Kendall et al., 2000; Stark et al., 1996). Emotional charades allow a youth to learn how to recognize the cues or triggers to his or her emotions (Stark et al., 1996).

Self-Monitoring

Self-monitoring involves the conscious act of observing oneself (Stark et al., 1996). In CBT, self-monitoring includes identifying one's thoughts, feelings, or behaviors (Friedberg & McClure, 2002; Stark, 1990; see also Hoff & Sawka-Miller, Chapter 20, this volume). Targeted behaviors can be self-monitored during treatment, such as engagement in pleasant events or amount of time spent performing a ritual. Self-monitoring is also used as a tool to identify patterns in thinking, with the goal of eventually helping the youth to develop and replace maladaptive thoughts with more realistic or adaptive thoughts. For example, a youth with depression or anxiety may be asked to write down his or her thoughts, feelings, and behaviors using a thought record (see Figure 26.3). Self-monitoring can be a difficult task, as the child or adolescent may feel too ashamed, fearful, or hopeless to report his or her thoughts, feelings, and behaviors. Therapists must take an active role in helping the child or adolescent self-monitor, if that is the case, by targeting the depressive symptom that is preventing him or her from engaging in self-monitoring. For example, if the client expresses that he or she is fearful about disclosing his or her thoughts, the therapist should query those beliefs (e.g., "What are you afraid will happen if you tell me your thoughts?"; Friedberg & McClure, 2002).

Date	Situation	Thought	Fear rating (1–10)	More realistic thought	Fear rating (1–10)
11/19	Reading in front of the class	I'm going to mess up.	7	I've done it before and it wasn't so bad. I actually did pretty well.	3

FIGURE 26.3. Sample thought record for a youth with anxiety.

Self-monitoring for children is not as straightforward as it is for most adolescents. Friedberg and McClure (2002) provide self-monitoring tasks that are creative ways for children to learn the relationship between their situations, thoughts, feelings, and behaviors (e.g., Tracks of My Fears worksheet; Friedberg & McClure, 2002). In addition to monitoring thoughts, feelings, and behaviors, it is beneficial for youths with depressive disorders to keep track of positive events based in reality in order to dispute their negative beliefs (Stark et al., 1996). Youths with anxiety disorders self-monitor their degrees of fear and anxiety (e.g., 1–10, 1–100) through the use of a fear thermometer (Friedberg & McClure, 2002) or SUDS ratings (Masters et al., 1987; see Figure 26.2).

Identifying Automatic Thoughts and Cognitive Distortions

It is important to teach youths to identify and change the maladaptive thought patterns that are reinforcing and exacerbating their depressive and anxious symptoms. There are times during session that automatic thoughts can be elicited and identified (e.g., when the therapist notices an affect shift during session). For more detailed techniques on eliciting automatic thoughts, see Beck (1995). Therapists should also engage in guided discovery, using Socratic questioning to guide the client to understand his or her maladaptive thought patterns (Reinecke & Ginsburg, 2008). By using Socratic questioning, the youth learns that his or her automatic thoughts are hypotheses to be tested (e.g., "What's the evidence to support that?" "On a scale of 0 to 100, how strongly do you believe that thought?" "What would you tell a friend in your situation?").

Once automatic thoughts have been identified, they are typically characterized by a negative bias or errors in thinking, called cognitive distortions. The therapist works with the client to identify his or her cognitive distortions at a developmentally appropriate level. Examples of cognitive distortions include fortune telling ("I won't be able to finish this assignment"), all-or-nothing thinking ("I have to get an A, or I'm a total loser"), personalization ("I must have made her mad, that's why she didn't wave at me"), labeling ("I'm a bad person"),

and discounting the positive ("I won that game, but it was just because I got lucky"). For a complete list of cognitive distortions, see Beck (1995).

Cognitive Restructuring

Cognitive restructuring involves identifying distorted thoughts and using strategies to evaluate and replace them with more rational or adaptive thoughts (Chorpita, 2007; Weissman et al., 2008). Cognitive restructuring for youths with depression serves to identify and change unrealistic, negative thinking about themselves, others, and the world around them. Cognitive restructuring for a youth with anxiety identifies negative thoughts and perceptions related to fears and perceptions of threat (Chorpita, 2007; Weissman et al., 2008). When it is determined that an automatic thought is dysfunctional, the therapist should then gauge how much the youth believes the automatic thought. Consider this case example of Sara, a 12-year-old female diagnosed with depression.

THERAPIST: Sara, I noticed your mood changed when you were describing moving to a new school. What was going through your mind?

SARA: That I'm not going to fit in.

THERAPIST: How much do you believe that thought, that you aren't going to fit in?

SARA: A lot, probably a 7.

THERAPIST: How does thinking that you won't fit in at your new school make you feel?

SARA: Worried, a 6 or 7.

Because Sara believes her thought and is distressed by it, the therapist continues to evaluate Sara's belief. Sara is taught that her thought is a hypothesis to be tested and is asked to look for evidence consistent and inconsistent with her thought.

THERAPIST: I can imagine that if you thought you weren't going to fit in at your new school that you might feel sad. Why don't we explore that thought a little and see if it really is true that you won't fit in.

SARA: OK.

THERAPIST: What evidence do you have that you won't fit in at your new school?

SARA: I don't know anyone there and they've probably all known each other for a long time.

THERAPIST: OK, so you might not fit in because you don't know anyone at your new school and they have probably known each other for a while?

SARA: Yeah.

THERAPIST: OK, let's write that in the "evidence for" column. What other evidence do you have that you won't fit in?

SARA: (pause) That's probably it, just that I don't know anyone.

THERAPIST: Well, let's see what evidence you have that you *will* fit in at your new school.

SARA: Maybe there will be someone who is nice there who will make friends with me.

THERAPIST: OK, let's add that there might be someone nice you can make friends with in the "evidence against" column. What else?

SARA: Well, it will be the beginning of the year, so there might be other new people.

THERAPIST: Let's add that to the list as well. Sara, you mentioned you joined a new soccer team this summer and are friends with the girls on the team. Do you think you made friends because everyone is nice or do you think you have an easy time making friends?

SARA: Well, not everyone on the team was that nice at first. I guess I make friends pretty easily. I was voted to be one of the team captains.

THERAPIST: OK, let's add that to our list. Has there been another time when you met new people and made friends with them?

SARA: I guess when I met Trish and Rebecca, the girls who live in my neighborhood.

THERAPIST: We'll put that in this column, too. How much do you believe the thought that you won't fit in at your new school now after gathering evidence for and against the thought?

SARA: Not that much anymore, like a 2.

THERAPIST: And what's your mood like now?

SARA: I don't feel that worried about it anymore. It might take some time, but I know I can make friends.

If Sara had still believed and been distressed by her thought, the therapist would have continued to logically analyze that thought by asking:

1. What's the evidence?
2. Is there another way of viewing the situation that has not been thought of before?
3. If the thought is true, what is the worst that could happen? Could you survive it? What is most likely to happen?
4. What would happen if you changed the way you thought about this?
5. What should you do about the situation?
6. What would you tell a friend to do to if he or she were in the same situation? (Beck, 1995)

Other cognitive restructuring strategies include identifying cognitive errors, reattribution, continuum technique, generating positive self-statements, thought stopping, and creating a coping plan (Friedberg & McClure, 2002; Kendall et al., 2000; Wright et al., 2006). A dysfunctional thought record (DTR) can also be used to aid a youth in evaluating and responding to his or her au-

Date	Situation	Automatic thought(s)	Emotion(s)	Adaptive response	Outcome
02/24	Moving to a new school	I won't fit in.	Worried (6–7)	I actually make friends pretty easily. It might take me a little time, but I know I can make friends here.	Less worried about first day of school.

FIGURE 26.4. Sara's dysfunctional thought record.

tomatic thoughts and can be an effective homework assignment. See Figure 26.4 for an example DTR (Beck, 1995). Also, see Beck (1995) for specific DTR guidelines.

Conclusions: Assessment and Treatment Implications for School Psychologists

School psychologists are the frontline professionals who are trained in the assessment, diagnosis, and treatment of depressive and anxiety disorders in youths. As Merrell and colleagues (2006) proposed, the roles and functions of school psychologists span the levels of prevention, risk reduction, intervention, and treatment. We also proposed that school psychologists sustain treatment gains by linking schools and families with community mental health agencies and community treatment providers. Cognitive-behavioral treatments have been proven effective and provide school psychologists with treatment strategies for use with depressed and anxious children and adolescents. Accurate assessment leads to accurate diagnosis, which informs best practices in the effective cognitive-behavioral treatment of anxiety and depression among school-age youths.

References

Albano, A. M., Chorpita, B. F., & Barlow, D. H. (1996). Childhood anxiety disorders. In E. J. Mash & R. A. Barkley (Eds.), *Child psychopathology* (pp. 279–329). New York: Guilford Press.

Albano, A. M., & DiBartolo, P. M. (2007). *Cognitive-behavioral therapy for social phobia in adolescents.* New York: Oxford University Press.

Albano, A. M., & Kendall, P. C. (2002). Cognitive behavioural therapy for children and adolescents with anxiety disorders: Clinical research advances. *International Review of Psychiatry, 14,* 129–134.

American Psychiatric Association. (2000). *Diagnostic and statistical manual of mental disorders* (4th ed., text rev.). Washington, DC: Author.

Anderson, J. C. (1994). Epidemiological issues. In T. H. Ollendick, N. King, & W. Yule (Eds.), *International handbook of phobic and anxiety disorders in children and adolescents* (pp. 43–65). New York: Plenum Press.

Avenevoli, S., Knight, E., Kessler, R. C., & Merikangas, K. R. (2008). Epidemiology of depression in children and adolescents. In J. R. Z. Abela & B. L. Hankin (Eds.), *Handbook of depression in children and adolescents* (pp. 6–32). New York: Guilford Press.

Bandura, A. (1986). *Social learning theory.* Englewood Cliffs, NJ: Prentice Hall.

Barrett, P. M., Dadds, M. R., & Rapee, R. M. (1996). Family treatment of childhood anxiety: A controlled trial. *Journal of Consulting and Clinical Psychology, 64,* 333–342.

Barrett, P. M., Rapee, R. M., Dadds, M. M., & Ryan, S. M. (1996). Family enhancement of cognitive style in anxious and aggressive children. *Journal of Abnormal Child Psychology, 24*(2), 187–203.

Beck, A. T., Rush, A. J., Shaw, B. F., & Emery, G. (1979). *Cognitive therapy of depression.* New York: Guilford Press.

Beck, J. S. (1995). *Cognitive therapy: Basics and beyond.* New York: Guilford Press.

Beidel, D. C. (1991). Social phobia and overanxious disorder in school-age children. *Journal of the American Academy of Child and Adolescent Psychiatry, 30,* 545–552.

Chorpita, B. F. (2007). *Modular cognitive-behavioral therapy for childhood anxiety disorders.* New York: Guilford Press.

Chorpita, B. F., & Southam-Gerow, M. A. (2006). Fears and anxieties. In E. J. Mash & R. A. Barkley (Eds.), *Treatment of childhood disorders* (3rd ed., pp. 271–335). New York: Guilford Press.

Compton, S. N., March, J. S., Brent, D., Albano, A. M., Weersing, V. R., & Curry, J. (2004). Cognitive-behavioral psychotherapy for anxiety and depressive disorders in children and adolescents: An evidence-based medicine review. *Journal of American Academy of Child and Adolescent Psychiatry, 43*(8), 930–959.

Costello, E. J., & Angold, A. (1995). Epidemiology. In J. S. March (Ed.), *Anxiety disorders in children and adolescents* (pp. 109–124). New York: Guilford Press.

Cowan, R. J., & Swearer, S. M. (2004). School–community partnerships. In C. Spielberger (Ed.), *Encyclopedia of applied psychology* (pp. 309–318). Oxford, UK: Elsevier.

Curry, J. F., Rohde, P., Simons, A., Silva, S., Vitiello, B., Kratochvil, C., et al. (2006). Predictors and moderators of acute outcome in the Treatment for Adolescents with Depression Study (TADS). *Journal of American Academy of Child and Adolescent Psychiatry, 45*(12), 1427–1439.

Curry, J. F., & Murphy, L. B. (1995). Comorbidity of anxiety disorders. In J. S. March (Ed.), *Anxiety disorders in children and adolescents* (pp. 301–317). New York: Guilford Press.

Emslie, G., Kratochvil, C., Vitiello, B., Silva, S., Mayes, T., McNulty, S., et al. (2006). Treatment for Adolescents with Depression Study (TADS): Safety results. *Journal of the American Academy of Child and Adolescent Psychiatry*, 45(12), 1440–1455.

Farris, A. M., & Jouriles, E. N. (1993). Separation anxiety disorder. In A. S. Bellack & M. Hersen (Eds.), *Handbook of behavior therapy in the psychiatric setting* (pp. 407–426). New York: Plenum Press.

Foa, E. B., Rothbaum, B. O., & Furr, J. M. (2003). Augmenting exposure therapy with other CBT procedures. *Psychiatric Annals*, 33(1), 47–53.

Friedberg, R. D., & McClure, J. M. (2002). *Clinical practice of cognitive therapy with children and adolescents: The nuts and bolts*. New York: Guilford Press.

Grills-Taquechel, A. & Ollendick, T. H. (2007). Introduction to special issue: Developments in the etiology and psychosocial treatments of anxiety disorders in children and adolescents. *Clinical Child and Family Psychology Review*, 10, 197–198.

Grover, R. L., Hughes, A. A., Bergman, R. L., & Kingery, J. N. (2006). Treatment modifications based on childhood anxiety diagnosis: Demonstrating the flexibility in manualized treatment. *Journal of Cognitive Psychotherapy: An International Quarterly*, 20, 275–286.

Harrington, R., Fudge, H., Rutter, M., Pickles, A., & Hill, J. (1991). Adult outcomes of childhood and adolescent depression: II. Links with antisocial disorders. *Journal of the American Academy of Child and Adolescent Psychiatry*, 30(3), 434–439.

Kahn, J. S., Kehle, T. J., Jenson, W. R., & Clark, E. (1990). Comparison of cognitive-behavioral, relaxation, and self-modeling interventions for depression among middle-school students. *School Psychology Review*, 19(2), 196–211.

Kazdin, A. E., & Weisz, J. R. (2003). *Evidence-based psychotherapies for children and adolescents*. New York: Guilford Press.

Kendall, P. C. (1992). *Coping Cat workbook*. Ardmore, PA: Workbook.

Kendall, P. C. (1994). Treating anxiety disorders in children: Results of a randomized clinical trial. *Journal of Consulting and Clinical Psychology*, 62, 100–110.

Kendall, P. C., Chu, B. C., Pimentel, S. S., & Choudhury, M. (2000). Treating anxiety disorders in youth. In P. C. Kendall (Ed.), *Child and adolescent therapy: Cognitive-behavioral procedures* (2nd ed., pp. 235–287). New York: Guilford Press.

Kendall, P. C., & Hedtke, K. A. (2006). *Coping Cat workbook* (2nd ed.). Ardmore, PA: Workbook.

Kendall, P. C., Hudson, J., & Webb, A. (2002). *"The C.A.T. Project": Workbook for the cognitive-behavioral treatment of anxious adolescents*. Ardmore, PA: Workbook.

Last, C. G., Strauss, C. C., & Francis, G. (1987). Comorbidity among childhood anxiety disorders. *Journal of Nervous and Mental Disease*, 175, 726–730.

Lewinsohn, P. M., Clarke, G. N., Hops, H., & Andrews, J. A. (1990). Cognitive-behavioral treatment for depressed adolescents. *Behavior Therapy*, 21(4), 385–401.

Lewinsohn, P. M., Rohde, P., & Seeley, J. R. (1998). Major depressive disorder in older adolescents: Prevalence, risk factors, and clinical implications. *Clinical Psychology Review*, 18, 765–794.

Lewinsohn, P. M., Zinbarg, R., Seeley, J. R., Lewinsohn, M., & Sack, W. (1997). Lifetime comorbidity among anxiety disorders and between anxiety disorders and other mental disorders in adolescents. *Journal of Anxiety Disorders*, 11, 377–394.

Maag, J. W., & Swearer, S. M. (2005). Cognitive-behavioral interventions for depression: Review and implications for school personnel. *Behavioral Disorders*, 30, 259–276.

Maag, J. W., Swearer, S. M., & Toland, M. D. (2009). Cognitive-behavioral interventions for depression in children and adolescents: Meta-analysis, promising programs, and implications for school personnel. In M. J. Mayer, R. Van Acker, J. E. Lochman, & F. M. Gresham (Eds.), *Cognitive-behavioral interventions for emotional and behavioral disorders: School-based practice* (pp. 235–265). New York: Guilford Press.

March, J. S., & Mulle, K. (1998). *OCD in children and adolescents: A cognitive-behavioral treatment manual*. New York: Guilford Press.

Masters, J. C., Burish, T. G., Hollon, S. D., & Rimm, D. C. (1987). *Behavior therapy: Techniques and empirical findings* (2nd ed.). San Diego, CA: Harcourt.

Meiser-Stedman, R., Yule, W., Smith, P., Glucksman, E., & Dalgleish, T. (2005). Acute stress disorder and posttraumatic stress disorder in children and adolescents involved in assaults or motor vehicle accidents. *American Journal of Psychiatry*, 162, 1381–1383.

Merrell, K. W. (2008). *Helping students overcome depression and anxiety: A practical guide* (2nd ed.). New York: Guilford Press.

Merrell, K. W., Ervin, R. A., & Gimpel Peacock, G. A. (2006). *School psychology for the 21st century: Foundations and practices*. New York: Guilford Press.

Mitchell, J., McCauley, E., Burke, P. M., & Moss, S. J. (1988). Phenomenology of depression in children and adolescents. *Journal of the American Academy of Child and Adolescent Psychiatry, 27,* 12–20.

Mufson, L., Dorta, K. P., Wickramaratne, P., Normura, Y., Oflson, M., & Weissman, M. M. (2004). A randomized effectiveness trial of interpersonal psychotherapy for depressed adolescents. *Archives of General Psychiatry, 63,* 577–584.

Mufson, L., Moreau, D., Weissman, M. M., & Klerman, G. L. (1993). *Interpersonal psychotherapy for depressed adolescents.* New York: Guilford Press.

Mufson, L., Moreau, D., Weissman, M. M., Wickramaratne, P., Martin, J., & Samoilov, A. (1994). The modification of interpersonal psychotherapy with depressed adolescents (IPT-A): Phase I and phase II studies. *Journal of the American Academy of Child and Adolescent Psychiatry, 33,* 695–705.

Mufson, L., Weissman, M. M., Moreau, D., & Garfinkel, R. (1999). Efficacy of interpersonal psychotherapy for depressed adolescents. *Archives of General Psychiatry, 56,* 573–579.

Nottelmann, E. D., & Jensen, P. S. (1995). Comorbidity of disorders in children and adolescents: Developmental perspectives. In T. H. Ollendick & R. J. Prinz (Eds.), *Advances in clinical child psychology* (Vol. 17, pp. 109–155). New York: Plenum Press.

Rapee, R. M., Wignall, A., Hudson, J. L., & Schniering, C. A. (2000). *Treating anxiety in children and adolescents: An evidence-based approach.* Oakland, CA: New Harbinger.

Reinecke, M. A., & Ginsburg, G. S. (2008). Cognitive-behavioral treatment of depression during childhood and adolescence. In J. R. Z. Abela & B. L. Hankin (Eds.), *Handbook of depression in children and adolescents* (pp. 179–206). New York: Guilford Press.

Rohde, P., Lewinsohn, P. M., Clarke, G. N., Hops, H., & Seeley, J. R. (2005). The adolescent coping with depression course: A cognitive-behavioral approach to the treatment of adolescent depression. In E. D. Hibbs & P. S. Jensen (Eds.), *Psychosocial treatments for child and adolescent disorders: Empirically based strategies for clinical practice* (2nd ed., pp. 219–237). Washington, DC: American Psychological Association.

Rosselló, J., & Bernal, G. (1999). The efficacy of cognitive-behavioral and interpersonal treatments for depression in Puerto Rican adolescents. *Journal of Consulting and Clinical Psychology, 67,* 734–745.

Schroeder, C. S., & Gordon, B. N. (2002). *Assessment and treatment of childhood problems: A clinician's guide* (2nd ed.). New York: Guilford Press.

Silverman, W. K., & Kurtines, W. M. (1996). *Anxiety and phobic disorders: A pragmatic approach.* New York: Plenum Press.

Silverman, W. K., & Kurtines, W. M. (2001). Anxiety disorders. In J. N. Hughes, A. M. La Greca, & J. C. Conoley (Eds.), *Handbook of psychological services for children and adolescents* (pp. 225–244). New York: Oxford University Press.

Stark, K. D. (1990). *Childhood depression: School-based intervention.* New York: Guilford Press.

Stark, K. D., Hargrave, J., Hersh, B., Greenberg, M., Herren, J., & Fisher, M. (2008). Treatment of childhood depression: The ACTION treatment program. In J. R. Z. Abela & B. L. Hankin (Eds.), *Handbook of depression in children and adolescents* (pp. 224–249). New York: Guilford Press.

Stark, K. D., & Kendall, P. C. (1996). *Treating depressed children: Therapist manual for "taking action."* Ardmore, PA: Workbook.

Stark, K. D., Sander, J. B., Hargrave, J., Schnoebelen, S., Simpson, J., & Molnar, J. (2006). Treatment of depression in children and adolescence: Cognitive-behavioral procedures for the individual and family. In P. C. Kendall (Ed.), *Cognitive-behavioral therapy with children and adolescents* (pp. 169–216). New York: Guilford Press.

Stark, K. D., Sander, J., Hauser, M., Simpson, J., Schnoebelen, S., Glenn, R., et al. (2006). Depressive disorders during childhood and adolescence. In E. Mash & R. A. Barkley (Eds.), *Treatment of childhood disorders* (3rd ed., pp. 336–410). New York: Guilford Press.

Stark, K. D., Schnoebelen, S., Simpson, J., Hargrave, J., Glenn, R., & Molnar, J. (2007). *Children's workbook for ACTION.* Ardmore, PA: Workbook.

Stark, K. D., Simpson, J., Schnoebelen, S., Hargrave, J., Glenn, R., & Molnar, J. (2007). *Therapist's manual for ACTION.* Ardmore, PA: Workbook.

Stark, K. D., Simpson, J., Yancy, M., & Molnar, J. (2007). *Parent training manual for ACTION.* Ardmore, PA: Workbook.

Stark, K. D., Swearer, S., Kurowski, D., Sommer, D., & Bowen, B. (1996). Targeting the child and the family: A holistic approach to treating child and adolescent depressive disorders. In E. D. Hibbs & P. S. Jensen (Eds.), *Psychosocial treatments for child and adolescent disorders: Empirically based strategies for clinical practice* (pp. 207–238). Washington, DC: American Psychological Association.

Treatment for Adolescents with Depression Study Team. (2004). Fluoxetine, cognitive-behavioral therapy, and their combination for adolescents with depression. *Journal of the American Medical Association, 292*(7), 807–820.

Treatment for Adolescents with Depression Study Team. (2005). The Treatment for Adolescents with Depression Study (TADS): Demographic and clinical characteristics. *Journal of the American Academy of Child and Adolescent Psychiatry, 44*(1), 28–40.

Treatment for Adolescents with Depression Study Team. (2007). The Treatment for Adolescents with Depression Study (TADS): Long-term effectiveness and safety outcomes. *Archives of General Psychiatry, 64*(10), 1132–1144.

Walkup, J. T., Albano, A. M., Piacenti, J., Birmaher, B., Compton, S. N., Sherrill, J. T., et al. (2008). Cognitive behavioral therapy, sertraline or a combination in childhood anxiety. *New England Journal of Medicine.* Retrieved November 10, 2008, from *www. mejm.org.*

Weissman, A. S., Antinoro, D., & Chu, B. C. (2008). Cognitive-behavioral therapy for anxious youth in school settings: Advances and challenges. In M. J. Mayer, R. Van Acker, J. E. Lochman, & F. M. Gresham (Eds.), *Cognitive-behavioral interventions for emotional and behavioral disorders* (pp. 173–203). New York: Guilford Press.

Weissman, M., Fendrich, M., Warner, V., & Wickramaratne, P. (2002). Incidence of psychiatric disorder in offspring at high and low risk for depression. *Journal of the Academy of Child and Adolescent Psychiatry, 31*, 640–648.

Weisz, J. R., McCarty, C. A., & Valeri, S. M. (2006). Effects of psychotherapy for depression in children and adolescents: A meta-analysis. *Psychological Bulletin, 132*(1), 132–149.

Wright, J. H., Basco, M. R., & Thase, M. E. (2006). *Learning cognitive-behavior therapy: An illustrated guide.* Washington, DC: American Psychiatric Press.

Young, J. F., & Mufson, L. (2008). Interpersonal psychotherapy for treatment and prevention of adolescent depression. In J. R. Z. Abela & B. L. Hankin (Eds.), *Handbook of depression in children and adolescents* (pp. 288–306). New York: Guilford Press.

Chapter 27

Strategies for Working with
Severe Challenging and Violent Behavior

Lee Kern
Jaime L. Benson
Nathan H. Clemens

Severe behavior problems pose particular challenges for educators. Teachers view their primary responsibility as providing academic instruction. When students engage in problem behaviors, this interferes with the job teachers have been trained to carry out. Further, teachers and other school personnel generally feel ill prepared to adequately intervene with severe behavior problems (e.g., Elam & Rose, 1995; Fink & Janssen, 1993; Mastropieri & Scruggs, 2002). In the absence of effective strategies to ameliorate challenges when they emerge, the trajectory of accelerating behavior problems is likely to continue (e.g., Dunlap et al., 2006).

Equally concerning is the overreliance on punitive, negative, and even coercive strategies used in many, if not most, school settings (Gunter & Coutinho, 1997; Gunter, Jack, Shores, Carrell, & Flowers, 1993; Shores et al., 1993). Such disciplinary procedures are commonly invoked in the case of severe problem behaviors. This can be seen in teacher–student interactions, as well as in school and district policies. A clear example is exclusionary policies—such as zero tolerance and related practices of automatic suspension, expulsion, or removal to an interim or alternative setting—that shift responsibility without considering how

a student's needs can be best met. In fact, frequently these discipline policies result in loss of available instruction time and place students at an increased risk for dropout (Eckstrom, Goertz, Pollack, & Rock, 1986; Wehlage & Rutter, 1986). Expelling a student who lacks the skills to obtain a profitable job is not in the best interest of the student or society. Likewise, when a student is placed in an alternative setting, adults are completely unfamiliar with the student's behavioral and mental health needs, yet they are responsible for identifying necessary and effective supports. These routine practices, endorsed through legislation, fail to provide meaningful interventions and supports that can lead to long-term resolution of severe problem behaviors, and, in fact, they often exacerbate school behavior problems (Mayer & Butterworth, 1979).

In spite of the aforementioned barriers, intervention has advanced considerably in recent years. Current preventive and problem-solving models hold great promise for averting and diminishing even the most difficult problems. Schools nationwide are beginning to adopt systemic changes that involve approaching problem behaviors in a positive and preventive manner and through multi-tiered support (e.g., Horner, Sugai, Todd, &

Lewis-Palmer, 2005). The result should be added availability of resources and expertise for students with the greatest needs. As these exciting changes ensue, school psychologists are perfectly positioned to guide important advances. In the remainder of this chapter, we describe how to design supports that successfully address intensive behavioral challenges. We begin with an overview of the nature of violent behaviors. We then describe key features of effective intervention, followed by essential support components. Finally, we discuss the importance of evaluating progress and outcomes.

The Complicated Nature of Severe Behaviors

Many problem behaviors, although distracting or disruptive to the environment, are not considered serious. Janney and Snell (2000) offer a useful heuristic system of prioritizing behavior problems. Behaviors that are *distracting* deviate from expected norms (e.g., inappropriate interactions, hand flapping) but do not substantially interfere with learning or typical activities. Distracting behaviors should be considered the lowest intervention priority. *Disruptive* behaviors (e.g., refusing to complete assignments, yelling), the next priority for intervention, do not pose immediate danger to the student or others but interfere with learning and the environment. Finally, *destructive* behaviors are harmful or threaten the safety of the student or others (e.g., aggression, property destruction, bringing weapons to school, self-harm), and are the first priority for intervention. Severe behavior problems fall within the latter category. Such behavior problems are complex for a number of reasons. First, they take many forms. For instance, overt behaviors may be seen in the form of aggression or property destruction. As the term implies, generally such behaviors are easily observed. Other times severe problem behaviors are covert in that they cannot be readily observed because of environmental context or timing of their occurrence. Behaviors such as vandalism, harassment, theft, self-injury, and substance abuse often occur in private circumstances. The use of a problem-solving approach to intervention requires understanding the environmental events that trigger, exacerbate, or reinforce problem behaviors. In the case of covert behaviors, associated events may never be observed. Thus they require a different approach to assessment and intervention development. Alternative assessment procedures may include analogue assessment, self-monitoring, self-report, and informant report (Skinner, Rhymer, & McDaniel, 2000). Also, intervention efforts may rely on additional community resources and collaboration among atypical intervention personnel, such as bus assistants and cafeteria workers, who may observe students in situations outside of the classroom.

In addition to diverse forms, the frequency of severe problem behaviors also adds to the complexity of assessment and intervention. Unlike more common behaviors, such as being off task, calling out, or disrupting instruction, that tend to occur regularly, severe problems often happen at relatively low frequencies. An adolescent may steal property a few times a year or engage in a fistfight every few months. As with covert behaviors, intervention becomes more difficult with low-frequency behavior, because it is not easy to determine the relationship between the behavior and events in the environment. Specifically, because few samples of the behavior are available, it is difficult to identify patterns of associated antecedent and subsequent events.

Another matter has to do with the resources required to resolve intensive behavior challenges. Generally, severe behaviors do not rapidly emerge but rather begin in a mild form and intensify over time (Dunlap et al., 2006). Given the history of such behavior problems, intervention must be accordingly intensive. Also, severe behavior problems typically result from a confluence of factors, among the most common being ineffective parenting practices, marginal life quality, poor academic achievement, and deficient communication skills. Hence, successful support must target the multiple domains that contribute to problem behavior. This means that comprehensive intervention efforts require collaboration and communication across systems of care, an enterprise that takes time and planning. Mental health providers, including school psychologists, seldom arrange for the resources that intensive intervention requires in the way of time, staff, and expertise.

A final problem is that the very intense nature of severe problem behaviors provokes reactions from others that may inadvertently contribute to maintaining the behaviors. For instance, in response to bullying or intimidation, peers may give in to an aggressive student's demands. Similarly, coercive cycles of interaction may occur in which a parent or other adult capitulates to the repeated inappropriate behaviors of a child, thereby reinforcing the problem behavior (e.g., Patterson, 1982; Patterson, Reid, & Dishion, 1992). In the classroom, teachers also may avoid situations that incite problems, such as requiring that a student complete an assignment he or she finds difficult. Over time, these somewhat natural reactions exacerbate the problems in that the child does not learn socially appropriate ways to negotiate the environment or deal productively with others (e.g., Walker, Colvin, & Ramsey, 1995). Further, the compromised environments that are often arranged, as in the case of classroom situations absent of demands, create students who lack the academic skills needed for later success.

General Features of Intervention for Intensive Behavior Problems

Decades of research have resulted in a better understanding of how to most effectively reduce behavior problems. We have learned a great deal from both intervention successes and failures. Based on research conducted, it appears that there are several essential components of interventions that are successful over the long term. One important feature is that the intervention must be *individualized*. In recent years, many schools, districts, and even entire states have adopted a multitiered preventive approach to discipline, known as schoolwide positive behavior support. As noted by Ervin, Gimpel Peacock, and Merrell, Chapter 1, and Hawkins, Barnett, Morrison, and Musti-Rao, Chapter 2, this volume, the primary tier of intervention occurs at the schoolwide level and is applied with all students. The majority of a school's student body, roughly 80%, will be responsive to the preventive strategies introduced at this level.

Students who continue to evidence behavior problems (about 15%) receive secondary interventions. At this level, interventions target small groups of students or specific problematic school settings. Examples of secondary interventions include small-group social skills instruction, academic skill practice, or a cafeteria incentive system to decrease noise.

When students are nonresponsive to both primary and secondary efforts, tertiary interventions are necessary. In addition, students with serious behavior problems (e.g., violent behavior, self-injury) require tertiary interventions immediately, regardless of whether less intensive interventions have been used. This level of intervention is individualized and tailored to address a student's specific deficits and capitalize on his or her strengths. Such interventions typically include preventive strategies (e.g., reduced number of required academic problems, periodic breaks), alternative skill and response instruction (e.g., prompt card reminding the student to request a break, academic skill instruction), and response strategies (e.g., calling home, losing points for aggression).

Another critical feature of tertiary-level intervention is that it must be *assessment-based*. That is, intervention should be derived from a functional behavioral assessment (FBA), as described by Jones and Wickstrom in Chapter 12 of this volume. An FBA yields several types of information important for intervention development (e.g., Bambara & Kern, 2005). First, it isolates immediate environmental variables associated with problem behavior. Events that precede problem behavior and those that follow it can be identified and later modified. For example, aggression or fighting might be preceded by teasing from peers, or self-injurious behavior may be followed by removal of a difficult task. Based on this important assessment information, intervention can be designed that is specific and efficient. Second, an FBA identifies skill deficits that need remediation. This may include social skills, academic skills, or self-control. Third, an FBA should include measures that examine overall life quality (e.g., Sacks & Kern, 2008). There are many qualities that make a life worth living, such as satisfaction with relationships, regular access to enjoyable activities, and self-determination. Inadequate life quality can contribute to the emergence and maintenance of severe problem behaviors.

The importance of an FBA for intervention development was illustrated in several recent studies that compared functional assessment-based interventions with non-assessment-based interventions. Newcomer and Lewis (2004) and Ingram, Lewis-Palmer, and Sugai (2005) conducted FBAs for problem behaviors and developed related interventions matched to the identified function. The effectiveness of those interventions was compared with that of interventions matched to an alternative function. The results showed that function-based interventions were superior to nonfunction-based interventions.

In addition to identifying the environmental factors that may make the problem behavior more likely, assessment of severe challenging behavior can identify precursor behaviors that precede the severe challenging behavior. These precursor behaviors may be less intense, but they can be extremely useful because they often occur at a higher frequency than severe behaviors. For example, although aggression may happen infrequently, peer problems, which routinely lead to aggression, may occur much more often. Focusing on precursors in this way makes it easier to identify the correlates of severe problems. In addition, precursors can indicate when the severe problem may occur or intensify. When staff members are aware of the precursor behaviors and can identify them readily, measures or interventions can be put into place to defuse a situation or prevent further escalation of the problem behavior.

Interventions for serious behavior problems also must be implemented *long term*. All too often practitioners look for a quick fix, considering interventions ineffective if they are not met with rapid decreases in problem behaviors. This is not surprising in light of the personal and environmental damage that severe problems usually cause. At the same time, it is important to keep in mind that serious behavior problems usually have evolved from minor problems and presumably have been subject to long histories of reinforcement. Over time, the student has learned that a particular form of behavior effectively obtains something very desirable or avoids something very undesirable. Hence, it is unreasonable to expect this history to be rapidly unlearned. New ways of communicating and dealing with disappointments must be shaped and practiced, which can take a considerable amount of time. Also, the course of skill development and quality-of-life improvements may be relatively slow. In all, emerging evidence suggests that supports usually need to be in place over long periods of time, along with appropriate adjustments to accommodate new environments, such as classroom changes across academic school years (e.g., Kern, Gallagher, Starosta, Hickman, & George, 2006).

Serious behavior problems also require *multicomponent* interventions. An abundance of research has clearly shown that the popular approach of simply responding to behavior, typically with punishment (e.g., suspension), has only short-lived effects (e.g., Mayer & Butterworth, 1979; Mayer, Butterworth, Nafpaktitis, & Sulzer-Azaroff, 1983). Rather, interventions that lead to long-term resolution of behavior problems must be multicomponent and must include strategies that prevent the likelihood of problems occurring, teach communication and other skill deficits, identify ways to respond to problems that will not be reinforcing, and consider lifestyle issues. Multicomponent interventions are described in added detail later in the chapter.

A final feature of effective intervention is that it should be implemented *across settings*. This is important for several reasons. First, when problem behaviors are allowed to occur in one setting (e.g., math class) but not another (e.g., English class), they often become more durable. For instance, if Oberto's math teacher allows him to play games on the computer to avoid his tantrums during math seatwork but his English teacher requires him to complete his assignments, problem behaviors are more likely to persist. More specifically, because it is not altogether clear when his problem behavior may get him what he wants (e.g., escape difficult work), Oberto will continue to test new situations.

A second reason that cross-setting implementation is important is that intervention is most effective when all variables contributing to problem behavior are addressed or eliminated. For example, Jenna engages in minor problem behavior whenever she is required to complete vocational activities. With intervention, including choice of activity sequence coupled with high rates of praise and the requirement of task completion, behavior problems are infrequent. Still, severe behavior problems, in the form of aggression and self-injury, occur any time she has not slept well the prior night. This happens when her parents do not see that she goes to bed at her usual time and she stays up late into the night watching television. Thus, until intervention is in place at home, as well as at school, her problem behaviors will not be fully addressed.

A third reason for intervention implementation across settings is that intervention components can be designed such that they complement one another. This cross-setting effort was successfully implemented with Tessa, a middle school student with internalizing problems. Tessa experienced extreme anxiety, often associated with self-injury (picking at her skin, causing bleeding and tissue damage), related to a fear of "looking stupid," as she put it, when called on in class. In her desire to avoid such situations, she began skipping classes in which she might be asked questions and hiding in the bathroom or school library. When the source of the problem was identified, an intervention package was developed that included an intensive reading intervention implemented daily at school to improve her oral reading fluency. In addition, each of Tessa's teachers provided her with a list of questions that she might be asked the following school day. Every night her mother worked with her to locate and practice responses to the questions. This combination of academic remediation and prepractice interventions, implemented at home and school, was sufficient to improve her class attendance and keep her engaged in academic activities in the same manner as her classmates.

Assessment of Severe Behavior Problems

Effective intervention begins with an assessment of behavior. In order to address the problem behavior most effectively, the assessment of severe challenging and violent behavior should be framed from an FBA methodology. Elements of an effective FBA have been described in several excellent sources (Jones & Wickstrom, Chapter 12, this volume; Kern, O'Neill, & Starosta,

2005; O'Neill et al., 1997) and are not detailed here. As discussed earlier, however, behavior that is severe and violent presents several unique challenges to assessment. During assessment, educators must consider new and different methods to gather data on the occurrence of the behavior and the variables surrounding it, particularly when the behavior occurs at very low rates or is typically displayed covertly. In the following sections, we describe considerations and adaptations that may need to be made when conducting an FBA for behaviors that are severe and violent.

Data Collection

The first consideration when assessing severe challenging and violent behavior is data collection methodology, particularly when the behavior occurs at low rates. In some cases, assessment may need to take place on a single occurrence of the behavior, such as weapon violations. Therefore, when an episode occurs, it is important to gather as much pertinent information as possible. Systematic record keeping of each instance of the problem behavior using a structured framework to gather information on several key variables is critical. An example of a data collection form is displayed in Figure 27.1. This form is not unlike those used in typical FBA procedures (e.g., Kern et al., 2005; O'Neill et al., 1997), but it includes important variations when considering severe challenging and violent behavior. First, the data collection system should allow the recording of the date, time, and location in which the behavior took place. Recording the location in which the problem behavior occurred, such as the school bus, hallway, cafeteria, or classroom, will provide important information regarding the settings or situations in which the behavior is more likely to occur. Also, noting behaviors the student displayed just prior to the severe challenging behavior, or precursor behaviors, allows staff to gather information on behaviors that can serve as warning signals that the student's behavior may escalate in severity. These precursor behaviors may be less intense forms of the severe challenging behavior or may be behaviors that the student exhibits when frustrated, uncomfortable, or stressed.

Date	Time	Location/Class Period	Antecedents: What happened just before?	Precursor Behaviors	Target Behavior	Immediate Staff Response	Disciplinary Action?
	Start: ____ End: ____	☐ Bus ☐ Arrival ☐ Homeroom ☐ Gym ☐ Reading ☐ Math ☐ Science ☐ Art ☐ Music ☐ Lunch ☐ Hallway ☐ Other _____	☐ Given command/direction ☐ Given academic task ☐ Peer conflict ☐ Alone/low attention ☐ Denied access to preferred object/activity ☐ Other _____	☐ Off task ☐ Crying ☐ Verbal threats ☐ Obscene gestures ☐ Other	Describe: _____ _____ _____ _____ _____ _____ _____	☐ Staff ignored ☐ Redirection ☐ Verbal reprimand ☐ Talked to student about behavior ☐ Time out ☐ Called parent ☐ Other:	☐ Detention ☐ Suspension (days: ___) ☐ Other: _____

FIGURE 27.1. Sample form for gathering data on severe problem behaviors.

An effective and thorough data collection system serves several purposes. First, it will aid in the assessment of the behavior toward the development of an effective intervention plan. In the case of low-frequency behavior, data collected across several incidents of behavior can be examined collectively to identify commonalities. For example, an antecedent–behavior–consequence (ABC) form could be used in which columns provide space to describe all of the events prior to the occurrence of behavior (e.g., setting, activity, students and teachers present, immediate precursor to behavior), a description of the topography of the behavior, and responses to the behavior. A well-designed data collection system also can serve as a means to collect ongoing information on the frequency or intensity of the behavior over time. This information can then be used to determine whether intervention strategies are successful in decreasing the occurrence of the behavior.

Interviews

When direct observational data on behavior cannot be collected, a greater emphasis may be placed on behavioral interviews, particularly interviews with students, provided they have the cognitive ability and insight to provide meaningful information. Structured interviews using an FBA approach are available, such as the Student-Assisted Functional Assessment Interview (Kern, Dunlap, Clarke, & Childs, 1994) and the Student-Completed Functional Assessment Interview (O'Neill et al., 1997). When using interviews in the assessment of severe behavior, certain factors may hold increased relevance. For some students and some forms of challenging behavior, stressful life events may act as setting events for severe challenging behavior. Life events such as parental divorce, moving to a new school, or parental substance abuse may cause emotional stress to the student and may increase the likelihood that a student will display severe challenging behavior in certain situations. On other occasions students may demonstrate a poor ability to cope appropriately with difficult situations or circumstances, such as the breakup of a relationship, completion of a long-term project, or family death. Thus it is important to ascertain from all interviewees

(including the student) whether there are significant life situations that are contributing to the student's difficulty.

Student interviews also may attempt to address mood, anxiety, and emotional states that may affect the occurrence or nonoccurrence of severe challenging behavior. Carr, McLaughlin, Giacobbe-Grieco, and Smith (2003) demonstrated that situations in which individuals with developmental disabilities rated themselves as being in a "bad mood" were highly associated with the incidence of severe problem behavior. Merrell (2001) described several methods for evaluating mood or emotional states associated with certain situations. One such method involves presenting the student with a series of incomplete statements, such as "I feel happy when ... " or "I get ___ when..." and asking the student to complete each statement with real examples from his or her life. The "emotional thermometer" is another exercise described by Merrell to help identify levels of emotionality in given situations. In this exercise, the practitioner presents a visual representation of a thermometer that includes various gradations such as *low*, *medium*, or *high* (smaller increments may be used for older students). The practitioner then asks the student to identify situations in which he or she experienced certain emotions (e.g., sadness, fear, anger) and indicate the level of intensity of the emotion experienced in that situation on the thermometer. These data collection methods may help to identify situations in which a student is likely to experience an elevated state of anxiety or frustration, information that can be used for intervention development.

In addition to evaluating variables such as mood or anxiety, interviewers may attempt to evaluate the presence of a hostile attribution bias. A hostile attribution bias is the tendency for an individual to infer negative intent from an ambiguous situation. Children who exhibit aggressive behaviors often show a greater tendency toward this pattern (Dodge, 1985). For example, Gerald was bumped in the hallway by another student. Immediately, Gerald assumed the student was trying to start a fight with him and turned around and tried to punch him. In actuality, the bump was merely an accident. During an interview, the interviewer may present several scenarios to the student containing both hypothetical and actual events to gauge his or her reactions. In the case of frequent hostile attributions, intervention may include cognitive-behavioral strategies to help the student accurately evaluate situations and interactions (see, e.g., Bushman & Gimpel Peacock, Chapter 25, this volume; Merrell, 2001).

Several considerations are important when conducting student interviews. First, level of functioning must be considered, as interviews may not be useful with students who have very low cognitive functioning. Second, given the extreme nature of some forms of severe challenging behavior, such as fighting, drug use, and vandalism, students may be particularly sensitive to discussing behaviors for fear that acknowledgement of such behaviors may lead to the involvement of the police or other authorities. In these cases, information shared by the student may not be reliable. It is important for the individual completing the assessment to spend time building rapport with the student in order to create a trusting and comfortable relationship. This also will help reduce the likelihood of problem behaviors during the interview. Students must be assured that the purpose of the interview is to help develop supports to make their lives better. If problem behaviors begin to occur, it is best to complete the interview at a later time. Third, individuals completing interviews should be aware of their responsibilities as mandatory reporters of any information students share that suggests that they may harm themselves or others. When a student provides information suggesting that he or she is in danger of hurting him- or herself or others, follow-up questions should be aimed at assessing the risk (i.e., seriousness and legitimacy of the threat). Specifically, these questions should assess the student's access to weapons or other materials for carrying out the threat, whether the student has a plan for carrying it out, and what other students or adults might be at risk or involved. See Figure 27.2 for some sample interview questions for assessing potential crisis situations. Reporting of such information to the appropriate authorities takes precedence over professional guidelines to protect confidentiality (National Association of School Psychologists, 2000). State guidelines should be consulted pertaining to mandatory reporting of information.

- Have you ever felt that life was not worth living?
- Have things ever reached the point at which you've thought of harming yourself?
- When did you first begin to have such thoughts?
- Describe things or events that led up to these thoughts.
- How often have you had those thoughts (including frequency, obsessional quality, controllability)?
- How close have you come to acting on those thoughts?
- How likely do you think it is that you will act on them in the future?
- Do you have a plan? Do you have access to the means necessary to carry out that plan?
- What things would make it more (or less) likely that you would try to hurt yourself and/or others?
- Are there others whom you think may be responsible for what you're experiencing (e.g., persecutory ideas, passivity experiences)?
- Are you having any thoughts of harming them?

FIGURE 27.2. Sample student interview questions for assessing potential crisis situations. For an extended list of questions, refer to American Psychiatric Association Practice Guidelines (American Psychiatric Association, 2003).

Record Reviews

Review of student records can provide important information in assessing severe challenging and violent behavior. School records may contain reports of prior instances of similar behavior, the situations or circumstances in which they occurred, and how others responded, thus providing information on setting events, antecedents, or consequences that may trigger or maintain the behavior. School records also may contain information pertaining to academic achievement, underlying disorders or diagnoses, or medications that might play a role in the occurrence of the severe challenging or violent behavior. A structured format can be used to facilitate record reviews, such as the School Archival Record Search (Walker, Block-Pedego, Todis, & Severson, 1991).

Evaluation of Communication Strategies

The notion that problem behaviors may serve a communicative function has a great deal of empirical support (Carr & Durand, 1985). Some students, particularly those without verbal language, may lack ways to communicate their needs and desires. In these instances, severe challenging or violent behavior, such as aggression or self-injury, may have been learned in order to obtain access to reinforcement or escape from aversive situations. For higher functioning students, severe problem behavior also can be viewed as serving a communicative function because its extremity makes it difficult for adults to ignored and is likely to produce some type of environmental response (e.g., obtaining adult or peer attention). Therefore, the assessment of severe challenging and violent behavior should include an evaluation of the student's skills in communicating needs and wants. Self-report can be used for higher functioning students, but for lower functioning and younger students, it is important to ask questions of the student's parents and teachers regarding the availability of modes of communication.

Evaluating Community Variables

Consideration of severe challenging and violent behavior within a broader context includes bearing in mind the community in which a student lives. Community variables, such as institutionalized poverty, gang and drug activity, or lack of activities or resources to positively engage young people, may not be a direct cause of severe challenging or violent behavior, but such variables create an environment with increased levels of stress. In such environments, severe and violent behavior may be considered more acceptable or even functional. If this is suspected, assessment information should ascertain who the student is associating with and the activities in which they engage. When asked directly, students often are forthright about disclosing drug use and other illegal activities, particularly when they understand that the purpose of obtaining information is to identify supports to improve their quality of life.

Considering Underlying Disorders

The evaluation of severe challenging and violent behaviors also should consider disorders or psychiatric diagnoses the student may have (e.g., Ervin et al., 2000). For instance, attention-deficit/hyperactivity disorder (ADHD) is associated with impulsiv-

ity and behavioral disinhibition (Barkley, 2006). Students with a history of ADHD commonly display difficulty in regulating their emotions, may be easily frustrated, and are prone to display more aggressive behavior than their peers without ADHD (DuPaul & Stoner, 2003). Evidence of an ADHD diagnosis carries implications for intervention to prevent severe challenging and violent behavior by ensuring that ADHD symptoms are appropriately managed through behavioral and/or pharmaceutical interventions. Disorders such as depression, oppositional defiant disorder, and conduct disorder present similar challenges. Evidence-based interventions specific to many of these underlying disorders are available and should be included among other supports for students (e.g., Hilt-Panahon, Kern, & Divatia, 2007).

Essential Intervention Components

Prevention

Perhaps the most important aspect of any behavior plan is the development of strategies to prevent problem behaviors. In the case of severe behaviors, prevention strategies are most critical given the intensity and potential danger of the behaviors. In order to prevent serious behavior problems in schools, efforts generally have to focus beyond the school environment. Collaboration among the school, parents, community systems (e.g., mental health, juvenile justice), and local organizations will make supports most effective. For example, intervention may include connecting a student with an after-school club or mentoring program, such as Big Brothers and Big Sisters. Given that severe behaviors are likely to occur in unsupervised settings, community supports may help provide additional supervision and positive activities in which the student can be engaged outside of the school.

On a more molecular level, because a major objective of an FBA is to identify functions of behavior, emergent information should be relied on to develop specific strategies to prevent behavior occurrence. For example, if the assessment revealed that the function of the student's severe problem behavior is to escape a task the student finds aversive, the intervention may include a number of strategies, such as modifying the task to incorporate preferred elements or offering choices of different ways to complete the task (e.g., on the computer, with a peer). Similarly, if the FBA indicates that drug use occurs primarily after school to escape boredom and obtain peer acceptance, preventive intervention may involve increasing adult supervision and scheduling preferred after-school activities and events.

Teaching Alternative Behaviors

Given that students with challenging behavior may lack the skills necessary to influence people in their environment in socially appropriate ways, teaching alternative behaviors and skills is an essential component to any intervention. Alternative behaviors may include academic skills, communication strategies, replacement behaviors, and self-control skills. These alternative behaviors help students learn to cope with difficult situations in order to become more independent and socially appropriate. For example, Becca, a middle school student, had extreme difficulties getting along with her peers and was suspended several times for physical altercations. Assessment data collected during lunch and transitions between classes indicated that Becca almost always initiated peer problems through name calling or false accusations. For instance, if she falsely believed that peers were talking about her in the hallway, she would yell at them, calling them condescending names. After documenting several specific types of situations that led to an inappropriate interaction by Becca, a peer of her choice was solicited to role-play alternative responses. Specifically, each situation was described, and Becca and the peer generated and role-played appropriate responses (e.g., ignoring the peers, approaching the peers and asking if they had a question). In addition, Becca was taught to self-monitor her use of appropriate interactions. This intervention resulted in significant reductions in peer problems and suspension, as well as increases in alternative behaviors.

Academic Skill Instruction

Children and adolescents with challenging behavior often have associated academic skill deficits. In fact, research has shown that children identified as having emotional and behavioral disorders (EBD) have the poorest academic outcomes of any disability group, including those with deficits in core academic areas (Kauffman, 2001; Wagner, Kutash, Duchnowski, Epstein, & Sumi, 2005). Intervention to remediate academic deficits is essential because problem behaviors frequently covary with academic skills problems. Further, the inclusion of instructional accommodations for children with severe behavioral disorders may result in improvements in both academics and classroom behavior (Penno, Frank, & Wacker, 2000). Once the associated skill deficits are resolved, problem behaviors may be irrelevant. For example, during writing class, Victor pinches his peers and makes disruptive noises when he is given an independent writing activity. An FBA indicated that behavior problems occur because he is unable to develop a response to a story starter. Instruction that provides Victor with strategies for generating ideas for stories gives him the skills to complete the task. Thus he no longer needs to engage in the problem behavior when confronted with this once difficult academic activity. Victor might also be taught other adaptive skills, such as methods for requesting help when he encounters difficulties with a task.

Assuring a good instructional match is an important approach to promote learning for any student, and particularly so for students with severe and challenging behaviors. Students should be taught at an appropriate level so that they are sufficiently challenged yet can succeed with a high level of accuracy. Mismatches between academic assignments and skill level are a frequent trigger for student misbehavior (Center, Deitz, & Kaufman, 1982; Gettinger & Seibert, 2002). The provision of assignments at students' appropriate instructional levels is an important strategy to promote appropriate behavior in the classroom.

Communication Strategies

Because challenging behavior generally serves as a method for conveying a message, communication on the part of the student, as well as the teacher, is another important aspect of intervention for students with severe and challenging behaviors. Without appropriate and effective means of communication, challenging behavior is likely to occur. Therefore, once the purpose of behavior is identified through an FBA, the results can help determine the focus of communication efforts. That is, assessment information is crucial in identifying specific areas in which communication needs to be improved. In particular, students must be taught replacement skills that achieve the same outcome as the problem behavior. For example, students who have academic skill deficits may not understand that asking for help is an adaptive skill when they encounter a difficult assignment. Instead of raising their hands, they may begin to exhibit off-task or disruptive behaviors that interfere with the teacher's or peers' activities. In order to encourage students to ask for help in the classroom, the teacher may develop an unobtrusive signal for the student. For example, the student could have a hand signal or card that she or he puts on her or his desk in order to indicate to the teacher that she or he is struggling with an assignment, without drawing undue attention to her- or himself. The student should learn how, when, and where to use the intervention and should also have sufficient opportunities to practice its use in the classroom.

Also important is that the teacher and others respond regularly to the student's appropriate communicative attempts. In order for the communication strategy to replace problem behavior, it must be as effective and efficient in producing the desired response as the disruptive behavior. Five criteria have been identified as important factors to consider for response effectiveness and efficiency: (1) the amount of effort the response requires, (2) the quality of the outcome, (3) the immediacy of the outcome, (4) the consistency of the outcome, and (5) the probability of punishment (Halle, Bambara, & Reichle, 2005). For example, if Jodi hits her peers in order to obtain their attention, then she must have another way to obtain that attention from her peers that is as easy as hitting and produces the same level of peer attention just as quickly. If a behavior serves multiple functions for a child, then replacement skills must be taught for each function. For example, if John kicks over his desk both to escape an assignment and to receive attention from his peers, then he

must be taught skills to replace both of these functions.

Self-Management

Self-management strategies are designed to help students change their own behavior and are an effective way to teach self-control during challenging situations (Shapiro & Cole, 1994). Self-management has been shown to increase appropriate behaviors, decrease disruptive behaviors, and enhance students' independence and self-reliance (Shapiro & Cole, 1994). Students may be taught to use goal setting, self-monitoring, and self-evaluation, either alone or in combination with each other, to manage problem behaviors, replacement skills, or adaptive behaviors (Halle et al., 2005). For example, Leon frequently arrived at school late because he stayed up at night watching movies and was too tired to get up when his alarm sounded. Leon was provided with a self-monitoring program to record what time he went to bed and whether he arrived at school on time. Working together with his mother, he also set goals for going to bed early and arriving to school on time, for which he earned rewards when achieved, such as movie passes to use on the weekend.

Social problem solving is another self-management strategy that attempts to develop "thinking" skills in students in order to remediate problem behavior (Shapiro & Cole, 1994). This procedure typically involves teaching a standardized way of dealing with problems by identifying the problem, generating potential solutions, considering the consequences of each solution, then choosing the best alternative solution (Halle et al., 2005). For example, Debra frequently punched classmates and destroyed property in the lunch room and hallways in response to teasing. After learning a social-problem-solving technique, Debra identified the problem as teasing and listed the potential solutions of informing a teacher, enlisting the support of a friend, walking into the nearest classroom, or confronting the peer. After determining the potential consequences to each of these actions, Debra decided that she would enter the nearest classroom and report the teasing to a teacher (Halle et al., 2005). When learning social-problem-solving techniques, students should be provided with explicit instructions, effective models, opportunities for role playing with feedback, and occasions to practice in multiple settings (Shapiro & Cole, 1994).

Self-management strategies also can be applied with internalizing problems, such as depression, anxiety, and negative mood. For example, students may monitor their moods across the day or within specific situations that pose increased challenges. When students identify heightened levels of mood during specific situations, they can be taught strategies to deescalate, seek help, or appropriately remove themselves from the situation. Recording internal states in this manner also can increase teachers' awareness of a student's current state so that they may intervene to prevent escalation of behavior. For example, Carl, an 8-year-old, experienced extreme anxiety that led to encopresis and frequent self-reports of feeling physically ill while at school (Divatia & Kern, 2007). Using an emotional thermometer, Carl was taught to evaluate and rate the level of anxiety he felt on a 1–10 scale when engaged in a variety of activities and events. His upcoming transition to a new school was one event associated with extremely high rates of anxiety. As a result, interventions were developed to decrease the aversiveness of this transition, such as touring the school prior to the transition, meeting with his new teacher, and exposing him to routines in his new classroom. Data collected after these activities and then subsequent to the transition indicted substantially reduced feelings of anxiety, as self-reported using the feeling thermometer.

Responding to Challenging Behaviors

Having antecedent strategies and teaching alternative skills are important intervention components for addressing challenging behavior. However, given the intense nature of the severe problems and the extensive learning histories that have shaped these behaviors, even with powerful antecedent interventions and intensive skill instruction, problem behaviors are still likely to occur on occasion. Thus it is also important to formulate a plan for responding to the challenging behavior.

When developing responses, an important consideration is to avoid reinforcing the behavior. It is not uncommon for educators to attempt to persuade a student to act appropriately through prompting or bargaining when they are confronted with severe behaviors. However, these responses provide attention to the student, which can inadvertently serve to maintain the student's disruptive behaviors. On the other hand, teachers' attempts to ignore problem behavior may also be ineffective if the students' behaviors produce desirable responses in the form of peer attention or escape from work. In addition to considering the function of the behavior, the response also should take into account the likelihood of escalation and any long-term implications (Kern, 2005). For example, Andrew frequently engaged in extremely disruptive classroom behaviors, including running around the classroom and jumping on the tables. His teacher was in the habit of containing him by using physical restraint. An FBA, however, found that the function of Andrew's behavior was to gain peer attention, and all eyes were on him during physical restraint. Instead, his teacher decided to clear the room, requesting classmates to move to an adjacent classroom. In the absence of peer attention, Andrew's problems quickly decreased, and restraint was not needed.

Intervention also can be planned just after precursors to challenging behavior. When teachers can effectively identify behaviors that occur early in an escalation cycle, problems are more easily deescalated, and crises often can be prevented (Kern, 2005). For example, when Kevin was presented with a difficult math activity, he refused to complete his work. He then cursed at the teacher and began teasing other students in the classroom. This behavior escalated to hopping from chair to chair around the classroom, verbally threatening the teacher, and physically assaulting peers. Thus a plan was put into place to intervene as soon as Kevin refused to begin an assignment. His teacher allowed him to work with a peer, use a calculator, or alternate easy and difficult problems.

Severe problem behaviors frequently pose crisis situations in which the individual or others are at risk of harm or in which severe property damage is foreseeable. In these cases, it is imperative that staff have a crisis plan in place in order to ensure the safety of the student, others, and the environment. It is important that crisis plans not be thought of as intervention to decrease severe problem behavior. Rather, the purpose of crisis plan is to ensure safety and protection. All key individuals should be involved in the development and approval of a crisis plan, including parents, teachers, other school staff, and, when appropriate, the student.

A crisis plan should clearly define the specific form and intensity of problem behavior that would initiate its use and delineate the specific actions staff members are to take (Kern, 2005). Effective deescalation strategies, such as using a calm, even tone, providing limited choices, utilizing active listening, avoiding coercion, and refraining from asking repeated questions or making demands should be included in the plan when precursors are observed (Walker & Walker, 1991). In addition, the plan should delineate actions to keep the environment and those present safe. An excellent discussion on crisis plan development is provided by Rock (2000). See Figure 27.3 for a sample crisis management plan.

A final caution about crisis plans pertains to restraint. Staff should carefully consider the role of physical restraint in a crisis plan. Far too often physical restraint is used as a first method of response when problem behavior occurs. There is no research demonstrating that physical restraint is effective for reducing problem behavior, and in some cases it can escalate problems and have lasting side effects (George, 2000; Ryan & Peterson, 2004). Restraint should be avoided whenever possible. Most school districts have policies that require use of the least restrictive behavioral interventions to address problem behaviors. These procedures should be carefully followed to ensure that student rights are protected and that minimally intrusive interventions are used. In unusual circumstances in which restrictive procedures must be used to prevent the student him- or herself or others from bodily harm, school committees that monitor their use (e.g., a Least Restrictive Behavior Intervention Committee) should approve the specific type of procedure and the circumstances under which it will be used. Further, if physical intervention is proposed, staff members must be fully trained and certified to use the

---

Crisis Management Plan

Student: Alina **Date:** March 17, 2008

Reason for plan: To avoid escalation of problem behavior. To keep Alina and others safe when she becomes aggressive/destructive.

Signs of escalation: Screaming, pacing around the classroom

Deescalation strategies: Stay calm and quietly ask Alina if she want to take a break in the back of the classroom until she cools down. Repeat this every 2–3 minutes.

Who will implement the plan: Mrs. Romano (classroom teacher), Mr. Levitt (classroom aide), Ms. McDermitt (school psychologist)

Crisis procedures:

1. If Alina begins to engage in aggression or destruction, stay between her and other students. Remove any materials that she could throw or destroy. Provide Alina with clear choices along with their consequences. Page Ms. McDermitt for assistance.
2. Instruct Alina that she needs to go to the counselor's office immediately. If she does not go, continue to provide this prompt once every minute while blocking any attempts at aggression or property destruction.
3. Two staff members should accompany her to the counselor's office, one on each side. Do not leave her by herself.
4. Ignore disruptive behaviors but block attempts to destroy property or endanger herself or others. Praise any attempts to self-soothe (e.g. "Alina, I like how you are sitting quietly"). Avoid other interactions until she appears to be calming down.
5. Once Alina has calmed down, as evidenced by speaking in a calm voice, lack of physical agitation (e.g. crying), and reporting that she is ready to return to the classroom, the counselor will complete a problem-solving sequence with her. Staff will then escort her back to the classroom. If she has not calmed down, repeat Step 4.

FIGURE 27.3. Sample crisis management plan.

strategies in a safe manner. Finally, parents should fully agree to the procedure and the situations for its use and should be informed whenever it has been used.

Evaluating Intervention Outcomes

Once a behavior intervention plan has been implemented, it is essential to determine whether it is effective. A system of ongoing data collection should be developed to measure student progress. Evaluating student progress requires measurement of the behavior both pre- and postintervention. Because direct observation may not be possible, a variety of alternative methods can be used, such as tracking student points, recording the frequency of critical incidents across time, or graphing self-monitoring data. When evaluating outcome data, it is important to keep in mind that severe behavior problems usually are not quickly resolved. Thus one should attempt to detect reductions in behavior problems, rather than their elimination. In the case of severe behavior problems, behavior change should be considered across multiple years to assure long-term resolution (e.g., Kern et al., 2006).

An important element in the evaluation of outcomes is the ongoing assessment of intervention integrity. If an intervention is not implemented consistently and according to the prescribed procedures, then student behavior problems may not decrease. Lapses in intervention integrity sometimes suggest that an intervention needs to be modified to accommodate a teacher's stylistic preference, to improve the contextual fit, and to enhance acceptability of the intervention. It may also be the case that additional training or reminders are necessary to assist in implementation. One should review intervention integrity data on a regular basis to determine whether modifications to the intervention would be beneficial.

Summary

Students who engage in severe and violent behavior problems require immediate, comprehensive, and intensive support. Fortunately, intervention has evolved considerably in recent years, and systemic changes, such as tiered support, hold promise for allocating the necessary resources to those students with the most intensive needs. Successful intervention requires a multicomponent approach that includes prevention, skill instruction, and carefully planned responses. Further, support must be implemented across settings and include multiple agents and care providers, most important educators and family members. There is an urgent need to deliver intensive, effective, and evidence-based interventions to students with serious problems. Without intervention, the cost of significant behavior problems to society is a tremendous.

References

American Psychiatric Association. (2003). *Practice guideline for the assessment and treatment of patients with suicidal behaviors.* Arlington, VA: American Psychiatric Association.

Bambara, L. M. & Kern, L. (2005). *Individualized supports for students with problem behaviors: Designing positive behavior plans.* New York: Guilford Press.

Barkley, R. A. (2006). *Attention-deficit hyperactivity disorder: A handbook for diagnosis and treatment* (3rd ed.). New York: Guilford Press.

Carr, E. G., & Durand, M. M. (1985). Reducing problem behaviors through functional communication training. *Journal of Applied Behavior Analysis, 18,* 111–126.

Carr, E. G., McLaughlin, D. M., Giacobbe-Grieco, T., & Smith, C. E. (2003). Using mood ratings and mood induction in assessment and intervention for severe problem behavior. *American Journal on Mental Retardation, 108,* 32–55.

Center, D. B., Deitz, S. M., & Kaufman, M. E. (1982). Student ability, task difficulty, and inappropriate classroom behavior: A study of children with behavior disorders. *Behavior Modification, 6,* 355–374.

Divatia, A., & Kern, L. (2007, March). *Putting the pieces together: Helping support teams to assess, intervene, and monitor.* Paper presented at the annual conference of the Association for Positive Behavior Support, Boston.

Dodge, K. A. (1985). Attributional bias in aggressive children. In P. C. Kendall (Ed.), *Advances in cognitive-behavioral research and therapy* (Vol. 4, pp. 73–110). New York: Academic Press.

Dunlap, G., Strain, P. S., Fox, L., Carta, J. J., Conroy, M., Smith, B. J., et al. (2006). Prevention and intervention with young children's challenging behavior: Perspectives regarding current knowledge. *Behavioral Disorders*, *32*(1), 29–45.

DuPaul, G. J., & Stoner, G. (2003). *ADHD in the schools: Assessment and intervention strategies*. New York: Guilford Press.

Eckstrom, R. B., Goertz, M. E., Pollack, J. M., & Rock, D. A. (1986). Who drops out of high school and why? Findings from a national study. *Teachers College Record*, *87*, 357–373.

Elam, S. M., & Rose, L. C. (1995). The 27th annual Phi Delta Kappa/Gallup Poll of the public's attitudes towards the public schools. *Phi Delta Kappan*, *73*, 41–56.

Ervin, R. A., Kern, L., Clarke, S., DuPaul, G. J., Dunlap, G., & Friman, P. C. (2000). Evaluating functional assessment-based intervention strategies for students with ADHD and comorbid disorders within the natural classroom context. *Behavioral Disorders*, *25*, 344–358.

Fink, A. H., & Janssen, K. N. (1993). Competencies for teaching students with emotional–behavioral disabilities. *Preventing School Failure*, *37*, 11–15.

George, M. (2000). Establishing and promoting disciplinary practices at the building level that ensure safe, effective, and nurturing school environments. In M. Bullock & R. A. Gable (Eds.), *Positive academic and behavioral supports: Creating safe, effective nurturing schools for all students* (pp. 11–15). Reston, VA: Council for Children with Behavioral Disorders.

Gettinger, M., & Seibert, J. K. (2002). Contributions of study skills to academic competence. *School Psychology Review*, *31*, 350–365.

Gunter, P. L., & Coutinho, M. J. (1997). Negative reinforcement in classrooms: What we're beginning to learn. *Teacher Education and Special Education*, *20*, 249–264.

Gunter, P. L., Jack, S. L., Shores, R. E., Carrell, D. E., & Flowers, J. (1993). Lag sequential analysis as a tool for functional analysis of student disruptive behavior in classrooms. *Journal of Emotional and Behavioral Disorders*, *3*, 138–148.

Halle, J., Bambara, L. M., & Reichle, J. (2005). Teaching alternative skills. In L. M. Bambara & L. Kern (Eds.), *Individualized supports for students with problem behaviors: Designing positive behavior plans* (pp. 237–274). New York: Guilford Press.

Hilt Panahon, A., Kern, L., & Divatia, A. (2007). School-based interventions for students with or at risk for depression: A review of the literature. *Advances in School Based Mental Health Promotion*, *1*, 32–41.

Horner, R. H., Sugai, G., Todd, A. W., & Lewis-Palmer, T. (2005). Schoolwide positive behavior support. In L. M. Bambara & L. Kern (Eds.), *Designing positive behavior supports for students* (pp. 359–390). New York: Guilford Press.

Ingram, K., Lewis-Palmer, T., & Sugai, G. (2005). Function-based intervention planning: Comparing the effectiveness of FBA indicated and contra-indicated intervention plans. *Journal of Positive Behavior Interventions*, *7*, 224–236.

Janney, R., & Snell, M. E. (2000). *Teachers' guide to inclusive practices: Behavioral support*. Baltimore: Brookes.

Kauffman, J. M. (2001). *Characteristics of emotional and behavioral disorders in children and youth.* (7th ed.). Upper Saddle River, NJ: Merrill/Prentice Hall.

Kern, L. (2005). Responding to problem behavior. In L. M. Bambara & L. Kern (Eds.), *Individualized supports for students with problem behaviors: Designing positive behavior.* New York: Guilford Press.

Kern, L., Dunlap, G., Clarke, S., & Childs, K. E. (1994). Student-Assisted Functional Assessment Interview. *Diagnostique*, *19*, 7–20.

Kern, L., Gallagher, P., Starosta, K., Hickman, W., & George, M. (2006). Longitudinal outcomes of functional behavioral assessment-based intervention. *Journal of Positive Behavior Interventions*, *8*, 67–78.

Kern, L., O'Neill, R. E., & Starosta, K. (2005). Gathering functional assessment information. In L. M. Bambara & L. Kern (Eds.), *Individualized supports for students with problem behaviors: Designing positive behavior plans* (pp. 129–164). New York: Guilford Press.

Mastropieri, M. A., & Scruggs, T. E. (2002). *Effective instruction for special education* (3rd ed.). Austin, TX: Pro-Ed.

Mayer, G. R., & Butterworth, T. (1979). A preventive approach to school violence and vandalism: An experimental study. *Personnel and Guidance Journal*, *57*, 436–441.

Mayer, G. R., Butterworth, T., Nafpaktitis, M., & Sulzer-Azaroff, B. (1983). Preventing school vandalism and improving discipline: A three-year study. *Journal of Applied Behavior Analysis*, *16*, 355–369.

Merrell, K. W. (2001). *Helping students overcome depression and anxiety: A practical guide*. New York: Guilford Press.

National Association of School Psychologists. (2000). *Professional conduct manual*. Bethesda, MD: Author.

Newcomer, L. L., & Lewis, T. J. (2004). Functional behavioral assessment: An investigation of assessment reliability and effectiveness of function-based interventions. *Journal of Emotional and Behavioral Disorders*, *12*, 168–181.

O'Neill, R. E., Horner, R. H., Albin, R. W., Sprague, J. R., Storey, K., & Newton, J. S. (1997). *Functional assessment and program development for problem behavior: A practical handbook* (2nd ed.). Pacific Grove, CA: Brooks/Cole.

Patterson, G. R. (1982). *Coercive family process.* Eugene, OR: Castalia.

Patterson, G. R., Reid, J. B., & Dishion, T. J. (1992). *Antisocial boys.* Eugene, OR: Castalia.

Penno, D. A., Frank, A. R., & Wacker, D. P. (2000). Instructional accommodations for adolescent students with severe emotional or behavioral disorders. *Behavior Disorders, 25,* 325–343.

Rock, M. L. (2000). Effective crisis management planning: Creating a collaborative framework. *Education and Treatment of Children, 23,* 248–264.

Ryan, J. B., & Peterson, R. L. (2004). Physical restraint in school. *Behavioral Disorders, 29,* 154–168.

Sacks, G., & Kern, L. (2008). A comparison of quality of life variables for students with emotional and behavioral disorders and students without disabilities. *Journal of Behavioral Education, 17,* 111–127.

Shapiro, E. S., & Cole, C. L. (1994). *Behavior change in the classroom: Self-management interventions.* New York: Guilford Press.

Shores, R. E., Jack, S. L., Gunter, P. L., Ellis, D. N., DeBriere, T. J., & Wehby, J. H. (1993). Classroom interactions of children with behavior disorders. *Journal of Emotional and Behavioral Disorders, 1,* 27–39.

Skinner, C. H., Rhymer, K. N., & McDaniel, E. C. (2000). Naturalistic direct observation in educational settings. In E. S. Shapiro & T. R. Kratochwill (Eds.), *Conducting school-based assessments of child and adolescent behavior.* New York: Guilford Press.

Wagner, M., Kutash, K., Duchnowski, A. J., Epstein, M. H., & Sumi, W. C. (2005). The children and youth we serve: A national picture of the characteristics of students with emotional disturbances receiving special education. *Journal of Emotional and Behavioral Disorders, 13,* 76–96.

Walker, H. M., Block-Pedego, A., Todis, B., & Severson, H. (1991). *School Archival Record Search (SARS).* Longmont, CO: Sopris West.

Walker, H. M., Colvin, G., & Ramsey, E. (1995). *Antisocial behavior in school: Strategies and best practices.* Pacific Grove, CA: Brooks/Cole.

Walker, H. M., & Walker, J. E. (1991). *Coping with noncompliance in the classroom: A positive approach for teachers.* Austin, TX: Pro-Ed.

Wehlage, G. G., & Rutter, R. A. (1986). Dropping out: How much do schools contribute to the problem? *Teachers College Record, 87,* 374–393.

Chapter 28

Psychopharmacological Interventions

George J. DuPaul
Lisa L. Weyandt
Genery D. Booster

Children and adolescents with behavior and social–emotional disorders make up a significant percentage of the school population. Epidemiological data indicate that 11.7–15% of children and adolescents in the United States exhibit significant symptoms of one or more psychiatric disorders during a given 3-month period, with approximately 36% of the population exhibiting a disorder by the age of 16 years (Costello, Mustillo, Erkanli, Keeler, & Angold, 2003). Lifetime prevalence of a behavior disorder prior to the age of 16 is higher in males (42%) than females (31%; Costello et al., 2003). Pediatricians have reported that, on average, 15% of their patients have behavior disorders (Williams, Klinepeter, Palmes, Pulley, & Foy, 2004). Some of these children are identified as having serious emotional disturbance, which is the fourth largest special education category, make up 8.1% of students receiving special education services (U.S. Department of Education Office of Special Education Programs, 2005).

Although students with behavior and social–emotional disorders may receive a variety of psychosocial and educational interventions, the use of psychotropic medication is one of the most common treatments in this population. In fact, it is estimated that between 3.4 and 4.6% of children under the age of 18 received psychotropic medica-

tion in 2002, and these rates are even higher among children in foster care (Safer, Zito, & Gardner, 2004; Zito et al., 2008). To put this percentage in perspective, approximately 2.8–3.8 million children and adolescents in the United States are treated with psychotropic medication. Over the past several decades, the use of psychotropic medication to treat behavior disorders in children has increased dramatically, particularly for preschool-age children (Zito et al., 2000). Inevitably, school psychologists and other educational professionals work with significant numbers of students who are being treated with medication.

The purpose of this chapter is to review the most critical issues relevant to the use of psychopharmacological interventions with children and adolescents. First, a rationale for the involvement of school psychologists in medication treatment is provided. This section is followed by an overview of the various classes of psychotropic medication that are used for treating child behavior disorders and the physiological bases for pharmacological effects. Next, medications used to treat symptoms of the two broad classes of psychopathology (i.e., externalizing and internalizing disorders) are reviewed. Finally, potential roles for school psychologists in psychopharmacological interventions are delineated with specific emphasis on (1) determining the need for medication and (2) monitoring medication effects on school performance. These roles are discussed in the context of a data-based problem-solving model.

Rationale for School Psychologist Involvement in Pharmacological Intervention

There are several reasons that it is critically important for school psychologists to be directly involved in pharmacological interventions. As mentioned previously, the use of medication to treat childhood social–emotional and behavioral disorders has increased exponentially over the past two decades. In addition, psychotropic medications have demonstrable effects, both positive and negative, on students' academic, social, and psychological functioning. Third, schools are an important source of data in determining the efficacy of medication treatment. Finally, school psychologists have training in assessment and intervention design processes that can aid physicians in making decisions regarding the initiation and effectiveness of pharmacotherapy.

Key areas of functioning (e.g., educational, social, and psychological) can be affected by treatment with psychotropic medication. For example, central nervous system (CNS) stimulants (e.g., methylphenidate) have been found not only to reduce attention-deficit/ hyperactivity disorder (ADHD) symptoms but also to enhance academic productivity, reduce negative interactions with peers, and promote positive relationships with authority figures (American Psychiatric Association, 2000; for a review, see Connor, 2006). Alternatively, antipsychotic medications (e.g., clozapine) used to treat schizophrenic disorder may reduce symptomatic behaviors but may also lead to adverse side effects, including cognitive impairment (Weyandt, 2006). Given the potential for positive and negative effects of medication on school functioning, school psychologists should be directly involved in assessing outcomes associated with this commonly used treatment modality.

Children and adolescents spend a significant proportion of their lives in the school setting. Thus schools are a very rich source of data about students' psychological, social, behavioral, and academic functioning. Assessment measures such as teacher behavior ratings, direct observations of classroom behavior, and peer interactions, as well as products of student behavior (e.g., classwork), can be invaluable in documenting medication effects. These data can be obtained before initiating and following receipt of medication in order to determine initial effects. Ongoing collection of these data can aid in determining whether medication continues to be effective and whether adjustments to dosage might be necessary.

School psychologists have extensive training in assessment of academic, psychosocial, and behavioral functioning, as well as in intervention design. Therefore, school psychologists are ideally suited to assist physicians and families in determining whether medication is necessary for a given student, as well as in evaluating the salutary and potentially adverse side effects of a specific medication regimen. The data-based problem-solving model that serves as a framework for school psychology services can be used as a context for making decisions about the use and effectiveness of pharmacotherapy. This model of service delivery serves as a context for later discussion of potential roles for school psychologists in medication treatment.

Overview of Psychotropic Medications

Psychotropic drugs are commonly prescribed to treat a wide range of disorders in children, including anxiety, mood, and disruptive behavior disorders. Studies indicate that the use of psychotropic medication has increased in children of all ages, particularly preschool-age children (e.g., DeBar, Lynch, Powell, & Gale, 2003; Olfson, Marcus, Weissman, & Jensen, 2002). The main classes of medications used to treat children and adolescents include stimulants, antianxiety medications, antidepressants, antipsychotics, and mood stabilizers. Less commonly prescribed medications include antihypertensives and anticonvulsants. It is important to note that empirical information concerning the safety, effectiveness, and long-term outcomes of children treated with psychotropic medication, with the exception of stimulant medication, is scant relative to the adult literature (Brown et al., 2007; Vitiello

& Swedo, 2004). In addition, the amount of medication needed to attain a therapeutic effect can vary widely among individuals, and side effects vary among individuals, as well as across types of medications (Trenton, Currier, & Zwemer, 2003). With respect to prescribing practices, stimulants and antidepressants are prescribed most frequently, followed by mood stabilizers (DeBar et al., 2003; Zito et al., 2003). Many children who are prescribed medication take more than one psychotropic medication (Safer, Zito, & dosReis, 2003).

The following section reviews the main classes of medication used to treat children with behavioral and social–emotional disorders and describes the purpose and mode of action of each medication. Information is also provided concerning the general prevalence rates of disorders for which these medications are prescribed. It is important to note that despite the increased use of psychotropic medication in children and adolescents (Olfson et al., 2002), the precise mode of action of these medications is unknown. What is known is that psychotropic medications affect cellular communication in the brain, primarily by altering chemical systems (i.e., neurotransmitter systems) by which cells (i.e., neurons) communicate. Medications can be classified into two main categories: agonists which facilitate the effects of neurotransmitters, and antagonists, which interfere with the effects of neurotransmitters. Part of the difficulty in understanding the precise effects of psychotropic medications is that variables such as genetic factors, individual differences, and sensitivity to medications are likely to influence cellular communication in ways that are not currently understood (for a review, see Weyandt, 2006).

Stimulant Medications

Stimulants are used primarily for the treatment of behavior disorders, particularly ADHD. ADHD is estimated to affect 3–7% of the school-age population (American Psychiatric Association, 2000). The Food and Drug Administration (FDA) has approved three stimulant medications for the treatment of ADHD: methylphenidate (Ritalin, Concerta, Metadate, Methylin), dextroamphetamine (Dexedrine), and mixed amphetamine compounds (Adderall). Pemoline (Cy-

lert) had been approved by the FDA and was used to treat children with ADHD but was pulled from the U.S. market in 2005 because of potential liver toxicity (Connor, 2006). Methylphenidate is the most commonly prescribed stimulant for ADHD, and it is used in the majority of childhood cases (Safer & Zito, 2000). In 2002, the FDA approved a nonstimulant drug, atomoxetine (Strattera), for the treatment of ADHD. When problems with depression, obsessive–compulsive disorder, or other disorders coexist, children are sometimes prescribed medications in addition to the stimulants. This process is known as augmentation and may include antidepressants such as fluoxetine (Prozac) or imipramine (Tofranil), antianxiety medications such as paroxetine (Paxil), or other types of medications depending on symptoms and history of the child.

The precise mechanisms by which stimulants improve ADHD symptoms (e.g., improve attention and decrease impulsivity) are not fully understood. Research indicates that stimulants increase the arousal level of the inhibitory components of the CNS, primarily by affecting the availability and efficiency of brain chemicals (i.e., neurotransmitters) such as dopamine and norepinephrine among neurons (Chamberlain, Robbins, & Sahakian, 2007). It may seem contradictory to prescribe a stimulant to an individual who appears overstimulated; however, stimulants activate systems in the brain that facilitate sustained attention and inhibition of impulsive responding. Ultimately, stimulants serve to enhance self-control and self-regulatory systems. Current research suggests that stimulants (methylphenidate) alter communication among neurons by affecting the reuptake process for dopamine and, to a lesser extent, norepinephrine (Grace, 2001).

Antidepressant Medications and Mood Stabilizers

Antidepressants are used most often to treat children suffering from mood disorders, which include depressive and bipolar disorders. Major depression is the most common type of mood disorder among children and adolescents, and approximately 0.4–8 % of children and adolescents suffer from depression (Lewinsohn, Rohde, & Seeley, 1998). Antidepressants used to treat children and adolescents with major depression include selective serotonin reuptake inhibitors (SSRIs) such as fluoxetine (Prozac), fluvoxamine (Luvox), and sertraline (Zoloft), as well as tricyclic antidepressants (e.g., anafranil, imipramine, amitriptyline, and desipramine). Fluoxetine (Prozac) was approved by the FDA in 2003 for the treatment of depression in children ages 7–17; however, this medication (as do other SSRIs) carries a "black box" label, warning patients of the potential increased risk of suicidal thoughts. Adverse events associated with these medications are discussed later in this chapter. Bipolar disorder, compared with major depression, rarely occurs in children and adolescents (i.e., 1%; Lewinsohn, Klein, & Seeley, 1995), but, when medicated, children with bipolar disorder are typically treated with mood stabilizers. Three main types of mood stabilizers used in the treatment of bipolar disorders include lithium carbonate, anticonvulsants (e.g., carbamazepine, and divalproex), and antipsychotic medications (e.g., risperidone). Lithium is approved by the FDA for use with children ages 12 and older, and in 2007 the FDA approved the use of risperidone (Risperdal) for the treatment of bipolar disorder in children ages 10–17.

Older, tricyclic antidepressants (e.g., imipramine and desipramine) are believed to block the reuptake of the neurotransmitter norepinephrine and, to a lesser degree, serotonin. Tricyclic antidepressants have more adverse side effects than the newer, atypical antidepressants and are therefore used less frequently with children and adolescents. Atypical antidepressants (e.g., SSRIs) primarily affect the neurotransmitter serotonin by preventing the reuptake of serotonin, increasing the amount of serotonin produced by the cell.

Despite the long history of lithium in the treatment of mood disorders, the manner in which lithium affects brain functioning is poorly understood. Current research suggests that lithium may have a number of effects; it may influence internal processes of cells, alter gene expression, or inhibit various cellular processes that result in the death of neurons and glial cells in the hippocampus and frontal cortex associated with individuals with bipolar disorder (Bown, Wang, & Young, 2003; Pardo, Andreolotti, Ramos, Picatoste, & Claro, 2003). The mode of action of anticonvulsants is also unclear, but studies suggest that anticonvulsants inhibit norepinephrine reuptake, block sodium channels, and enhance the action of gamma-aminobutyric acid (Perrine, 1996).

Antianxiety Medications

Antianxiety medications are used to treat a variety of anxiety disorders (e.g., generalized anxiety disorder, obsessive–compulsive disorder, and phobias) in children and adolescents. It has been estimated that 12–20% of children suffer from some type of anxiety disorder, and specific phobias are commonly diagnosed in children and adolescents (Albano, Chorpita, & Barlow, 2003; King, Muris, & Ollendick, 2004). Anxiety disorders frequently co-occur, and several studies suggest that they occur more frequently in girls than boys (Verduin & Kendall, 2003). The most commonly prescribed medications to treat anxiety disorders in children are antidepressants such as the SSRIs and clomipramine (anafranil), a tricyclic antidepressant. Less often, benzodiazepines (e.g., diazepam [Valium], alprazolam [Xanax]) are used to treat anxiety disorders (Stein & Seedat, 2004; Wittchen, 2002). Other types of medication sometimes used to treat anxiety in children include buspirone (BuSpar), clonidine (Catapres), and diphenhydramine (Benadryl), but it is important to note that these medications are used "off label" and are not currently approved by the FDA for the treatment of anxiety disorders in children. In fact, antidepressants are the only medications approved by the FDA for the treatment of anxiety disorders in children.

Antipsychotic Medications

Antipsychotic medications are primarily used to treat psychotic disorders in children (e.g., schizophrenia), although they are sometimes used to treat nonpsychotic disorders such as Tourette syndrome (Gaffney et al., 2002). The prevalence of psychotic disorders, such as schizophrenia, in children is uncertain but believed to be quite rare (< 1%; Eggers, Bunk, & Krause, 2000). Antipsychotic medications used to treat psychotic symptoms in children include risperidone (Risperdal), ziprasidone (Geodon), chlorpromazine (Thorazine), clozapine (Clozaril), and haloperidol (Haldol). The only FDA-approved antipsychotic medication for the treatment of schizophrenia in children is risperidone (Risperdal). One of the most disturbing side effects of some antipsychotic medications (e.g., chlorpromazine and haloperidol) is tardive dyskinesia, characterized by involuntary muscle movements, and, consequently, these medications tend to be reserved for more severe cases that do not respond to other forms of treatment.

Antipsychotic medications primarily affect the neurotransmitter dopamine by blocking the receptor sites for dopamine, thereby interfering with or diminishing the effects of dopamine on the cell. Depending on the medication, one or several types of dopamine receptors may be blocked. For example, chlorpromazine blocks D2 receptors, whereas clozapine is believed to block D4 and serotonin receptors (Strange, 2001). Grunder et al. (2003) recently reported that antipsychotic medications also reduce the level of dopamine that is synthesized by neurons.

Effects of Medications Used to Treat Externalizing Disorders

Stimulants

Numerous double-blind, placebo-controlled trials have demonstrated the effectiveness of psychostimulants such as methylphenidate and dextroamphetamine in the treatment of ADHD (for review, see Connor, 2006), and current best practices support the use of combined treatment, including both medication and behavioral management strategies. A randomized clinical trial conducted by the MTA Cooperative Group (1999), for example, compared the effectiveness of medication management with methylphenidate, behavior modification, and combined treatment with routine community care for 597 children ages 7–9 who met criteria for ADHD, combined type. Results indicated significantly greater improvement in ADHD symptoms for children who received either the medication management or combined treatment compared with those who received behavior management only or community care. In addition, a 24-month follow-up (MTA Cooperative Group, 2004) showed continued greater improvement of ADHD symptoms in those children who received medication management over those

in the behavior-management-only and community care groups. It is important to note that the combined treatment was superior in addressing deficits associated with ADHD (e.g., social behavior), particularly for those children with comorbid conduct and anxiety disorders, as well as for children from lower socioeconomic status (SES) backgrounds (Arnold et al., 2003).

In addition to traditional stimulants such as methylphenidate, there is emerging support for amphetamine compounds and atomoxetine. A meta-analysis conducted by Kratochvil, Wilens, et al. (2006) pooled data from seven double-blind placebo-controlled and six open-label studies examining the effectiveness of atomoxetine with 6- and 7-year-old children who met DSM-IV (American Psychiatric Association, 2000) criteria for ADHD. Results showed that 74.4% of participants had at least a 25% reduction in their ADHD symptoms, as measured by parent ratings of ADHD symptoms. There is preliminary evidence, however, that amphetamine compounds are superior to atomoxetine. A recent randomized, double-blind forced-dose-escalation study of children with ADHD found that children who received an amphetamine compound (MAS-XR) showed greater improvement in attention, academic performance, and overall clinical functioning than those who received atomoxetine (Faraone, Wigal, & Hodgkins, 2007). Additional evidence suggests that atomoxetine may also be less effective than methylphenidate. An open-label study by Starr and Kemner (2005), for example, found that although both methylphenidate and atomoxetine resulted in significant improvements in ADHD symptomatology, children who received methyphenidate showed significantly greater treatment responses than those who received atomoxetine.

Although the majority of pharmacological studies do not directly assess the impact of medication on children's functioning in the classroom, research by Rapport, Denney, DuPaul, and Gardner (1994) suggest that methylphenidate may have a positive impact on students' classroom behaviors. Their double-blind placebo-controlled study evaluated the effects of methylphenidate on 76 children who met DSM-III (American Psychiatric Association, 1980) criteria for ADHD in terms of their attention, academic functioning, and behavior in regular classroom settings. Results revealed significant improvements in the children's observed time on task, academic efficiency (as measured by the number of correct problems completed), and teacher ratings of classroom behavior. Importantly, however, an evaluation of clinically significant treatment effects revealed that only 53% of students showed improvement in academic functioning compared with attention and classroom behavior, which showed improvements in 76 and 94% of students, respectively. This finding suggests that for some students, supplemental interventions (e.g., direct instruction) may be required to address academic functioning. Finally, it should be noted that stimulant medications are often associated with side effects such as headaches, insomnia, decreased appetite, abdominal pain, and tics (Connor, 2006).

Medications Used to Treat Disruptive Behavior Disorders

Although there are currently no FDA-approved pharmacological treatments for aggression and conduct problems, a recent meta-analysis conducted by Ipser and Stein (2007) provides some evidence to support the pharmacological treatment of disruptive behavior disorders. Their analysis of 14 medication trials found lithium and risperidone to be effective in reducing symptoms of conduct disorder. Although pharmacological interventions resulted in significantly more adverse events, such as nausea, dizziness, fatigue, and loss of appetite, there were no significant differences in dropout rates between those children who received medication and those in the placebo groups.

In addition, stimulant medications are used to treat aggression in children and adolescents, most commonly in children with comorbid ADHD and severe aggression or conduct disorder. Methylphenidate has also been used to treat aggression in children with autism (Parikh, Kolevzon, & Hollander, 2008), mental retardation (Aman, Marks, Turbott, Wilsher, & Merry, 1991; Pearson et al., 2003), and conduct disorder without ADHD (Klein et al., 1997). A recent meta-analysis of randomized, placebo-controlled trials by Pappadopulos and colleagues (2006) found that stimulants exerted a me-

dium to large effect on aggressive symptoms (mean effect size = 0.78), with higher doses linked to stronger effect sizes. It should be noted, however, that stimulants alone may not produce a clinically significant reduction in symptoms for all children (Barzman & Findling, 2008). Researchers from the Multimodal Treatment Study of Children with ADHD (MTA), for example, found that 44% of children who received methylphenidate treatment continued to exhibit high levels of aggression after 14 months of treatment (MTA Cooperative Group, 1999; Jensen et al., 2007). As a result, treatment may need to be augmented with additional interventions for these children (Barzman & Findling, 2008).

Effects of Medications Used to Treat Internalizing Disorders

Antidepressants

Although effective in treating adult depression, tricyclic antidepressants (TCAs) have not been shown to be superior to placebo in the treatment of children and adolescents with major depression. A meta-analysis of 12 placebo-controlled trials with TCAs in children ages 6–18 found that the difference between treatment groups was too small to achieve clinical significance (Hazell, O'Connell, Heathcote, Robertson, & Henry, 1995). These findings have been replicated in more recent double-blind placebo-controlled trials in which treatment with TCAs such as amitriptyline was not superior to placebo (Birmaher et al., 1998; Keller, Ryan, & Strober, 2001; Kye et al., 1996). As a result, TCAs are not recommended as a first-line treatment for children and adolescents with major depression (Birmaher et al., 1998; Wagner, 2005).

In contrast to the studies examining TCAs, several double-blind placebo-controlled studies examining the effectiveness of SSRIs have revealed positive results for fluoxetine (Emslie et al., 1997; Emslie et al., 2002; Treatment for Adolescents with Depression Study [TADS] Team, 2004), sertraline (Wagner et al., 2003), and citalopram (Wagner et al., 2004). Emslie and colleagues (2002), for example, compared the effects of fluoxetine (10 mg/day for 1 week, then 20 mg/day for 8 weeks) and placebo in 219 youths ages 8–17 who met DSM-IV criteria for major depression. Although there was no significant difference between children who received fluoxetine and those who received a placebo in terms of the authors' prospectively defined response criteria (> 30% decrease in self-report of depressive symptoms), participants who received fluoxetine showed significantly greater improvement according to self-report ratings. Furthermore, significantly more fluoxetine-treated patients met criteria for remission than those who received placebo.

Fluoxetine also has been compared with psychotherapeutic interventions in the treatment of childhood depression. Members of the TADS team (2004) compared fluoxetine alone, fluoxetine with cognitive-behavioral therapy (CBT), CBT alone, and a pill placebo in a multicenter trial with 439 adolescent outpatients ages 12–17 who met DSM-IV criteria for major depression. Results showed that although fluoxetine alone was superior to CBT alone and to placebo with regard to self-report of depressive symptoms, adolescents who received both fluoxetine and CBT showed greater improvement than either treatment alone. In addition, a more recent study examining data from TADS (Kratochvil, Emslie, et al., 2006) found that participants receiving combined treatment showed faster onset of benefit (as measured by clinician ratings of global improvement) than those who received either treatment alone.

In addition to depression, SSRIs have been used treat children and adolescents with anxiety disorders. The majority of placebo-controlled trials have examined youths with obsessive–compulsive disorder (OCD), and a meta-analysis of 13 studies of SSRIs in the treatment of pediatric OCD demonstrated a small effect size (0.46), with no significant difference between the types of SSRI (fluoxetine, paroxetine, sertraline, and fluvoxamine; Geller et al., 2003). Geller and colleagues (2001), for example, conducted a 13-week double-blind placebo-controlled study examining the effects of fluoxetine (10 mg/daily for 2 weeks, then 20 mg daily for 11 weeks) for 103 participants who met DSM-IV criteria for OCD, ages 7–17. Intent-to-treat analyses revealed that fluoxetine was associated with significantly greater symptom improvement (as measured by

self-report ratings of OCD symptoms) than placebo. In addition, the occurrence of side effects in the treatment group was not significantly greater than in the placebo group.

Studies examining SSRIs in the treatment of other anxiety disorders (e.g., separation anxiety disorder [SAD], social phobia, and generalized anxiety disorder [GAD]) commonly group these children together due to the high levels of comorbidity among these disorders (Reinblatt & Walkup, 2005). Birmaher and colleagues (2003), for example, examined the efficacy of fluoxetine for the acute treatment of 74 children and adolescents who met DSM-IV criteria for GAD, SAD, and/or social phobia. Intent-to-treat analyses revealed that significantly more of the participants taking fluoxetine (61%) showed "very much improvement" (based on clinician ratings of global improvement). Significant results were found for all anxiety diagnoses when analyzed by group. Headaches and gastrointestinal difficulties were the only significant side effects experienced by those taking fluoxetine. Another study examining SSRIs found similar positive results for fluvoxamine (Pine et al., 2001). It is important to note, however, that few randomized clinical trials have been conducted with children and adolescents for individual anxiety disorders other than OCD (Reinblatt & Walkup, 2005).

Mood Stabilizers

Psychopharmacological treatment with mood stabilizers such as lithium, carbamazepine, and oxcarbazepine is often the first line of treatment for children and adolescents with bipolar disorder (McIntosh & Trotter, 2006; Weckerly, 2002). The efficacy of such treatment is difficult to determine given the lack of controlled trials examining the use of mood stabilizers and antipsychotic medications for children and adolescents; the majority of research reports are case studies, retrospective chart reviews, or open-label trials. Although several open-label trials reported significant short-term improvement of bipolar symptoms after treatment with risperidone (Biederman, Mick, Wozniak, et al., 2005; Pavuluri et al., 2004), lithium (Pavuluri et al., 2004), divalproex (Wagner et al., 2002), and olanzapine (Biederman, Mick,

Hammerness, et al., 2005), recent studies comparing the effects of several mood stabilizers with placebo have produced equivocal results (e.g., Delbello et al., 2005; Kafantaris et al., 2004; Wagner et al., 2006).

Wagner and colleagues (2006), for example, examined the efficacy and safety of oxcarbazepine in a double-blind, randomized, placebo-controlled, multicenter trial with 116 outpatients ages 7–18 who met DSM-IV criteria for bipolar I disorder. Results after 7 weeks of treatment revealed no difference in improvement (as measured by self-report ratings of bipolar symptoms) between the treatment and placebo groups. In addition, significantly more participants who received oxcarbazepine discontinued treatment due to adverse events, including dizziness, nausea, somnolence, fatigue, and rash. An earlier double-blind and placebo-controlled study by Geller and colleagues (1998) examined the effects of lithium for adolescents with bipolar disorder and comorbid secondary substance dependency. After 6 weeks of treatment, adolescents who had been randomly assigned to receive lithium showed significantly better symptom improvement (as measured by clinician ratings of global improvement) and had significantly fewer positive drug tests. No significant differences in symptoms based on child diagnostic interview data, however, were found. In addition, adolescents receiving lithium reported significantly more side effects including thirst, nausea, vomiting, and dizziness.

Antianxiety Medications

Although SSRIs are most commonly used to treat pediatric anxiety disorders, benzodiazepines are also prescribed. The efficacy of benzodiazepines for use with children and adolescents, however, is unclear. A double-blind placebo-controlled study by Simeon and colleagues (1992), for example, examined the efficacy of alprazolam in 30 outpatients ages 8–16 who were diagnosed with overanxious disorder or avoidant disorder. Although clinical global improvement ratings following 28 days of medication showed a trend favoring alprazolam, the results did not meet clinical significance due to a high level of improvement in the placebo group. Similarly, another double-blind crossover trial of clonazepam for children with anxiety

disorders showed a trend toward clinical improvement, but the results following 4 weeks of medication did not differ significantly from the placebo phase (Graae, Milner, Rizzotto, & Klein, 1994). The small sample size ($n = 12$), however, may have contributed to the lack of statistically significant findings.

Risk and Adverse Events

There has been recent concern regarding adverse side effects of the medications used to treat internalizing disorders in children. Mood stabilizers, for example, have been associated with dizziness, nausea, somnolence, fatigue, thirst, and rash (Wagner et al., 2006). In addition, headaches, nausea, abdominal pain, insomnia, somnolence, tremor, and agitation have been noted to occur with the use of antidepressants. Approximately 2% of adolescents taking fluoxetine in the TADS, for example, reported sedation, insomnia, vomiting, and upper abdominal pain (Emslie et al., 2006).

Although SSRIs have been shown to have fewer and less severe side effects than TCAs (Wagner, 2005), there has been recent concern regarding suicidality (suicidal thoughts and attempts) in children and adolescents taking SSRIs. A review by Rey and Martin (2006) suggests that rates of suicidality may be affected by the method of data collection. When data regarding adverse events are gathered via general inquiry (e.g., "Have you had any problems since your last visit?"), results suggest that SSRIs increase suicidality. When questionnaires are systematically used, however, no comparable increase in suicidality was noted. The safety results from the Treatment for Adolescents with Depression Study (Emslie et al., 2006) examined systematically administered rating scales, as well as individually reported adverse events. Results revealed significantly more suicide-related events (defined as attempts, preparatory actions, self-injurious behavior with intent unknown, or suicidal ideation) in adolescents taking fluoxetine than those on placebo. It should be noted, however, that only five suicide attempts were reported during the trial, which included 439 adolescents. The low base rate of suicidal events requires extremely large samples for study, which have yet to be conducted. In sum, the currently available data indicate that SSRIs do not increase the risk for completed suicide in children, but there is some evidence to suggest that SSRIs may be associated with higher rates of suicidal thoughts and self-injurious behaviors. As a result of these concerns, the FDA recently announced a request to manufacturers of all antidepressant medications to update the "black box" on their product labeling to include warnings about increased risks of suicidal thinking and behavior.

Effects of Medication on School Functioning

Although not extensively studied, medication treatment of childhood disorders is presumed to have an impact on the academic, behavioral, and social functioning of treated children in school settings. In some cases, medications have led to significant improvements in critical performance areas beyond intended symptom reduction effects. For example, methylphenidate and other psychostimulants have been found to enhance academic productivity and accuracy for many students with ADHD (Rapport et al., 1994). Although stimulant-induced improvements in academic performance are noted over the short term, effects on long-term academic achievement are small to nonexistent (e.g., MTA Cooperative Group, 1999, 2004). In other cases, medications have led to adverse side effects wherein functioning is deleteriously affected despite symptom reduction. For example, antipsychotic medications (e.g., clozapine and haloperidol) used to reduce symptoms of schizophrenia or Tourette syndrome can lead to social withdrawal and/or adverse effects on cognition and learning (Brown et al., 2007).

An exclusive focus on symptom reduction as a treatment outcome is problematic because changes in symptoms are not necessarily correlated with improvements in school functioning. In fact, in a classic study, Sprague and Sleator (1977) showed that attention and activity difficulties associated with ADHD were optimally reduced at higher dosages of stimulants, whereas the impact on cognitive functioning was optimized at lower dosages. Sprague and Sleator (1977) further found that performance on a cognitive task was impaired at the dosage levels that optimized behavioral improve-

ments. Thus a comprehensive evaluation of medication effects must not only focus on reduction of target symptoms but also assess changes to academic, social, and behavioral functioning.

Limitations of the Research Literature

Although the studies discussed previously provide some evidence suggesting that certain pharmacological treatments can be efficacious in the treatment of child psychopathology, a number of limitations to the body of literature must be considered. First, the majority of participants in the studies are Caucasian, and many did not report socioeconomic data. The results of these studies, therefore, cannot be generalized to populations from diverse racial and/or socioeconomic backgrounds. Second, it is important to note that although the positive studies presented here showed treatment effects that were statistically significant, many studies did not include effect sizes, and it is unclear whether these effects were clinically significant. As many participants in these pharmacological studies showed some positive results with placebo, the inclusion of effect-size calculations in the analyses would aid in the interpretation of the results. There is also a paucity of research examining the long-term effects of psychopharmacological treatment in children and adolescents. In addition to psychological functioning, longitudinal research would provide important information regarding the long-term effects of adverse events. Finally, it must be noted that the majority of clinical trials do not provide information regarding the effects of medication across settings. As children and adolescents spend a significant portion of their time in school, and as academic functioning is an important correlate of mental health, future studies should assess medication effects via multiple methods and multiple informants, beyond parent and clinician reports.

Potential Roles for School Psychologists in Pharmacological Treatment

Given the increasing use of psychotropic medication to treat childhood social–emotional and behavioral disorders, as well as the potential impact of this treatment on academic, socioemotional, and cognitive functioning, it is critical for school psychologists to play two major roles (cf. DuPaul & Carlson, 2005; Power, DuPaul, Shapiro, & Kazak, 2003). First, school psychologists can collaborate with physicians, school personnel, and parents to determine whether medication is needed as part of a student's intervention plan. In particular, school-based assessment data may be helpful in deciding whether medication is needed immediately or whether psychosocial and/or educational interventions should be implemented before considering pharmacotherapy. Second, school psychologists can collect and interpret data that will aid physicians in deciding whether a specific medication is effective and, if so, in identifying the optimal dosage. Further, monitoring the safety and effectiveness of medication over time (e.g., across school years) may be warranted in the treatment of chronic disorders (e.g., ADHD).

Determining Need for Medication

The first step in the pharmacological treatment process is to collect data that will help to determine whether medication treatment is, in fact, necessary. Specifically, school psychologists can provide data and input to physicians that are helpful in making the decision to initiate medication; however, the child's physician and parents will ultimately make this decision. Some states (e.g., Connecticut, Utah) have passed laws that restrict school personnel from discussing or recommending medication treatment. Thus it is critical for school psychologists to know relevant state regulations and their school district's interpretation of such laws so that their participation in medication treatment is consistent with legal guidelines.

As is the case for educational and behavioral interventions, a data-based problem-solving model can be used to reach decisions about the necessity of medication to treat one or more specific target behaviors. Specifically, several steps should be followed, including (1) determining the target behavior(s) occasioning a referral for treatment, (2) collecting data regarding all areas of functioning (e.g., behavioral, social, psychological, and educational) that may be affected by the identified problem(s), (3) considering response to prior and/or current interventions, and (4) delineating treatment components based on obtained data and empirical support.

Potential targets for intervention should be identified through a collaborative problem-solving process with the child's parent(s) and/or teacher(s) (Sheridan, Kratochwill, & Bergan, 1996). Once one or more problem behaviors are identified, data are then collected to provide a comprehensive evaluation of the child's functioning. Beyond consideration of specific behaviors, thorough evaluations of relevant areas of functioning should be undertaken. In many cases, this would include completion of a comprehensive assessment of behavior, academic skills, and psychological functioning (see Mash & Barkley, 2007, as well as the following chapters in this volume: Marcotte & Hintze, Chapter 5; Burns & Klingbeil, Chapter 6; Gansle & Noell, Chapter 7, on academic problems; Martens & Ardoin, Chapter 10, on disruptive behaviors; and Miller, Chapter 11, on internalizing problems).

Evaluation data will aid in the diagnostic decision-making process that must be undertaken if pharmacological treatment is going to be considered. Although the data-based decision-making process does not typically involve a diagnostic evaluation, it is important to assess behaviors relevant to psychiatric diagnoses when the possible use of medication is being considered. Information about behaviors symptomatic of various psychopathological disorders will facilitate evaluation of the degree to which a child's functioning meets criteria for a DSM-IV-TR (American Psychiatric Association, 2000) diagnosis. This is particularly important when communicating data regarding school functioning to physicians and other mental health professionals (e.g., clinical psychologists). From a medical perspective, the student's diagnostic status (i.e., severity, chronicity, and presence of comorbid disorders) will be a critical determinant of whether medication will be considered as a first-line treatment, later in the treatment process, or not at all. In some cases, the school psychologist will directly participate in the diagnostic decision-making process, whereas in others data regarding behavioral, social, and educational functioning will be communicated to physicians without attaching a diagnostic "label." What is most important is that the school psychologist and/or other school personnel provide data about school functioning that can be used by the physician and family to determine whether medication is necessary.

Prior to a physician referral for possible medication treatment, data should be collected regarding the student's response to prior and/or current interventions. Interviews with parents and teachers can identify specific prior attempts to address the target behaviors, as well as their degree of success. It is particularly helpful to consider written reports or other documentation of prior treatment outcomes, particularly the results of interventions implemented as part of a response-to-intervention (RTI)/tiered-intervention protocol. When interventions are being implemented in the classroom or other school settings, the student's behavior should be observed both with and without the intervention, if possible. These data would be particularly helpful in deciding whether medication (which, in most, cases, would be considered a Tier 3 intervention) would be needed.

In some cases, psychosocial, behavioral, and/or academic interventions will be implemented initially prior to a referral for medication treatment. Several factors are relevant to this decision. First, the nature of the child's disorder and the likelihood that nonpharmacological treatments will be effective should be considered. For example, behavioral and psychosocial interventions have strong empirical support for the treatment of some disorders (e.g., oppositional defiant disorder, conduct disorder) but have less support as a primary treatment for other disorders (e.g., schizophrenia). Second, the severity of a child's symptoms is an important consideration. In general, if symptoms are mild to moderate, the higher the probability is that psychosocial and educational interventions will be sufficient, thus precluding the need for medication. Conversely, when symptomatic behaviors are relatively severe, frequent, and chronic, then medication should be considered as a first-line treatment in combination with nonpharmacological strategies. Finally, assessment data should be examined

to delineate environmental factors (e.g., antecedent and consequent events, or instructional level of the curriculum) that can be modified in the context of psychosocial or educational approaches. To the extent that data indicate that symptomatic behaviors are associated with specific settings and environmental factors, then nonpharmacological approaches may be more appropriate as an initial treatment approach. When symptomatic behaviors are more pervasive across settings and associated with a variety of environmental factors, then initial treatment with medication may be warranted (Power et al., 2003).

Sharing evaluation results with physicians to assist in the determination of potential treatment options and ultimate treatment goals is an important part of the consultation process (American Academy of Pediatrics, 2001; HaileMariam, Bradley-Johnson, & Johnson, 2002; Kainz, 2002). Specifically, a brief report can be sent to the primary care physician that summarizes the key findings and recommendations of the school-based problem-solving process and/or evaluation. This written report should be followed by a telephone call to facilitate emphasis of major findings and to discuss the next steps in a potential treatment collaboration process. The participation of physicians (or representatives of their practice) in problem-solving team discussions centered on medical treatment components should be encouraged either through telephone conference call or by holding meetings at physicians' offices. Team decision making allows the consideration of alternate treatment options and cooperation in evaluating medication effects. Examples of a collaborative approach to medication decision making are provided in the current guidelines for the treatment of ADHD published by the American Academy of Pediatrics (2001). One of the primary recommendations of this report is that the treating physician, the parents, and the child should collaborate with school personnel in determining appropriate targets for treatment. Further, parental and child acceptability of the potential pharmacotherapy regimen should be assessed prior to conducting a medication trial. In particular, whether or not the parents perceive the need for medication and understand the potential effects and side effects of drug therapy should be assessed.

Monitoring Medication Effects

Once the physician prescribes a specific medication, the school psychologist and other school personnel (e.g., nurse, teacher, counselor) can collaborate to collect data that can help evaluate whether a specific medication dosage is effective. In fact, a recent survey of National Association of School Psychologists members indicates that the majority (55%) of school psychologists are involved in monitoring the effects of medication, primarily for students with ADHD (Gureasko-Moore, DuPaul, & Power, 2005).

Multiple models for school-based medication evaluation have been proposed (e.g., Gadow, Nolan, Paolicelli, & Sprafkin, 1991; Power et al., 2003; Volpe, Heick, & Gureasko-Moore, 2005). For example, Volpe et al. (2005) propose a monitoring protocol in the context of a behavioral problem-solving framework. The Agile Consultative Model of Medication Evaluation (ACMME) involves several steps. First, feedback is obtained from key stakeholders (e.g., parent, teacher, physician) to assess the acceptability and feasibility of various medication evaluation components (e.g., behavior ratings, direct observations) a priori. Next, the standard initial two phases of consultative problem-solving (i.e., problem identification and problem analysis) are completed to determine whether a medication trial is necessary as an adjunctive treatment to any classroom or school interventions. Then a medication trial is conducted in the context of the treatment implementation and evaluation stages of consultative problem solving. Stated differently, the same problem-solving process is followed as in the case of a behavioral or academic intervention; however, in this case the treatment being evaluated is medication. The acceptability and feasibility of evaluation components are assessed in a continuous fashion, and adjustments are made to data gathering as a function of feasibility and accessibility information. For example, if a particular assessment component (e.g., observation) is not feasible to obtain on a regular basis, then the teacher and school psychologist would work collaboratively to

identify an alternative assessment measure that is deemed more feasible to complete (e.g., a brief rating scale). Although this model has not been empirically investigated to date, it may have advantages over other monitoring protocols given the emphasis on feasibility and consultative problem solving.

Most proposed medication monitoring protocols (Gadow et al., 1991; Power et al., 2003; Volpe et al., 2005) have several important features in common (see Table 28.1). In particular, critical components include (1) timelines, procedures, and measures specified prior to the evaluation; (2) brief, psychometrically sound measures to assess targeted areas of functioning; (3) data obtained to guide medication and/or dosage decisions; (4) potential adverse side effects assessed prior to and following receipt of medication; (5) data on both nonmedication and medication conditions; and (6) data communicated in a clear, concise fashion to physicians and parents (Power et al., 2003).

Power and colleagues (2003) describe an example of a medication monitoring protocol for the case of Barry, a 7-year-old, second-

---

TABLE 28.1. Important Features of Medication Evaluation Procedures

1. Medication trial is designed through consultation between school-based or clinic-based team and the prescribing physician.
2. Specific timelines, measures, and procedures are identified and agreed on.
3. Areas of functioning (e.g., cognitive, academic, and behavioral) to assess are identified and measures to assess these are utilized.
4. Objective, psychometrically sound measures (e.g., behavior rating scales and direct observations) are highly desirable.
5. Potential side-effects are identified and measures to assess these are utilized.
6. Data are collected during both nonmedication and medication conditions in as controlled a fashion as possible.
7. Data are summarized through graphic display and/or tabular presentation of statistics to facilitate interpretation.
8. Interpretation of outcomes is made collaboratively with the child's physician, and recommendations are clearly communicated to the child's parents.

Note. From Power, DuPaul, Shapiro, and Kazak (2003). Copyright 2003 by The Guilford Press. Reprinted by permission.

grade student who was placed in a general education classroom in a moderately sized, suburban elementary school. He had been diagnosed with ADHD, combined type, by a child psychiatrist using DSM-IV-TR (American Psychiatric Association, 2000) criteria. Barry exhibited significant difficulties with work completion and accuracy, as well as in following classroom rules, despite the implementation of school- and home-based contingency management systems. Therefore, his physician, parents, teachers, school psychologist, and school nurse decided to evaluate Barry's response to several dosages of AdderallXR, a psychostimulant medication found to be effective in reducing ADHD symptoms (Pelham et al., 2000).

Barry's team conducted an assessment across a 4-week period, wherein he received a different dosage (0, 5, 10, and 15 mg) of AdderallXR each week. Medication was administered once per day (prior to his leaving home for school) under parental supervision. The order of medication conditions was randomly determined, and his teacher was blind to the dosage conditions. Weekly ratings on the ADHD Rating Scale–IV (DuPaul, Power, Anastopoulos, & Reid, 1998) and a side-effect rating scale (Barkley, 1990) were obtained from Barry's parents and teacher. The school psychologist observed Barry's on-task behavior and activity level two or three times per week during a 20-minute independent-seatwork period in his regular classroom. Barry's teacher collected samples of his schoolwork so that the team could monitor possible improvements in the completion and accuracy of his work.

Barry exhibited clinically significant increases in the completion and accuracy of his work during the 10 and 15-mg conditions relative to the no-medication condition (see Figure 28.1). Adverse side effects (e.g., mild appetite reduction and insomnia) were relatively mild for the 10-mg dosage. The school psychologist recommended to his physician that Barry receive 10 mg of AdderallXR on a regular basis and provided suggestions to Barry's parents to help address his mild appetite and sleep difficulties (e.g., preparing a meal for him later in the evening when his appetite returned).

As was the case for Barry, assessment measures should be chosen based on the

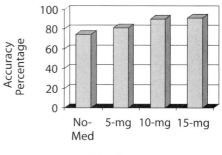

FIGURE 28.1. Percentage of schoolwork completed accurately by a 7-year-old boy treated with several dosages of AdderallXR for ADHD. From Power, DuPaul, Shapiro, and Kazak (2003). Copyright 2003 by The Guilford Press. Reprinted by permission.

areas of functioning and specific behaviors that will presumably be affected by the medication. Because measures will be collected in a repeated fashion (e.g., daily or weekly) throughout the medication trial, relatively brief instruments are preferred. Typically, assessment measures will include brief behavior ratings completed by teachers and parents, self-report questionnaires, direct observations of classroom and/or playground behavior, and permanent products (e.g., completion and accuracy on assigned schoolwork).

Measures addressing side effects (e.g., brief ratings completed by parent, teacher, and student) should be included, especially if possible adverse events (e.g., impairment of cognitive functioning) could occur during the school day. A popular method to detect side effects is to ask teachers, parents, or children about the frequency and/or severity of physical symptoms, behaviors, emotions, or cognitions that have been found associated with a specific medication in prior cases. For example, Barkley (1990) developed a brief rating scale for evaluating possible side effects of stimulant medication that has been used for both clinical and research purposes. It is important to note that the side-effect profile in a specific case may differ depending on who is asked to report these. DuPaul, Anastopoulos, Kwasnik, Barkley, and McMurray (1996) found that children reported more severe side effects of methylphenidate (relative to placebo conditions) than did parents or teachers. The ideal strategy would be to obtain side-effect ratings from parents, teachers, *and* students, although this is not feasible in all cases. In the case of potential adverse effects on academic or cognitive functioning, assessment measures might include brief cognitive tests, academic achievement tests, curriculum-based measurement probes, or permanent products reflecting these domains (e.g., classwork completed by the student). Further, side effects need to be assessed during both medication and nonmedication conditions, as behaviors or symptoms that could be interpreted as "side effects" may, in some cases, be present prior to treatment.

Data need to be collected during baseline (or nonmedication) conditions, as well as during each active dosage condition. Further, it is important to consider the time-response properties of a medication when scheduling data collection. For example, the behavioral effects of short-acting stimulants (e.g., methylphenidate) are typically evident beginning about 30–45 minutes after ingestion, with peak behavioral effects occurring between 1.5 and 3 hours postingestion. Thus classroom observations would be timed to occur during the "window" of peak effects. In contrast to stimulants, most psychotropic medications (e.g., fluoxetine) need to be taken for several days or weeks before behavioral effects can be observed (for details, see Brown, Carpenter, & Simerly, 2005), so the assessment protocol should be designed accordingly.

Once data collection across the prescribed dosage conditions is complete, information should be summarized in a graph or table (i.e., as concisely as possible) for communication to the physician and parents. Data are used to identify the optimal dosage, which is generally the lowest dose associated with the greatest improvement and fewest side effects (see Power et al., 2003). Typically, the school psychologist would highlight medication effects on one or two keystone measures that may best represent academic (e.g., curriculum-based measurement probes) and behavioral (e.g., brief teacher behavior ratings) functioning. If treatment with medication is implemented following the initial evaluation trial, then long-term effects should

be assessed by periodically repeating data collection. For example, children placed on medication across several school years might undergo an annual reevaluation of this treatment by assessing current and alternate dosages (possibly including no medication) some time during the middle of the school year after the student has adjusted to the new classroom and the teacher is familiar with his or her behavior. Another alternative would be to assess medication effects in a more continuous fashion through ongoing brief monitoring of symptomatic behaviors and school functioning.

Summary and Conclusions

Psychotropic medication is increasingly used to treat a variety of behavior and social–emotional disorders in children and adolescents. Although the neurophysiological effects of psychoactive compounds are not fully known, there is a growing literature documenting their impact on various neurotransmitters. Psychopharmacological interventions have been found successful in treating a variety of externalizing and internalizing disorders, with the most extensive evidence supporting the use of stimulants to treat ADHD. The specific effects of psychotropic medication on school performance, particularly regarding academic achievement, are essentially unknown, except, again, with respect to stimulants.

School psychologists can support the effective use of psychopharmacological interventions in at least two ways. First, school psychologists can assist physicians and parents in determining whether medication is a necessary treatment for a specific student, particularly in the context of other (e.g., psychosocial and educational) interventions that might be warranted. Second, school psychologists can collect data to document whether a specific medication is effective in changing behavior and functional impairments, as well as to determine which dosage is optimal with respect to both behavioral change and minimal adverse side effects. Given that medication treatment has an important impact on school performance, it will be critical for the field of school psychology to increase attention to this issue from both a research and training perspective.

Acknowledgment

Preparation of this chapter was supported, in part, by National Institute of Mental Health grant No. R01-MH62941.

References

Albano, A. M., Chorpita, B. F., & Barlow, D. H. (2003). *Childhood anxiety disorders*. New York: Guilford Press.

Aman, M. G., Marks, R. E., Turbott, S. H., Wilsher, C. P., & Merry S. N. (1991). Clinical effects of methylphenidate and thioridazine in intellectually subaverage children. *Journal of the American Academy of Child and Adolescent Psychiatry, 30,* 246–256.

American Academy of Pediatrics. (2001). Clinical practice guideline: Treatment of the school-aged child with attention-deficit/hyperactivity disorder. *Pediatrics, 108,* 1033–1044.

American Psychiatric Association. (1980). *Diagnostic and statistical manual of mental disorders* (3rd ed.). Washington, DC: Author.

American Psychiatric Association. (2000). *Diagnostic and statistical manual of mental disorders* (4th ed., text rev,). Washington, DC: Author.

Arnold, L. E., Elliott, M., Sachs, L., Bird, H., Kraemer, H. C., Wells, K. C., et al. (2003). Effects of ethnicity on treatment attendance, stimulant response/dose, and 14-month outcome in ADHD. *Journal of Consulting and Clinical Psychology, 71,* 713–727.

Barkley, R. A. (1990). *Attention-deficit/hyperactivity disorder: A clinical workbook*. New York: Guilford Press.

Barzman, D. H., & Findling, R. L. (2008). Pharmacological treatment of pathologic aggression in children. *International Review of Psychiatry, 20,* 151–157.

Biederman, J., Mick, E., Hammerness, P., Harpold, T., Aleardi, M., Dougherty, M., et al. (2005). Open-label, 8-week trial of olanzapine and risperidone for the treatment of bipolar disorder in preschool children. *Biological Psychiatry, 58,* 589–594.

Biederman, J., Mick, E., Wozniak, M. A., Aleardi, M., Spencer, T., & Faraone, S. V. (2005). An open-label trial of risperidone in children and adolescents with bipolar disorder. *Journal of Child and Adolescent Psychopharmacology, 15,* 311–317.

Birmaher, B., Axelson, D. A., Monk, K., Kalas, C., Clark, D. B., Ehmann, M., et al. (2003). Fluoxetine for the treatment of childhood anxiety disorders. *Journal of the American Academy of Child and Adolescent Psychiatry, 42,* 415–423.

Birmaher, B., Waterman, S., Ryan, N. D., Perel, J., McNabb, J., Balach, L., et al. (1998). Randomized, controlled trial of amitriptyline versus placebo for adolescents with treatment-resistant major depression. *Journal of the American Academy of Child and Adolescent Psychiatry, 37,* 527–535.

Bown, C. D., Wang, J. F., & Young, L. T. (2003). Attenuation of N-methyl-D-aspartate-mediated cytoplasmic vacuolization in primary rat hippocampal neurons by mood stabilizers. *Neuroscience, 117,* 949–955.

Brown, R. T., Antonuccio, D. O., DuPaul, G. J., Fristad, M. A., King, C. A., Leslie, L. K., et al. (2007). *Childhood mental health disorders: Evidence base and contextual factors for psychosocial, psychopharmacological, and combined interventions*. Washington, DC: American Psychological Association.

Brown, R. T., Carpenter, L. A., & Simerly, E. (2005). *Mental health medications for children*. New York: Guilford Press.

Chamberlain, S. R., Robbins, T. W., & Sahakian, B. J. (2007). The neurobiology of attention-deficit/hyperactivity disorder. *Biological Psychiatry, 61,* 1317–1319.

Connor, D. F. (2006). Stimulants. In R. A. Barkley (Ed.), *Attention-deficit/hyperactivity disorder: A handbook for diagnosis and treatment* (3rd ed., pp. 608–647). New York: Guilford Press.

Costello, E. J., Mustillo, S., Erkanli, A., Keeler, G., & Angold, A. (2003). Prevalence and development of psychiatric disorders in childhood and adolescence. *Archives of General Psychiatry, 60,* 837–844.

DeBar, L. L., Lynch, F., Powell, J., & Gale, J. (2003). Use of psychotropic agents in preschool children: Associated symptoms, diagnoses, and health care services in a health maintenance organization. *Archives of Pediatric and Adolescent Medicine, 157,* 150–157.

Delbello, M. P., Findling, R. L., Kushner, S., Wang, D., Olson, W. H., Capece, J. A., et al. (2005). A pilot controlled trial of topiramate for mania in children and adolescents with bipolar disorder. *Journal of the American Academy of Child and Adolescent Psychiatry, 44,* 539–547.

DuPaul, G. J., Anastopoulos, A. D., Kwasnik, D., Barkley, R. A., & McMurray, M. B. (1996). Methylphenidate effects on children with attention-deficit/hyperactivity disorder: Self-report of symptoms, side effects, and self-esteem. *Journal of Attention Disorders, 1,* 3–15.

DuPaul, G. J., & Carlson, J. S. (2005). Child psychopharmacology: How school psychologists can contribute to effective outcomes. *School Psychology Quarterly, 20,* 206–221.

DuPaul, G. J., Power, T. J., Anastopoulos, A. D., & Reid, R. (1998). *ADHD Rating Scale-IV: Checklists, norms, and clinical interpretation.* New York: Guilford Press.

Eggers, C., Bunk, D., & Krause, D. (2000). Schizophrenia with onset before the age of eleven: Clinical characteristics of onset and course. *Journal of Autism and Developmental Disorders, 30,* 29–38.

Emslie, G. J., Kratochvil, C., Vitello, B., Silva, S., Mayes, T., McNulty, S., et al. (2006). Treatment for Adolescents with Depression Study (TADS): Safety results. *Journal of the American Academy of Child and Adolescent Psychiatry, 45,* 1440–1445.

Emslie, G. J., Heiligenstein, J. H., Wagner, K. D., Hoog, S. L., Ernsest, D. E., Brown, E., et al. (2002). Fluoxetine for acute treatment of depression in children and adolescents: A placebo-controlled, randomized clinical trial. *Journal of the American Academy of Child and Adolescent Psychiatry, 41,* 1205–1214.

Emslie, G. J., Rust, A., Weinberg, W. A., Kowatch, R. A., Hughes, C. W., Carmody, T., et al. (1997). A double-blind, randomized, placebo-controlled trial of fluoxetine in children and adolescents with depression. *Archives of General Psychiatry, 54,* 1031–1037.

Faraone, S. V., Wigal, S. B., & Hodgkins, P. (2007). Forecasting three-month outcomes in a laboratory school comparison of mixed amphetamine salts and extended release (Adderall XR) and atomoxetine (Strattera) in school-aged children with ADHD. *Journal of Attention Disorders, 11,* 74–82.

Gadow, K. D., Nolan, E. E., Paolicelli, L. M., & Sprafkin, J. (1991). A procedure for assessing the effects of methylphenidate on hyperactive children in public school settings. *Journal of Clinical Child Psychology, 20,* 268–276.

Gaffney, G. R., Perry, P. J., Lund, B. C., Bever-Stille, K. A., Arndt, S., & Kuperman, S. (2002). Risperidone versus clonidine in the treatment of children and adolescents with Tourette's syndrome. *Journal of the American Academy of Child and Adolescent Psychiatry, 41,* 330–336.

Geller, B., Cooper, T. B., Sun, K., Zimerman, B., Frazier, J., Williams, M., et al. (1998). Double-blind and placebo-controlled study of lithium for adolescent bipolar disorders with secondary substance dependency. *Journal of the American Academy of Child and Adolescent Psychiatry, 37,* 171–178.

Geller, D. A., Biederman, J., Stewart, S. E., Mullin, B., Martin, A., Spencer, T., et al. (2003). Which SSRI? A meta-analysis of pharmacotherapy trials in pediatric obsessive–compulsive disorder. *American Journal of Psychiatry, 160,* 1919–1928.

Geller, D. A., Hoog, S. L., Heiligenstein, J. H., Ricardi, R. K., Tamura, R., Kluszynski, S., et al. (2001). Fluoxetine treatment for obsessive–compulsive disorder in children and adolescents: A placebo-controlled trial. *Journal of the American Academy of Child and Adolescent Psychiatry, 40,* 773–779.

Graae, F., Milner, J., Rizzotto, L., & Klein, R. G. (1994). Clonazepam in childhood anxiety. *Journal of the American Academy of Child and Adolescent Psychiatry, 33,* 372–376.

Grace, A. A. (2001). Psychostimulant actions on dopamine and limbic system function: Relevance to the pathophysiology and treatment of ADHD. In M. V. Solanto, A. F. T. Arnsten, & F. X. Castellanos (Eds.), *Stimulant drugs and ADHD: Basic and clinical neuroscience* (pp. 134–157). New York: Oxford University Press.

Grunder, G., Vernaleken, I., Muller, M. J., Davids, E., Heydari, N., Buchholz, H. G., et al. (2003). Subchronic haloperidol downregulates dopamine synthesis capacity in the brain of schizophrenic patients in vivo. *Neurosychopharmacology, 28,* 787–794.

Gureasko-Moore, D., DuPaul, G. J., & Power, T. J. (2005). Stimulant treatment for attention-deficit/hyperactivity disorder: Medication monitoring practices of school psychologists. *School Psychology Review, 34,* 232–245.

HaileMariam, A., Bradley-Johnson, S., & Johnson, C. M. (2002). Pediatricians' preferences for ADHD information from schools. *School Psychology Review, 31,* 94–105.

Hazell, P., O'Connell, D., Heathcote, D., Robertson, J., & Henry, D. (1995). Efficacy of tricyclic drugs in treating child and adolescent depression: A meta-analysis. *British Journal of Psychiatry, 310,* 897–901.

Ipser, J., & Stein, D. J. (2007). Systematic review of pharmacotherapy of disruptive behavior disorders in children and adolescents. *Psychopharmacology, 191,* 127–140.

Jensen, P. S., Youngstrom, E. A., Steiner, H., Findling, R. L., Meyer, R. E., Malone, R. P., et al. (2007). Consensus report on impulsive aggression as a symptom across diagnostic categories in child psychiatry: Implications for medication studies. *Journal of the American Academy of Child and Adolescent Psychiatry, 46,* 309–322.

Kafantaris, V., Coletti, D. J., Dicker, R., Padula, G., Pleak, R. R., Alvir, J., et al. (2004). Lithium treatment of acute mania in adolescents: A placebo-controlled discontinuation study. *Journal of the American Academy of Child and Adolescent Psychiatry, 43,* 984–993.

Kainz, K. (2002). Barriers and enhancements to physician–psychologist collaboration. *Profes-

sional Psychology: Research and Practice, 33, 169–175.

Keller, M. G., Ryan, N. D., & Strober, M. (2001). Efficacy of paroxetine in the treatment of adolescent major depression: A randomized, controlled trial. *Journal of the American Academy of Child and Adolescent Psychiatry, 40*, 762–772.

King, N. J., Muris, P., & Ollendick, T. H. (2004). *Specific phobia.* In T. L. Morris & J. S. March (Eds.), *Anxiety disorders in children and adolescents* (2nd ed., pp. 263–279). New York: Guilford Press.

Klein, R. G., Abikoff, H., Klass, E., Gancles, D., Seese, L. M., & Pollack, S. (1997). Clinical efficacy of methylphenidate in conduct disorder with and without attention-deficit/hyperactivity disorder. *Archives of General Psychiatry, 54*, 1073–1080.

Kratochvil, C., Emslie, G., Silva, S., McNulty, S., Walkup, J., Curry, J., et al. (2006). Acute time to response in the Treatment for Adolescents with Depression Study (TADS). *Journal of the American Academy of Child and Adolescent Psychiatry, 45*, 1412–1418.

Kratochvil, C. J., Wilens, T. E., Greenhill, L. L., Gao, H., Baker, K. D., Feldman, P. D., et al. (2006). Effects of long-term atomoxetine treatment for young children with attention-deficit/hyperactivity disorder. *Journal of the American Academy of Child and Adolescent Psychiatry, 45*, 919–927.

Kye, C. H., Waterman, G. S., Ryan, N. D., Birmaher, B., Williamson, E., Iyengar, S., et al. (1996). A randomized, controlled trial of amitriptyline in the acute treatment of adolescent major depression. *Journal of the American Academy of Child and Adolescent Psychiatry, 35*, 1139–1144.

Lewinsohn, P. M., Klein, D. N., & Seeley, J. R. (1995). Bipolar disorders in a community sample of older adolescents: Prevalence, phenomenology, comorbidity, and course. *Journal of the American Academy of Child and Adolescent Psychiatry, 34*, 454–463.

Lewinsohn, P. M., Rohde, P., & Seeley, J. R. (1998). Major depressive disorder in older adolescents: Prevalence, risk factors, and clinical implications. *Clinical Psychology Review, 18*, 765–794.

Mash, E. J., & Barkley, R. A. (2007). *Assessment of childhood disorders* (4th ed.). New York: Guilford Press.

McIntosh, D. E., & Trotter, J. S. (2006). Early onset bipolar spectrum disorder: Psychopharmacological, psychological, and educational management. *Psychology in the Schools, 43*, 451–460.

MTA Cooperative Group. (1999). A 14-month randomized clinical trial of treatment strategies for attention-deficit/hyperactivity disorder. *Archives of General Psychiatry, 56*, 1073–1086.

MTA Cooperative Group. (2004). National Institute of Mental Health multimodal treatment study of ADHD follow-up: 24-month outcomes of treatment strategies for attention-deficit/hyperactivity disorder. *Pediatrics, 113*, 754–761.

Olfson, M., Marcus, S. C., Weissman, M. M., & Jensen, P. S. (2002). National trends in the use of psychotropic medications by children. *Journal of the American Academy of Child and Adolescent Psychiatry, 41*, 514–521.

Pappadopulos, E., Woolston, S., Chait, A., Perkins, M., Connor, D. F., & Jensen, P. S. (2006). Pharmacotherapy of aggression in children and adolescents: Efficacy and effect size. *Journal of the Canadian Academy of Child and Adolescent Psychiatry, 15*, 27–36.

Pardo, R., Andreolotti, A. G., Ramos, B., Picatoste, F., & Claro, E. (2003). Opposed effects of lithium on the MEK–ERK pathway in neural cells: Inhibition in astrocytes and stimulation in neurons by GSK3 independent mechanisms. *Journal of Neurochemistry, 87*, 417–426.

Parikh, M. S., Kolevzon, A., & Hollander, E. (2008). Psychopharmacology of aggression in children and adolescents with autism: A critical review of efficacy and tolerability. *Journal of Child and Adolescent Psychopharmacology, 18*, 157–178.

Pavuluri, M. N., Henry, D. B., Carbray, J. A., Sampson, G., Naylor, M. W., & Janicak, P. G. (2004). Open-label prospective trial of risperidone in combination with lithium or divalproex sodium in pediatric mania. *Journal of Affective Disorders, 82S*, S103–S111.

Pearson, D. A., Santos, C. W., Roache, J. D., Casat, C. D., Loveland, K. A., Lachar, D., et al. (2003). Treatment effects of methylphenidate on behavioral adjustment in children with mental retardation and ADHD. *Journal of the American Academy of Child and Adolescent Psychiatry, 42*, 209–216.

Pelham, W. E., Gnagy, E. M., Greiner, A. R., Hoza, B., Hinshaw, S. P., Swanson, J. M., et al. (2000). Behavioral versus behavioral and pharmacological treatment in ADHD children attending a summer camp program. *Journal of Abnormal Child Psychology, 28*, 507–525.

Perrine, D. M. (1996). *The chemistry of mind-altering drugs: History, pharmacology, and cultural context.* Washington, DC: American Chemical Society.

Physicians' desk reference (58th ed.). (2004). Montvale, NJ: Thomson PDR.

Pine, D. S., Walkup, J. T., Labellarte, M. J., Riddle, M. A., Greenhill, L., Klein, R., et al. (2001). Fluvoxamine for the treatment of anxiety disorders in children and adolescents. *New England Journal of Medicine, 344,* 1279–1285.

Power, T. J., DuPaul, G. J., Shapiro, E. S., & Kazak, A. E. (2003). *Promoting children's health: Integrating health, school, family, and community systems.* New York: Guilford Press.

Rapport, M. D., Denney, C., DuPaul, G. J., & Gardner, M. J. (1994). Attention-deficit disorder and methylphenidate: Normalization rates, clinical effectiveness, and response prediction in 76 children. *Journal of the American Academy of Child and Adolescent Psychiatry, 33,* 883–893.

Reinblatt, S. P., & Walkup, J. T. (2005). Psychopharmacologic treatment of pediatric anxiety disorders. *Child and Adolescent Psychiatric Clinics of North America, 14,* 877–908.

Rey, J. M., & Martin, A. (2006). Selective serotonin reuptake inhibitors and suicidality in juveniles: Review of the evidence and implications for clinical practice. *Child and Adolescent Psychiatric Clinics of North America, 15,* 221–237.

Safer, D. J., & Zito, J. M. (2000). Pharmacoepidemiology of methylphenidate and other stimulants for the treatment of attention-deficit/hyperactivity disorder. In L. L. Greenhill & B. B. Osman (Eds.), *Ritalin: Theory and practice* (2nd ed., pp. 7–26). New York: Mary Ann Liebert.

Safer, D. J., Zito, J. M., & dosReis, S. (2003). Concomitant psychotropic medication for youths. *American Journal of Psychiatry, 160,* 438–449.

Safer, D. J., Zito, J. M., & Gardner, J. F. (2004). Comparative prevalence of psychotropic medications among youths enrolled in the SCHIP and privately insured youths. *Psychiatric Services, 55,* 1049–1051.

Sheridan, S. M., Kratochwill, T. R., & Bergan, J. (1996). *Conjoint behavioral consultation: A procedural manual.* New York: Plenum.

Simeon, J. G., Ferguson, H. B., Knott, V., Roberts, N., Gauthier, B., Dubois, C., et al. (1992). Clinical, cognitive, and neurophysiological effects of alprazolam in children and adolescents with overanxious and avoidant disorders. *Journal of the American Academy of Child and Adolescent Psychiatry, 31,* 29–33.

Sprague, R. K., & Sleator, E. K. (1977). Methylphenidate in hyperkinetic children: Differences in dose effects on learning and social behavior. *Science, 198,* 1274–1276.

Starr, H. L., & Kemner, J. (2005). Multicenter, randomized, open-label study of OROS methyphenidate versus atomoxetine: Treatment

outcomes in African-American children with ADHD. *Journal of the National Medical Association, 97,* S11–S16.

Stein, D. J., & Seedat, S. (2004). Unresolved questions about treatment-resistant anxiety disorders. *CNS Spectrums, 9,* 715.

Strange, P. G. (2001). Antipsychotic drugs: Importance of dopamine receptors for mechanisms of therapeutic actions and side effects. *Pharmacology Review, 53,* 119–133.

Treatment for Adolescents with Depression Study Team. (2004). Fluoxetine, cognitive-behavioral therapy, and their combination for adolescents with depression: TADS randomized controlled trial. *Journal of the American Medical Association, 292,* 807–820.

Trenton, A., Currier, G., & Zwemer, F. (2003). Fatalities associated with therapeutic use and overdose of atypical antipsychotics. *CNS Drugs, 17,* 307–324.

U.S. Department of Education Office of Special Education Programs. (2005). *25th annual report to Congress on the implementation of the Individuals with Disabilities Education Act.* Washington, DC: Author.

Verduin, T. L., & Kendall, P. C. (2003). Differential occurrence of comorbidity within childhood anxiety disorders. *Journal of Clinical Child and Adolescent Psychology, 32,* 290–295.

Vitiello, B., & Swedo, S. (2004). Antidepressant medications in children. *New England Journal of Medicine, 350,* 1489–1491.

Volpe, R. J., Heick, P. F., & Gureasko-Moore, D. (2005). An agile behavioral model for monitoring the effects of stimulant medication in school settings. *Psychology in the Schools, 42,* 509–523.

Wagner, K. D. (2005). Pharmacotherapy for major depression in children and adolescents. *Progress in Neuro-Psychopharmacology and Biological Psychiatry, 29,* 819–826.

Wagner, K. D., Ambrosini, P., Rynn, M., Wohlberg, C., Yang, R., Greenbaum, M., et al. (2003). Efficacy of sertraline in the treatment of children and adolescents with major depressive disorder. *Journal of the American Medical Association, 290,* 1033–1041.

Wagner, K. D., Kowatch, R. A., Emslie, G. J., Findling, R. L., Wilens, T. E., McCague, K., et al. (2006). A double-blind, randomized, placebo-controlled trial of oxcarbazepine in the treatment of bipolar disorder in children and adolescents. *American Journal of Psychiatry, 163,* 1179–1186.

Wagner, K. D., Robb, A. S., Findling, R. L., Jin, J., Gutierrez, M., & Heydorn, W. E. (2004). A randomized, placebo-controlled trial of citalopram for the treatment of major depression in children and adolescents. *American Journal of Psychiatry, 161*, 1079–1083.

Wagner, K. D., Weller, E. B., Carlson, G. A., Sachs, G., Biederman, J., Frazier, J. A., et al. (2002). An open-label trial of divalproex in children and adolescents with bipolar disorder. *Journal of the American Academy of Child and Adolescent Psychiatry, 41*, 1224–1230.

Weckerly, J. (2002). Pediatric bipolar mood disorder. *Developmental and Behavioral Pediatrics, 23*, 42–56.

Weyandt, L. L. (2006). *The physiological bases of cognitive and behavioral disorders.* Mahwah, NJ: Erlbaum.

Williams, J., Klinepeter, K., Palmes, G., Pulley, A., & Foy, J. M. (2004). Diagnosis and treatment of behavioral health disorders in pediatric practice. *Pediatrics, 114*, 601–606.

Wittchen, H.-U. (2002). Generalized anxiety disorder: Prevalence, burden, and cost to society. *Depression and Anxiety, 16*, 162–171.

Zito, J. M., Safer, D. J., dosReis, S., Gardner, J. F., Boles, M., & Lynch, F. (2000). Trends in the prescribing of psychotropic medications to preschoolers. *Journal of the American Medical Association, 283*, 1025–1030.

Zito, J. M., Safer, D. J., dosReis, S., Gardner, J. F., Magder, L., Soeken, K., et al. (2003). Psychotropic practice patterns for youth: A 10-year perspective. *Archives of Pediatric and Adolescent Medicine, 157*, 17–25.

Zito, J. M., Safer, D. J., Sai, D., Gardner, J. F., Thomas, D., Coombes, P., et al. (2008). Psychotropic medication practice patterns among youth in foster care. *Pediatrics, 121*, 157–163.

PART V

EVALUATING INTERVENTIONS

Chapter 29

Summarizing, Evaluating, and Drawing Inferences from Intervention Data

Edward J. Daly III
David W. Barnett
Sara Kupzyk
Kristi L. Hofstadter
Elizabeth Barkley

School psychologists bring specialized knowledge to intervention planning by assisting school teams with problem solving, which is an inquiry process that requires a series of decisions. Decision *reliability* refers to consistency of decisions from problem solving and data analysis. Decision *validity* is about marshaling evidence to support professional actions and evaluating actions by their outcomes and consequences (e.g., Messick, 1995). The behavioral practice methods discussed in this chapter can improve decisions concerning students' needs by improving inferences about intervention data. The difference between a sound and an unsound plan creates *consequences* for children and those who help them. Effective plans reduce or even eliminate the need for more intensive, individualized, sometimes stigmatizing, and costly services or placements. Plans not well carried out or that do not work may move children further away from the objectives of schooling and cost all concerned, such as parents and teachers, in time and trust in and enthusiasm for future efforts at intervention. Questions about instructional and behavioral plans are addressed by organizing and analyzing technically adequate intervention data and improving data-based inferences about the data.

Many of the foundations of behavioral practice also are key characteristics of response to intervention (RTI), a service delivery option intended to improve decisions about students' education appearing in the Individuals with Disabilities Education Act of 2004 (IDEA; see Ervin, Gimpel Peacock, & Merrell, Chapter 1, and Hawkins, Barnett, Morrison, & Musti-Rao, Chapter 2, this volume). In RTI, decision reliability and validity are based on tiered and sequential interventions, ruling out questions about a lack of effective instruction as an alternative explanation to specific learning disability, finding and applying an optimal amount of intervention strength to bring about desired changes in a child's performance or behavior, and then using that information as evaluation data (Batsche et al., 2005; Gresham, 2007).

Both behavioral practice and RTI include step-by-step approaches to intervention planning and evaluation that require use of the data analysis methods discussed in this chapter. The basics serve as a general model: (1) current performance is measured through universal screening to evaluate risk status; (2) a prevention or intervention plan is developed; (3) data collection is organized to evaluate specific prevention or intervention questions; (4) the plan is evaluated by comparing results with baseline data and benchmarks for success; and (5) the information is used to decide next steps and needed resources. Even if a student is deemed "responsive," teams want to see whether and how rapidly students can "catch up" to peers and be successful in typical environments. If a student's data show a lack of positive response, teams may want to evaluate functional hypotheses related to the student's skill or performance that require different instructional strategies. Teams may want to try out several interventions to look for the strongest intervention alternative. Through problem solving, teams select, modify, or change interventions to maximize success. Shared between behavioral practice and RTI is the basic question of how students *respond* to an intervention to move to the next decision point or tier.

Once intervention data have been generated, meaning is ascribed to the results. This is the *interpretive task* within the problem-solving model. The way this is done is fundamentally different from the interpretive task for other forms of assessment. For example, a psychodiagnostic approach generates data that have very different qualities from those of data from direct assessment to attempt to answer questions about the child's status with regard to constructs such as learning disabilities. In the psychodiagnostic assessment process, emphasis is placed on whether one arrives at a correct classification at one point in time: Does the child have a learning disability or not? Alternately, when intervention data are interpreted, inferences are explicitly tied to actions that should lead to problem resolution for an educational setting (rather than just determining whether a child has a condition or not). There are two direct benefits of high-quality intervention data. Teams can carefully evaluate problem-solving efforts, and RTI allows intervention outcome data from tiers and problem solving to be used as evaluation data to help directly with special education decisions.

The interpretive task dealt with in this chapter builds on all steps in the problem-solving sequence but is specific to the point at which the school psychologist is ready to evaluate the effectiveness of an intervention. Therefore, the assumption is that a sound data set already exists for interpreta-

tion drawing on other chapters dealing with selecting variables for change (i.e., target variables; Hawkins et al., Chapter 2, this volume) and specific considerations for academic and social intervention (the topics of other chapters in this volume).

The purpose of this chapter is to provide guidance on data interpretation and to highlight issues that increase or decrease the reliability and validity of decisions regarding intervention effect so that school psychologists have the knowledge to plan in advance, to react appropriately when problems arise, and to plan what to do next based on the intervention dataset. A focal point of the chapter is how to establish a design prior to data collection so that the results are interpretable. With an appropriate design and high-quality data in place, interpretation of intervention data can be framed as four questions that guide subsequent professional actions. These questions, which appear in Table 29.1, reveal different aspects of the data to which school psychologists must pay attention if they want to help solve the problem.

Question 1: Is There an Effect?

The first question is whether a change in behavior occurred (the effect), which needs to be answered either "yes" or "no." The school psychologist may look at a graph containing measures of behavior prior to intervention (referred to as a baseline or control condition) and during intervention and decide either that behavior changed in the desired direction or it did not. The reality, however, is that this decision may or may not correspond to the actual state of affairs; whether it is correct or not is affected by a number of factors. Therefore, decision errors may occur if the data do not accurately represent what is really happening or if the school psychologist pays attention to the wrong characteris-

TABLE 29.1. The Interpretive Task

1. Is there an effect?
2. What produced the effect?
3. How generalizable is the effect?
4. What should be done next?

tics when "reading" the data. The accuracy of decision outcomes can be represented as a two-by-two contingency table (see Table 29.2). The most desirable situation is one in which the problem-solving or RTI team correctly decides that an intervention is effective when it is indeed effective (Cell A in Table 29.2). It is important, although a less desirable outcome, that the team decide that an intervention is ineffective when it is, in fact, ineffective (Cell D). These decisions are valid ones and serve as a point of departure for decisions about whether to withdraw an intervention, keep it in place, modify it in some way, or change the intervention altogether (a topic discussed in relation to Question 4, "What should be done next?").

Unfortunately, error can always creep in when psychosocial variables are measured and judgments are made based on those measurements. In some cases, the school psychologist may determine that there was an effect when, in fact, none occurred (Cell B, a Type I error in hypothesis-testing terms), or he or she may decide that there was no effect when in fact one occurred (Cell C, a Type II error in hypothesis-testing terms). The goal is to minimize these errors so that one can arrive at correct decisions about (1) the size and significance of the effect, (2) what caused the effect (or lack of effect), (3) how widespread the effect is (generalization of the effect across time and to all relevant situations), and (4) what should be done next. The risk of making inaccurate, invalid, and incorrect decisions that adversely affect children's educational opportunities (and therefore their learning trajectories) is the reason that it is critical to make valid decisions, which can be done by carefully following established interpretive guidelines prior to taking action.

Two prominent factors that influence the accuracy of decisions are the *design* one uses for detecting behavioral effects and the interpretive *method* for estimating effects. A poor choice of design diminishes one's chances of finding a true effect and will cause educators to have to change or intensify interventions unnecessarily, whereas a good choice will prompt educators to make necessary instructional adjustments. Therefore, a good design is sensitive to intervention effects when they truly occur (Lipsey, 1990). A good design choice with the right intervention might even reduce efforts in the long run. For example, finding that a simple intervention such as a parent practicing reading at home with his or her child is effective may reduce the need for a more complex intervention, such as a small group outside the classroom.

The Role of Design Choice in Interpreting Effect

Single-case designs (Bailey & Burch, 2002; Kazdin, 1982; Kennedy, 2005; Sidman, 1960), including the A/B design and a variety of experimental designs, are especially well suited to detecting behavioral effects when they occur. When reliable and valid indicators of important educational and developmental behavioral targets are chosen, repeated measures allow school psychologists to react to data over time by maintaining, changing, or withdrawing interventions. The use of these designs for making decisions about what caused the effect is discussed in the next section. Our purpose here is to examine their use for determining whether an effect actually occurred.

The simplest version of the single-case design is a case-study design, commonly referred to as the A/B design, which involves two phases. In the first phase, A baseline, the target behavior is measured repeatedly prior to treatment. In the second phase, B, an intervention is introduced and the target response is again continuously measured. The purpose of the baseline phase is to predict what the natural course of behavior would be if the treatment were not introduced. It should contain (and therefore control for) all the same variables as those present in the intervention phase except for the intervention

TABLE 29.2. Decision Outcomes: Correct and Incorrect Interpretations of Intervention Data for Behavioral Effect

Interpretive conclusion	True effect ("reality")	
	Yes	No
Yes	Correct	Incorrect (Type I error)
	A	B
No	Incorrect (Type II error)	Correct
	C	D

itself. When an intervention is introduced, the intervention should be the only factor that changes between phases.

A/B designs are often used in applied settings because practitioners are more concerned about whether a change in behavior occurred than about demonstrating that the treatment caused the change in behavior (Miltenberger, 2008). Although it is not a true research design, it is the "workhorse" of basic accountability (Bloom, Fischer, & Orme, 2005). The A/B design provides a good means of evaluating whether an empirically established treatment is working for an individual. According to Bushell and Baer (1994), "measurably superior instruction means close, continual contact with outcome data that are made relevant by attentive, responsive audiences" (p. 9). The requirements of the A/B design—use of repeated measures over time with systematic changes in intervention conditions as warranted by the results—allows one to stay in close, continual contact with outcome data. The team's *attentiveness and responsiveness* to the results is vital to producing superior instruction, as well as to making meaningful changes in social behaviors. Responsiveness to results should not be merely a reactive and haphazard process. The school psychologist should draw from available tools for data interpretation, including structured guidelines for visual interpretation of data and, where appropriate, statistical methods for evaluating effects, each of which is discussed next.

Visual Analysis of Effects

Plotting results directly on a graph allows educators and stakeholders (e.g., parents) to obtain a firsthand view of the raw data for themselves without any mediating influences or need for understanding complex statistical assumptions (Bailey & Burch, 2002). There are important steps and contextual guidelines for visual analysis, but not rigid or formal decision rules for interpretation (Brossart, Parker, Olson, & Mahadevan, 2006). Graphed data should be inspected for changes in level, trend, and/or variability both within (e.g., What are the data like in baseline?) and across phases (e.g., How do data in intervention compare with baseline?; Cooper, Heron, & Heward, 2007; Parsonson & Baer, 1986, 1992). *Level* refers to the

central location of data within a phase and is often represented as the mean or median (Franklin, Gorman, Beasley, & Allison, 1996). Drawing a horizontal line through the mean of the results in a baseline or intervention phase generally gives the clearest depiction of the central location of data (if the data are sufficient and there are not one or several "odd" data points). One needs to be careful, however, about overinterpreting level, because trend(s) and variability in the data may be more important characteristics of a given dataset. *Trend* refers to how the central location shifts over time within a phase (Franklin et al., 1996). Trend is readily seen when there is acceleration (consistent increases) or deceleration (consistent decreases) in the data points within the phase. If a line is drawn to represent the data such that variability in the data points is temporarily ignored and the line is projecting upward (acceleration) or downward (deceleration), the data have a trend. Data on graphs usually represent trend using the least-squares regression method with spreadsheets like Microsoft Excel. *Variability* refers to deviations above and below level (Franklin et al., 1996). When data points are close to the mean, there is little variability in the phase. When data points vary considerably from the mean and from one another, variability becomes a dominating feature of the dataset, and understanding the reason for variability may be a goal (e.g., speculating about why both high and low performance occur in the same condition).

Characteristics of the data within phases are interesting and important. But the purpose of intervention is to change behavior by changing conditions, which means that level, trend, and, in some cases, variability should change *across* phases in desired directions (Cooper et al., 2007). Therefore, level, trend, and variability of the data should be directly compared across baseline and intervention phases (Parsonson & Baer, 1992). For academic interventions, an increase in level between baseline and intervention is desirable. However, because academic interventions target skilled behaviors that usually grow slowly and cumulatively over time, an increasing trend during the intervention is often a more realistic expectation. The same is true of appropriate behaviors such as social skills, which usually require explicit instruction. For appropriate social behaviors that are already in the student's repertoire but do not occur frequently enough during baseline, a more immediate change in behavior might be achievable. In this case, a successful intervention would lead to a change in level between conditions. Some behavioral interventions will target reductions in inappropriate behavior. Because these behaviors are generally under the direct control of environmental contingencies, a strong intervention should be capable of producing a relatively immediate change in level of responding. Some interventions may simply produce slower effects and result in a changing trend over time toward desirable levels of behavior.

Variability within and across phases may be a prominent feature of the data that needs to be addressed. For example, an intervention that reduces variability in such a way that behavior occurs more consistently at a desirable level is judged to be effective. On the other hand, a less effective intervention is one that increases variability such that some data points reach or approach desirable levels whereas other data points deviate substantially in the undesired direction. This latter scenario should lead to an investigation of the reasons that behavior is so variable (Parsonson & Baer, 1992). Inconsistent implementation of the intervention, unreliable measurement, and fluctuating motivating conditions as a result of satiation (e.g., rewards have become stale or uninteresting) or deprivation (e.g., lack of attention or stimulation prior to problem situations) are major culprits when this happens. The key is to figure out why the intervention is effective at some times and not effective at others. Variable data generally complicate matters and make it difficult to interpret level and trend (Franklin et al., 1996). The ideal is to obtain stable data within each phase, but this is not always achieved in practice partly due to limited control of conditions (Kennedy, 2005).

Statistical Analysis through Structured Criteria for Visual Inspection

Visual analysis is a holistic approach that can address the question of whether a reliable change in performance occurs and the amount of that change. Visual analysis re-

lies on an interpreter who can simultaneously attend to trend, repeating patterns, delayed or temporary effects, within-phase changes in variability, and changes in *both* level and trend, as well as sudden changes across phases. Unfortunately, the virtues of the visual-analysis method may also be sources of vulnerabilities. Visual interpretations of treatment effect with A/B graphs may be inconsistent across judges, raising questions about the reliability of decisions (Franklin et al., 1996; but see Fisher, Kelly, & Lomas, 2003). Different interpreters may attend to different features of the data. Fisher et al. (2003) developed an objective and easy-to-use method for determining whether a reliable treatment effect has been achieved that does a relatively good job of controlling for Type I and Type II errors. Fisher et al. (2003) demonstrated that training in the use of the method substantially increased consistency and accuracy of treatment outcome decisions. The method also has the advantage of accounting for both level and trend simultaneously in the data. The result of the analysis is a statistical decision regarding effectiveness. The data point requirements are minimal (2 baseline data points and at least 5 intervention data points), and no statistical assumptions must be met.

The logic of Fisher et al.'s (2003) structured criteria is based on projecting the level (calculated as a mean line) and trend (calculated as a least-squares regression line) from baseline into the intervention phase. The logic is that the baseline level and trend should not change during the intervention phase if the intervention is not effective (the equivalent of the null hypothesis in the hypothesis-testing framework; Kazdin, 1982). Therefore, if a significant number of data points fall above both lines for a behavior acquisition intervention (e.g., improving oral reading fluency), then the effect is judged to be significant because the level, trend, or both deviate from baseline level and trend. For a behavior reduction intervention (e.g., reducing disruptive behavior), if a significant number of data points fall below both lines, then the effect is judged to be significant. If the criterion for a sufficient number of data points falling above (acquisition) or below (reduction) is not met, the intervention is judged to have not been effective. With this method, the number of intervention data points needed to achieve significance is based on the binomial sampling distribution, which expresses probability when there are only two possible outcomes—above a mean or trend line or below a mean or trend line, in this case.

The program for calculating whether there is a reliable treatment effect based on Fisher et al.'s (2003) criteria is in a Microsoft Excel file that can be downloaded (with instructions) from the Internet under the "Behavior Analysis Tools" link on the Munroe–Meyer Institute for Genetics and Rehabilitation website (available at the time of this writing at *www.unmc.edu/dept/mmi/index.cfm?L2_ID=82&L1_ID=29&L3_ID=89&CONREF=97*). The program does all of the calculations. The program reports the number of intervention data points above or below both lines that must be obtained to reach the criterion for effectiveness. It also displays the actual number of data points that do fall above or below both lines so that a decision regarding effect can be made. In addition, it displays the results on a Microsoft Excel graph containing the mean and trend lines from baseline extended into the intervention phase to facilitate visual inspection. In our experience using the program, we have found that it tends to be conservative, but conservatism may prompt educators to strive for stronger interventions (Parsonson & Baer, 1992).

Statistical Analysis through Effect Sizes

Another basic approach to summarizing treatment effect is estimating the size of effect independent of statistical significance. For example, two treatments may produce statistically significant effects, but those effects (e.g., By how much do students improve?) may be very different in size. Effect sizes provide an objective, continuous index of behavioral effect across conditions (Parker & Hagan-Burke, 2006). For single-case designs, the most common methods of calculating effect sizes are based on dividing the difference of the means for each condition (e.g., treatment minus baseline) by a standard deviation (either of the baseline condition or pooled across baseline and intervention phases), which produces a result akin to a z-score (in which the difference between a score and the mean is divided by the standard deviation of the sample). These types

of effect sizes are referred to as standardized mean differences effect sizes (or Cohen's d; Parker & Hagan-Burke, 2006). A wide variety of statistical methods for calculating effect sizes with different methods, assumptions, and requirements has appeared in the research literature (Brossart et al., 2006; Busk & Serlin, 1992; Busse, Kratochwill, & Elliott, 1995; Parker et al., 2005; Parker & Hagan-Burke, 2006). Although effect sizes can aid in evaluating the magnitude and meaningfulness of a change, there are also a number of limitations to the use of effect sizes (Parker et al., 2005; Parker & Hagan-Burke, 2006). The results vary by large margins according to the formula used, which makes it difficult to determine whether an effect is truly large or not. Factors such as intervention intensity levels, time frame within phases, types of participants, and reliability and sensitivity to growth in the outcome measure also affect outcomes. Results vary according to whether level or trend is analyzed and whether trend is controlled statistically. Some formulas require more data points than practitioners can often gather during an evaluation of an intervention (e.g., more than 20 data points), or they require statistical assumptions that often cannot be met in practice. Finally, there is a lack of clear and objective guidelines for interpretation. Therefore, until these limitations are worked out in the research literature, one should proceed very cautiously when comparing effect sizes based on single-case datasets across studies. When a consistent effect size is used and when other conditions (e.g., treatment intensity and participant characteristics) are constant across individual cases, their use for descriptive purposes may be more justified.

How Important Are the Changes or Goals?

We have progressed through addressing whether a change is reliable and has some magnitude of effect. Final questions are how close the performance or behavior is to that of typical and successful peers or benchmarks showing reduced risk. These final questions must be addressed by teams in order to consider next steps. Conceptually, a change may be reliable and show meaningful effects but not move the child out of risk without further planning. Common terms are social or clinical significance. Ways to address the importance of changes include using (1) measures or criteria for setting goals and judging attainment, (2) benchmarks for short- and/or long-term goals, (3) typical peer performance as comparisons, and (4) judgments of teachers or other consumers about goals, methods, and outcomes (Kennedy, 2005; Wolf, 1978).

In conclusion, to answer the question of whether there is an effect, a design that is sensitive to relevant behavior changes is needed even before any measurements are taken. Practitioners are advised to rely primarily on visual analysis and to use an objective index of treatment effect as an adjunct where possible. Fisher et al.'s (2003) structured criteria for visual inspection appears to be the best and easiest to use method available at this time. Estimating size of effect, although complicated, is considered a basic way of analyzing and comparing treatments in research. Confidence in decisions can be increased by adding further single-case design elements to the A/B design (discussed later) because they increase the number of times the treatment effect is replicated while ruling out other possible interpretations. Last but certainly not least, one must consider the importance of both the goals and amount of behavior change.

Question 2: What Produced the Effect?

A behavioral effect may occur (and may be correctly detected), but it may not be the intervention that produces it. In other words, one cannot simply assume that the intervention is responsible for behavior change just because behavior changed in the desired direction. Also, many interventions are "packages" of separate components (i.e., more practice *and* more reinforcement), some of which may be more influential than others. Question 2 raises the issue of determining what actually changed behavior: Was it the intervention, an intervention component, or something else? Fundamentally, it is a question about inferring *causation*. For example, if a teacher assumes that a child's academic performance improved as a result of taking stimulant medication when, in fact, the child began a newly instituted instructional strat-

egy at the very same time (e.g., more practice with feedback and reinforcement), resulting in an unplanned package, then the teacher may incorrectly infer that medication was effective and recommend its use in the future when it may have been due to instructional changes or a mix of the interventions.

Internal Validity and Hypotheses about Change

Two Ways Internal Validity Is Important

Internal validity is about producing evidence that the intervention and not other extraneous factors caused the change in behavior or performance. Examples of evidence for causation are immediate level and/or trend changes that appear when the intervention is introduced, with these changes replicated in other, similar conditions in the selected design. First, internal validity comes into play as problem-solving teams consider which interventions may be used in a situation (e.g., Horner, Carr, McGee, Odom, & Wolery, 2005). Interventions that have been used before with strong evidence for internal validity (i.e., that have been shown to cause behavior change in published investigations that used experimental designs) are preferred in many circumstances. Second, internally valid single-case designs are important if teams want to argue convincingly that a selected intervention is individually effective for a student or to see whether a novel intervention may have "caused" the outcome.

The Conceptual Basis of Planning: How Construct Validity Fits In

Hypotheses about change (what to change, how to change it) come from constructs about educational risk, such as students' problems with school achievement and social behavior. A well-developed construct includes valid models of how student risk "works": what produces and can alleviate reading failure or socially disruptive behavior. The use of educational constructs also means that careful decisions need to be made about how to best measure critical features of the construct, select students, sample behavior or performance, set goals, and intervene. Thus construct validity requires the careful alignment of students, measurement, and intervention and enables meaningful analysis of cause-and-effect relationships. School psychologists improve inferences about the constructs (high reading risk, reduced social risk) from assessment and intervention results by making sure the measure is strongly linked both to the construct and to the intervention. For example, curriculum-based measurement (CBM) is a good candidate for intervention measurement because of valid links to reading success and intervention outcomes. Construct measures need to win at least three competitions to be selected by teams: (1) demonstrating strong links to school risk, (2) showing sensitivity to intervention effects, and (3) having feasibility as progress monitoring measures.

Strengthening Conclusions through Single-Case Experimental Designs

Although the A/B design, consisting of a simple phase change (see Panel A in Figure 29.1 for an example), is the core of all versions of single-case designs, its primary limitation is that it cannot be used to identify for sure what caused a change in behavior. The baseline provides the only means of estimating what would have happened if no intervention were applied, and it does not account for possible extraneous variables that might have coincided with the introduction of the intervention. The various single-case experimental designs that provide appropriate experimental controls increase replications of conditions and vary the timing of phase changes (e.g., baseline to intervention) to rule out possible threats to interpretation. They all involve comparisons of data series that contain repeated measures over time. The difference is in whether the comparisons are within the same series or between different data series. Some single-case designs combine within data series and between data series comparisons. The reader is referred to recent and classic textbooks (Bailey & Burch, 2002; Cooper, Heron, & Heward, 2007; Kazdin, 1982; Kennedy, 2005) for a complete account of the logic and methods and the variations that are available. Here, the three most common types of designs are discussed—the A/B/A/B design, the multi-element design, and the multiple-baseline design.

The A/B/A/B design involves the introduction and removal of treatment across separate phases (baseline, treatment, baseline, treatment). An example is displayed in Panel B of Figure 29.1. The data are compared within the series for changes in level, trend, and/or variability both within and across phases. When behavior changes clearly across phases and results are replicated for each condition, the A/B/A/B design provides a powerful demonstration that the treatment is responsible for behavior change and not other variables. For the demonstration to be convincing, it is important to have a fairly stable, steady state of responding in each phase before moving on to the next phase to be able to show contrasts. The A/B/A/B design is often used by sequentially adding and withdrawing a treatment (e.g., praise for appropriate behavior). Another application of the A/B/A/B design involves sequentially reversing the contingencies. For example, Broussard and Northup (1995) found during baseline that a participant's problem behavior was maintained by teacher attention (the baseline, or A phase). The intervention involved providing attention noncontingently to the student (i.e., independently of problem behavior), which led to an increase in work completion and a decrease in disruptive behavior during the intervention phase (i.e., B). In the second A phase (the reversal), the contingency (teacher attention) was reversed by having the teacher again pay attention to the student when he or she acted up. A final treatment phase (i.e., the second B phase) replicated the original treatment effects. More complex versions can be created by adding additional or combining treatments (with additional treatments designated as sequential alphabetical letters: C, D, etc.). For example, a practitioner may be interested in the effects of a token economy (B) and performance feedback (C), as well as the combination of the two (B+C), as compared with baseline levels.

Although the A/B/A/B design provides a strong basis for inferring causation, it has several limitations. First, it cannot be used if the target behavior is irreversible, as would be the case for a skilled behavior such as reading, writing, or math. Although durable change is positive from a clinical standpoint, a problem arises if the goal is to show a functional relationship between the treatment and the behavior change. The practitioner or researcher should consider other designs when dealing with irreversible behaviors.

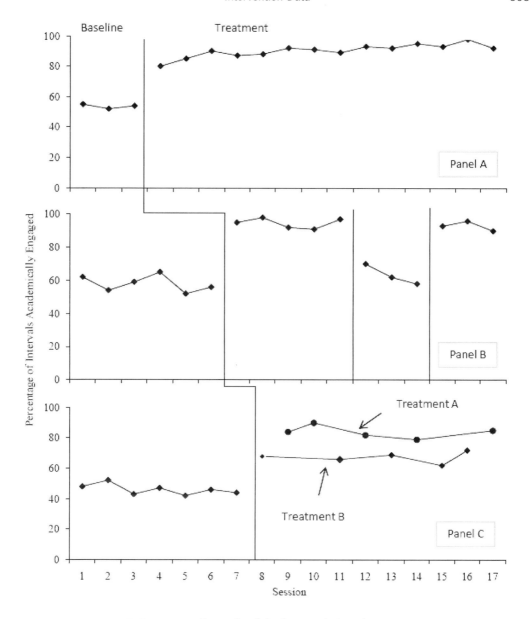

FIGURE 29.1. Example of single-case design elements.

Second, each phase must be run long enough to establish stability and to draw conclusions about the effects of the treatment. Third, sequence effects (the order in which the phases are presented) may influence the behavior when treatments are compared using this design (e.g., A/B/C/B/C). One way to overcome this limitation is to counterbalance the phases across participants (e.g., have one or more participants for whom the design sequence is A/C/B/C/B). Finally, withdrawing an effec-

tive intervention may be ethically (e.g., behavior is harmful to the individual), socially, or educationally (e.g., loss of instructional time) indefensible in some situations.

A very common design for comparing treatments is the multielement design (Ulman & Sulzer-Azaroff, 1975), also commonly called the alternating treatment design (Barlow & Hayes, 1979). The multielement design is essentially a fast-paced reversal design (Higgins-Hains & Baer,

1989) that incorporates multiple replications of different treatment conditions so that comparisons can be made across data series, with each data series associated with a different condition. An example can be found in Panel C of Figure 29.1. In the example, a baseline condition is displayed, although this is not a necessary requirement of the design. Experimental control is established when the data reveal clearly discriminable differences between conditions in the intervention comparison phase to the right of the baseline (e.g., Treatment A is shown to be more effective than Treatment B in Figure 29.1). The goal of this design is to identify in a short time period which treatment is most effective for the individual. The design can be used without a baseline and without withdrawing treatment (Cooper, Heron, & Heward, 2007). The multielement design is also not without its limitations, however. Rapidly alternating and counterbalancing treatments in a way that allows the participant to discriminate which treatment is in effect is complex and may not be feasible. Also, multiple treatment interference may confound the results: The treatments may not produce the same effects if they are implemented alone as they do when preceded and followed by other treatments. However, the treatments that are found to be the most effective can be further evaluated by using a reversal or multiple-baseline design during a follow-up period (Wacker et al., 1990).

The multiple-baseline design (Baer, Wolf, & Risley, 1968) involves the successive introduction of a treatment across established baselines. It is perhaps the most versatile because it can compare performance across behaviors, participants, or settings. The essential components of a multiple-baseline design are displayed in Figure 29.1 as the total combination of Panels A, B, and C. At least two functionally related baselines are established over the same time period, but generally three or four are preferred. After the baselines have stabilized, the treatment is applied to one behavior, participant, or setting, but not to the others. Once a stable change is seen in the first response, the treatment is then applied to the next behavior, participant, or setting, and so on. The treatment is said to be responsible for the behavioral effect when behavior changes with the introduction of treatment and remains stable across the other data series. Therefore, this design relies on comparisons across data series. First, one looks within the series to determine whether behavior change occurs at the point of a phase change (i.e., baseline to treatment); then one looks to determine whether behavior remained stable across subsequent baselines (i.e., as yet untreated behaviors, participants, or settings). Although the effects may not be convincing when looking at one individual, behavior, or setting, to the extent that effects are replicated, treatment results are more believable.

Multiple-baseline designs are used when the behavior is irreversible or when it is not preferable or ethical to return to baseline. Additionally, the behaviors, participants, and settings must be independent of one another but are predicted to respond to the same treatment. If the targets are dependent, then a change in one target may cause a change in one of the other targets prior to the implementation of the treatment for the second target. For example, if a teacher begins praising a child for work completion in math, work completion in writing may also increase, even though the teacher has not begun praising work completion in writing. The main limitation of multiple-baseline designs is that the treatment is delayed for some behaviors, settings, or participants. Another limitation is the possible emergence of a changing trend in a data series as behavior is measured repeatedly over time. A trend in a desirable direction will complicate interpretation. A trend in an undesirable direction may indicate that the repeated measurements are adversely affecting the student. A variation of the multiple-baseline design is the multiple-probe design (Horner & Baer, 1978), which is particularly well suited to examining instructional interventions (Wolery, Bailey, & Sugai, 1988). If stability in performance is expected, fewer measures rather than continuous measurement are needed overall with this design. The multiple-probe design is strengthened by intensified measurement introduced before and after interventions and then by continuing with sparser probes. This savings in unneeded measurement may be considerable and may also reduce a student's reactivity to being repeatedly tested.

Question 3: How Generalizable Is the Effect?

Question 3 assumes that affirmative responses have been obtained for the first two questions and that there is a significant and meaningful effect and a good degree of confidence about what produced the behavioral effect. In addressing Question 3, the school psychologist inquires about the degree to which the child's behavior change generalizes to other settings (e.g., across classrooms), conditions (e.g., when instructional tasks become harder or when using a newly learned skill with other skills), responses (e.g., to other socially appropriate responses as an alternative to verbal aggression), time (e.g., maintenance of academic intervention effects), and/or behavior change agents (e.g., to the reading teacher as well as the math teacher). Generalized improvements in behavior are not likely to occur without plans to measure and intervene during those times (Stokes & Baer, 1977). Johnston and Pennypacker (1993) state:

> Behavioral practitioners must consider extending the initial behavior change to other settings as a necessary and integral part of the overall project, which must receive the same care and attention in environmental design and arrangement as is given to the setting and behavior or primary interest. ... It is simply that the behavior modifier's job is not finished until the subject is behaving appropriately in all of the desired settings. (pp. 174–175)

The basic point is that one cannot merely assume that desired behavior changes will generalize to all relevant settings. An intervention will be incomplete if it does not program for generalization, which usually requires adding additional intervention components or extending the intervention to other settings or conditions.

A list of generalization strategies based on several reviews of the research literature for academic and behavior problems (Miltenberger, 2008; Daly, Martens, Barnett, Witt, & Olson, 2007; Daly, Martens, Skinner, & Noell, 2009; Stokes & Baer, 1977) appear in Table 29.3. The reader is referred to the reviews for an in-depth discussion of each strategy. As with planning measurement in advance, target behaviors and intervention components should be selected in advance

to increase the likelihood of producing generalized improvements in behavior. Evaluating generalized effects requires that areas in which generalization is important are identified prior to intervention (e.g., generalizing reading fluency across all third-grade reading texts) and there is a plan to measure behavior change in the generalization setting (e.g., sampling reading fluency in a wide variety of third-grade reading passages). Plans then can readily include methods for improving chances for generalization.

In some cases, perhaps rarely if the problem comes to the attention of a school team, generalization might not be an important issue. For example, if the goal is simply to resolve an out-of-seat problem during math and the behavior is not a problem elsewhere, generalized effects are not a concern. On the other hand, if an intervention targets reduction of aggressive behavior on the playground during recess, it is desirable to see a similar reduction of aggressive behavior on the playground before and after school as well (if problems are occurring during those times, too). Therefore, it should be measured at all three times.

Question 4: What Should Be Done Next?

There are five possible "next steps" when sufficient intervention data have been gathered to establish a reliable trend: (1) continuing the intervention, (2) extending the same or a modified version of the intervention to other settings or conditions, (3) strengthening the intervention, (4) changing the intervention (and/or goal) altogether by redoing problem-solving steps, or (5) discontinuing the intervention. The decision about which avenue to pursue depends in large part on answers to the prior questions (i.e., Questions 1, 2, and 3).

To decide the next steps, the team must evaluate behavior change, variability (or stability) in current levels of performance following intervention, and the degree to which the child is performing as expected at the end of the intervention phase (referred to as goal attainment). Judgment about whether the child is achieving or even approaching criterion levels of behavior (e.g., improved reading fluency levels, reduced self-injurious

TABLE 29.3. Intervention Strategies for Producing Generalized Effects

Generalization strategy	Example
Selecting skills that allow the student to generalize	
Teach skills that will be naturally reinforced.	Teach a student to appropriately recruit attention from a teacher (the teacher is likely to naturally attend to the student).
Teach skills that are generalizable.	Teach a student to segment and blend words because it makes decoding easier.
Teach a range of skills that will produce the same result.	Teach students various ways to initiate social contacts with peers.
Designing the training situation to promote generalization	
Provide training in the natural environment or maximize the similarities between the training and natural environments; consider people, relevant materials, and settings.	Teach appropriate manners in the lunchroom, where problems were occurring in the first place.
When skills are taught in isolation, have the student also practice the skill under natural conditions.	Teach a student to read words on flash cards, followed by having the student practice reading those words in connected text.
Incorporate many varied examples of situations in which the skill should be used.	Teach compliance while using various behavioral and academic requests.
Provide rationales and teach self-management strategies.	Teach a student to self-record skill use with a checklist; use self-instructions.
Sequentially teach to high fluency levels.	Teach using appropriate difficulty level materials, use repeated practice to criterion levels, give performance feedback, and move sequentially to harder materials as the student achieves criterion levels.
Supporting the skill outside of training	
Reinforce the skill when it is used outside of training.	Praise a child for not responding to a stranger on the playground following skills training.
Make the natural environment more reinforcing.	Have both the teacher and peers praise the school bully for appropriate social behaviors.
Delay or fade the frequency of reinforcement when adequate skill level has been achieved.	Thin the schedule of praise for on-task behavior.

behavior) consistently, inconsistently, or not at all should influence recommendations for what to do next.

This process is individualized for every child. For example, although a child might be part of a group intervention (e.g., a Tier 2 supplementary reading intervention), this decision is made for every child receiving intervention by considering his or her patterns of scores alone. In reality, the *degree of effect*, including change in performance close to that of typical or successful peers, may more heavily influence decisions about what to do next. Data-based judgments play an essential role here, as both how much be-

havior change has occurred in light of goals and the sustainability of the intervention are weighed against costs associated with the intervention (which includes both material and human resources). Counterbalancing factors include teams finding ways to reduce the intensity of interventions by changing plans or eliminating or reducing unneeded components while still maintaining or making needed gains (Barnett, Daly, Jones, & Lentz, 2004). Other unique circumstances include stakeholder preferences or reactions to the intervention that are often difficult to predict in schools or other applied settings. A large initial effect for an intervention that is not sustainable as carried out may require more creative and efficient solutions by the team. A small but detectable effect may be important in some cases.

Choosing a next step (e.g., continuing an intervention) depends also on how confident the team is about *why* behavior changed or did not change (Question 2). If behavior is at or approaching desired levels, if there is reason to believe that the intervention is responsible for the change, and if the team believes that the student is unlikely to continue to be successful without the intervention, it is probably best to *continue the intervention* in most cases. If all of these things are true but there is a lack of generalized improvements in behavior, then *extending the intervention* in some form to settings or conditions to which behavior change should generalize is recommended. For example, a successful token economy plus response cost for appropriate and aggressive behaviors may be extended to other times of the day or other settings.

If behavior is not progressing as rapidly as expected, but the team believes that parts of the intervention are important, the existing *intervention may be strengthened*. For example, the school psychologist or teacher might discover that a poor reader who is progressing slowly with increased reading practice has a high error rate and might decide to add an error correction strategy prior to practice time. If behavior is not progressing as rapidly as expected or is changing in the undesired direction, the *intervention may be completely changed*. For example, if planned ignoring in the classroom is not reducing classroom disruptions, it may be that the intervention is not a relevant one. In this case, it may be the peers' behavior (e.g., laughing, snickering) that is reinforcing the problem behavior, in which case the planned-ignoring procedure has not addressed the cause of the problem. Alternately, an intervention might be appropriately targeting the cause of behavior change, but the change agent might not be able to implement it appropriately. For example, praising appropriate behavior and redirecting inappropriate behavior may be effective temporarily as long as a teacher is able to sustain higher rates of praise initially but may lose its effectiveness when new demands on the

teacher oblige him or her to rearrange class time in ways that make it harder to praise appropriate behavior. In this case, the intervention could be changed to reward accurate work completion based on permanent products instead.

If the intervention has achieved desired effects and the team thinks that it is no longer needed to support behavior change in the natural setting, the *intervention may be discontinued*. For example, a young child whose previously aggressive behavior with peers was replaced with appropriate social interactions may no longer need explicit support from the teacher because peer social interactions maintain appropriate behavior. Also, reward schedules can be thinned by increasing requirements for meeting criteria (e.g., offering free time contingent on completing more math problems) or by lengthening the delay before rewards can be accessed (e.g., offering an end-of-the-week reward instead of a daily reward), a process referred to as *fading* of the contingencies. Discontinuing an intervention may occur by degrees, and brief classroom observations and consultation checks with a teacher can confirm outcomes.

The goal when answering the question of what to do next is to achieve the appropriate treatment strength to assure that behavior change continues in the desired direction (e.g., child continues to catch up to peers in math performance) or is maintained at desired levels (e.g., a youth's quiz and test scores in science are now at an acceptable level) without unduly taxing available resources. Of course, this is the goal prior to intervention as well. But, at this point in the problem-solving process, the issue is one of adjusting the intervention to assure the appropriate balance between treatment strength and sustainability of the intervention. A multi-component intervention that appears to be a strong treatment is weak if the behavior change agent cannot carry it out consistently. Increasing treatment strength comes at a cost in terms of resources, effort, and time, and decreasing an intervention prematurely reintroduces risk; increasing and decreasing intervention strength appropriately are both significant data-based tactics used by teams (Barnett et al., 2004). Sometimes it is difficult to decide clearly about an effect and what to do next, and if this situation arises, more or better data are needed to improve accuracy, and to better understand trend or variability, or to improve intervention selection through another try at problem solving. Table 29.4 provides recommendations for interpretation and next steps for various behavioral outcomes.

Conclusions

Instructional design and evaluation are the basic questions in decision making by schools. Instead of one-point-in-time measurement, a very different dataset is used to improve instructional decision validity in behavioral practice and RTI. The basics

TABLE 29.4. Reading Your Data

Data pattern	Suggested interpretation	Possible next steps
Level, trend, and variability approximate or exceed desired level and rate of growth prior to goal date.	Desired degree of effect is achieved.	Continue the intervention until desired level is achieved consistently.
Data reach predetermined level at or before specified goal date.	Intervention is effective.	• Extend the intervention to other settings or conditions. Or • Discontinue intervention.
Data are highly variable.	Performance is not under control of the intervention.	• Reward compliance. • Provide performance feedback. • Improve treatment integrity. • Check for satiation with rewards. And/or • Check for possible outside factors that may be attenuating intervention effects.
Level and/or trend indistinguishable from baseline data, or desired level is not met by specified goal date.	Intervention is ineffective and possibly not relevant to the source of the problem.	For skill-based interventions: • Ensure prerequisite skills have been mastered. • Add modeling of correct responding. • Teach components of larger skill set. And/or • Change difficulty level. For contingency-based interventions: • Ensure that rewards are truly motivating. • Ensure that rewards target correct function of behavior. And/or • Ensure that rewards for appropriate behavior compete effectively with whatever is reinforcing inappropriate behavior.
Level, trend, and or variability in the undesired direction.	Intervention is having a possible negative effect on behavior.	• Consider possible extinction burst if inappropriate behavior is no longer being rewarded. • Improve treatment integrity. • Consider potentially aversive intervention components. • Consider interventions matched to other possible functions of the problem. And/or • Change the intervention altogether.
Adequate level under training conditions, but variable performance under other conditions.	Student is not generalizing use of the skill.	See Table 29.3.

serve as a general model. They include a baseline of current performance and criteria for success. Data are organized by single-case design elements to evaluate specific intervention questions. An intervention plan is implemented and evaluated, and information is used to decide next steps and needed resources. These plans may be carried out with classrooms, smaller groups, and individuals serving as units of analysis.

Similarly, RTI uses tiers of prevention and intervention to increase the accuracy of educational decisions. RTI starts with the premise of scientifically sound instruction and allows teams to refine educational decisions and to demonstrate outcomes step by step, progressing through tiers of services as needed. Single-case designs discussed in this chapter may be used to improve the accuracy of team inferences and decisions about what students need. They are at the heart of school intervention support practices and may fit questions (Kennedy, 2005) such as, Is this intervention working? Which intervention works best? and Which instructional components are needed? at any tier. Single-case designs can be used for evaluating common interventions used by school teams, as well as intensive function-based interventions that involve severe exigencies in school planning.

References

Baer, D., Wolf, M., & Risley, T. (1968). Some current dimensions of applied behavior analysis. *Journal of Applied Behavior Analysis, 1,* 91–97.

Bailey, J., & Burch, M. (2002). *Research methods in applied behavior analysis.* Thousand Oaks, CA: Sage.

Barlow, D., & Hayes, S. (1979). Alternating treatments design: One strategy for comparing the effects of two treatments in a single subject. *Journal of Applied Behavior Analysis, 12,* 199–210.

Barnett, D. W., Daly, E. J., III, Jones, K. M., & Lentz, F. E., Jr. (2004). Response to intervention: Empirically-based special service decisions from increasing and decreasing intensity single-case designs. *Journal of Special Education, 38,* 66–79.

Batsche, G., Elliott, J., Graden, J. L., Grimes, J., Kovaleski, J. F., Prasse, D., et al. (2005). *Response to intervention: Policy considerations and implementation.* Alexandria, VA: National Association of State Board of Directors of Special Education.

Bloom, M., Fischer, J., & Orme, J. G. (2005). *Evaluating practice: Guidelines for the accountable professional* (5th ed.). Boston: Allyn & Bacon.

Brossart, D. F., Parker, R. I., Olson, E. A., & Mahadevan, L. (2006). The relationship between visual analysis and five statistical analyses in a simple AB single-case research design. *Behavior Modification, 30,* 531–563.

Broussard, C., & Northup, J. (1995). An approach to functional assessment and analysis of disruptive behavior in regular education classrooms. *School Psychology Quarterly, 10,* 151–164.

Bushell, D., & Baer, D. M. (1994). Measurably superior instruction means close, continual contact with the relevant outcome data. Revolutionary! In R. Gardner, III, D. M. Sainato, J. O. Cooper, T. E. Heron, W. L. Heward, J. W. Eshleman, et al. (Eds.), *Behavior analysis in education: Focus on measurably superior instruction* (pp. 3–10). Pacific Grove, CA: Brooks/Cole.

Busk, P. L., & Serlin, R. C. (1992). Meta-analysis for single-case research. In T. R. Kratochwill & J. R. Levin (Eds.), *Single-case research design and analysis: Applications in psychology and education* (pp. 187–212). Hillsdale, NJ: Erlbaum.

Busse, R. T., Kratochwill, T. R., & Elliott, S. N. (1995). Meta-analysis for single-case consultation outcomes: Applications to research and practice. *Journal of School Psychology, 33,* 269–285.

Cooper, J. O., Heron, T. E., & Heward, W. L. (2007). *Applied behavior analysis* (2nd ed.). Upper Saddle River, NJ: Prentice Hall.

Daly, E. J., III, Martens, B. K., Barnett, D., Witt, J. C., & Olson, S. C. (2007). Varying intervention delivery in response-to-intervention: Confronting and resolving challenges with measurement, instruction, and intensity. *School Psychology Review, 36,* 562–581.

Daly, E. J., III, Martens, B. K., Skinner, C. H., & Noell, G. H. (2009). Contributions of applied behavior analysis. In T. B. Gutkin & C. R. Reynolds (Eds.), *The handbook of school psychology* (4th ed.). New York: Wiley.

Fisher, W. W., Kelley, M. E., & Lomas, J. E. (2003). Visual aids and structured criteria for improving visual inspection and interpretation of single-case designs. *Journal of Applied Behavior Analysis, 36,* 387–406.

Franklin, R. D., Gorman, B. S., Beasley, T. M., & Allison, D. B. (1996). Graphic display and visual analysis. In R. D. Franklin, D. B. Allison, & B. S. Gorman (Eds.), *Design and analysis of single-case research* (pp. 119–158). Mahwah, NJ: Erlbaum.

Gresham, F. M. (2007). Evolution of the response-to-intervention concept: Empirical foundations and recent developments. In S. Jimerson, M. Burns, & A. VanDerHeyden (Eds.), *The handbook of response to intervention: The science and practice of assessment and intervention* (pp. 10–24). New York: Springer Science.

Higgins-Hains, A., & Baer, D. (1989). Interaction effects in multielement designs: Inevitable, desirable, and ignorable. *Journal of Applied Behavior Analysis, 22,* 57–69.

Horner, R., & Baer, D. (1978). Multi-probe technique: A variation of the multiple baseline design. *Journal of Applied Behavior Analysis, 11,* 189–196.

Horner, R. H., Carr, E. G., McGee, G., Odom, S., & Wolery, M. (2005). The use of single-subject research to identify evidence-based practice in special education. *Exceptional Children, 71,* 165–179.

Johnston, J. M., & Pennypacker, H. S. (1993). *Readings for strategies and tactics of behavioral research* (2nd ed.). Hillsdale, NJ: Erlbaum.

Kazdin, A. E. (1982). *Single-case research designs: Methods for clinical and applied settings.* New York: Oxford University Press.

Kennedy, C. H. (2005). *Single-case designs for educational research.* Boston: Allyn & Bacon.

Lipsey, M. W. (1990). *Design sensitivity: Statistical power for experimental research.* Newbury Park, CA: Sage.

Messick, S. (1995). Validity of psychological assessment. *American Psychologist, 50,* 741–749.

Miltenberger, R. G. (2008). *Behavior modification: Principles and procedures* (4th ed.). Belmont, CA: Wadsworth/Thomson Learning.

Parker, R. I., Brossart, D. F., Vannest, K. J., Long, J. R., Garcia de Alba, R., Baugh, F.

G., et al. (2005). Effect sizes in single case research: How large is large? *School Psychology Review, 34,* 116–132.

Parker, R. I., & Hagan-Burke, S. (2006). Useful effect size interpretations for single-case research. *Behavior Therapy, 38,* 95–105.

Parsonson, B. S., & Baer, D. M. (1986). The graphic analysis of data. In A. Poling & R. W. Fuqua (Eds.), *Research methods in applied behavior analysis: Issues and advances* (pp. 157–186). New York: Plenum Press.

Parsonson, B. S., & Baer, D. M. (1992). The visual analysis of data, and current research into the stimuli controlling it. In T. R. Kratochwill & J. R. Levin (Eds.), *Single-case research design and analysis* (pp. 15–40). Hillsdale, NJ: Erlbaum.

Sidman, M. (1960). *Tactics of scientific research: Evaluating experimental data in psychology.* New York: Basic Books.

Stokes, T. F., & Baer, D. M. (1977). An implicit technology of generalization. *Journal of Applied Behavior Analysis, 10,* 349–367.

Ulman, J., & Sulzer-Azaroff, B. (1975). Multielement baseline design in educational research. In E. Ramp & G. Semb (Eds.), *Behavior analysis: Areas of research and application* (pp. 377–391). Englewood Cliffs, NJ: Prentice Hall.

Wacker, D., McMahon, C., Steege, M., Berg, W., Sasso, G., & Melloy, K. (1990). Applications of a sequential alternating treatments design. *Journal of Applied Behavior Analysis, 23,* 333–339.

Wolery, M., Bailey, D. B., Jr., & Sugai, G. M. (1988). *Effective teaching: Principles and procedures of applied behavior analysis with exceptional children.* Boston: Allyn & Bacon.

Wolf, M. M. (1978). Social validity: The case for subjective measurement or how applied behavior analysis is finding its heart. *Journal of Applied Behavior Analysis, 11,* 203–214.

Chapter 30

Empirical and Pragmatic Issues in Assessing and Supporting Intervention Implementation in Schools

George H. Noell

School psychologists have diverse roles in schools, including student assessment, counseling, consultation, administration, staff development, and program evaluation, among many others (Hosp & Reschly, 2002). It may be reasonable to describe school psychological services as existing on two continua: individual–systemic and indirect–direct. The first continuum is the extent to which services are either student focused or systemic in nature. Student-level services appear to be the traditional dominant focus within school psychology. They include services such as psychoeducational assessments, counseling, and consultation regarding educational programming. The passage of the Individuals with Disabilities Education Improvement Act (IDEIA, 1975), easily the most significant development in the provision of psychological services in schools, created a tremendous need for student-focused services. In particular, IDEIA led to an explosive increase in the provision of psychoeducational assessments in schools.

At the opposite end of the individual-versus-system continuum is the provision of system-focused services. Systemic services would include activities such as program development, program evaluation, policy development, training, and supervision. The critical feature of the systemic end of the continuum is that the services are designed to affect many students rather than one individual. At one end of the continuum, system-level intervention would be designed to affect all students across many schools over a considerable period of time. School reform efforts, policy development, and program development efforts would all be examples of systemic intervention (e.g., Shapiro, 2006; Sheridan & Gutkin, 2000; Stollar, Poth, Curtis, & Cohen, 2006). Although dichotomies are attractive because they are simpler than continuous variables, in conceptualizing the directness versus indirectness of school psychological services, it is probably most productive to think of them in a continuous fashion. For example, work for a single student with autism related to that student's access to discrete-trial applied behavior analysis instruction may have both an individual component that is relevant to only that student and systemic policy implications for other students with autism. Similarly, intervention in a classroom relevant to classroom management is not systemic in the broad sense of the word but certainly extends beyond the individual focus.

A second major continuum that may be used to describe school psychological services is the distinction between direct and indirect services. Direct services are those services that a school psychologist provides directly to the student. These include counseling and psychoeducational assessments. Indirect services are those services that school psychologists provide to a third party, with the intent that the third party will in turn provide services to the student. Indirect services include consultation with teachers and parents, program evaluation services, and staff development training. As with the degree to which services are systemic, the degree to which services are direct or indirect is clearly continuous. For example, consultations regarding individual students can vary considerably in the degree to which they include direct services (Barnett et al., 1997; Noell, Gansle, & Allison, 1999). At one end of the continuum are consultations that are brief and consist entirely of a teacher and a school psychologist soliciting and providing advice, respectively. In these brief informal contacts, the psychologist may not have any direct contact with the student, and the services provided are clearly entirely indirect. In contrast, consultation with a teacher regarding an individual student can frequently require a range of activities beyond simply meeting with the teacher. Consultation may frequently include direct assessment of the student, preparation of intervention materials, student training, and conversations with the student regarding his or her concerns (e.g., Barnett et al., 1997; Noell et al., 2005). In these instances, services will be partially indirect (the intervention provided by the teacher to the student) and partially direct.

In describing the evolution of school psychology, it might be fair to describe the profession as gradually and consistently moving from direct services that were predominantly at the individual end of the continuum—exemplified by individual assessments and counseling—to services that are indirect and that vary tremendously in the degree to which they are individually focused versus systemic in nature. There have certainly been increasing calls for school psychologists to become actively involved in policy, prevention, and systems change (Shapiro, 2006; Sheridan & Gutkin, 2000; Stollar et al., 2006). In each of these instances, services will be largely indirect, in addition to being systemic. Additionally, an increasing emphasis on consultation at the individual and small-group levels is clearly evident in the school psychological professional literature (e.g., Sheridan, Welch, & Orme, 1996). The general and increasing emphasis on prevention, intervention in general education, mainstream support, problem solving, and response-to-intervention (RTI) within school psychology all result in an increasing emphasis on indirect services as a core element of school psychology.

Although this evolutionary change from a profession emphasizing direct services to individual students toward indirect services to individual students, groups of students, and systems may be healthy for students, schools, and psychologists, it has important implications for the practice and preparation of school psychologists that have not been articulated clearly and frequently enough. An important feature of direct services such as assessment and counseling is that school psychologists can control the implementation of the services because they are responsible for implementing them. However, in the shift to consultation, intervention, problem solving, RTI, prevention, and policy-level intervention services become largely and increasingly indirect (Barnett, Daly, Jones, & Lentz, 2004; Sheridan et al., 1996). In these activities, school psychologists are moving from being service providers to service multipliers. The idea is that by contributing psychological knowledge, evaluation skills, and research expertise, school psychologists can enhance the effectiveness of existing resources to help educators use those resources in a more focused, effective, efficient, and equitable fashion. The possibility of schools using resources in an increasingly effective, efficient, and equitable fashion is broadly appealing, as is evident both in the school psychological literature and the broader school reform and effective-schools literatures (Cook, Gerber, & Semmel, 1997; Kim & Crasco, 2006).

Although the adoption of service models that increase the availability of psychological services to all students is attractive, this move has profound implications for school psychology that may have been underappreciated and that are clearly insufficiently considered in the professional literature.

Traditional direct services permit school psychologists to control the service that is provided and to alter it as they deem appropriate to the context. In a counseling context, for instance, the school psychologist can choose to adopt a cognitive-behavioral framework, an emotionally supportive approach, or a life-skills curriculum in their work with students (Prout & Prout, 1998). The extent to which services are delivered as designed is directly in the control of the school psychologist, and their evaluation is directly traceable to their impact on students.

In contrast, within an indirect-services model such as problem-solving consultation, RTI, or policy consultation, the school psychologist has little or no direct control over the services that are provided to students (Ardoin, Witt, Connell, & Koenig, 2005; Sheridan, Kratochwill, & Bergan, 1996). In these cases, the extent to which services are provided to students is determined by the extent to which other educators, typically teachers, implement the intended intervention. This is a tremendously more complicated service delivery system than direct services. Direct services simply require that the school psychologist identify a professionally indicated course of action, implement that course, and then evaluate that outcome. More simply, all that is required is knowing what to do, doing it, and evaluating its effects. Although knowing what to do, having the skills needed to do it, and having the evaluation skills needed to assess its efficacy are no small feats, they are substantially simpler tasks than what is required of the psychologist engaged in indirect service delivery such as consultation. Indirect services require the same three fundamental elements that direct services require, plus three additional elements that are tremendously underresearched and poorly understood within school psychology. First, how does one get parents and educators to implement the desired intervention, innovation, or systems change? Second, how does one assess the degree to which parents and educators have implemented the desired intervention, innovation, or systems change? Third, how does one assess whether the level of implementation is sufficient?

Scholars in school psychology have advanced theories about how various factors might influence implementation, but data ex-

amining the proposed mediators and models has largely been absent (Noell, 2008). It is also important to acknowledge that for the most part the hypotheses were developed based on the assumption that human beings behave primarily in a rational manner. For example, it was argued that teachers would be more likely to implement interventions that are simple and acceptable (Eckert & Hintze, 2000). However, these hypotheses did not account for the abundance of data suggesting that rational acceptability and plan simplicity are not sufficient to account for human behavior in other domains. For example, assuming that simplicity and acceptability are key determinants of behavior would suggest that most adults would have significant saved assets to prepare them for future needs, such as emergencies, major purchases, and retirement, because little could be simpler than depositing funds in a savings account, and most adults would be expected to report that saving for the future is not only acceptable but desirable. Despite this obvious linear connection, numerous sources are available documenting that Americans do not save or invest at a level that economists would project to be prudent (Farrell, 2004). Human behavior is more complicated than is accounted for through a model based on simple rational comparison of relative desirability and response cost or effort. It would seem reasonable to assume that, in fact, human behavior, including intervention implementation, is a complex, multiply determined behavior that is influenced by biological, environmental, cognitive, and emotional factors whose sum effect may or may not be judged to be rational by a third party.

This chapter focuses on how school psychologists can influence students, parents, and educators to implement interventions designed to improve student functioning. This is a critical consideration for school psychologists engaging in consultation, RTI, or systemic intervention because ample evidence demonstrates that educators will infrequently sustain interventions in the absence of systematic follow-up (Noell et al., 2005; Noell, 2008). School psychologists can only be effective consultants and system-change agents to the extent to which they can induce change in other adults. Interventions that are not implemented are unlikely to benefit anyone. This chapter does not address direct-service models in which school psychologists directly control service because the issues addressed herein would obviously not be relevant. Generally, the discussion emphasizes intervention implementation following consultation for individuals or small groups but touches on systemic issues selectively. This focus reflects the bulk of referrals that school psychologists are called on to address in practice: individuals and classes.

The following sections of this chapter examine issues in terminology, assessing intervention implementation, supporting implementation, evaluating implementation, and practical implications for practice. At the outset it is important to acknowledge that research examining intervention implementation is nascent in comparison with the instructional, intervention, and psychometric literatures that are fundamental to school psychology. Systematic research examining intervention implementation following indirect services such as consultation emerged in school psychology only about a decade ago. As a result, what we know is a small fraction of what we need to know. However, a scientific basis does exist for identifying some things that are effective, as well as practices that are ineffective.

Intervention Integrity, Implementation, and Fidelity

One of the challenges in gaining a solid understanding of intervention implementation within the psychological literature is the array of terms that commonly have been used to describe intervention implementation. A variety of terms have been used to describe what is being implemented, including *treatment*, *intervention*, *program*, *practice*, and *innovation*. The meanings of those words and the traditions of their use vary across literatures. For example, the term *treatment* is most likely to appear in clinical and experimental contexts, whereas the terms *intervention* and *program* are most likely to appear in the educational literature. Many terms have also been used to describe the extent to which the treatment is implemented as planned. For example, researchers have used the terms *integrity*, *fidelity*, *reliability*, *adherence*, and *implementation* (Dusenbury, Brannigan, Falco, & Hansen,

2003; Henggeler, Melton, Brondino, Scherer, & Hanley, 1997; Peterson, Homer, & Wonderlich, 1982). No theme other than author preference is readily apparent that clarifies the reasons that such a diverse array of terms has emerged.

In all likelihood, *treatment integrity* has emerged as the most frequently used combination of terms, but due to its experimental roots it is problematic. Treatment integrity is to the extent to which an independent variable (IV) is implemented as designed in an experiment (Peterson et al., 1982). The parallel between this and the implementation of an intervention in a school is not difficult to grasp; the intervention is like an IV. However, it is not an IV. For example, in much of the research reviewed in this chapter, the outcome that was studied was implementation of interventions by teachers. As a result, implementation of interventions in these experimental studies was actually the dependent variable (DV). In the context of indirect services within schools, terms such as *treatment integrity* or *procedural fidelity* are simply too imprecise to have a great deal of utility. They can refer to the extent to which a consultation process was followed, the extent to which an experimental manipulation was effected within consultation, or the degree to which the resulting intervention was implemented.

To establish consistency in the discussion of interventions, treatments, and their implementation, this chapter adapts the use of three terms recommended by Noell (2008). Treatment integrity is used to refer to the accuracy of implementation of the IV in an experimental study, but not using it to describe practice. Intervention plan implementation (IPI) is used to describe the degree to which an intervention plan developed within consultation is implemented as designed. *Intervention* was adopted over *treatment* because that is the most common term used in schools. This is the term that would typically be used to describe practice and would commonly describe implementation when it is the DV targeted in research. Finally, Noell (2008) recommended using consultation procedural integrity (CPI) to describe the extent to which consultation procedures were implemented as designed. These general recommendations are followed throughout this chapter.

Measuring IPI

At a conceptual level, assessing IPI is not much different from assessing any other behavior. It is readily amenable to the same three common means of behavioral assessment that have been extensively discussed in the behavioral assessment literature for decades: self-reports, observations, and rating scales (Haynes & O'Brien, 2000). However, when one attempts to move from the concept of assessing IPI to its actual assessment, the issues become a bit more complex. One issue that will arise as one prepares to assess IPI is the level of specification of the intervention (Gresham, 1989). It is possible to define interventions at a very molecular level using exceedingly discrete behaviors. This approach can result in a definition of the intervention that includes hundreds of steps. For practical reasons, this seems an unworkable solution and is not represented in the research literature to any degree. An alternative strategy is to define the steps of intervention at a relatively molar level, with observable outcomes such as providing rewards, grading assignments, and providing prompts (e.g., Noell et al., 2000). This is clearly the level of definition that has predominated in the research literature. This intermediate to mildly molar level of definition has also provided a sufficient level of specificity to demonstrate a relationship between implementation and outcome in some studies and to demonstrate a sensitivity of implementation to experimental manipulation (Noell et al., 2000; Noell et al., 2005).

At a practical level, it is important to recognize that a tension will always exist between molecular definitions that provide detailed information that may be useful for debugging implementation problems and molecular definitions that are practical to measure. I recommend a relatively molar strategy that ensures that the major active elements of the intervention are distinct and measured. For example, as an element of a classwide behavior management strategy, a teacher might be asked to review the classroom expectations each morning as a prompt. A simple assessment might define this as that the teacher either did or did not review the classroom rules. An alternative definition might include prompting the class to attend, waiting to speak until students are quiet and oriented toward the teacher, speaking in a clear loud voice, stating each rule in succession, and offering encouragement that the teacher expects that the students will be able to meet these expectations. Although the latter definition provides richer behavioral detail, as each step in an intervention plan is defined with this level of detail, the measurement problem will quickly become unsolvable. My research team has found that molar assessments are commonly effective and sufficient (Noell et al., 1997; Noell, Duhon, Gatti, & Connell, 2002). In the unusual case in which molar-level implementation data are positive but RTI is poor, a more fine-grained analysis may be needed.

Once an intervention definition has been selected, the remaining major task is selecting a measurement approach. Direct observation is likely to be very appealing due to the unambiguous data produced. However, as a practical reality, few practitioners are likely to have the extensive time available that may be necessary to obtain a representative sample of implementation and to overcome issues such as reactivity to observation (Hintze & Mathews, 2004). It is worth noting that schoolwide systemic interventions may be particularly amenable to observational assessment. A schoolwide behavior management initiative that included prompting, monitoring, and consequence strategies might be a good candidate for observational assessment. A simple walk through the school using momentary time sampling across teachers might be able to capture a great deal of information in an efficient manner.

An intuitively appealing alternative approach is to use self-reports. Simply asking teachers, parents, and students if they have implemented intervention plans via interviews or rating scales has the virtues of being simply implemented, adaptable to a range interventions, and avoiding sampling issues inherent in observational methods. Unfortunately, the limited extant data should give any psychologist pause in accepting school consultees' reports of the degree to which they have implemented interventions. Research evidence suggests that teachers report substantially higher levels of implementation than assessment by direct observation or permanent products would suggest and that there is little relationship between the levels reported by the teacher and the levels obtained by more direct assessment (Noell et al., 2005; Wickstrom, Jones, LaFleur, & Witt, 1998).

A third option for the assessment of IPI is the use of permanent products. Permanent product measurement means assessing the physical products of the behavior. For example, in assessing IPI, a consultant might review the daily behavior monitoring cards for a behavioral intervention or the daily academic work materials that students complete as part of compensatory reciprocal peer tutoring for an academic intervention. Permanent products have both striking advantages and disadvantages. Permanent products are an unobtrusive measurement strategy that should create limited reactivity and that have the advantage of permitting of collection data that reflect an entire day without having to have an observer present (Mortenson & Witt, 1998; Noell et al., 1997). Additionally, permanent products do not rely on the implementers' memory or self-evaluation, as with self-reports. Permanent products are potentially subject to data fabrication if an intervention participant is motivated to appear to have implemented an intervention without actually having done so. On a practical level, though, having implemented or supervised far more than 100 consultation cases using a permanent-product-assessment strategy, I have never had the issue of faked data emerge. It appears that for most teachers that sort of dishonest behavior is not appealing. Additionally, the work required to fake the data is frequently nearly as great as is implementing the intervention itself. Additionally, if the consultant remains in contact with the student, the chances of the faked data being discovered become exceedingly high. The most important weakness of permanent-product data collection methods is their inability to detect intervention elements that do not produce a physical product, such as contingent praise. In these cases, direct observation and self-report appear to be the only viable options at present.

Devising an IPI assessment approach in a practice context will require consideration of the resources at hand, the design of the intervention, and the goals of the assessment. There will be very few cases in which it will be possible to know everything about implementation that a school psychologist might want to know. A number of authors have recommended mixed assessments that could include observation, permanent products, and self-reports (Dusenbury et al., 2003; Gresham, 1989); however, a research literature that examines how to integrate these measurement technologies has not yet emerged. The limited available literature does suggest that assessing implementation is a critical component of ensuring implementation and that relying on self-report alone is exceedingly unlikely to be sufficient.

Enhancing IPI

One of the critical challenges for practicing school psychologists is how to support IPI by parents and teachers. This is a particularly daunting challenge given that many school psychologists have no training in this domain and the common perception that many things might affect IPI. It is important to recognize three features that are fundamental to supporting IPI. First, having a teacher or parent implement an intervention represents a behavior change like any other. Second, any behavior change will require active programming. Third, the likelihood of successful behavior change will be strongly influenced by the degree to which data that monitor the behavior change are collected (Fuchs & Fuchs, 1986). Psychologists and educators have developed a massive literature regarding behavior change, with very little data regarding how effective or important those factors are in supporting implementation of educational interventions in schools by educators. This section briefly reviews some of the more commonly appealing and intuitive strategies that have been the targets of research.

Perhaps the most obvious and widely discussed strategy for supporting behavior change in teachers has been to ask them to change their behavior and to present acceptable and appealing strategies. Although some studies have reported positive results for implementation using such a strategy, the literature is fairly bleak regarding the effectiveness of this behavior change strategy (Noell et al., 1997; Noell et al., 2000; Noell et al., 2005; Witt, Noell, LaFleur, & Mortenson, 1997). It is interesting to note that one study that used a fairly elaborate verbal social influence strategy derived from the adult behavior change literature (e.g., Gonzales,

Aronson, & Costanzo, 1988; Howard, 1995; Lipsitz, Kallmeyer, Ferguson, & Abas, 1989) and achieved mildly encouraging results (Noell et al., 2005). The procedure was described as commitment emphasis and included a number of key elements. The consultant discussed how common it is for people to fail to complete commitments they make sincerely, the importance of the intervention as a commitment to the student and his or her parents, and the loss of credibility that would accompany failure to follow through. The script also discussed the importance of implementation to permit evaluation of the intervention and planning for resolving barriers to implementation. Although the study found that mean differences for the social influence condition were higher than for the traditional consultation condition, the result did not achieve statistical significance (Noell et al., 2005). The authors hypothesized that this may be due to a lack of statistical power combined with a much smaller magnitude of effect for social influence as compared with strategies for supporting IPI, such as performance feedback.

Despite previously advanced hypotheses, research data have suggested that acceptability may not be strongly related to implementation and may not be sufficient to ensure implementation (Noell et al., 2005). In a surprising way, it may be comforting to know that the data for IPI align with other research findings regarding behavior change in that simply agreeing that a behavior is desirable does not mean that a person will behave in that way. For example, engaging in regular exercise would commonly be perceived as a highly acceptable behavior, but the extent to which individuals actually engage in exercise appears to be the product of a complex interaction of variables, including issues such as environmental opportunity, schedules, and social influence (e.g., Gabriele, Walker, Gill, Harber, & Fisher, 2005). Intervention implementation in schools might parallel the literature relevant to health behaviors in several ways. Teachers may perceive interventions for students positively and intend to implement them when they are discussed in consultation. However, when they return to their classrooms with the existing routines and the many competing time demands, the intention may not be acted on because environmental supports for the new behavior (intervention) are not sufficient either to get

started or to persist within the demands of the classroom. I would argue that a critical role for consultants is providing the support educators need to help them implement new practices.

Another recurrent theme in the consultation literature in education has been the proposal that poor IPI may largely be a function of inadequate training in how to implement interventions (Watson & Robinson, 1996). For example, it has been demonstrated that implementation of a time-out procedure following a didactic training procedure was poor, but that it improved dramatically following an extensive *in vivo* training procedure (Taylor & Miller, 1997). A similar positive effect has also been demonstrated for direct instruction over didactic instruction in an analogue study of intervention implementation, but there are strong reasons to question the external validity of this study (Sterling-Turner, Watson, Wildmon, Watkins, & Little, 2001). This study examined undergraduates acting as teachers in a one-to-one teaching analogue situation with a research confederate playing the part of the student. In contrast, other research has suggested that training that includes enacting the intervention may not be necessary for other supports to sustain implementation (Noell et al., 1997). A rational appraisal of the literature in juxtaposition with other existing evidence regarding behavior change suggests that training would be critical in some instances and nearly irrelevant in others. When educators already possess the skills that are needed to implement the targeted intervention or innovation, then extensive training should not be necessary. When the targeted intervention or innovation includes skills that are not currently in their repertoires, training may be critically important. However, it is important to recognize that training can be necessary but insufficient. Generalization from training to actual application is certainly not ensured without active programming (Lentz & Daly, 1996).

Performance feedback is by far the most studied procedure for ensuring IPI in schools following consultation. The studies supporting the efficacy of performance feedback are fairly numerous at this point and are consistent in their finding that performance feedback works (Jones, Wickstrom, & Friman, 1997; Martens, Hiralall, & Bradley,

1997; Mortenson & Witt, 1998; Noell et al., 2002; Noell et al., 1997; Noell et al., 2000; Noell et al., 2005; Witt et al., 1997). Performance feedback has been demonstrated to be effective across diverse populations of teachers, students, interventions, and referral concerns. These studies have demonstrated poor implementation for both relatively simple interventions and complex ones that have both improved when performance feedback was provided (Witt et al., 1997; Noell et al., 2000). It is worth noting that this finding suggests that intervention simplicity may not be sufficient to ensure implementation. Studies have also demonstrated that performance feedback was more effective than brief follow-up meetings that did not include feedback and that the provision of materials and extensive training was not necessary for feedback to work (Noell et al., 1997; Noell et al., 2002). Performance feedback also has been demonstrated to be effective across varying schedules for its delivery and can be systematically faded without compromising IPI or intervention effects (e.g., Noell et al., 2005). Readers interested in a more detailed review of these studies can consult Noell (2008).

Cumulatively, the data suggest that brief, typically 5–10 minute, meetings once per week between a school psychologist and a teacher are sufficient to support behavior change if that meeting includes a number of critical elements. First, the meeting needs to include review of objective data regarding implementation (observations or permanent products). It is highly desirable that the data include both student and teacher behavior and that it be graphed to show the time course of the behavior (Noell et al., 2000). The meeting should include a brief discussion of what is going well with implementation and its impact on the student and what is going poorly. This, in turn, should occasion problem solving to modify the intervention and to support implementation where needed. Research has also demonstrated that intervention implementation can be sustained when the frequency of follow-up meetings is thinned to a more infrequent schedule (Noell et al., 2000).

Some readers will read the preceding paragraph and be concerned that teachers will be offended at having their behavior measured and receiving feedback on it. Our experience at Louisiana State University has indicated that this is an exceedingly rare case. Teachers consistently rate consultants who provide performance feedback very positively (Noell et al., 2000; Noell et al., 2005) and continue to make new referrals. Additionally, it is important to note that the approach used in meeting with teachers emphasizes shared work, support, respect for the teacher, and an overt commitment to helping the teacher and student succeed. Anecdotal comments from teachers exposed to performance feedback have included observations about how supported they felt, how committed to the case the consultant was, and how much more beneficial this approach was than the common consultation without systematic follow-up to which they were accustomed.

Systemic interventions that are schoolwide or that use structures such as grade-level teams provide a unique context for the implementation of the fundamental principles of objective assessment and feedback described earlier. In systemic intervention, it may be possible that a faculty member could have responsibility both for implementing some aspect of the intervention and for supporting another faculty member's implementation. In this type of context, in addition to implementing the intervention, the faculty member would check in on and provide feedback to a peer regarding his or her implementation. In this type of design, all faculty members are not only service providers but also support providers. It may be somewhat analogous to reciprocal peer tutoring, in which students serve in multiple roles within the intervention.

In summary, high acceptability, simplicity of interventions, and requests to implement the intervention do not appear to be sufficient to ensure consistent or sustained implementation (Noell et al., 2000; Noell et al., 2005). In contrast, performance feedback that includes review of objective implementation data with graphing of outcomes has been found to be effective across diverse settings, students, and referral concerns. Additionally, teachers rate consultants who provide performance feedback very positively. Although it seems certain that performance feedback is not the only implementation support strategy that will work, it is the only one that has accumulated a substantial literature base.

Evaluating IPI

One question that has confronted every psychologist who has monitored IPI and tried to improve it is, How much implementation is enough? Unfortunately, a number of initially plausible answers do not survive closer scrutiny very well. One logical initial response might be that the goal should be complete implementation. Although that may be desirable in the abstract, it is likely to set implementation standards that are not obtainable for intervention agents who have many alternative competing demands (Noell & Gresham, 1993). It may also be a substantially inefficient strategy in that perfect implementation may not be necessary to achieve a positive outcome. As it turns out, a number of studies demonstrate positive intervention outcomes with imperfect implementation (e.g., Gansle & McMahon, 1997; Holcombe, Wolery, & Snyder, 1994; Vollmer, Roane, Ringdahl, & Marcus, 1999). If imperfect implementation can be effective, then requiring perfect implementation will alienate some potential consumers by setting unattainable or unnecessarily burdensome goals and will increase the opportunity cost of providing interventions to students, with the net effect of reducing the number of students who receive services. It is also interesting to consider that the standards for sufficient implementation are likely to be quite different for systemic interventions than for individually targeted interventions. Generally, it would be reasonable to expect that it will be harder to obtain nearly ideal implementation for an intervention implemented by a whole faculty but that for many systemic interventions it may not be as necessary.

A logical alternative would be to argue that some implementation is better than none, so any implementation is a good thing. Unfortunately, this standard also will not withstand even modest empirical scrutiny. Research evidence is readily available demonstrating dramatically attenuated intervention benefits and complete intervention failure when implementation falls to sufficiently low levels (Greenwood, Terry, Arreaga-Mayer, & Finney, 1992; Henggler et al., 1997; Noell et al., 2002). Additionally, when interventions are part of services that carry the weight of due process or civil rights protections for students, such as is the case with RTI or special education services, low IPI may result in the loss of civil rights protections that have been guaranteed to students (Gansle & Noell, 2007).

A logical alternative to the intuitive, but poor, standards described previously would be to expect "enough" IPI. Unfortunately, the research base is woefully inadequate to define what that level of IPI would be. Noell (2008) argued that general a priori specification of sufficient IPI may be an unattainable goal because of the complexity of interventions, the variety of ways in which implementation can be degraded, the heterogeneity of environments in which interventions are embedded, and variations in students' and clients' needs. However, in practice, school psychologists will rarely need to specify the level of IPI a priori but can choose targets ad hoc based on the data that are emerging in specific cases. For example, if a teacher is implementing a new reading intervention with only 66% integrity but students are making excellent gains that meet the levels obtained in the published field trails for that intervention, then 66% may be enough for this intervention with these students. That is not to argue that improved implementation might not provide additional benefit but that it may not be necessary to provide an appropriate education and meet the intervention goals.

When students do not make sufficient progress and implementation is imperfect, the decision-making cycle is much more complex. Poor progress suggests a number of plausible hypotheses. It is possible that the intervention would be effective if it were implemented with a higher level of accuracy. However, near-perfect implementation may not be an attainable goal because the intervention is too complex or because competing environmental demands for intervention agents are numerous and salient. For example, a teacher may commit to spending 10 minutes per day working with a small group of referred students on phonemic awareness with the complete intention of doing so but may actually implement the intervention only intermittently due to a tight daily schedule of activities and unplanned classroom disruptions, such as visitors. It may also be the case that the intervention could be highly effective but that one of the components that is not being implemented is critical to that students' needs. For example, omitting the reinforcement component could be particularly problematic (e.g., Noell et al., 2000). For some students, nearly perfect implementation overall that omits just the motivational element of the intervention will fail. It is also worth noting that even interventions that are effective for most students may fail for individual students. For example, competing contingencies in the classroom may overwhelm the programmed reinforcement in the intervention. Similarly, the same prompting schedule that works for many students may not be efficient for a particular student (Heckaman, Alber, Hooper, & Heward, 1998). Unfortunately, in practice, it is not necessarily clear which components are critical for an individual student or which specific intervention might be most effective. These realities of practice highlight the need to continually assess implementation and student RTI so that interventions can be formatively revised.

It is important to recognize that implementation problems are not the only reason that interventions can produce poor results. The interventions themselves may be poorly designed or may be mismatched to students' needs. Additionally, poor progress monitoring data may be the result of selecting an insufficiently sensitive outcome measure or selecting one that is an indirect indicator of the student's behavior. In practice, many school psychologists will be confronted with imperfect implementation of interventions that are unlikely to be optimal in design and whose effect is being monitored with a measure that was readily obtainable rather than one that is ideal to the target. When students do not make adequate progress, interpreting the data at hand to determine where to focus efforts to improve student outcomes is a complex task. I would argue that it is similar in complexity to assessing and intervening with poor early reading (see Snow, Burns, & Griffin, 1998).

A considerable number of factors may be implicated, and assessment may need to consider multiple dimensions of the problem, but effective solutions are frequently attainable with some care, analysis, and data. For example, a student who is a poor reader might be provided with an intervention that included oral passage preview and repeated readings

(e.g., Noell et al., 1998). If that student did not exhibit adequate progress, a number of factors might be implicated. It might be the wrong intervention for the student's needs. The intervention is a fluency-building intervention, and further assessment data might reveal that the student has more fundamental decoding needs, such as the alphabetic principle and phonics skills. Further assessment that examined progress monitoring in varied levels of reading materials might yet reveal that the student is indeed progressing but that the grade-level materials being used to assess progress are too difficult to be sensitive to his growth. Review of implementation data may reveal—and unfortunately does so too commonly—that the tutoring sessions simply are rarely implemented. Alternatively, the sessions may reveal that the passages are being previewed at too fast a reading rate and that the repeated readings are being skipped to "squeeze sessions into a busy schedule." The key is that simply recognizing that the student is not progressing rapidly is a beginning that should occasion a systematic data-based process to dismantle the entire intervention to see where the breakdown is. Some practical recommendations for engaging in the problem-solving process relative to IPI are provided in the following section.

Some Practical Considerations and Recommendations for Practice

The goal of this section is to provide readers with practical recommendations regarding approaches to assess and support intervention implementation in schools. The recommendations are derived from a review of the literature and my experiences as a researcher, practitioner, and trainer across many cases of examining implementation issues in schools. As a result, some of the recommendations are based on the experience of working in schools rather than on hypotheses that have withstood the crucibles of empirical test and peer review.

Entry

Although we have not submitted it to an empirical test, I believe that the ways in which school psychologists manage entry into consulting, program development, and systems development play an important role in determining the success of those activities. From my experience as a supervisor, it would appear that the most common mistakes that graduate students and early career professionals make are underspecifying their role and overpromising outcomes. It is important to recognize that educators generally have prior experience with problem-solving work and as a result have considerable expectations prior to our contact with them. When engaging with a new service consumer, it is important to clarify what the planned course of action is, what the school psychologist will be contributing, what will be expected of consultees, and what the expected outcomes are (Sheridan, Kratochwill, & Bergan, 1996). My primary practical recommendations are to be specific, to be brief, and to promise a bit less than you think you can deliver. It is almost always better to exceed expectations than to either meet them or fall short.

Shared Work

Educators and parents are busy people with many simultaneous competing demands on their time. What they frequently need more than advice is help. Similarly, school psychologists are busy people with many simultaneous competing demands on their time who often cannot spend long periods of time with individual students, parents, teachers, or administrators to help. This would seem to create an insoluble problem, but that may not be the case. Educators who have many competing needs seem to be frequently appreciative of other professionals who will lend a hand, even if the help is modest. This may be particularly so when the instrumental help is unexpected. Direct assistance rather than mere advice giving from a school psychologist, as it turns out, is a surprise for some teachers in our experience at Louisiana State University.

For most school-based systemic initiatives and interventions, the reality is that teachers will carry the bulk of the responsibility and do the bulk of the work. Because the school psychologist cannot be in class all day to run the response-cost system or supervise the peer-tutoring intervention, the question is what instrumental help school psycholo-

gists can contribute. As it turns out, there is a great deal we can do, if we conceptualize helping to implement interventions as part of our work scope and function. I would recommend that school psychologists generally assume responsibility for preparatory and support roles in the intervention, as they cannot implement most interventions directly. These activities would include writing up the intervention plan, materials preparation, contacting parents, training peer tutors, training teachers (where needed), and arranging progress monitoring materials.

Assessment

My research team at Louisiana State University has developed an approach to consulting that requires *direct* assessment of *all* referred students. Direct assessment in this context means that the school psychologist assesses academic skills (typically curriculum-based measurement [ECBM]; Shinn, 1989), observes the student in relevant contexts, and interviews the student. Our reasoning is this: Teachers may be highly successful with many students in their classes, but the ones they refer are the ones with whom they are struggling. It seems imprudent to base intervention plans primarily or exclusively on the information the teacher has at hand. It is also the case that if school psychologists have no direct experience with students it is exceedingly difficult for them to provide an informed second opinion, and they have little credible basis for making recommendations or questioning teachers' assumptions regarding the factors maintaining current concerns. As a result I would suggest that school psychologists make a routine practice of completing at least brief direct assessments of referred students themselves prior to making any intervention recommendations. Additionally, the information gained about how the referring teacher teaches and manages the class can be invaluable.

Intervention Initiation

The process of devising interventions and developing systemic initiatives is complex, and adequately addressing it is beyond the scope of this chapter. However, some general recommendations regarding how to develop and initiate interventions that have a better chance of being implemented are provided. It is a general reality of human behavior that people like to know why things work as they do and why they are being asked to behave in a particular way. Toward this end, developing interventions that are overtly linked to assessment data and about which a school psychologist can specify the reason that these intervention elements are indicated for this student can be exceedingly helpful in reducing initial resistance and attending to consultees' questions. Additionally, interventions that are guided by prior assessment data will generally have a better chance of being effective.

It is also important to recognize that for any concern a range of intervention options will typically be viable and that these may range from relatively straightforward, simple interventions to ones that are exceedingly complex. One of the tremendous challenges confronting school psychologists who are attempting to bring about systems change or to support implementation of interventions is that it is very difficult to know what is practical and tolerable for individual teachers. Additionally, the same intervention that was practical for a teacher with one constellation of students can become impractical subsequently if new students with different needs join the class. The most appropriate approach to this dilemma may be talking about this issue directly with teachers, acknowledging that fitting an intervention to a classroom is sometimes an iterative process that requires revisions, and *pilot testing* ideas before concluding that the intervention is appropriate. Pilot testing appears to be the most important element of our strategy at LSU. We set up a time to begin implementation, and the school psychologist is in the classroom to observe and interact with the teacher as the teacher tries the intervention out (e.g., Noell et al., 2005). If the intervention appears to be impractical or if there is confusion about how to carry it out, those issues can be addressed immediately. It is a terrible waste of time and strain on rapport to wait days or a week to find out that the intervention that was planned was completely impractical in reality, despite everyone's best intentions, or that there was confusion regarding how it was to be implemented.

For many of the children referred to my team for in-class disruptive behavior prob-lems, we set up a behavior management intervention that includes student self-monitoring of target behaviors, teacher review of the record, goal setting, and contingent rewards, among other elements. Critical elements of the intervention appear to be (1) how many behaviors can be kept up with, (2) how many blocks the day will be broken up into, (3) what the goals are, (4) how frequently the teacher reviews the record, and (5) how often the student can earn a reward (once, twice, or three times daily). While observing implementation and talking with teachers, we have frequently found that one or more of these values was poorly chosen, despite having sounded plausible in the consultation meeting. As a result of this ongoing formative assessment, we routinely make adjustments to ensure that the teacher can actually implement the intervention and still teach and that the student is getting enough feedback that his or her behavior changes.

Follow-up and Support

Two of the fundamental decisions that any practicing school psychologist will have to make regarding support for any intervention or innovative systemic practice are how frequently to follow up and what form that follow-up should take. Although more frequent contact may be necessary initially, research suggests that brief weekly contacts that include a structured review of implementation and outcome data are typically sufficient to support implementation and obtain positive outcomes for students (Noell et al., 2005). Given that these follow-up contacts are frequently of 10 minutes' duration, they appear to be a reasonable and manageable format. Additionally, weekly contact helps prevent the development of long windows in which things are not going well in the classroom. It is also highly recommended that consultees and educators have quick, reliable means of reaching school psychologists who are working with them when unexpected issues arise. Typically, phone or e-mail contact information is sufficient.

A final issue in approaching follow-up is the inevitable breakdowns in intervention ef-fects. It may be most productive to approach cases expecting that issues will emerge for nearly all cases sooner or later. Health is-sues can create implementation problems for teachers; reinforcer satiation can erode intervention effectiveness; misplacing materials can disrupt interventions; students' improvement can make the initial intervention irrelevant or unworkable; and so on. For example, some years ago, when working with a student who was academically disengaged and disruptive, the teacher and I devised an intervention that included a visual cue to remind him to raise his hand and participate in class discussions, self-monitoring positive participation, and rewards for meeting participation benchmarks. However, at the end of the first week of implementation, the student was asking so many questions and making so many comments and was so engaged in the class discussion that it actually had become problematic in itself. As we revised the intervention to adjust to the students' improved behavior, implementation of the intervention began to fall apart. It was striking when the student described how frustrated he was because he was doing his part, but the teacher "was not holding up her end." That course of events and the resultant discussions in turn led to renewed implementation with a systematic plan for fading the intervention. A critical aspect of being realistic in approaching practice is recognizing that we cannot just give intervention and system change in schools to educator colleagues, then walk away and come back in 8 weeks to see how it is working. In those cases we should expect to fail. Intervention and system change is an ongoing iterative process that will normally require ongoing contributions by school psychologists.

Summary and Conclusions

It is frequently far harder to get effective interventions and valuable systemic reforms implemented than it is to identify them (Foxx, 1996; Noell et al., 2004). This reality evolves from a number of facts. Insight does not necessarily equal behavior change, and it certainly does not make behavior change easy (Cautela, 1993). School psychology has been characterized by a research literature that is vastly underdeveloped regarding how to help teachers, parents, and schools implement effective interventions or move systemic reforms from planning to implementation (Noell et al., 2002; Sheridan & Gutkin,

2000). Additionally, much of the existing professional literature has talked about implementation as if it consisted of simple rational exchanges that occur in a vacuum. The general suggestion has seemed to be to identify an effective acceptable intervention, tell teachers about it, and assume that they will or should do it. Interestingly, given what we know about human behavior in virtually every other context, this seems a very unrealistic approach. Despite these barriers, initial work has emerged demonstrating that if implementation is measured, graphed, and shared with educators in supportive professional meetings, then reasonable levels of implementation that lead to improved student outcomes can be obtained. Adapting this general model to schoolwide reforms in which educators provide the environmental support for one another seems a promising adaptation of this approach. Although I am quite certain that other methods will be discovered that can support implementation, that is what has been developed to date. The critical features are really not different from what we know about changing behavior in many other contexts: Define the behavior of interest, measure it, and create environmental feedback that reinforces implementation of the behavior of interest. The key is recognizing that teachers will need environmental supports to change behavior, just as students need supports to change behavior.

References

Ardoin, S. P., Witt, J. C., Connell, J. E., & Koenig, J. L. (2005). Application of a three-tiered response to intervention model for instructional planning, decision making, and the identification of children in need of services. *Journal of Psychoeducational Assessment, 23*, 362–380.

Barnett, D. W., Bell, S. H., Bauer, A., Lentz, F. E., Petrelli, S., Air, A., et al. (1997). The Early Childhood Intervention Project: Building capacity for service delivery. *School Psychology Quarterly, 12*, 293–315.

Barnett, D. W., Daly, E. J., Jones, K. M., & Lentz, F. E. (2004). Response to intervention: Empirically based special service decisions from single-case designs of increasing and decreasing intensity. *Journal of Special Education, 38*, 66–79.

Cautela, J. R. (1993). Insight in behavior therapy. *Journal of Behavior Therapy and Experimental Psychiatry, 24*, 155–159.

Cook, B. G., Gerber, M. M., & Semmel, M. I. (1997). Reflections on "Are effective school reforms effective for all students? The implications of joint outcome production for school reform." *Exceptionality, 7,* 131–137.

Dusenbury, L., Brannigan, R., Falco, M., & Hansen, W. B. (2003). A review of research on fidelity of implementation: Implications for drug abuse prevention in school settings. *Health Education Research, 18*(2), 237–256.

Eckert, T. L., & Hintze, J. M. (2000). Behavioral conceptions and applications of acceptability: Issues related to service delivery and research methodology. *School Psychology Quarterly, 15,* 123–148.

Farrell, P. B. (2004). *The lazy person's guide to investing.* New York: Warner Business Books.

Foxx, R. M. (1996). Twenty years of applied behavior analysis in treating the most severe problem behavior: Lessons learned. *Behavior Analyst, 19,* 225–236.

Fuchs, L. S., & Fuchs, D. (1986). Effects of systematic formative evaluation on student achievement: A meta-analysis. *Exceptional Children, 53,* 199–208.

Gabriele, J. M., Walker, M. S., Gill, D. L., Harber, K. D., & Fisher, E. B. (2005). Differentiated roles of social encouragement and social constraint on physical activity behavior. *Annals of Behavioral Medicine, 29,* 210–215.

Gansle, K. A., & McMahon, C. M. (1997). Component integrity of teacher intervention management behavior using a student self-monitoring treatment: An experimental analysis. *Journal of Behavioral Education, 7,* 405–419.

Gansle, K. A., & Noell, G. H. (2007). The fundamental role of intervention implementation in assessing resistance to intervention. In S. R. Jimerson, M. K. Burns, & A. M. VanDerHeyden (Eds.), *The handbook of response to intervention: The science and practice of assessment and intervention* (pp. 244–251). New York: Springer Science.

Gonzales, M. H., Aronson, E., & Costanzo, M. A. (1988). Using social cognition and persuasion to promote energy conservation: A quasi-experiment. *Journal of Applied Social Psychology, 18,* 1049–1066.

Gresham, F. M. (1989). Assessment of treatment integrity in school consultation and prereferral intervention. *School Psychology Review, 18,* 37–50.

Greenwood, C. R., Terry, B., Arreaga-Mayer, C., & Finney, R. (1992). The classwide peer tutoring program: Implementation factors moderating students' achievement. *Journal of Applied Behavior Analysis, 25,* 101–116.

Haynes, S. N., & O'Brien, W. H. (2000). *Principles and practices of behavioral assessment.* New York: Kluwer Academic/Plenum.

Heckaman, K. A., Alber, S., Hooper, S., & Heward, W. L. (1998). A comparison of least-to-most prompts and progressive time delay on the disruptive behavior of students with autism. *Journal of Behavioral Education, 8,* 171–201.

Henggeler, S. W., Melton, G. B., Brondino, M. J., Scherer, D. G., & Hanley, J. H. (1997). Multisystemic therapy with violent and chronic juvenile offenders and their families: The role of treatment fidelity in successful dissemination. *Journal of Consulting and Clinical Psychology, 65,* 821–833.

Hintze, J. M., & Matthews, W. J. (2004). The generalizability of systematic direct observations across time and setting: A preliminary investigation of the psychometrics of behavioral observation. *School Psychology Review, 33,* 258–270.

Holcombe, A., Wolery, M., & Snyder, E. (1994). Effects of two levels of procedural fidelity with constant time delay on children's learning. *Journal of Behavioral Education, 4,* 49–73.

Hosp, J. L., & Reschly, D. J. (2002). Regional differences in school psychology practice. *School Psychology Review, 31,* 11–29.

Howard, D. J. (1995). "Chaining" the use of influence strategies for producing compliance behavior. *Journal of Social Behavior and Personality, 10,* 169–185.

Individuals with Disabilities Education Improvement Act of 1975, Publ. L. No. 94-142, §1400 et seq.

Jones, K. M., Wickstrom, K. F., & Friman, P. C. (1997). The effects of observational feedback on treatment integrity in school-based behavioral consultation. *School Psychology Quarterly, 12,* 316–326.

Kim, J. J., & Crasco, L. M. (2006). Best policies and practices in urban educational reform: A summary of empirical analysis focusing on student achievements and equity. *Journal of Education for Students Placed at Risk, 11,* 19–37.

Lentz, F. E., & Daly, E. J., III. (1996). Is the behavior of academic change agents controlled metaphysically? An analysis of the behavior of those who change behavior. *School Psychology Quarterly, 11,* 337–352.

Lipsitz, A., Kallmeyer, K., Ferguson, M., & Abas, A. (1989). Counting on blood donors: Increasing the impact of reminder calls. *Journal of Applied Social Psychology, 19,* 1057–1067.

Martens, B. K., Hiralall, A. S., & Bradley, T. A. (1997). A note to teacher: Improving student behavior through goal setting and feedback. *School Psychology Quarterly, 12,* 33–41.

Mortenson, B. P., & Witt, J. C. (1998). The use of weekly performance feedback to increase teacher implementation of a prereferral academic intervention. *School Psychology Review*, 27, 613–627.

Noell, G. H. (2008). Research examining the relationships among consultation process, treatment integrity, and outcomes. In W. P. Erchul & S. M. Sheridan (Eds.), *Handbook of research in school consultation: Empirical foundations for the field* (pp. 323–342). Mahwah, NJ: Erlbaum.

Noell, G. H., Duhon, G. J., Gatti, S. L., & Connell, J. E. (2002). Consultation, follow-up, and behavior management intervention implementation in general education. *School Psychology Review*, 31, 217–234.

Noell, G. H., Gansle, K. A., & Allison, R. (1999). Do you see what I see? Teachers' and school psychologists' evaluations of naturally occurring consultation cases. *Journal of Educational and Psychological Consultation*, 10, 107–128.

Noell, G. H., Gansle, K. A., Witt, J. C., Whitmarsh, E. L., Freeland, J. T., LaFleur, L. H., et al. (1998). Effects of contingent reward and instruction on oral reading performance at differing levels of passage difficulty. *Journal of Applied Behavior Analysis*, 31, 659–664.

Noell, G. H., & Gresham, F. M. (1993). Functional outcome analysis: Do the benefits of consultation and prereferral intervention justify the costs? *School Psychology Quarterly*, 8, 200–226.

Noell, G. H., & Witt, J. C. (1998). Toward a behavior analytic approach to consultation. In T. S. Watson & F. M. Gresham (Eds.), *Handbook of child behavior therapy* (pp. 41–57). New York: Plenum.

Noell, G. H., Witt, J. C., Gilbertson, D. N., Ranier, D. D., & Freeland, J. T. (1997). Increasing teacher intervention implementation in general education settings through consultation and performance feedback. *School Psychology Quarterly*, 12, 77–88.

Noell, G. H., Witt, J. C., LaFleur, L. H., Mortenson, B. P., Ranier, D. D., & LeVelle, J. (2000). A comparison of two follow-up strategies to increase teacher intervention implementation in general education following consultation. *Journal of Applied Behavior Analysis*, 33, 271–284.

Noell, G. H., Witt, J. C., Slider, N. J., Connell, J. E., Gatti, S. L., Williams, K. L., et al. (2005). Treatment implementation following behavioral consultation in schools: A comparison of three follow-up strategies. *School Psychology Review*, 34, 87–106.

Peterson, L., Homer, A. L., & Wonderlich, S. A. (1982). The integrity of independent variables in behavior analysis. *Journal of Applied Behavior Analysis*, 15, 477–492.

Prout, S. M., & Prout, H. T. (1998). A meta-analysis of school-based studies of counseling and psychotherapy: An update. *Journal of School Psychology*, 36, 121–136.

Shapiro, E. S. (2006). Are we solving the big problems? *School Psychology Review*, 35, 260–265.

Sheridan, S., Welch, M., & Orme, S. (1996). Is consultation effective? A review of outcome research. *Remedial and Special Education*, 17, 341–354.

Sheridan, S. M., & Gutkin, T. B. (2000). The ecology of school psychology: Examining and changing our paradigm for the 21st century. *School Psychology Review*, 29, 485–502.

Sheridan, S. M., Kratochwill, T. R., & Bergan, J. R. (1996). *Conjoint behavioral consultation: A procedural manual*. New York: Springer.

Shinn, M. R. (1989). *Curriculum-based measurement: Assessing special children*. New York: Guilford Press.

Snow, C. E., Burns, M. S., & Griffin, P. (Eds.). (1998). *Preventing reading difficulties in young children*. Washington, DC: National Academy Press.

Sterling-Turner, H. E., Watson, T. S., Wildmon, M., Watkins, C., & Little, E. (2001). Investigating the relationship between training type and treatment integrity. *School Psychology Quarterly*, 16, 56–67.

Stollar, S. A., Poth, R. L., Curtis, M. J., & Cohen, R. M. (2006). Collaborative strategic planning as illustration of the principles of systems change. *School Psychology Review*, 35, 181–197.

Taylor, J., & Miller, M. (1997). When timeout works some of the time: The importance of treatment integrity and functional assessment. *School Psychology Quarterly*, 12, 4–22.

Vollmer, T. R., Roane, H. S., Ringdahl, J. E., & Marcus, B. A. (1999). Evaluating treatment challenges with differential reinforcement of alternative behavior. *Journal of Applied Behavior Analysis*, 32, 9–23.

Watson, T. S., & Robinson, S. L. (1996). Direct behavioral consultation: An alternative to traditional behavioral consultation. *School Psychology Quarterly*, 11, 267–278.

Wickstrom, K. F., Jones, K. M., LaFleur, L. H., & Witt, J. C. (1998). An analysis of treatment integrity in school-based consultation. *School Psychology Quarterly*, 13, 141–154.

Witt, J. C., Noell, G. H., LaFleur, L. H., & Mortenson, B. P. (1997). Teacher usage of interventions in general education: Measurement and analysis of the independent variable. *Journal of Applied Behavior Analysis*, 30, 693–696.

PART VI

BUILDING SYSTEMS TO SUPPORT
THE PROBLEM-SOLVING MODEL

Chapter 31

Collaboration across Systems
to Support Children and Families

Susan M. Sheridan
Katie L. Magee
Carrie A. Blevins
Michelle S. Swanger-Gagné

Schools are social places embedded in communities with a range of individuals who collectively share the responsibility for achieving one overarching goal—socializing and educating children. Indeed, within and beyond the walls of school buildings, a vast array of individuals contribute to children's instruction, support, and overall care. The most effective methods for achieving the far-reaching goals of schools are those that bring together all the key players in collaboration with one another.

This chapter presents the important topic of cross-system collaboration and provides concrete examples of how professionals can weave partnerships into their practice. First, the defining characteristics and benefits of cross-system collaboration are outlined. Second, different models of school-based problem-solving teams are presented to demonstrate how cross-system collaboration can be implemented. Third, specific relationship-building strategies are discussed to help professionals create a framework to carry out cross-system collaboration. One model of cross-system collaboration, conjoint behavioral consultation, is discussed in detail to illustrate the features and stag-

es of cross-system collaboration within a problem-solving framework. Fourth, potential challenges to cross-system collaboration are addressed with strategies professionals can use to address these challenges.

Introduction to Collaboration

Definition of Cross-System Collaboration

Collaboration is not a new concept, nor is it specific to education or psychology. It has been defined in several ways. In a generic sense, collaboration is a structured, recursive process in which two or more people work together toward a common goal—typically an intellectual endeavor—by sharing knowledge and building consensus (*Merriam-Webster's Online Dictionary*, 2007). In educational circles, it is often defined in a manner similar to that posited by Cowan, Swearer, and Sheridan (2004), who stated that collaboration is "a reciprocal dynamic process that occurs among systems, schools/classrooms, and/or individuals (e.g., parents, educators, administrators, psychologists) who share in decision making toward common goals and solutions related to students"

(p. 201). In practice, collaboration allows individuals to pool resources to create cooperative interdependent relationships on behalf of children, ensuring the availability and provision of appropriate and effective services. The joint work of families, educators, and specialists who work together (i.e., *co-labor*; *Merriam-Webster's New Collegiate Dictionary*, 1981) to promote the academic and social development of students may result in stronger and integrated support systems, contributing to children's learning and development.

Children's development is influenced by many systems, including but not limited to schools. Thus children's adaptation and functioning is a product of interactions within and between these systems. Collaboration among the major systems of influence in children's lives (e.g., families, schools, religious, health systems) is advantageous in that it can lead to better prevention, identification, and management of children's conditions (American Academy of Pediatrics [AAP], 2000, 2001). We define *cross-system collaboration* as a process by which providers across multiple support systems join together to identify needs, pool resources, and achieve goals for enhancing outcomes for children.

Implicit in the adoption of cross-system collaboration is the recognition by both professionals and family members that the unique perspectives and expertise of each individual contributes meaningfully to a child's learning experience. Prerequisite to specific collaborative actions are *attitudes and beliefs* that families and other providers have important roles throughout the problem-solving process and that they will participate to their fullest capacity if given the opportunity. Conveying these beliefs in a genuine and sincere manner is the responsibility of school personnel early on and throughout the collaborative process. This is accomplished through frequent, open communication and predictable, consistent follow-through (e.g., through phone calls, e-mail communications, notes, brief but frequent meetings), which go far in building trust and relationships among participants. Parents' involvement is heightened by specific invitations to be involved (Green, Walker, Hoover-Dempsey, & Sandler, 2007). Genuine invitations and outreach to parents can include information on specific roles they can play and sources of information they can provide. Highlighting their previous efforts and examples of positive actions they have taken on their child's behalf communicates respect and validation and increases their potential acceptance and trust. Detailed accounts of strategies for promoting involvement, building relationships, and implementing collaborative strategies across systems (including home and school systems) are summarized in later sections of this chapter. In addition, readers are referred to Clarke, Sheridan, and Woods (in press) for recommendations on strengthening relationships with families.

Common to all definitions of collaboration are notions that collaboration is interactive and dynamic. It is a *process*, not an event or activity. Participants (i.e., partners) share mutual goals and work together to make decisions and solve identified problems (Welch & Sheridan, 1995). In many ways, collaboration is an approach, an ethos (Phillips & McCullough, 1990), or an overarching philosophical framework for educating students. As such, collaborative efforts can take many structures or formats. Examples include interdisciplinary teaming efforts within schools and consultation within and across systems. The context, needs, and available resources in large part determine the form or structure that collaboration will take.

Regardless of structure, collaborative efforts share common characteristics. Collaboration is characterized by a *relationship* among players that is mutually collegial, interdependent, and coequal. At a fundamental level, collaboration involves both *equality*, the willingness to listen to, respect, and learn from one another, and *parity*, the blending of knowledge, skills, and ideas to enhance outcomes for children (Welch & Sheridan, 1995). Collaborative efforts require that *communication channels* be open and bidirectional. There is *joint ownership* of the issue or problem being addressed, with personal resources and expertise shared and pooled to create optimal solutions. Decisions are made in a *consensual* manner among participants. In sum, collaboration requires that participants "share joint responsibilities and rights, are seen as equals, and can jointly contribute to the process" (Vosler-Hunter, 1989, p. 15).

Rationale for Cross-System Collaboration

Educational, psychological, and health/mental health needs of children often require the expertise of multiple professionals across many disciplines (Hoagwood, Kelleher, Feil, & Comer, 2000), including (but not limited to) educators, psychologists, medical specialists, and parents. The potential effectiveness of treatment programs for children may be maximized to the extent that these experts work together to identify a child's strengths and primary needs and to develop, support, and implement coordinated treatment plans. Collaboration across systems supports "processes for monitoring and evaluating children's adjustment ... by combining perspectives from persons and information from school, family, and health care contexts" (Shapiro & Manz, 2004, p. 60). As such, information can be shared and discussed in ways that promote broader perspectives and understandings of problems and solutions. Through collaborative ventures, family, school, and other support systems (e.g., health, justice, social systems) align to facilitate comprehensive problem solving and mutual decision making for meeting children's needs (Power, DuPaul, Shapiro, & Kazak, 2003).

The benefits of cross-system collaboration among professionals and family members are many. Information from families and educators can help health and mental health professionals make diagnoses based on knowledge and observations of children's functioning in home and school environments. Educators and family members can monitor treatment efficacy and report on the influence of interventions on children's cognitive, social, and behavioral functioning (Kline & Rubel, 2001). Health professionals can provide pertinent information about children's health, prognosis, and physical abilities, all of which can have a direct impact on children's educational performance and psychological well-being. Indeed, the focus of a particular situation will determine the composition of a collaborative team (i.e., the specific individuals who serve as participants) and their most appropriate roles. In certain situations involving mental health issues, behavioral problems, or unique developmental concerns, a school psychologist may take a primary lead and guide the team

TABLE 31.1. Potential Benefits of Collaborative Approaches to Practice

1. Increased communication and collaboration among school personnel and other support systems
2. Increased ownership and commitment to program goals
3. Increased understanding of the complexities of a situation
4. Greater conceptualization of a problem
5. Increased range of solutions generated
6. Diversity of expertise and resources available
7. Superiority of solutions generated
8. Integrity in plan implementation and maintenance of treatment gains
9. Successful implementation of innovation and change

by outlining relevant questions, pooling information from multiple sources, and sharing recommendations based on all available data. In cases involving family or domestic issues, similar roles may be assumed by a social worker, and in cases involving communication delays, a speech–language pathologist may take the lead role. A summary of the benefits of collaboration is provided in Table 31.1.

Operationalizing Cross-System Collaboration through School-Based Teams

All too often, efforts to meet children's needs occur via services that are disjointed and fragmented. To provide the best care for students, cross-system collaboration is necessary to create continuity among the many services and supports that exist in children's lives (Anderson-Butcher & Ashton, 2004). Problem-solving, team-based approaches in schools have emerged to provide a comprehensive, integrated approach to service delivery and to operationalize cross-system collaboration (Gravois & Rosenfield, 2006; Rosenfield, Silva, & Gravois, 2007).

Collaborative teams can create opportunities for key stakeholders to enhance their understanding of students' difficulties and work together toward common goals (Rosenfield et al., 2007). Additionally, teaming can lead to increased feelings of support among professionals during the design and implementation of effective interventions (Tourse

& Sulick, 1999). The teaming model serves as an ideal framework for professionals to collectively navigate through the problem-solving process to better meet children's needs.

Process elements within collaborative teams require attention to achieve their full benefits. Specifically, it is important that teams are developed in ways that support clarity of roles and responsibilities, mutual goal setting, shared responsibility and ownership, and regular communication. Structural elements of teams are also important. One structural feature of teams concerns their membership. Team membership varies depending on the purpose and structure of the team. Membership of school-based teams can include a variety of individuals from home, school, and community settings. Traditional teaming involves the engagement of all parties jointly to exchange relevant information to support a child's learning, adaptation, or adjustment. When professionals are housed outside the school, however, it is not always possible to achieve full membership and attendance at team meetings. In these cases, school personnel are encouraged to find ways to include these professional perspectives within the collaborative process, even in cases in which their physical involvement is not possible. Scheduled phone calls, Web meetings, e-mails, and interactive memos all represent ways to achieve bidirectional information sharing and increase relevant participation. Various process and structural elements of teams and their potential benefits are given in Table 31.2.

Teams also vary in the levels at which they facilitate interdisciplinary collaboration. The most basic level of teaming includes professionals from a number of different disciplines who assess and provide parallel services to students. There is unidirectional communication from team members to the team leader, who then integrates all of the information. At this level there are often built-in formal mechanisms for communication (e.g., formal meetings, calling outside professionals to gather information). Professionals relay important information and observations to the team leader without much discussion or interaction among members. Each step of the problem-solving process is carried out by individual professionals within their specific discipline (Friend & Cook, 2007). For example, physicians, mental health professionals, and other community professionals may pose questions and share valuable information regarding a child's performance and needs but not be present at school-based meetings. To ensure access to that information, the team leader is typically responsible for eliciting information from these professionals prior to meetings (e.g., through e-mail, phone calls, or notes) and for sharing their perspectives with the school-based team.

The next level of teaming adopts a more collaborative approach to problem solving and decision making. All team members make a strong commitment to frequent communication by collaborating to design, implement, and evaluate interventions. Team members share information with each other and engage in open discussion about their observations. Services are carried out by individual service providers, however, making coordinated services an exception (Friend & Cook, 2007). Collaborative teaming at this level is useful when planning interventions for children who are being treated with medication, for example. School professionals are often asked by doctors to complete behavior rating scales and checklists before and after the medication changes to inform medication decisions. School psychologists can also

TABLE 31.2. Elements and Benefits of Effective Teams

Element	Benefit
• Clear roles and expectations	• Prevents replication of services.
• Mutual goals	• Defines and drives the team's primary purpose.
• Shared responsibility and ownership	• Maximizes team productivity.
• Regular communication among team members	• Information is shared across disciplines leading to better provision of services.
• Supportive leadership	• Gives team members a sense of ongoing support.

gather valuable information that contributes to treatment planning by conducting classroom observations and sharing this information with the child's health-care provider. Optimal outcomes occur when school and medical professionals keep each other informed about treatment changes, challenges, and successes (Power et al., 2003).

A more collaborative approach to teaming creates shared responsibility for the provision of services, with professionals working together throughout the assessment, treatment planning, and treatment implementation stages. These activities are often conducted simultaneously by individuals from more than one discipline. Areas of overlap among various disciplines are frequently used as the springboard for other shared activities. This approach to collaborative teaming is often found in early childhood home visit models. Teachers, physical therapists, occupational therapists, school psychologists, parents, and other specialists work as a cohesive team to assess the child's needs and to design and deliver services. Within this context, the entire team takes part in planning the intervention components from each discipline, but only one or two professionals may be responsible for delivering all of the services to the child during home visits.

Finally, in the highest level of collaborative teaming, no one person or professional is assumed to have adequate knowledge or sufficient expertise to execute all the functions associated with the provision of services for students. Team members share ownership and responsibility for planning and monitoring all goals and strategies, as well as intervention objectives (Wilcox, Kouri, & Caswell, 1991).

The teaming model provides an optimal framework for meeting children's complex needs and fostering cross-system collaboration. However, it is important that teams have clear roles, expectations, and agreed-upon goals to maximize the time and resources spent in collaborative efforts. Team members work most efficiently when they feel supported and part of a collective group that has taken on shared responsibility for meeting children's needs. Garnering the support of the leadership, holding regular meetings with adequate time allotted, and implementing the effective use of communication and collaboration skills (Wolery & Odom,

2000) increase effective interdisciplinary teaming.

Building Relationships for Cross-System Collaboration

Certain conditions must be present when working across systems to promote positive relationships and collaborative partnerships. These conditions are created when participants engage in practices that promote relationships and partnerships across settings and participants involved in cross-system collaboration. Relationship-building objectives and strategies are described next, with examples illustrated in Table 31.3.

Promote and Improve Understanding and Communication across Settings

A key objective of cross-system collaboration concerns the improvement of knowledge, understanding, and communication across settings (Sheridan & Kratochwill, 2008). Opportunities for learning are present across all contexts in which children are immersed, and outcomes are enhanced when persons across settings actively partner during intervention planning and implementation. This "essential partners" attitude by all participants is a vital part of collaboration (Christenson & Sheridan, 2001). To meet this objective, a positive and strength-based orientation is beneficial to both increase acceptance among participants (including parents and other team members) and maximize desirable outcomes. This can be accomplished by highlighting the expertise of all participants, eliciting information, and creating opportunities for participants to share in the responsibility for serving children. In addition, offering coaching, training, and parent support groups is a possible mechanism for increasing information sharing and providing support. For example, during the intervention implementation phase, team members can coach (i.e., observe, provide feedback, model for) parents in their home, which not only builds parenting skills but also offers an opportunity for communication across systems.

Communication is a cornerstone of effective collaboration. Regular communication procedures, such as scheduled phone calls

TABLE 31.3. Relationship-Building Objectives, Strategies, and Examples

Objective	Strategies	Examples
Promote and improve understanding and communication across settings	Communicate an "essential partners" attitude.	• Highlight expertise of all participants. • Elicit ideals, information, and perspectives from all participants. • Paraphrase and validate messages.
	Exhibit a positive and strength-based orientation.	• Always start with positive message. • Encourage positive communications such as good-news phone calls. • Reframe negative messages into positive messages. • Focus on child's abilities and skills. • Focus on team members' abilities to help the child.
	Provide support.	• Coach participants. • Facilitate support groups. • Conduct training. • Communicate regularly. • Thank team members for their efforts.
	Use regular communication systems.	• Schedule phone calls, notes, e-mails. • Use handbooks, newsletters, folders for exchanging notes.
	Use strategic questioning.	• Follow problem-solving structure to guide questions. • "When does he follow directions?" • "What does he gain by talking to his friends in class?" • "What is happening before he is off task?"
	Use clarifying statements.	• "So, what you are saying is. ... "
	Summarize and paraphrase.	• "It sounds like. ... " • "To summarize, Jon is more off task during math time when the work is more difficult for him. ... " • Use team members' words when paraphrasing.
	Use reflective and empathetic statements.	• "It seems like you are frustrated." • "It must be hard to. ... "
	Use open questioning (questions that cannot be answered with a single word such as "yes" or "no").	• "What does the morning routine look like?" • "What ideas do you have?"
	Follow shared decision making orientation.	• Clarify rationales for collaboration. • Specify expectations and roles of team members. • Avoid "being the expert" and giving unsolicited advice, unless it is given in a highly supportive, facilitative manner.
Promote shared ownership and joint responsibility for child success	Make process "overt."	• Provide rationales and expectations for collaboration. • Clearly describe roles and expectations.
	Reinforce and encourage all participants to participate.	• Paraphrase and validate the team member's messages. • Verbally encourage sharing by saying such things such as "uh-huh." • Nonverbally encourage sharing with body language such as nodding or leaning head toward speaker. • Structure interventions that require cooperation.
	Facilitate relationships and partnerships.	• Point out similarities across settings. • Reinforce problem solving across settings.
	Invite others to share their perspectives.	• "What do you think?"

(cont.)

TABLE 13.3. *(cont.)*

Objective	Strategies	Examples
Increase perspective taking	Use active listening skills.	• Use minimal encouragers such as nodding, sharing eye contact.
	Verbally acknowledge different points of view.	• "I see your point." • "That is important to help us see the whole picture."
	Emphasize joint expectations and responsibilities.	• State expectations. • "We all need to work together to help Jon be successful and build his skills."
	Structure specific efforts to strengthen relationships.	• Arrange room to encourage dialogue by placing chairs in a circle so members face each other; remove physical barriers such as tables. • Encourage members to sit next to each other. • Use language to unify group, such as "we," "us," "our."
Strengthen relationships within and across systems	Model positive communication.	• Say "concern" or "need" instead of "problem." • Remind team of child's strengths and ability to build skills. • Emphasize positive efforts by all members. • Point out strengths of all. • View system differences as strengths. • Refrain from blaming or finding fault. • Attribute success to efforts of team members. • Focus on child's performance.
	Reframe negative messages.	• Reframe problems into opportunities for growth. • Reframe negative comments into areas of shared concern.
	Discuss shared experiences across systems.	• Point out and discuss similarities in each system. • Discuss strengths in each setting.
	Create opportunities for open communication.	• Focus on shared goal of improving child's performance. • Focus on mutual interest across settings. • Share resources and information.
	Point out importance of creating opportunities for children to experience success.	• Highlight opportunities for similar interventions across settings. • Discuss importance of continuity across settings.
Maximize opportunities to address needs across settings	Provide rationale and benefits of congruence and continuity of experiences.	• Discuss importance of systems to support consistent goal setting, expectations, and plan development.
	Emphasize team concept.	• Use inclusive language such as "we." • State that all members contribute unique knowledge and expertise. • State that all members have the responsibility for contributing and for seeking help from other members.
Increase shared commitment to goals	Involve all members in discussion.	• Ask questions of all members and ask for opinions from all. • Involve all important members of the child's life (e.g., caregiving grandparents). • Involve students when possible.
	Be open to all contributions of ideas.	• Validate all member's treatment ideas.
	Emphasize shared commitment in treatment.	• Discuss how to make treatment consistent across settings. • Develop intervention plans that can be implemented successfully across settings.

or written communications (notes, memos, brief progress reports), allow information to be shared continuously. Specific effective communication techniques, such as the use of strategic questioning (questions that guide participants through structured problem solving), encourage sharing and improve communication across systems (Friend & Cook, 2007; Sheridan & Kratochwill, 2008; see Table 31.3). Open questions (i.e., questions that cannot be answered with "yes" or "no") are a form of strategic questioning that elicits ideas, information, and perspectives from participants. For example, an open question such as, "What are some intervention ideas to help Joe meet his goals?" will elicit more information than a closed question such as "Do you have any ideas that can help Joe meet his goals?" Reframing negative messages into positive messages keeps the team focused on the abilities and attributes (not just deficits) of the child and team members. For example, a comment focusing on a child's social skill problems can be reframed to a statement such as "Jeremy's high energy level with peers shows his desire to participate in group activities. I wonder how we can help him channel this energy to interact socially in ways his peers will accept."

Team members can also summarize and paraphrase statements to check for understanding, provide structure, and identify themes evident in team meetings. Additionally, reflecting statements, such as, "It sounds like you are frustrated," reinforce participation by responding to the emotional tone of the participant and conveying support. Together, paraphrasing, summarizing, and reflecting allow participants to confirm clarity in communication, thus improving relationships. Additional examples of communication-building techniques are illustrated in Table 31.3.

Promote Shared Ownership and Joint Responsibility for Child Success

Shared ownership in decision making and joint responsibility within a team are essential to children's success (Sheridan & Kratochwill, 2008). Throughout the collaborative process, discussions regarding the problem-solving process should be considered a shared decision-making venture. At the beginning of the process, it is useful to clarify rationales (why it is important) and expectations for collaboration (behaviors that make it effective). The contribution of all participants can be encouraged by paraphrasing and validating their messages (e.g., repeating back key ideas or phrases, reinforcing members for their contributions). It is also helpful to point out similarities and to build cohesion, to verbally encourage sharing and open communication, and to reinforce problem solving across settings (see Table 31.3 for examples).

Increase Perspective Taking

A benefit of cross-system collaboration is the fact that different, and unique, perspectives are brought to the table. This serves as a strength only if participants are willing to consider the various perspectives on a particular issue. Thus, when bringing together multiple systems and professionals, it is important to create a safe climate wherein varied perspectives among team members can be voiced and shared understandings encouraged (Sheridan & Kratochwill, 2008). For example, team members can openly invite others to share their opinions and observations on relevant matters. Perspective taking is further encouraged by verbally acknowledging different points of view using statements such as, "I see your point," or "That's an important perspective." The use of active listening skills such as minimal encouragers (e.g., nodding head, body leaning toward person speaking, making eye contact; Friend & Cook, 2007) can increase active information and opinion sharing by participants.

Strengthen Relationships within and across Systems

Relationships may be strained when individuals with diverse goals from multiple systems join together; therefore, it is important to structure specific efforts to strengthen relationships across settings (Sheridan & Kratochwill, 2008). Simple strategies such as (1) arranging the room to encourage dialogue (e.g., in a circle so participants face each other), (2) modeling positive communication (e.g., pointing out strengths and validating opinions and efforts of participants), and (3) using language to unify the group (e.g., terms such as *we*, *us*, or *our*, rather than *I* or *my*) can foster positive relationships across systems. Techniques such as reframing problems into opportunities for growth and development and negative comments into areas of shared concern provide a means of addressing concerns in a positive and nonthreatening manner. Sometimes team members do not realize the similarities that exist across systems. It is important for team members to recognize and discuss similarities and strengths across settings to empower participants and create opportunities for open communication. Empowerment can also be facilitated by promoting joint responsibility for children's school success and focusing on the shared goal of improving children's performance. These techniques may help manage potential conflict during cross-setting team meetings.

Maximize Opportunities to Address Needs across Settings

Continuity across settings supports children's positive adaptation through the establishment of mutual goals and consistent implementation of responsive, effective interventions (Sheridan & Kratochwill, 2008). The potential for addressing needs across settings can be maximized by pointing out the importance of creating opportunities for children to experience success. It is pertinent to highlight opportunities for similar interventions across settings to provide a sense of continuity for children (e.g., plans targeting similar behaviors across home and school and providing agreed-upon rewards for positive performance in both settings). Providing a rationale for and explaining the benefits of continuity across home and school for the child's benefit will support consistent goal setting and plan development, thereby enhancing children's services.

Increase Shared Commitment to Goals

Team members typically desire similar successes for children, and retaining a focus on congruent goals helps build cohesion. A shared commitment to goals facilitates collaborative relationships within the team (Christenson & Sheridan, 2001; Sheridan & Kratochwill, 2008). To increase shared commitment, team members can emphasize a team concept by using inclusive language (e.g., *we*), and incorporating the unique

knowledge of and expertise regarding children that each brings to the table. The active recognition of unique contributions to the team's efforts allows opportunities to seek help and learn from one another. For example, parents and teachers know the child's behaviors and interests in various settings and strategies that may lead to improvements for the child. Other family members involved in the child's life, as well as the child him- or herself, can also be involved in the process to diversify expertise in the group. During treatment development, open contribution of ideas for treatment implementation and its consistent use across settings also increases shared commitment. For example, if the child is working on following directions at bedtime, he or she could also focus on following directions during structured times at school.

For different systems to collaborate effectively, relationships must be supported and partnerships promoted. Thus facilitators are advised to use strategies such as effective communication and problem solving and to emphasize the group's shared goals and joint responsibility to help the child progress toward his or her goals.

Structures and Procedures for Cross-System Collaboration

Relationships between systems are relevant only to the extent that they lead to improved outcomes for children. Structured means for delivering cross-system services are necessary to optimize child outcomes. Behavioral consultation was one of the first structured models of service delivery that utilized a problem-solving process in which consultants and consultees work together to develop and implement interventions aimed at indirectly benefiting student behavior change. In traditional behavioral consultation, a consultant guides the consultee (i.e., parent or teacher) through the stages of a structured problem-solving process. Behavioral consultation (Kratochwill & Bergan, 1990) is widely utilized in school settings to address children's social–emotional, behavioral, and academic concerns (Martens & DiGennaro, 2008).

Given that children's development and learning take place across and are affected by numerous systems, including only one consultee in services limits their scope and impact. Conjoint behavioral consultation (CBC) is one model of cross-system collaboration. CBC emerged as an extension of behavioral consultation (Sheridan, Kratochwill, & Bergan, 1996; Sheridan & Kratochwill, 2008) in an effort to articulate a collaborative approach within the structured, data-based behavioral consultation framework. CBC is defined as "a strength-based, cross-system problem-solving and decision-making model wherein parents, teachers, and other caregivers or service providers work as partners and share responsibility for promoting positive and consistent outcomes related to a child's academic, behavioral, and social–emotional development" (Sheridan & Kratochwill, 2008, p. 25). In CBC, important individuals in children's lives work collaboratively in a consultative process. A distinct feature of CBC is the active role of parents, teachers, and other service providers as appropriate in joint problem solving and decision making. CBC has been found to be useful and effective in numerous experimental small-n studies (Sheridan, Clarke, & Burt, 2008) and meta-analyses (Sheridan, Eagle, Cowan, & Mickelson, 2001), and recently it has been promoted in the work of broader cross-system (i.e., home, school, pediatric health care setting) collaboration (Burt, Clarke, Dowd-Eagle, & Sheridan, 2008; Power et al., 2003; Sheridan, Warnes, Woods, Blevins, Magee, & Ellis, in press). There are three main goals of CBC: (1) to promote positive outcomes for children, (2) to promote parent engagement, and (3) to establish and strengthen partnerships (Sheridan & Kratochwill, 2008). These goals and related objectives are listed in Table 31.4.

Parents, teachers, and other professionals and service providers are potential team members in the CBC process. Features inherent in CBC (i.e., practices designed to increase perspective taking, relationship building, cultural acceptance, and collaborative problem solving) allow the recognition of individual and cultural differences among participants and elucidate their role in a child's functioning. Partnerships among home, school, and medical systems are fostered through open lines of communication in CBC, allowing each party to share relevant expertise. Shared responsibility for

TABLE 31.4. Overarching Goals and Objectives of Conjoint Behavioral Consultation

Goals

1. Promote academic, socioemotional, and behavioral *outcomes for children* through joint, mutual, cross-system planning.
2. Promote *parent engagement* wherein parental roles, beliefs, and opportunities for meaningful participation are clear within a developmental, culturally sensitive context.
3. Establish and strengthen *home–school partnerships* on behalf of children's learning and development, immediately and over time.

Outcome objectives

1. Obtain comprehensive and functional data over extended temporal and contextual bases.
2. Establish consistent intervention programs across settings.
3. Improve the skills, knowledge, or behaviors of all parties (i.e., family members, school personnel, and the child client).
4. Monitor behavioral contrast and side effects systematically via cross-setting intervention agents.
5. Enhance generalization and maintenance of intervention effects via consistent programming across sources and settings.
6. Develop skills and competencies to promote further independent conjoint problem solving between the family and school personnel.

Process objectives

1. Improve communication, knowledge, and understanding about family, child, and school.
2. Promote shared ownership and joint responsibility for problem solution.
3. Promote greater conceptualization of needs and concerns and increase perspective taking.
4. Strengthen relationships within and across systems.
5. Maximize opportunities to address needs and concerns across, rather than within, settings.
6. Increase shared (parent and teacher) commitments to educational goals.
7. Increase the diversity of expertise and resources available.

Note. From Sheridan and Kratochwill (2008). Copyright 2008 by Springer Science and Business Media. Reprinted by permission.

collaboratively identifying primary foci for services and components of comprehensive intervention plans is an additional cornerstone of the model.

CBC consultants play a vital role in creating and maintaining cross-system partnerships as liaisons between the home, school, and medical systems. School-based CBC consultants are in an ideal position to educate medical service providers about educational and school-related issues, as well as to educate school professionals about medication and medically related issues that may affect the child's functioning at school. It is essential to communicate with medical professionals to gather information about medication changes and the impact of medical conditions on the child. Because consultants understand the child's strengths, needs, and current performance at home and school, they are in an optimal position to gather information from physicians about medical issues and to bring them back to the team. Other consultant roles include: channeling information among school, family, and health-care providers; synthesizing important case issues from multiple perspectives; educating each system about issues and plans for intervention or placement changes; coconstructing and coordinating cross-system intervention plans; and inviting community professionals such as therapists, case workers, and health liaisons (e.g., nurses, physicians assistants) to attend CBC meetings. CBC services may be initiated by parents, teachers, or consultants (e.g., situations in which problem behaviors are interfering with school and/or home functioning). The CBC consultant guides all parties through a systematic and collaborative problem-solving process, as specified later.

By developing a collaborative partnership across systems, it is possible to promote consistency among service providers and families, thereby promoting maintenance and generalization of treatment effects. Throughout all stages, facilitators work to develop an infrastructure for communication, information sharing, and decision making across educational, medical, psychological, and family systems. A structured problem-solving framework that guides the interactions of multiple systems in a structured and goal-focused manner is necessary to realize the benefits of cross-system collaboration. This framework promotes consistency across service providers and allows participants to remain focused on and achieve a common goal that is determined through the problem-solving process. Through this structure, consultants and consultees are able to systematically and mutually identify and prioritize concerns, establish goals, analyze factors that contribute to the presence of the concern, develop treatment strategies, and evaluate progress. The unique variables that make up the collaborative problem-solving model are described in detail by Sheridan and Kratochwill (2008) and are summarized here.

At each stage of the collaborative problem-solving process, relevant individuals from multiple systems (e.g., parents, teachers, psychologists, day care providers, nutritionists, physical therapists) are invited to meet together to engage in collaborative problem-solving. The nature of the specific concerns determines the main participants in the process. All participants are encouraged to contribute their unique expertise, observations, and suggestions in a common effort to address the pervasive needs of the child. A team facilitator will be important to coordinate and guide the problem-solving process. The facilitator (e.g., school psychologist, clinical social worker, special education coordinator) should be in a position to link individuals between and across systems and to facilitate the problem-solving process by organizing meetings, inviting participants, directing discussions, and summarizing procedures.

Identify/Prioritize Concerns

First, it is necessary for individuals investing in cross-system collaboration to determine shared goals. Participants should gain a unified conceptualization of the foremost needs relevant to children's success across all contexts. Additionally, it is important to identify the strengths of the child, as well as those of the systems in which the child is embedded, as these strengths will be beneficial in successfully targeting key concerns. This can be done by asking what the child likes to do, how he or she performs certain tasks, and what the relevant adults (parents, teachers, physical therapists, nurses) do to support the child. After all meeting participants have shared their concerns, the facilitator should encourage team members to prioritize the child's precise concerns and target one objective at a time. The primary concern is selected based on the greatest benefit to the child, and team members should consider the priority behavior based on data they have collected (through direct observations, work samples, and permanent products), on goals for the child across environments, on severity of the behavior, and on its association to other behaviors. Once the priority behavior is agreed upon, group members collectively develop an operational definition by describing what the target concern "looks like" in a typical instance, using clear and measurable terms to ensure a consistent understanding across all participants and contexts.

In some cases, data regarding concerns of parents, teachers, and other team members (e.g., occupational therapists, speech and language pathologists, reading specialists) are readily available and used in the context of the first problem-solving meeting. This is the case in which direct observations are conducted by school psychologists, academic work samples are provided by teachers, or historical information is given by parents. In other cases, additional data are necessary, and team members are recruited to gather further information regarding the specified target concern. A cross-system framework (i.e., home–school–community) provides an ideal structure in which to gain a comprehensive account of the child's behavior. It naturally allows thorough data collection from multiple sources (e.g., parents, teachers, peers, the child), using multiple methods (e.g., rating scales, direct observations, interviews) from multiple settings (e.g., home, classroom, community settings). Data may be collected through a variety of means, including direct observations, assessments, and permanent products. The team facilitator should ensure that data collection is conducted in the most reasonable and meaningful manner achievable. This can be accomplished through open dialogue wherein the facilitator and participants determine together what data are necessary to inform the problem-solving process and the easiest, most appropriate way to collect them. Specific individuals, methods, and settings are determined based on the relevant presentation (i.e., time and place) of the specified target behavior. For example, the child's day care provider, teacher, and parents may each collect data on the number of words spoken by a nonverbal child through a simple system of transferring tokens from one pocket to another. Regardless of the system used, data collection will be an ongoing process,

continually collected before, during, and following plan implementation to inform treatment decision making and to monitor progress toward goals.

Together, all team members who have observed the target concern should assess the environmental conditions that may be functionally related to problem behaviors. The facilitator should ask team members who are knowledgeable about the child's behavior to identify environmental events that occur directly before and after the target behavior and conditions in the child's environment that may contribute to or account for target concerns (for a detailed description of functional behavioral assessment, refer to Jones & Wickstrom, Chapter 12, this volume). This information will inform a theory regarding the purpose (i.e., function) of the problem behavior, help identify points of intervention (e.g., targeting antecedents to a behavior), and alter environmental conditions that influence a behavior so as to control its recurrence in the future.

Analyze Concerns

Following cross-system information gathering, the team is prepared to mutually analyze the data and to formulate strategies to address the needs of the child. Analyzing the data involves conducting a functional and skills assessment to determine environmental conditions that may affect the prioritized concern. The behavior of concern is typically enacted to serve a particular purpose, or it may indicate a skill deficit in the child. To better understand the purpose of the behavior, data from home and school settings are evaluated. The facilitator should ask each participant to share observations of environmental events that occur in relation to the target behavior in each appropriate setting. For example, the facilitator may elicit information from a child's teacher by asking, "What do you notice that triggers John's fighting on the playground?" or asking family members, "Describe what takes place when John and his brother get into arguments." Additionally, it is important to determine whether the primary concern is due to a lack of prerequisite skills necessary to demonstrate a more highly desired behavior. For example, a health professional may have insight regarding typical developmental trends or a child's health conditions that influence his or her ability to engage in fine motor activities or to acquire certain academic skills.

Based on the functional and skills assessment, a plan is devised directly linking functional hypotheses to specific plan strategies. Hypothesis generation and plan development are collaborative in nature and should meet the needs of the child across multiple environments. The facilitator should encourage all participants to share suggestions for plan development. Plan components should consist of evidence-based strategies that address the previously identified function of the behavior. Consideration should be given to the feasibility and acceptability of the plan components and their implementation across home and school settings. Mutual involvement of team members as the plan is being developed will facilitate a sense of ownership and promote the successful execution of plan strategies. Additionally, establishing similar strategies across home, school, and other treatment settings promotes consistency for the child, which may produce greater success.

Plan Implementation

In a collaborative framework, participants continue to communicate regarding plan procedures and to troubleshoot difficulties during plan implementation. Likewise, participants' responsibilities for data collection allow initial assessment of treatment effects. Self-report, permanent product, or observational data are often useful to determine the ease with which treatment plans are being implemented. Monitoring intervention fidelity in this way will allow team members to assist parents, teachers, and other treatment agents to implement important plan tactics as designed, to improve child outcomes, and to promote an accurate interpretation of program effects.

Plan Evaluation

Lastly, the effects of the intervention are assessed across settings, and progress toward overall team goals is evaluated. The facilitator should collect data from all sources (e.g., parent, day care provider) and graph the results across the stages of the problem-solving process. Intervention effectiveness is determined by analyzing data collected during treatment in relation to baseline data (see Daly, Barnett, Kupzyk, Hofstadter, & Barkley, Chapter 29, this volume). The team reconsiders the shared goals of consultation in relation to child performance and determines whether objectives have been met. Based on this information, participants should discuss the need to extend, modify, or terminate the current plan and develop strategies accordingly.

Collaboration and communication across important systems in children's lives are essential to their healthy emotional, social, academic, and behavioral growth and development. When the identified goals for behavior change have been met and problem resolution occurs, it is necessary to identify ways to continue keep channels of communication open (e.g., establishing specific times and methods for exchanging information and progress updates) and to reengage in joint problem solving as necessary to maximize ongoing child success.

Challenges to Cross-System Collaboration

Despite the numerous potential benefits of joining systems in children's lives in collaborative interactions, team members are faced with many challenges in reaching their mutual goals. Common barriers include (1) time required to meet together to address concerns, (2) forging relationships among diverse individuals, (3) ineffective communication, (4) divergent perspectives and expectations among participants, and (5) systemic variables. Each of these challenges and strategies for addressing them are summarized in Table 31.5 (Christenson & Sheridan, 2001; Johnson, Zorn, Tam, Lamontagne, & Johnson, 2003; Sheridan & Kratochwill, 2008). The challenges are also described in more detail below.

Time

A major challenge of cross-system collaboration is finding time for meaningful and productive interactions (Christenson & Sheridan, 2001; Friend & Cook, 2007; Johnson et al., 2003; Sheridan & Kratochwill, 2008). Collaboration is a time-consuming process,

TABLE 31.5. Challenges to Collaboration and Strategies to Address Them

Challenge	Strategy
Time	• Provide many options for meeting times. • Hold meetings in a central location. • Keep meetings focused. • Allow specific time in the day for collaborative interactions.
Impaired relationships	• Look for areas of agreement. • Emphasize relationships over roles. • Avoid judgments. • Separate the person from the problem. • Focus on mutual interests. • Base decisions on objective criteria. • Eliminate "turf" issues.
Communication	• Talk about differences. • Keep open lines of communication. • Encourage informal communication to foster relationships. • Create frequent opportunities for communication.
Divergent perspectives	• Define goals in more detail. • Promote a shared understanding of participants' rights, roles, and responsibilities from the start. • Learn about collaborating systems' customs and missions.
Systemic variables	• Involve upper management earlier, especially during the planning phase. • Advocate for financial resources to support collaboration.

as individuals must make time for activities such as planning and preparation, multiple meetings, travel, data collection, and plan implementation to promote successful child outcomes. Synchronizing numerous schedules to plan meetings hinders the involvement of many participants. Nevertheless, time spent in structured, data-based problem-solving meetings, which result in the implementation of effective interventions to minimize problems, can reduce ongoing efforts to address unresolved behavioral concerns. Thus commitment to the collaborative process may be highly time- and cost-effective in the long run.

Strategies must be utilized to increase time commitment for collaborative processes by influential individuals in children's lives. Friend and Cook (2007) suggest that meeting facilitators provide many options for meeting times, hold meetings at a central location convenient to all participants, and keep meetings focused and succinct. Additionally, meeting participants should prioritize opportunities to collaborate by scheduling a specific time in the day or week for collaborative interactions (Friend & Cook, 2007). Lastly, dissemination of successful examples of collaborative interactions (e.g., "real life" case examples in which cross-

system collaboration paid off) will increase acceptance and improve the likelihood of time commitment to preventative efforts up front (Johnson et al., 2003).

Impaired Relationships

The joining of diverse individuals with varying opinions and personalities to support positive relationships presents another important challenge. As multiple systems join together, difficult relationships are likely to develop due to attitudinal barriers, history of conflict, and resistance. It is not uncommon for participants on problem-solving teams to dwell on existing problems, which may contribute to strained relationships between systems (Christenson & Sheridan, 2001). Although certain attitudes promote healthy interactions, others may impair them. Counterproductive attitudes include stereotypical views of people, events, conditions, or actions; failure to view differences as strengths; lack of belief in a partnership orientation; placing blame; and lack of perspective taking (Christenson & Sheridan, 2001). Friend and Cook (2007) add that conflict may also result from differing goals and expectations for child outcomes, from power struggles, and from variations in conflict responses. Moreover, some individuals may simply demonstrate resistance to collaboration, evidenced by refusing to take part in collaborative efforts, advocating for change without following through, displacing responsibility, putting off efforts to a future time, or relying on past practice (Friend & Cook, 2007).

Fostering strong relationships is a principal goal of collaboration. Therefore, impaired relationships should be improved by the effective utilization of aforementioned process variables. Additionally, the facilitator can continuously look for and draw attention to areas of agreement and mutual interests among all team members. This will help center discussion on common goals and prevent negative or conflictual interactions (Sheridan & Kratochwill, 2008). The facilitator should also endorse objective decisions and positively reframe judgmental statements to keep the tone collaborative and constructive (Sheridan & Kratochwill, 2008). Lastly, an effort should be made to hold collaborative meetings at neutral locations (e.g., meeting rooms in local libraries or neighborhood community centers) to avoid defensive "turf" issues (Johnson et al., 2003) that may result in a perceived imbalance of power.

Communication

Communication is a critical component in the success of collaboration. However, communication can be challenging when it is initiated during times of crisis or conflict (Christenson & Sheridan, 2001; Friend & Cook, 2007). Frequent communication is a time-consuming process and requires numerous meetings, e-mails, and phone calls, especially when traversing multiple people and systems. Johnson et al. (2003) found that communication was the most often reported problem encountered during the collaboration process by departments and agencies working with children with disabilities and their families. Ineffective communication (e.g., receiving inaccurate information, using various uncoordinated data systems, speaking different languages) has been found to be a contributor to unsuccessful interagency collaboration (Johnson et al., 2003).

Maintaining effective communication can be enhanced by openly discussing differences among settings, group members, or opinions. For example, sharing an observation that some members may be holding back on expressing opinions can help create a norm for encouraging others to ask questions and to listen to all parties. The facilitator should encourage all group members to keep lines of communication open by purposefully scheduling frequent opportunities to communicate through e-mail, phone calls, notes, or other practical strategies (Christenson & Sheridan, 2001; Johnson et al., 2003). Due to the important emphasis on relationship building in collaborative interactions, the facilitator should also exercise and support informal communication to foster relationships.

Divergent Perspectives

When individuals from multiple systems collaborate, difficulties may arise related to the differing perspectives of each contributor. There may be overlap or confusion regarding the responsibilities of each participant. When unfamiliar systems converge, knowledge regarding the roles and expectations of participants may be erroneous or discrepant, leading to conflict, repetition, or confusion. Additionally, ineffective collaboration may result from a lack of shared vision or mismatch of goals (Johnson et al., 2003). If the goals for collaboration are divergent, opinions may also differ regarding the plan to address them.

The facilitator can promote more unified perspectives by ensuring that participants' rights, roles, and responsibilities are clarified and defined at the initiation of collaboration (Christenson & Sheridan, 2001). An open discussion about how the team can best work together is often necessary to minimize discrepancies or erroneous assumptions. Additionally, it will be essential for participants to actively learn about each others' cultures, customs, and values to enhance and strengthen future collaborative relationships (Johnson et al., 2003).

Systemic Variables

Lastly, the structure and influence of larger systemic variables present challenges to collaborating effectively. Participants may face lack of systemic support, both managerial and financial. Time-consuming partnering efforts may not be supported or understood by administration within organizations. Additionally, cross-system collaboration often requires additional funding to reimburse staffing needs or to meet expenses or other costs associated with collaborative efforts. Likewise, maintaining access to adequate resources can be difficult. For example, health reimbursement systems (i.e., third-party payers) may not support interdisciplinary care (Power et al., 2003).

Because of the wide range of benefits gained from collaborative interactions, it is necessary for those individuals concerned with child success to advocate for financial resources to support multisystemic collaboration. If needed, team members should look for supplemental funding resources. Additionally, it is beneficial to involve upper management during initial planning phases and to disseminate instances of successful collaboration (Johnson et al., 2003).

Uniting a diverse group of individuals to address a joint goal is a complex endeavor. Collaboration can fail when there is no consideration of the challenges that accompany it; however, preventative measures can be taken to avoid possible pitfalls of cross-system collaboration. Proper utilization of process and procedural variables aimed at fostering relationships and mutual problem solving, as well as maintaining flexibility, will help ensure a successful collaborative experience.

Summary and Conclusions

Children live in multiple, sometimes diverse systems embedded within settings that influence and are influenced by one another. Continuity within and across these systems is a stabilizing factor that promotes positive adaptation. Cross-system interdisciplinary collaboration provides the context for coordinated, consistent planning for children with unique needs. Although cross-system collaboration is not a new concept in education, new opportunities and models warrant careful consideration of such approaches in professional practice. Important process and structural variables define effective collaborative practices, highlighting the importance of attending to procedures ("what" is done

in efforts to deliver effective problem-solving services) and relationships ("how" services are provided to facilitate engagement and active participation in all aspects of the process). Collaborative models, including teaming and conjoint behavioral consultation, have promoted a structure and process for bringing parties together to address a child's needs in a comprehensive manner. Despite its potential utility, however, challenges to collaboration exist. Intentional efforts to promote cross-system relationships, to develop functional structures for ongoing collaboration, and to address potential barriers will allow the realization of its potential.

Acknowledgments

This chapter was developed with partial support from grants awarded to Susan M. Sheridan (U.S. Department of Education Grant Nos. H325D030050 and R305F05284). The opinions expressed herein are those of the authors and do not reflect positions or policies of the funding agencies.

References

American Academy of Pediatrics. (2000). Clinical practice guideline: Diagnosis and evaluation of the child with attention-deficit/hyperactivity disorder. *Pediatrics, 95,* 301–304.

American Academy of Pediatrics. (2001). Clinical practice guidelines: Treatment of the school-aged child with attention-deficit/hyperactivity disorder. *Pediatrics, 108,* 1033–1044.

Anderson-Butcher, D., & Ashton, D. (2004). Innovative models of collaboration to serve children, youths, families, and communities. *Children and Schools, 26,* 39–53.

Burt, J. B., Clarke, B. L., Dowd-Eagle, S., & Sheridan, S. M. (2008). Conjoint behavioral consultation in unique practice contexts. In S. M. Sheridan & T. R. Kratochwill, *Conjoint behavioral consultation: Promoting family–school connections and interventions* (pp. 97–128). New York: Springer.

Christenson, S. L., & Sheridan, S. M. (2001). *Schools and families: Creating essential connections for learning.* New York: Guilford Press.

Clarke, B. L., Sheridan, S. M., & Woods, K. L. (in press). Elements of healthy family–school relationships. In S. Christenson & A. Reschly (Eds.), *Handbook of family–school partnerships.* New York: Springer.

Cowan, R., Swearer, S. M., & Sheridan, S. M. (2004). Home–school collaboration. In C. Spielberger (Ed.), *Encyclopedia of applied psychology* (Vol. 2, pp. 201–208). San Diego, CA: Academic Press.

Friend, M., & Cook, L. (2007). *Interactions: Collaboration skills for school professionals* (5th ed.). Boston: Pearson Education.

Gravois, T. A., & Rosenfield, S. A. (2006). Impact of instructional consultation teams on the disproportionate referral and placement of minority students in special education. *Remedial and Special Education, 27,* 42–52.

Green, C. L., Walker, J. M. T., Hoover-Dempsey, K. V., & Sandler, H. (2007). Parents' motivations for involvement in children's education: An empirical test of a theoretical model of parental involvement. *Journal of Educational Psychology, 99,* 532–544.

Hoagwood, K., Kelleher, K. J., Feil, M., & Comer, D. M. (2000). Treatment services for children with ADHD: A national perspective. *Journal of the American Academy of Child and Adolescent Psychiatry, 39,* 198–206.

Johnson, L. J., Zorn, D., Tam, B. D. Y., Lamontagne, M., & Johnson, S. A. (2003). Stakeholders' views of factors that impact successful interagency collaboration. *Exceptional Children, 69,* 195–209.

Kline, F. M., & Rubel, L. (2001). Why this book? Collaboration between school and medical communities. In F. M. Kline, L. B. Silver, & S. C. Russell (Eds.), *The educator's guide to medical issues in the classroom* (pp. 1–12). Baltimore: Brookes.

Kratochwill, T. R., & Bergan, J. R. (1990). *Behavioral consultation in applied settings: An individual guide.* New York: Plenum.

Martens, B. K., & DiGennaro, F. D. (2008). Behavioral consultation. In W. P. Erchul & S. M. Sheridan (Eds.), *Handbook of research in school consultation.* New York: Erlbaum.

Merriam-Webster's new collegiate dictionary. (1981). Springfield, MA: Merriam.

Merriam-Webster's Online Dictionary (2007). Available at *www.webster.com/.*

Phillips, V., & McCullough, L. (1990). Consultation-based programming: Instituting the collaborative ethic. *Exceptional Children, 56,* 291–304.

Power, T. J., DuPaul, G. J., Shapiro, E. S., & Kazak, A. E. (2003). *Promoting children's health: Integrating school, family, and community.* New York: Guilford Press.

Rosenfield, S. A., Silva, A., & Gravois, T. A. (2007). Bringing instructional consultation to scale: Research and development of IC and IC teams. In W. P. Erchul & S. M. Sheridan (Eds.), *Handbook of research in school consultation* (pp. 203–223). Mahwah, NJ: Erlbaum.

Shapiro, E. S., & Manz, P. H. (2004). Collaborating with schools in the provision of pediatric psychological services. In R. T. Brown (Ed.), *The handbook of pediatric psychology in school settings* (pp. 49–64). Mahwah, NJ: Erlbaum.

Sheridan, S. M., Clarke, B. L., & Burt, J. D. (2008). Conjoint behavioral consultation: What do we know and what do we need to know? In W. P. Erchul & S. M. Sheridan (Eds.), *Handbook of research in school consultation: Empirical foundations for the field* (pp. 171–202). Mahwah, NJ: Erlbaum.

Sheridan, S. M., Eagle, J. W., Cowan, R. J., & Mickelson, W. (2001). The effects of conjoint behavioral consultation: Results of a 4-year investigation. *Journal of School Psychology, 39,* 361–385.

Sheridan, S. M., & Kratochwill, T. R. (2008). *Conjoint behavioral consultation: Promoting family–school connections and interventions* (2nd ed.). New York: Springer.

Sheridan, S. M., Kratochwill, T. R., & Bergan, J. R. (1996). *Conjoint behavioral consultation: A procedural manual.* New York: Kluwer Academic/Plenum.

Sheridan, S. M., Warnes, E. D., Woods, K. E., Blevins, C. A., Magee, K. L., & Ellis, C. (in press). An exploratory evaluation of conjoint behavioral consultation to promote collaboration among family, school, and pediatric systems: A role for pediatric school psychologists. *Journal of Educational and Psychological Consultation.*

Tourse, R. W. C., & Sulick, J. (1999). The collaboration alliance: Supporting vulnerable children in school. In R. W. C. Tourse & J. F. Mooney (Eds.), *Collaborative practice: School and human service partnerships* (pp. 59–78). Westport, CT: Praeger.

Vosler-Hunter, R. W. (1989). *Changing roles, changing relationships: Parent and professional collaboration on behalf of children with emotional disabilities.* Portland, OR: Portland State University, Research and Training Center on Family Support and Children's Mental Health.

Welch, M., & Sheridan, S. M. (1995). *Educational partnerships: Serving students at-risk.* San Antonio, TX: Harcourt-Brace Jovanovich.

Wilcox, M. J., Kouri, T. A., & Caswell, S. B. (1991). Early language intervention: A comparison of classroom and individual treatment. *American Journal of Speech–Language Pathology, 1,* 49–61.

Wolery, R. A., & Odom, S. L. (2000). *An administrator's guide to preschool inclusion.* Chapel Hill: University of North Carolina, Frank Porter Graham Child Development Center, Early Childhood Research Institute on Inclusion.

Chapter 32

The School Psychologist's Role in Assisting School Staff in Establishing Systems to Manage, Understand, and Use Data

Elizabeth Schaughency
Brent Alsop
Anna Dawson

The document *School Psychology: A Blueprint for Training and Practice III* builds upon its predecessors and the Conference on the Future of School Psychology held in 2002 to provide a framework for the profession (Ysseldyke et al., 2006). Blueprint III specifies two major outcomes for school psychologists' work in schools: improved competencies for all children and improved delivery-system capacity (Ysseldyke et al., 2006). *Data-based decision making* is considered key to achieving improved outcomes (e.g., Thomas & Grimes, 2008), but it requires systems to manage, understand, and use data. This is important at a number of levels. For individual students, assessment can support and enhance learning in general education (Pellegrino, Chudowsky, & Glaser, 2001) and special education (Stecker, Fuchs, & Fuchs, 2005). Similarly, for organizations, data-based decision making is part of continuous quality improvement models, with assessment integral to efforts to improve education (Pellegrino et al., 2001). Data-based decision making is foundational to multi-tiered service delivery using response to intervention (RTI) to determine need for further intervention (Gresham, 2004) and has been applied to academic (Coyne, Kame'enui, & Simmons,

2004) and behavioral (Horner, Sugai, Todd, & Lewis-Palmer, 2005) targets. School psychologists have a pivotal role in this process. They are *knowledge brokers* communicating information about using evidence-based assessment and practices (EBPs) to educators as instructional, mental health, and systems consultants (Ervin & Schaughency, 2008). This chapter considers the rationale for using data collection, organization, and availability of data to aid decision making and how characteristics of the user and the context relate to taking on these tasks.

Why Data?

In applied settings, data and results are often equated with research or administrative activities rather than professional decision making and service delivery. However, data can be functional. Data support decision making and service delivery in two general ways: evaluation for continued program development and communication with internal (e.g., parents, teachers) and external (e.g., district administrators) stakeholders. This *functionality* should be conveyed to users (Rolfsen & Torvatn, 2005) because it can improve professional decision making for individuals (Swets, Dawes, & Mona-han, 2000) or teams (Barnett, Macmann, & Lentz, 2003).

Two types of evaluation are relevant to improving capacity to provide evidence-based competence-building practices. *Summative evaluation* is conducted after the assessment is complete and answers the question, Was the intervention program effective? This serves two purposes. First, summative evaluation is used to meet demands for accountability (e.g., No Child Left Behind). Second, summative evaluation provides the basis for selecting evidence-based practices because it forms the practice literature (see Stoiber & DeSmet, Chapter 13, this volume). Results from previous outcome studies guide hypotheses about what might work because the interventions worked in the past. However, results from summative evaluation studies were obtained in particular settings under particular conditions, and results may not generalize to the local situation.

Formative evaluation is conducted during the course of intervention implementation. It informs educators whether the intervention is having the desired effect, and so assists in adapting EBPs to better meet local needs (Ervin & Schaughency, 2008; Schaughency & Ervin, 2006). In general, through the process of formative evaluation, professionals make one of three decisions: (1) programs are working, and issues become those of sustaining intervention integrity or programming for maintenance and generalization (see Noell, Chapter 30, this volume); (2) programs show some success, but further adaptations might better address remaining needs; or (3) programs are not working, and additional or different strategies are indicated.

Without data and appropriate evaluation designs (see Daly, Barnett, Kupzyk, Hofstadter, & Barkley, Chapter 29, this volume), professionals may reach inaccurate conclusions (Dawes, 1994). They may overlook improvements that have occurred but that have not reached the desired level. For example, if school report card data were aggregated across the entire school population, including both younger students who benefited from a beginning reading initiative and older students who had not participated in the initiative, then these data may suggest that overall achievement has not yet reached the desired level for all students. If data at this level were reviewed to evaluate the beginning reading initiative, professionals may conclude that beginning reading initiatives were unsuccessful, even though students who participated in the initiative did show improvement. However, this level of analysis would be inappropriate for evaluating the effectiveness of a beginning reading initiative that targeted only a subgroup of students, that is, students who were in the early grades at the time the initiative was implemented.

Professionals may also fail to see problems that continue to occur, because their attention has shifted elsewhere. For example, literacy problems may remain in a school but are overlooked because improvement priorities have changed to numeracy; now numeracy problems are noticed. Finally, professionals may make misattributions about the cause of a problem. For example, if higher levels of bullying are reported in schools that introduce antibullying initiatives, then one conclusion may be that the antibullying initiatives caused more bullying. However, it is also possible that schools with a bullying problem were more likely to participate in antibullying initiatives or that the initiatives led to increased perception and reports of bullying rather than to more bullying behavior per se.

Evaluation data also support communication with internal and external stakeholders (see Figure 32.1). For example, adequacy of the initial stage of problem solving (i.e., problem identification) is a predictor of the outcome of consultation (Gresham, 2004). Collaborative discussions among internal stakeholders or team members (e.g., parents, teachers) to select appropriate outcome measures provide a mechanism for addressing this issue (Noell, Chapter 30, this volume). Following implementation, formative evaluation data help communicate to school personnel the outcome of their efforts. Seeing that their efforts are making a difference (e.g., reduced behavioral difficulties, improved academic performance) may reinforce personnel and prompt continued problem-solving efforts (Ervin & Schaughency, 2008; Schaughency & Ervin, 2006). Finally, evaluation data support communication with external stakeholders, such as district or state administrators. Not only can these data meet accountability requirements

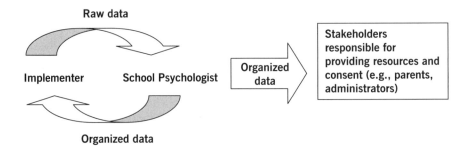

FIGURE 32.1. Different directions and functions of communication. Communication is particularly important between the program or intervention designer and its implementers because program integrity requires cooperation and vigilance; the psychologist needs not only their careful implementation of the program but also their care in collecting raw data. In this context, communication is not only about information; it can also provide both positive (we hope) feedback concerning the implementers' past efforts and support and encouragement for future efforts.

(Gibbons & Silberglitt, 2008), but they may also garner financial and political support for school initiatives by showing how schools are working toward priorities set by these external bodies (Ervin & Schaughency, 2008).

The Challenge: Having and Using Data

It is not enough simply to collect data. The *use* of data is the active ingredient in achieving improvements (Stecker et al., 2005). Readily available and evidence-based assessment information is necessary but not sufficient to promote data-informed decision making. Unfortunately, professionals do not always have appropriate data available, nor do they always use it to inform their decision making.

For example, the Texas Department of Mental Health and Mental Retardation was interested in promoting best practices in pharmacological interventions for children with attention-deficit/hyperactivity disorder (ADHD). They developed a medication algorithm to inform decision making regarding medication dosage that required parent and teacher ratings during each medication condition (Pliszka et al., 2003). The researchers struggled to obtain the appropriate data. Only 61.9% of treatment conditions included parent-rating data, and only a handful of teacher ratings were obtained (seven teachers returned ratings for both baseline and

treatment conditions; Pliszka et al., 2003). In their discussion, Pliszka et al. (2003) recommended strategies to increase likelihood of data collection, including using information technology to reduce the response effort necessary to obtain and collate assessment results.

Consistent with these recommendations, another research group created a Web-based care coordination system in which password-protected student assessment information would be available to parents, teachers, and physicians (Evans, Green, & Serpell, 2005). Although developed in response to a stated need by stakeholders and in collaboration with them (Evans, 2007; Evans et al., 2005), website visit counts showed that the system was rarely used (Evans, 2007).

To enhance and support student outcomes, assessment—and use of assessment information—should be embedded in practice (Ercikan, 2006). To this end, Power, Mautone, Manz, Frye, and Blum (2007) worked with primary care physicians to develop standardized, interactive electronic protocols in which assessment data were available for use during contacts with child patients with ADHD. To facilitate use of these data in decision making, prompts were built into the electronic protocol to guide physicians' consideration of assessment results in treatment decisions. These researchers are currently evaluating whether physicians used available data in treatment of their patients with ADHD. In school settings, surveys similarly indicate that data collection and data-based decision making are among the most difficult components of reform initiatives such as schoolwide positive behavior support (SWPBS; Scott & Martinek, 2006).

Other chapters in this volume focus on technical issues pertaining to assessment methodologies and evaluation design (see, e.g., VanDerHeyden, Chapter 3; McIntosh, Reinke, & Herman, Chapter, 9; Daly et al., Chapter 29). We approach this chapter from an implementation perspective (Graczyk, Domitrovich, Small, & Zins, 2006). From this perspective, data-informed decision making may be seen as an innovation, a new idea or new way of doing things for school personnel. Our task is to consider factors that influence adoption (decision to use an innovation), implementation (using the innovation in the field), and sustainability (continued use at the end of the initiative) and, from this, to consider how to facilitate development of implementation support systems (see Graczyk et al., 2006) to promote use of data for problem solving.

Research has identified factors that influence adoption and likelihood of implementation. These include characteristics of the innovation, the user, the context, and the interactions between these factors (Ervin & Schaughency, 2008). Next we discuss each of these factors as they might apply to the task of promoting data-informed problem solving. Adoption likelihood appears specifically related to whether the innovation "fits"—or is perceived to "fit" (Aarons, 2005)—the practice context (Ervin & Schaughency, 2008), so we consider this especially.

Characteristics of the Innovation: Data for Decision Making

Assessment skills have long been part of school psychologists' professional expertise. To guide practice, Blueprint III charges psychologists to use these skills to develop prevention and intervention efforts for students and to provide technical assistance to school personnel. In this chapter, we limit discussion to general considerations for collecting and interpreting data to support school-based prevention and intervention program development and evaluation, and we refer readers to other chapters in this volume that focus specifically on assessment of academic (VanDerHeyden, Chapter 3) and behavioral (McIntosh et al., Chapter 9) domains.

Recently, implementation research has begun to identify characteristics associated with likelihood that innovations (programs, processes, or practices) will be adopted and implemented with integrity (Ervin & Schaughency, 2008). The components include: *content* (e.g., what data are collected), *timing* (when data are available), *structure* (how data are presented), and *dosage* (how much support is provided to assist in interpretation and decision making; Graczyk et al., 2006). In this section, we limit discussion of "support" to material supports, such as technological resources. Interpersonal supports, such as professional development and consultation, are discussed later.

What Data Should Be Collected?

Data are needed that inform, foster, and document the effectiveness of prevention and intervention strategies to improve outcomes for children (Shapiro & Elliott, 1999), and methods are required to link assessment to intervention. These methods should be evidence-based (Mash & Hunsley, 2005; U.S. Department of Health and Human Services [DHHS], 2002), with validity evidence to support their use for a given purpose (e.g., screening, instructional planning, evaluating response to treatment; see American Educational Research Association, American Psychological Association, & National Council on Measurement in Education [AERA, APA, & NCME], 1999).

Two types of data guide prevention and intervention program development and evaluation activities: information concerning students' functioning in the academic or social domain of interest, and the instructional or socialization contexts relevant to those domains (Blueprint III). Measures for assessing student growth in important academic and social domains should be based on developmental theory and research (e.g., on developing literacy and reading difficulties), related to important outcomes (e.g., academic success), sensitive to development (i.e., show change over time or following instruction), efficient (i.e., consider time demands on practitioner and child), and instructionally useful (i.e., help to inform educational problem solving; U.S. DHHS, 2002). Moreover, to assist in problem solving within particular contexts (e.g., classrooms), domains assessed should reflect performance in the natural environment and consider the alignment of curriculum and context with domain being assessed (i.e., have the skills been taught?), possible skill deficits (i.e., have the skills been learned?), and possible performance deficits (i.e., is performance adversely affected by other factors, such as a lack of motivation?; Shapiro & Elliott, 1999).

Information about instructional context is vital for problem solving and consultation activities. For example, functional assessment to select behavioral interventions (Jones & Wickstrom, Chapter 12, this volume) focuses on understanding the problem in context and improving the instructional environment to support student learning. Information about instructional context also informs whether recommended instructional or environmental changes are being implemented (i.e., implementation integrity; Noell, Chapter 30, this volume), foundational to RTI decision making and service delivery (Gresham, 2004). Furthermore, information about instructional context may provide performance feedback, which may support implementation and practice change. Most feedback in professional practice is neither systematic nor reliable, and many professionals may not accurately perceive their performance nor recognize discrepancies between current and desired practice (Riemer, Rosof-Williams, & Bickman, 2005). Progress monitoring combined with performance feedback to the implementer (e.g., teacher) can improve intervention integrity and student outcomes (Noell et al., 2005).

Many professional decision-making and problem-solving activities happen in the context of work groups or teams, whether focused on individuals (student assistance teams), groups of students (grade-level teams), or the school as a whole (school improvement teams). A systems consultant working to facilitate team use of data for problem solving will need appropriate student performance and relevant contextual data, as well as information on team use of data for decision making (Rosenfield, Silva, & Gravois, 2008). For example, a systems consultant working with a grade-level team

on a three-tiered approach to reading support might want the team to consider appropriate student performance data, implementation integrity data at each of the tiers, and methods to encourage and monitor team use of these data for problem solving in the context of grade-level meetings.

When Should Data Be Collected and Available for Use?

For professionals to use data in decision making, data need to be available at the time that decisions are being made. Student achievement test data sent away for processing in January, with results not returned until after school year's end in July, are useless for formative evaluation by those students' teachers.

When Should Data Be Collected?

When data should be collected depends on the purpose of data collection, the desired time frame for decision making, and issues of feasibility. As discussed by VanDerHeyden in Chapter 3, this volume, schoolwide screening is a large undertaking, and many, if not most, students should be on track and meeting developmental expectations (see also Gibbons & Silberglitt, 2008). Therefore, such screenings may occur relatively infrequently, with many systems recommending three assessments per year, at roughly the beginning, middle, and end of the year (Gibbons & Silberglitt, 2008). In this way, individual students or cohorts who have not yet met expected developmental competencies may be identified during the year. This creates an opportunity to provide instructional or curricular supports and to evaluate whether these efforts are bringing growth trajectories in line with expected developmental competence.

However, if students are not on track, more frequent assessment can inform decision making regarding instructional modifications and supports. For example, the Dynamic Indicators of Basic Early Literacy Skills (DIBELS; Kaminski, Cummings, Powell-Smith, & Good, 2008) assessment system places scores into risk categories based on literacy development and statistical analysis. DIBELS benchmarks were established such that 80% of students attaining that performance level achieved subsequent early literacy goals (Kaminski et al., 2008). The "intensive support" category was derived such that fewer than 20% of students performing at that level attained subsequent literacy goals (Kaminski et al., 2008). However, DIBELS also includes an intermediary ("strategic") group, in which approximately 50% of students achieve subsequent literacy goals, because it recognizes that scores close to cutoffs are more likely to be misclassified (Ercikan, 2006). It might be expected that many students will achieve benchmark levels. For these students, current instruction appears effective, and schoolwide screenings are likely sufficient. A smaller proportion would be expected to fall into the "strategic" category in which outcome is uncertain, and the remaining small percentage of students appear unlikely to achieve developmental competence in literacy without further support ("intensive support" category). Because students in these latter categories may be at risk of reading difficulties, additional assessment and perhaps supplemental reading supports may be appropriate (see Linan-Thompson & Vaughn, Chapter 16, this volume).

Organizational routines and feasibility are both considerations when embedding practices in applied settings (Ervin & Schaughency, 2008; Gibbons & Silberglitt, 2008). For students in the "strategic" category, outcome is uncertain, and more frequent monitoring could inform professionals as to whether students' reading progress is coming on track *before* half the school year has elapsed. In many school settings, the academic year is broken into four grading periods, forming four naturally occurring decision points regarding student progress. Therefore, it might be useful for educators to have information regarding reading trajectories of students in the "strategic" category over the grading period so that additional supports can be provided during the next grading period, if indicated. Conducting one reading probe per month, for example, could feasibly provide educators with information with which to examine trends in the students' reading growth at meaningful decision points (Gibbons & Silberglitt, 2008).

For students in the "intensive" category, individualized intervention is indicated (Coyne et al., 2004), and progress monitoring provides the basis for inducing whether the intervention has met student needs (Kavale & Forness, 1999). More frequent review is indicated because students at this level are unlikely to meet developmental expectations without a change in their reading trajectory. Again considering routines and best practices, if student assistance teams meet monthly, progress monitoring probes at least once per week would allow teams to examine trends in reading performance in light of intervention efforts (Gibbons & Silberglitt, 2008).

How Can Availability of Data Be Facilitated?

To be useful, data not only need to be collected, but they also need to be available in ways that facilitate their interpretation. By making assessment results accessible as soon as they are entered, databases such as those available for DIBELS and the School-Wide Information System (SWIS; Todd, Sampson, & Horner, 2005) potentially afford school personnel timely access to data for use in decision making, provided that data are entered into the Web system.

Data entry presents challenges for schools that should not be overlooked, however. For example, SWIS is a Web-based information system for monitoring ongoing patterns of office discipline referrals (see Irvin et al., 2006), including type, frequency, location, and time of problem behavior, as well as who received the referral. In a study of school teams implementing SWPBS and using data management systems such as SWIS, requests for assistance with data entry were the most frequent and the only SWPBS component for which assistance was requested by the majority of schools (Scott & Martinek, 2006). Moreover, electronic management systems for data that have been collected by hand initially can reduce efficiency when they entail additional steps for teachers (going to computers, loading software, entering data, etc.; Fuchs & Fuchs, 2001).

Alternative approaches are lower technology options, such as manually plotting results on prepared graphs (see the next section), or technological resources that bypass data entry. Computers may be used to generate, administer, and score academic assessments, increasing efficiency and satisfaction (Fuchs & Fuchs, 2001; Stecker et al., 2005).

For example, software is now available to allow administration of DIBELS using handheld computers. Assessment results may then be synchronized with the DIBELS database, providing instant access to interpretative information (Wireless Generation, n.d.). Other technology tools for progress monitoring are reviewed in resources such as Thomas and Grimes (2008, Vol. 5, Section 8) and Ysseldyke and McLeod (2007).

How Should Data Be Presented?

The interpretation of data, such as test scores, has long been part of psychologists' armamentarium. However, not everyone can readily interpret and use data. Research has consistently found that high school students have substantial difficulties in two important aspects of scientific reasoning—interpreting data and generating or revising theories in light of those data (Mayer, 2004). We have observed similar difficulties at the preservice (undergraduate and graduate) and inservice levels. Daly and colleagues (Chapter 29, this volume) consider data analysis in some detail, so here we focus on means of displaying data for effective communication with internal and external stakeholders.

Effective communication requires a common language. Before presenting data, it is important to determine whether the audience (internal or external stakeholders) is familiar with the metric used to report academic or social functioning. To illustrate, as part of our measurement development work, we routinely provide feedback to school personnel. We quickly learned that statistical concepts basic to psychologists (e.g., correlation) were not always fully understood by school personnel. To develop a common language, we now include a primer covering the statistics (e.g., correlations) used in our reports and try to convey statistical information in user-friendly ways. For example, rather than presenting overwhelming tables of correlation coefficients, we used stars to denote significant correlations with different strengths of association (e.g., * minimal, ** modest, *** robust). This display was similar to other commonly used metrics (e.g., movie ratings), and staff seemed to appreciate and readily comprehend our findings.

Understanding the questions asked of data also aids communication, and this should be reflected in the display. Psychological research often frames responses to evaluation questions as a comparison. The question might involve a nomothetic comparison (e.g., comparing a student's performance with that of a group), a criterion-referenced comparison (e.g., comparing a student's performance with a standard of performance), or an idiographic comparison (e.g., comparing a student's performance with his or her own performance over time or as a function of intervention). These comparisons are not mutually exclusive and can be combined within displays. For example, formative evaluations typically focus on idiographic questions of change, but determination of outcome may be based on whether those receiving instructional strategies achieved certain nomothetic (e.g., percentile) or mastery levels. Labeling these criteria on displays can aid interpretation.

For some evaluations, in particular summative evaluations, the question simply may be whether or not performance differs between start and finish of implementation. In this case, the data presentation may simply be two numbers or a bar chart. However, even here, some care is required for effective communication. For example, is the change better presented as an absolute number—such as a 10-point increase in reading performance—or as a percentage change—such as a 20% increase—since the beginning of implementation? It might be more meaningful that a reading program has increased performance by 20% than by 10 points on some scale.

In many evaluations, especially formative evaluations, the question involves understanding trends in performance. In other words, is the implementation moving performance in the right direction? If so, how quickly is it moving? Does it look as though improvements will continue, or that performance has reached a plateau? Trends are typically easier to see in graphs than in tables. Figure 32.2 plots some hypothetical data collected three times a week during a baseline week and then over 6 weeks of an intervention or program. The score (dependent variable) is on the y-axis, and successive measurements or assessments are on the x-axis.

Panel A and Panel B of Figure 32.2 show the data in their rawest form. The two pan-

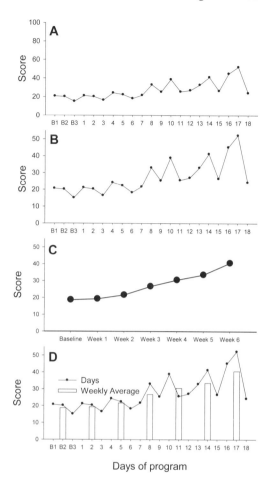

FIGURE 32.2. Different presentations of the same hypothetical data set. Panels A and B both plot the raw data; however, Panel B depicts only the actual range of scores and thereby may better depict gains. Panels C and D aggregate data weekly to illustrate average weekly gain, with Panel D illustrating both daily variability and weekly averages.

els differ in only one way; the *y*-axis of Panel A extends over a greater range of scores than those obtained in the program. As a result, the progressive gains are less apparent in Panel A than in Panel B, which scales its *y*-axis more appropriately for the intervention. A simple formatting change to the data presentation in Panel B improves our ability to communicate the results. Panels A and B also illustrate a common issue in presenting and interpreting data, that is, the natural variability of performance. The challenge is

to highlight important performance aspects underlying this variation. Aggregating data can reduce effects of variability. Instead of presenting data from each collection period separately, for example, we can calculate the mean or median over a number of data collection periods. Panel C replots these data, presenting them in terms of each week's average (mean) score. The steady increase in scores as a function of instructional intervention is readily apparent to viewers. Smoothing data's natural variability has its downside, however. The results simply will not reflect implementers' firsthand experience of good days and bad days, and stakeholders may be skeptical of data that draw a straight path out of a very winding road. Furthermore, variability in performance may cause school personnel to search for the reasons that performance is good or bad on some days, potentially helping them to strengthen intervention programs through needed adjustments. In such situations, data presentations that acknowledge variability in performance but that also illustrate underlying success might communicate more effectively than those that overly smooth bumps in performance. Panel D tries to capture benefits of both Panels B and C. It shows the raw data, but it overlays weekly averages. Data trends are clear without losing realities of inherent variability. The crucial point is to choose a display that most effectively communicates the important characteristics of the data for a particular audience or implementer. General recommendations for communicating about data are presented in Table 32.1. Further information on presenting data and on use of technology to support data displays is provided in Hood and Dorman (2008). Information on other issues, such as goal setting, is available elsewhere (e.g., Gibbons & Silberglitt, 2008).

How Much Support Is Needed to Facilitate Using Data in Decision Making?

Access to quality materials and resources such as technological supports seems to facilitate implementation generally (Graczyk et al., 2006) and, in particular, to increase teacher use of data for decision making (Stecker et al., 2005). For example, computer applications, especially those that facilitate data collection and management (e.g.,

TABLE 32.1. Guidelines for Communicating about Data

What not to do	Recommendation
Don't assume everyone is familiar with interpreting graphs and tables.	Take time to convey what is illustrated by the display. For example, giving a clear explanation of the units on the axes of graphs can be time well spent.
Don't dazzle them with technical jargon (i.e., avoid obfuscation).	Our task is to communicate effectively and build capacity for problem solving. Consider how you can best convey what you're trying to get across and teach the big ideas.
Don't lose sight of the forest for the trees (i.e., avoid pointless detail).	Help the audience understand the heart of the issue, with discussion of relevant factors related to this.
Don't write a murder mystery. (i.e., avoid slowly unfolding the evidence until the moment of truth when the logical and insightful deductions reveal all).	Be up front with the conclusions of your analysis, and then support them with the evidence.

graphing), and decision rules for interpreting when data indicate warranted instructional modification facilitate teachers' data use (Stecker et al., 2005). Computerized skill analyses can aid teachers' identification of specific instructional targets across academic domains, and expert systems software can help teachers identify alternative strategies for teaching material within some domains (e.g., math; Fuchs & Fuchs, 2001). However, resources and technology alone are unlikely to build capacity for data-informed problem solving (Fuchs & Fuchs, 2001; Stecker et al., 2005).

Conclusions and Recommendations for Making Data User Friendly

In general, characteristics associated with the likelihood of adoption and implementation integrity include ease, efficiency, and effectiveness of the innovation and access to quality materials and resources necessary for implementation (Gresham, 2004; Graczyk et al., 2006). Potential barriers to data collection and data-based decision making are time (e.g., time for data collection, entry, collation, and reflection on results), implementer factors (e.g., attitudes and skills), and contextual factors (e.g., organizational support). Strategies to address these barriers include efforts to reduce the time necessary to perform these tasks (Fuchs & Fuchs, 2001), professional and organizational de-

velopment activities to provide requisite skills, and a host environment that supports implementation. We turn to these latter considerations in the next section.

Characteristics of the User and the Context

To promote innovation implementation and professional development (Salas & Cannon-Bowers, 2001), professional and organizational context should be considered, along with characteristics of the innovation. Rather than viewing training on how to do the innovation as a stand-alone event, professional development and support for implementation should be integrated into the organization (Salas & Cannon-Bowers, 2001). Psychologists can facilitate organizational development via activities such as educative and skill-building professional development, problem and systems analysis, and team development (Ervin & Schaughency, 2008; George, White, & Schlaffer, 2007). Therefore, we consider these organizational development activities to assist staff use of data in the sections to follow. First, however, we briefly review two social–contextual dimensions that are relevant to understanding and promoting implementation of innovations. These are the *nested ecology*, which recognizes that professionals and teams exist in larger systemic contexts, and *course of implementation*, which acknowledges that practice or systems change occurs over time (Ervin & Schaughency, 2008).

The Nested Ecology

A systems perspective recognizes that the individual implementer (e.g., teacher) works within a social context (Ervin & Schaughency, 2008). The individual is a member of one or more groups or subsystems (e.g., one of several grade-level teachers, a member of a school-based team) nested within broader social contexts or systems such as schools, districts, or states (see Figure 32.3). These levels—individual, microsocial (e.g., interpersonal and interprofessional), and macrosocial (organizational)—are likely interrelated, with individual characteristics and organizational variables influencing professional practice (cf. Glisson, 2002; Riemer et al., 2005).

The Individual Implementer

At the individual level, cognitive and affective variables can influence the adoption of new practices (Ervin & Schaughency, 2008). The professional development literature refers to these variables as the knowledge, skills, and attitudes necessary to perform the task (Salas & Cannon-Bowers, 2001).

When the task is promoting data use for decision making, several attitudinal factors are relevant. Whether one is motivated to participate in professional development, to learn new skills, or to try something new in general relates to whether skills are acquired, retained, and applied on the job (Aarons, 2005; Salas & Cannon-Bowers, 2001). Motivation for professional development and willingness to try new professional activities is multifaceted and influenced by individual (e.g., self-efficacy, anxiety) and situational characteristics, including previous experience with professional development and organizational initiatives (Aarons, 2005; Salas

& Cannon-Bowers, 2001). When "trying something new" involves managing and using data, additional, potentially interrelated, attitudinal factors may come into play: (1) investment in philosophical or theoretical approaches perceived to be at odds with the scientific method and EBPs, (2) limited understanding of potential contributions of the scientific method and evidence base within domains, and (3) apprehension or reluctance about data and technology.

When working in schools, psychologists should consider what factors hinder adoption for personnel and should employ strategies to address them. At times these potential barriers may be identified in the context of a needs assessment or in preliminary discussions with relevant personnel. In other instances, these may be identified over the course of the problem-solving consultation process. We discuss potential factors relevant to the use of data and evidence-based practice in this section to alert to the psychologist to the issues and to introduce general approaches to addressing them.

Ideological issues underlying resistance to adoption of EBPs have been discussed elsewhere (e.g., Schaughency & Ervin, 2006). To promote data-based decision making, it is useful to distinguish between causative theories and action models (Graczyk et al., 2006). Causative theory underlies specific intervention strategies or approaches; for example, applied behavioral analysis underlies SWPBS (Horner et al., 2005). The action model provides guidelines for implementation. Formative evaluation and data-based decision making may be considered tools of the action model without dictating particular causative theories and intervention strategies. Emphasizing the *principle* of evidence-based assessment and decision making, rather than adoption of specific data systems, provides participatory roles for educational personnel in selecting interventions and evolution of practices within

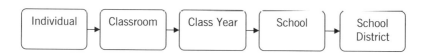

FIGURE 32.3. The nested ecology of implementation.

the setting as new technologies develop (see later in the chapter). It also may help offset the perception that this is just another discrete initiative to be discarded at a later date (Ervin & Schaughency, 2008).

Understanding the basis of resistance allows psychologists to seek common ground with school personnel. For example, although some practitioners fear that EBP presents a prescriptive approach, EBPs and principles of self-determination or empowerment are not necessarily antithetical or mutually exclusive; they can be integrated in building capacity for *localized* service delivery (Schaughency & Ervin, 2006). To convey functionality, formative evaluation can be presented as a means to localize service delivery by iteratively adapting and refining research-based interventions to meet local needs (Schaughency & Ervin, 2006). Similarly, to offset notions that data-oriented psychologists do not care about children, psychologists promoting data use should convey a shared primary concern with promoting children's well-being; data-based decision making is a tool to that end, rather than an end in itself (Blueprint III).

Implementers need knowledge to implement innovations (Ervin & Schaughency, 2008; Salas & Cannon-Bowers, 2001). When considering data-based decision making, this includes professional content knowledge (e.g., reading development and reading difficulties), knowledge of assessment strategies and their limitations, and recognition of discrepancies between current and desired practice (Riemer et al., 2005). However, school personnel may be less aware of these issues and may overestimate their knowledge within a domain (Cunningham, Perry, Stanovich, & Stanovich, 2004). Moreover, although progress monitoring and performance feedback provide means of facilitating practice change (Noell et al., 2005), feedback should be more effective if data are perceived to be credible and valuable (Riemer et al., 2005). Finally, the degree to which new practices are perceived to diverge from current practices, particularly when existing practices have a positive affective valence, relates to practice adoption (Aarons, 2005).

To address these issues, we should consider how data collection and use are perceived to fit within current practice. School personnel can hold strong opinions about best educational practice, which may or may not be consistent with moves toward data-based decision making. Some personnel may perceive that they are already making informed decisions based on qualitative observations and see no need to shift to other assessment strategies. Others may question the proposed assessment's validity. For example, best practice in promoting literacy has been controversial, as evidenced by the so-called "reading wars" (Stanovich, 2000). In assessing literacy growth, some authors note the utility of oral reading fluency (ORF) as a general outcome measure of reading competence in young children (Fuchs, 2004; Kame'enui & Simmons, 2001). Other practitioners, however, question ORF's validity (Roberts, Good, & Corcoran, 2005). This issue might be addressed by taking a social validity approach to adoption of new indices, in which a new measure (e.g., ORF) is evaluated locally for correspondence with evaluative indices from significant others (e.g., teachers), social systems (e.g., team decisions), or measures currently used for decision making (Gresham, 2002). For example, in our preliminary evaluation of DIBELS in New Zealand, we have been collecting DIBELS data alongside school concerns about literacy progress and school-used measures of literacy progress (e.g., book level; Schaughency & Suggate, 2008). By seeing the new tasks in action and learning of their correspondence with locally used measures and perceptions, over time teachers may gain confidence in the new measure's validity and appreciate its increased efficiency. In addition, local data may be used to develop local norms (Stewart & Silberglitt, 2008) and goals (Gibbons & Silberglitt, 2008).

Finally, there are individual differences in levels of technology uptake, requiring different levels of support (e.g., Anderson-Inman, Knox-Quinn, & Horney, 1996; Fuchs & Fuchs, 2001; Scott & Martinek, 2006). Some personnel may readily use technology independently, others may require interpersonal supports such as prompting, and others may continue to be "reluctant users" of the technology (Anderson-Inman et al., 1996; Scott & Martinek, 2006). For example, Scott and Martinek (2006) used a multiple-baseline-across-subjects (schools) design to examine the relative effects of different coaching actions—weekly phone contact to prompt data entry versus visiting the school, modeling, and assisting relevant school personnel with data entry—on amount of data entered by four schools. For one school, weekly phone contact was sufficient to prompt data entry. For two schools, physical guidance and modeling, followed by weekly phone contact, was successful in obtaining data entry. For the fourth school, however, even these efforts were insufficient. Limited self-efficacy regarding the use of data or technology may contribute to the difficulties in uptake in the latter groups. Self-efficacy refers to the belief that one can perform specific tasks and behaviors and is strongly related to performance of those tasks and behaviors (Salas & Cannon-Bowers, 2001). It is related to teachers' professional practice (Gettinger & Stoiber, 1999) and is a predictor of learning and subsequent performance of professional development skills (Salas & Cannon-Bowers, 2001). Thus personnel in the latter groups may benefit from more direct assistance to develop the skills and efficacy to implement the innovation. Alternatively, they may be more comfortable with lower tech options to perform these functions.

Group- or organizational-level variables also affect whether professionals are likely to adopt new practices (Ervin & Schaughency, 2008; Ilgen, Hollenbeck, Johnson, & Jundt, 2005; Salas & Cannon-Bowers, 2001). These include climate, referring to the positive or negative impact of the work environment on employee well-being, and culture, behavioral expectations and the way things are done in an organization (i.e., norms; Glisson, Dukes, & Green, 2006). Therefore, these issues are considered in more detail in the following sections.

Working with Teams

Work in schools is often conducted by teams (Rosenfield & Gravois, 1999, Chapter 31), and school-based steering teams are commonly used in initiatives to implement data-based decision making in multi-tiered service delivery (Ervin & Schaughency, 2008). In working with teams, psychologists should recognize that teams are complex; they exist in particular contexts (schools and communities), and they adapt and change across time (Ilgen et al., 2005).

When teams are *forming*, the sense that the team is competent enough to accomplish the task (sometimes referred to as "collective efficacy"; Ilgen et al., 2005; Salas & Cannon-Barrows, 2001) relates to team performance, speaking to the potentially important role of professional development to promote use of data. Both shared understanding, as might be gathered through team-based professional development (discussed later), and specialized knowledge, as represented in a multidisciplinary team, can contribute to team performance (Ilgen et al., 2005). The sense that the team is a psychologically safe environment in which to forward potential solutions to problems or to try out new professional behaviors also relates to team performance, a finding again relevant to what may be perceived as a professionally sensitive task of interpreting and using data for systemic problem solving (Ilgen et al., 2005).

Team formation involves developing and maintaining roles and interaction patterns among team members (Ilgen et al., 2005), determining who is going to do what and how they are going to interact in the task of managing and using data for systemic problem solving. Whether a team arrives at an effective initial behavioral action plan seems to be key to team success and viability (Ilgen et al., 2005). Effective planning has two related, yet distinct components (Ilgen et al., 2005), both of which have direct relevance to this chapter's focus. First, the team needs to collate information relevant to their task and constituencies. Second, they must evaluate and use this information to arrive at a strategy for accomplishing their task.

Clarity in level of analysis of the intended intervention target and its outcome is important for multi-tiered service delivery and problem solving (Ervin & Schaughency, 2008; Schaughency & Ervin, 2006). When collating information, teams should consider data appropriately aggregated for their decision layer. For example, individual teachers or student assistance teams may evaluate learning trajectories of individual students; grade-level teams may track progress of students in their grade level (e.g., percentage achieving a target); and school improvement teams may examine data at the schoolwide level (e.g., percentage achieving targets at building level; Gibbons & Silberglitt, 2008; McGlinchey & Goodman, 2008).

School personnel may experience difficulties in considering alternative strategies to solve a problem (Fuchs & Fuchs, 2001). The psychologist may help teams explore alternative solutions and serve as knowledge broker or consultant to assist teams in developing action plans (McGlinchey & Goodman, 2008). Action plans should be appropriate to the team's mission (individual students, a grade level, a whole school). They should specify outcomes for those targeted for intervention and how implementation integrity will be monitored so that appropriate inferences can be reached about response to intervention and need for more intensive assessment or supports.

Over time, the team's task becomes learning to adapt when task conditions change. To this end, team development activities should focus on establishing constructive communication and interaction routines around interpreting and using data for formative evaluation and systemic problem solving to maintain a sense of rapport and enhance team performance (Ilgen et al., 2005).

Organizational Considerations

Context—the environment into which the innovation is to be implemented—matters (Schaughency & Ervin, 2006; Salas & Cannon-Bowers, 2001). It influences motivations, expectations, and attitudes for implementation and affects whether skills taught in professional development are used in practice (Salas & Cannon-Bowers, 2001). Implementation likelihood depends on the congruence between the innovation and organizational factors such as organizational mission ("fit" or alignment), available resources, constraints, and support for implementation (Ervin & Schaughency, 2008; Salas & Cannon-Bowers, 2001). Therefore, when working with staff to establish systems for data management and use, the psychologist should consider fit and resource constraints, striving for efficiency and alignment with the organizational context.

Course of Implementation

Practice and systems change is a dynamic process, often described by stages or phases of change (Ervin & Schaughency, 2008). The terminologies used to refer to these stages vary but point to common themes. This sequence of phases should not be thought of as linear but as overlapping and recursive, a sequence in which experience and formative evaluation influence future course. Moreover, implementation course varies across people or work units within organizations and across innovations within an organization.

Getting Ready

It is important to lay the groundwork for the innovation (Ervin & Schaughency, 2008; Salas & Cannon-Bowers, 2001). Conducting a training needs analysis is an important first step (Salas & Cannon-Bowers, 2001). Like a task analysis, a training needs analysis must consider requirements of the tasks (data collection, entry, collation, interpretation, problem solving). It must also specify who will implement these tasks (which teachers, teams, or other professionals), what skill development may be required, and systemwide components of the organization that can potentially affect implementation for these persons or teams (Salas & Cannon-Bowers, 2001). A training needs analysis, then, provides opportunities to identify challenges and consider how these may be addressed.

Contextual factors prior to professional development, including framing of the initiative, can affect motivation, learning, and skill retention (Salas & Cannon-Bowers, 2001). For example, feedback's emotional valence may influence its effectiveness (Riemer et al., 2005). Overemphasizing accountability, especially early in an initiative, may lead to negative reactions, may negatively affect climate, and may misguide decision making (Earl & Fullan, 2002; Ervin & Schaughency, 2008). Instead, one should emphasize formative evaluation, framing professional development as an opportunity to develop problem-solving skills, with benefits for personnel as well as students (Lau et al., 2006).

Teaching New Professional Skills

In general, effective professional development includes four basic principles: (1) presentation of relevant information or concepts to be learned (e.g., interpretation of data for academic problem solving; Gibbons & Silberglitt, 2008; Daly et al., Chapter 29, this volume); (2) demonstration of skills to be learned (e.g., data collation, interpretation); (3) creation of opportunities for personnel to practice skills (e.g., using technology, interpreting data, professional decision making based on data); and (4) provision of feedback to personnel during and after practice (Salas & Cannon-Bowers, 2001). For example, Codding, Skowron, and Pace (2005) successfully taught educators the skills to interpret assessment results and translate these into measurable objectives using an instructional approach that included modeling, practice, and performance feedback.

Social conditions within the learning process may facilitate learning and retention. Collaborative training, in which instructional methods include interactive activities between personnel (but not necessarily to perform a team task), has some potential benefits—opportunities for observational learning and reduced need for instructional time, resources, and practice. However, the effectiveness of collaborative training activities may interact with other factors, such as individual characteristics (Salas & Bower-Cannon, 2001). For example, in one study, trainees who experienced anxiety in social interactions did not benefit from collaborative training protocols (Arthur, Young, Jordan, & Shebilske, 1996). Thus group activities are not necessarily beneficial for everyone. In team training, team members are trained to perform a team task. Consistent with professional development research generally, team training is most likely to be effective when it is theoretically guided, focuses on requisite skills, and provides trainees with realistic opportunities for practice and feedback (Salas & Cannon-Bowers, 2001). Strategies that enhance generalization and transfer of skills to the work setting include integrating more challenging tasks during training and moving to those that approximate the work environment (Salas & Bower-Cannon, 2001).

Facilitating Implementation

Events that occur after training are important for increasing the likelihood that skills will be applied, generalized, and maintained (Salas & Cannon-Bowers, 2001). Such factors include situational cues for performing the skills; opportunities to perform the skills shortly after professional development has occurred; social support from peers, supervisors, and/or subordinates; and reinforcement (or punishment) for applying skills in the work setting (Salas & Cannon-Bowers, 2001). For example, ensuring that data review is on the agenda of relevant consultation and team meetings would provide a cue to perform the task, and rotating responsibility for this task across personnel or team members would provide opportunities to practice new skills (Ilgen et al., 2005).

Providing Ongoing Support

Over time, the change agent's task shifts from facilitating implementation to fostering the innovation's sustained use. This includes integrating the innovation into the organization and building capacity for continued evolution and adaptation in response to changing circumstances (Ervin & Schaughency, 2008). Possible strategies may involve fading change-agent involvement in primary data management, review, and problem-solving activities and having school personnel assume these responsibilities scaffolded with ongoing communication and resource support from the change agent (Ervin & Schaughency, 2008). This should also include infrastructure for ongoing sustained relationships with school personnel to provide support and technical assistance for program development, intervention planning, and data collection and review as new technologies or needs arise (Fuchs & Fuchs, 2001; Spoth, Greenberg, Bierman, & Redmond, 2004; Stecker et al., 2005).

Concluding Thoughts and Future Directions

Organizational development and systems change research support a broad, multifaceted approach that views technical and strategic change efforts within the organization's social contexts (Glisson et al., 2006). Promoting data management and use involves both *technical* (data entry, analysis) and *strategic* (professional decision making) aspects. The latter may be thought of as a "soft" technology, vulnerable to adaptation (Glisson, 2002). Adaptations may be positive, reworking the strategy to better meet local needs, or they can render the innovation useless (Ervin & Schaughency, 2008). Remembering the charge to build delivery system capacity to improve children's competencies (Blueprint III), when developing an implementation system to support data use, the psychologist's challenge is to maintain focus on the relationships between indices of student performance, strategies implemented to target performance, and systems and routines for examining these data in problem solving.

Implementation science and means of changing or introducing practices in a specific setting are newly emerging (Ervin & Schaughency, 2008). Practitioners need research to support their efforts in managing and using data to inform service delivery for children. Fuchs and Fuchs's (2001) research to promote teacher use of academic performance data provides an exemplar to guide technical research, and Rosenfield et al.'s (2008) work on instructional consultation a model to guide strategic efforts. Further work is needed to address these issues at multiple levels in multi-tiered service delivery. Psychologists can contribute through careful documentation of the change process, implementation integrity, lessons learned regarding barriers to implementation and how to address these, and the relationship of these efforts to student and systemic outcomes. Finally, if psychologists are to be effective systems consultants in building capacity for data-based decision making, then they will need professional development opportunities at the preservice, internship, and inservice levels that develop the skill sets needed to monitor outcomes at individual and systems levels and to integrate this information for problem solving (Blueprint III; Schaughency & Ervin, 2006).

Acknowledgments

Portions of this chapter were drafted while Elizabeth Schaughency was on sabbatical leave at the Department of Educational and Counselling Psychology and Special Education, University of British Columbia, Vancouver, British Columbia, Canada. Our work in schools has been supported by the Department of Psychology and University of Otago Research Grants. We also wish to thank the students and school personnel with whom we have worked. They have shaped our appreciation of the issues over the years.

References

Aarons, G. A. (2005). Measuring provider attitudes toward adoption of evidence-based practice: Consideration of organizational context and individual differences. *Child and Adolescent Psychiatric Clinics of North America, 14,* 255–271.

American Educational Research Association, American Psychological Association, & National Council on Measurement in Education. (1999). *Standards for educational and psychological testing.* Washington, DC: American Psychological Association.

Anderson-Inman, L., Knox-Quinn, C., & Horney, M. A. (1996). Computer-based study strategies for students with learning disabilities: Individual differences associated with adoption level. *Journal of Learning Disabilities, 29,* 461–484.

Arthur, W., Young, B., Jordan, J. A., & Shebilske, W. L. (1996). Effectiveness and individual and dyadic training protocols: The influence of trainee interaction anxiety. *Human Factors, 38,* 79–86.

Barnett, D. W., Macmann, G., & Lentz, F. E. (2003). Personality assessment research: Applying criteria of confidence and helpfulness. In C. R. Reynolds & R. W. Kamphaus (Eds.), *Handbook of psychological and educational assessment of children: Personality, behavior and context* (2nd ed., (pp. 3–29). New York: Guilford Press.

Codding, R. S., Skowron, J., & Pace, G. M. (2005). Back to basics: Training teachers to interpret curriculum-based measurement data and create observable and measurable objectives. *Behavioral Interventions, 20,* 165–176.

Coyne, M. D., Kame'enui, E. J., & Simmons, D. C. (2004). Improving beginning reading instruction and intervention for students with LD: Reconciling "all" with "each." *Journal of Learning Disabilities, 37,* 231–239.

Cunningham, A. E., Perry, K. E., Stanovich, K. E., & Stanovich, P. J. (2004). Disciplinary knowledge of K–3 teachers and their knowledge calibration in the domain of early literacy. *Annals of Dyslexia, 54,* 139–167.

Dawes, R. M. (1994). *House of cards: Psychology and psychotherapy built on myth.* New York: Free Press.

Earl, L., & Fullan, M. (2002). Using data in leadership for learning. *Cambridge Journal of Education, 33,* 383–394.

Ercikan, K. (2006). Developments in assessment of student learning and achievement. In P. A. Alexander & P. H. Winne (Eds.), *Handbook of educational psychology* (2nd ed., pp. 929–953). London: Erlbaum.

Ervin, R. A., & Schaughency, E. (2008). Best practices in accessing the systems change literature. In A. Thomas & J. P. Grimes (Eds.), *Best practices in school psychology* (5th ed., Vol. 3, pp. 853–874). Bethesda, MD: National Association of School Psychologists.

Evans, S. W. (2007, August). Discussant. In T. J. Power (Chair), *Linking schools and primary care practices for children with ADHD.* Symposium conducted at the annual convention of the American Psychological Association, San Francisco.

Evans, S. W., Green, A. L., & Serpell, Z. N. (2005). Community participation in the treatment development process using community development teams. *Journal of Clinical Child and Adolescent Psychology, 34,* 765–771.

Fuchs, L. S. (2004). The past, present, and future of curriculum-based measurement research. *School Psychology Review, 33*(2), 188–192.

Fuchs, L. S., & Fuchs, D. (2001). Computer applications to curriculum-based measurement. *Special Services in the Schools, 17,* 1–14.

George, M. P., White, G. P., & Schlaffer, J. J. (2007). Implementing school-wide behavior change: Lessons from the field. *Psychology in the Schools, 44,* 41–51.

Gettinger, M., & Stoiber, K. C. (1999). Excellence in teaching: Review of instructional and environmental variables. In C. R. Reynolds & T. B. Gutkin (Eds.), *Handbook of school psychology* (3rd ed., pp. 984–1024). New York: Wiley.

Gibbons, K. A., & Silberglitt, B. (2008). Best practices in evaluating psychoeducational services based on student outcome data. In A. Thomas & J. P. Grimes (Eds.), *Best practices in school psychology* (5th ed., Vol. 6, pp. 2103–2116). Bethesda, MD: National Association of School Psychologists.

Glisson, C. (2002). The organizational context of children's mental health services. *Clinical Child and Family Psychology Review, 5,* 233–253.

Glisson, C., Dukes, D., & Green, P. (2006). The effects of the ARC organizational intervention on caseworker, climate, and culture in children's service systems. *Child Abuse and Neglect, 30,* 855–880.

Graczyk, P. A., Domitrovich, C. E., Small, M., & Zins, J. E. (2006). Serving all children: An implementation model framework. *School Psychology Review, 35,* 266–274.

Gresham, F. M. (2002). Teaching social skills to high-risk children and youth: Preventive and remedial strategies. In M. R. Shinn, H. M. Walker, & G. Stoner (Eds.), *Interventions for academic and behavior problems: 2. Preventive and remedial strategies* (pp. 403–432). Bethesda, MD: National Association of School Psychologists.

Gresham, F. M. (2004). Current status and future directions of school-based behavioral interventions. *School Psychology Review, 33,* 326–343.

Hood, C., & Dorman, C. (2008). Best practices in the display of data. In A. Thomas & J. P. Grimes (Eds.), *Best practices in school psychology* (5th ed., Vol. 6, pp. 2117–2132). Bethesda, MD: National Association of School Psychologists.

Horner, R. H., Sugai, G., Todd, A. W., & Lewis-Palmer, T. (2005). Schoolwide positive behavior support: An alternative approach to discipline in schools. In L. Bambara & L. Kern (Eds.), *Individualized supports for students with problem behaviors: Designing positive behavior plans* (pp. 359–390). New York: Guilford Press.

Ilgen, D. R., Hollenbeck, J. R., Johnson, M., & Jundt, D. (2005). Teams in organizations: From input–process–output models to IMOI models. *Annual Review of Psychology, 56,* 517–543.

Irvin, L. K., Horner, R. H., Ingram, K., Todd, A. W., Sugai, G., Sampson, N. K., et al. (2006). Using office discipline referral data for decision making about student behavior in elementary and middle schools: An empirical evaluation of validity. *Journal of Positive Behavior Interventions, 8,* 10–23.

Kame'enui, E. J., & Simmons, D. C. (2001). Introduction to this special issue: The DNA of reading fluency. *Scientific Studies of Reading, 5,* 203–210.

Kaminski, R., Cummings, K. D., Powell-Smith, K. A., & Good, R. H., III. (2008). Best practices in using Dynamic Indicators of Basic Early Literacy Skills (DIBELS) for formative assessment and evaluation. In A. Thomas & J. P. Grimes (Eds.), *Best practices in school psychology* (5th ed., Vol. 4, pp. 1181–1204). Bethesda, MD: National Association of School Psychologists.

Kavale, K. A., & Forness, S. R. (1999). Effectiveness of special education. In C. R. Reynolds & T. B. Gutkin (Eds.), *Handbook of school psychology* (3rd ed., pp. 984–1024). New York: Wiley.

Lau, M. W., Sieler, J. D., Muyksens, P., Canter, A., Vankeuren, B., & Marston, D. (2006). Perspectives on the use on the problem-solving model from the school psychologist, administrator, and teacher from a large midwest urban school district. *Psychology in the Schools, 43*, 117–127.

Mash, E. J., & Hunsley, J. (2005). Evidence-based assessment of child and adolescent disorders: Issues and challenges. *Journal of Clinical Child and Adolescent Psychology, 34*, 362–279.

Mayer, R. E. (2004). Teaching of subject matter. *Annual Review of Psychology, 55*, 715–744.

McGlinchey, M. T., & Goodman, S. (2008). Best practices in implementing school reform. In A. Thomas & J. P. Grimes (Eds.), *Best practices in school psychology* (5th ed., Vol. 3, pp. 983–994). Bethesda, MD: National Association of School Psychologists.

Noell, G. H., Witt, J. C., Slider, N. J., Connell, J. E., Gatti, S. L., Williams, K. L., et al. (2005). Treatment implementation following behavioral consultation in schools: A comparison of three follow-up strategies. *School Psychology Review, 34*, 87–106.

Pellegrino, J. W., Chudowsky, N., & Glaser, R. (Eds.). (2001). *Knowing what students know: The science and design of educational assessment.* Washington, DC: National Academy Press.

Pliszka, S. R., Lopez, M., Crimson, L., Toprac, M. G., Hughes, C. W., Emslie, G. J., et al. (2003). A feasibility study of the Children's Medication Algorithm Project (CMAP) for the treatment of ADHD. *Journal of the American Academy of Child and Adolescent Psychology, 42*, 279–287.

Power, T. J., Mautone, J. A., Manz, P. H., Frye, L., & Blum, N. J. (2007, August). Managing ADHD in primary care: The role of primary care providers. In T. J. Power (Chair), *Linking schools and primary care practices for children with ADHD.* Symposium conducted at the annual convention of the American Psychological Association, San Francisco.

Riemer, M., Rosof-Williams, J., & Bickman, L. (2005). Theories related to changing clinician practice. *Child and Adolescent Psychiatric Clinics of North America, 14*, 241–254.

Roberts, G., Good, R., & Corcoran, S. (2005). Story retell: A fluency-based indicator of reading comprehension. *School Psychology Quarterly, 20*, 304–317.

Rolfsen, M., & Torvatn, H. (2005). How to "get through": Communication challenges in formative evaluation. *Evaluation, 11*, 297–309.

Rosenfield, S., & Gravois, T. (1999). Working with teams in the school. In C. R. Reynolds & T. B. Gutkin (Eds.), *Handbook of school psychology* (3rd ed., pp. 1025–1040). Hoboken, NJ: Wiley.

Rosenfield, S., Silva, A., & Gravois, T. A. (2008). Bringing instructional consultation to scale: Research and development of IC and IC teams. In W. P. Erchul & S. M. Sheridan (Eds.), *Handbook of research in school consultation: Empirical foundations for the field* (pp. 203–223). Mahwah, NJ: Erlbaum.

Salas, E., & Cannon-Bowers, J. A. (2001). The science of training: A decade of progress. *Annual Review of Psychology, 52*, 471–499.

Schaughency, E., & Ervin, R. (2006). Building capacity to implement and sustain effective practices to better serve children. *School Psychology Review, 35*, 155–166.

Schaughency, E., & Suggate, S. (2008). Measuring basic early literacy skills amongst year 1 students in New Zealand. *New Zealand Journal of Education Studies, 43*, 85–106.

Scott, T. M., & Martinek, G. (2006). Coaching positive behavior support in school settings: Tactics and data-based decision making. *Journal of Positive Behavior Interventions, 8*, 165–173.

Shapiro, E. S., & Elliott, S. N. (1999). Curriculum-based assessment and other performance assessment strategies. In C. R. Reynolds & T. B. Gutkin (Eds.), *Handbook of school psychology* (3rd ed., pp. 383–409). New York: Wiley.

Spoth, R., Greenberg, M., Bierman, K., & Redmond, C. (2004). PROSPER community-university partnership model for public education systems: Capacity-building for evidence-based, competence-building prevention. *Prevention Science, 5*, 31–39.

Stanovich, K. E. (2000). *Progress in understanding reading: Scientific foundations and new frontiers.* New York: Guilford Press.

Stecker, P. M., Fuchs, L. S., & Fuchs, D. (2005). Using curriculum-based measurement to improve student achievement: Review of the research. *Psychology in the Schools, 42*, 795–819.

Stewart, L. H., & Silberglitt, B. (2008). Best practices in developing academic local norms. In A. Thomas & J. Grimes (Eds.), *Best practices in school psychology* (5th ed., Vol. 2, pp. 225–242). Bethesda, MD: National Association of School Psychologists.

Swets, J. A., Dawes, R. M., & Monahan, J. (2000). Psychological science can improve diagnostic decisions. *Psychological Science in the Public Interest, 1,* 1–26.

Thomas, A., & Grimes, J. P. (Eds.). (2008). *Best practices in school psychology* (5th ed.). Bethesda, MD: National Association of School Psychologists.

Todd, A. W., Sampson, N. K., & Horner, R. (2005). Data-based decision making using office discipline referral data from the schoolwide information system (SWIS). *Journal of Positive Behavior Interventions, 7,* 3.

U.S. Department of Health and Human Services. (2002). *Early childhood education and school readiness: Conceptual models, constructs, and measures.* Washington, DC: Author.

Wireless Generation. (n.d.). Retrieved October 3, 2007, from *wirelessgeneration.com/products. html.*

Ysseldyke, J. E., Burns, M., Dawson, P., Kelley, B., Morrison, D., Ortiz, S., et al. (2006). *School psychology: A blueprint for training and practice: III.* Bethesda, MD: National Association of School Psychologists.

Ysseldyke, J. E., & McLeod, S. (2007). Using technology tools to monitor response to intervention. In S. R. Jimerson, M. K. Burns, & A. M. VanDerHeyden (Eds.), *Handbook of response to intervention: The science and practice of assessment and intervention* (pp. 396–407). New York: Springer.

Chapter 33

Implementing the Problem-Solving Model with Culturally and Linguistically Diverse Students

Robert L. Rhodes

The recent growth of the culturally and linguistically diverse (CLD) population within the United States and changing legislative requirements have placed the educational and assessment needs of CLD students squarely and unavoidably in the public eye. States and individual school districts around the nation are working to align their instruction, intervention, and assessment practices with federal requirements related to research-based interventions, student response to intervention, and nondiscriminatory assessment. Driven by both altruistic motives and a desire to make adequate yearly progress, many states and districts are carefully evaluating how curriculum-based assessment methods such as a response-to-intervention (RTI) model within a problem-solving framework are best implemented with CLD students.

Curriculum-based methods of assessing student response to intervention have generated a great deal of interest over the past several years. Because of the difficulties inherent in the use of norm-referenced measures of academic achievement with students in general and with culturally and linguistically diverse students in particular, researchers and practitioners have advocated for the use of alternative procedures to assess the skills and abilities children have acquired through either direct intervention or instruction (e.g., Shinn, 2002; Fuchs & Fuchs, 1997). Because numerous factors must be considered when evaluating the academic progress of students who are culturally and linguistically diverse, the problem-solving model offers several potential advantages in comparison with traditional assessment approaches.

Students who are English language learners (ELLs), for example, often display characteristics and behaviors that are similar but unrelated to disorders and disabilities that require special education intervention. Students who are learning English as a second language may often be slow to begin and to finish tasks and appear to be inattentive, impulsive, easily distracted, disruptive, and disorganized as a result of the time required to translate instruction and directions, the partial or incomplete understanding of instruction and directions, and the mental fatigue associated with language acquisition (Ortiz, 2005). Roseberry-McKibbin (2002) identified several potential issues related to second language acquisition. She cautions that there are "normal processes of second language acquisition [that] ... need to be recognized as normal behaviors for students who are not yet proficient in English" (p. 193). Without careful consideration and evaluation, CLD students displaying these and other characteristics either may be inappropriately identified as having a need for special education intervention or may have the true nature of their concern masked by extraneous variables.

The CLD Student Population

The education of diverse student populations is an international concern. Wan (2008), in an examination of the education of diverse students worldwide, notes that countries such as the United Kingdom, Canada, South Africa, China, Singapore, Australia, and New Zealand are unique but similar in the challenges they face in teaching CLD students. The CLD student population in the United States, for example, includes speakers of more than 400 different languages (Kindler, 2002). The majority of students who speak a language other than English (77%) are Spanish speakers (National Clearinghouse for English Language Acquisition and Language Instruction Educational Programs [NCELA], 2002). Vietnamese (2.3%), Hmong (2.2%), Haitian Creole (1.1%), Korean (1.1%), Cantonese (1.0%), Arabic (0.9%), Russian (0.9%), Navajo (0.9%), and Tagalog (0.8%) round out the list of top 10 languages spoken by students in the United States (NCELA, 2002).

The most recent nationwide census (U.S. Census Bureau, 2001) revealed that among the 48.7 million students in the United States, 1 in 10 (11%) students were born outside of the United States and that 1 in 5 (20%) had a parent born outside of the United States. During the past decade, the overall student population within the nation increased by only 2.6%. The ELL student population in kindergarten through twelfth grade increased by 60.8% during this same period (National Clearinghouse for English Language Acquisition and Language Instruction Educational Programs [NCELA], 2006). Interestingly, the highest rate of ELL student growth has been in states that, historically, have not had high numbers of ELL students (NCELA, 2006).

Watson, Rinaldi, Navarrete, Bianco, and Samson (2007) point out that this increase in the number of students with limited English proficiency necessitates that there be a structure in place when referring, assessing, and identifying ELL students for special education services. They note that each school should have well-developed referral guidelines and procedures, as well as knowledgeable professionals who can examine academic and behavioral concerns in the context of language, culture, and disability. Unfortunately, many schools lack this necessary structure and are unable to differentiate between culture and language differences and actual disabilities (Rueda & Windmueller, 2006; Sanchez & Brisk, 2004).

History of Difference versus Disability Differentiation Attempts

The differentiation between culture and language difference and actual disability is a multifaceted task that has been attempted for decades. One of the most debated and long-standing concerns in this area is the potential overrepresentation of diverse students across various special education categories (Perez, Skiba, & Chung, 2008; Artiles, Trent, & Palmer, 2004; Losen & Orfield, 2002; Artiles & Trent, 2000). Diverse students with disabilities and those suspected of having disabilities often participate in an inconsistent system of referral, assessment, and intervention in which they may or may not receive the quality of service they need, depending on whom they are served by and where they are served. This unintended but all too real situation does not occur because of a lack of effort or interest. Numerous practitioners, researchers, and theorists have provided excellent guidelines and have advanced the methods and models of assessment and intervention for all students.

A good example of this advancement of assessment and intervention procedures for CLD students is the Screening to Enhance Equitable Placement (STEEP) model by Witt (2002). The STEEP model uses a problem-solving approach not only to develop intervention strategies but also to screen students to determine the need for further brainstorming and evaluation. Under the framework of this model, students who are identified as being "at risk" during the screening process are referred to a school-based team to determine appropriate intervention procedures. Following the development of an intervention plan, progress monitoring is used to adjust the intervention procedures and evaluate effectiveness. Noell, Gilbertson, VanDerHeyden, and Witt (2005) report that although the STEEP screening model has been evaluated with African American populations, such evaluation efforts have not been conducted with ELL students. Although more data are clearly needed, it seems likely that such an approach would be appropriate for ELL and other CLD students.

To date, methods and models that take into account the unique circumstances and experiences of culturally and linguistically diverse students have not been consistently and widely implemented. The minimal standards of practice mandated by federal law (e.g., nondiscriminatory assessment procedures, monitoring of disproportional representation) have helped but have largely been reactionary (designed to right or avoid repeating a wrong) rather than providing aspirational standards of practice that incorporates the broad knowledge base developed over the past several decades.

As the field of school psychology continues to develop, opportunities exist to establish a more thoughtful and comprehensive model of assessment and intervention. The problem-solving model incorporates many of the prereferral considerations, classroom and instructional evaluation strategies, and alternative diagnostic procedures long recommended for CLD students. Merrell, Ervin, and Gimpel (2006) share the hope of many in their statement that the problem-solving model's movement away from a focus on within-child pathology and toward a focus on environments, contexts, desired outcomes, and assets has the potential to greatly enhance the ability of school psychologists to respond effectively to students, families, and school systems.

Legislative History
Related to Nondiscriminatory Assessment

Fuchs, Mock, Morgan, and Young (2003) provide a brief history of the development of the problem-solving model within the public school setting, noting that the rapid expansion of the special education population from the 1970s through the 1990s sparked concern about the apparent overidentifica-

tion of students across various disability areas and the unmet educational needs of many students prior to referral for special education evaluation. Efforts to meet the individual needs of students prior to special education referral or "prereferral intervention" is defined as a teacher's modification of instruction or some other aspect of the learning environment to better accommodate a difficult-to-teach student prior to formal referral of the student for testing and possible special education placement (Fuchs et al., 2003, p. 160).

The structured approach and classroom-based emphasis of problem identification and intervention offered the problem-solving model has been viewed by many researchers and practitioners as an effective method of prereferral intervention for diverse students experiencing academic difficulties. Tharp and Wetzel (1969), Bergan (1970), and Bergan and Kratochwill (1990) considered the inductive nature of the model to be a key feature in identifying and meeting the individual needs of students. They observed that supporters of the model believe that no student characteristic (e.g., disability label, race, socioeconomic status) dictates a priori what intervention will work. Nor will a given intervention be effective for all students of a particular group, no matter how homogenous the group may appear to be. Instead, solutions to instructional and behavioral problems are induced by evaluating students' responsiveness to a multistage process comprising problem identification, problem analysis, plan implementation, and problem evaluation (Fuchs et al., 2003).

Recently, application of the problem-solving model in the schools has been bolstered by legislation allowing for an RTI approach to the identification of learning disabilities. The movement to expand beyond the discrepancy model in the identification of learning disabilities was fueled in part by growing dissatisfaction with the use of this model with CLD students. The following section provides a summary of legislation related to nondiscriminatory assessment.

Public Law 94-142: Education of All Handicapped Children Act

The need to differentiate difference from disability among CLD students was addressed in this first federal law requiring special education services. Section 4 of the exclusionary clause for Public Law 94-142 states that a child should not be identified as learning disabled if the "discrepancy between ability and achievement is primarily the result of environmental, cultural, or economic disadvantage" (U.S. Department of Education, 1977, p. 65083). Although students who have unique environmental, cultural, or economic circumstances may be identified as having learning disabilities, the extent to which these external factors affect their academic performance must be established and may not be the primary cause of the performance deficit in question.

Public Law 105-17: Individuals with Disabilities Education Act (IDEA '97)

Each successive revision of the special education law has addressed the appropriate identification of CLD students suspected of having a disability and the continued mislabeling and disproportionate identification of these same students. Public Law 105-17 concluded that "greater efforts are needed to prevent the intensification of problems connected with mislabeling minority children with disabilities" [601 (c) (8) (A)] and that "more minority children continue to be served in special education than would be expected given the percentage of minority students in the general population" [601 (c) (8) (B)]. Public Law 105-17 added provisions related to lack of effective instruction and limited English proficiency as a safeguard against these concerns, stating that "in making a determination of eligibility under paragraph 4(A), a child shall not be determined to be a child with a disability if the determinant factor for such determination is lack of instruction in reading or math or limited English proficiency" [Section 614 (b) (5)]. Within this law, congress further required states to (1) collect ethnic data by type of disability; (2) determine whether disproportionality exists; and (3) address the problem via corrective action measures.

Public Law 108-446: Individuals with Disabilities Education Act (IDEA 2004)

According to IDEA 2004, states must work to prevent the inappropriate overidentifica-

tion or disproportionate representation in disability categories by race and ethnicity of children, including children with disabilities with a particular impairment (U.S. Department of Education, 2007). Public Law 108-466 further establishes policies and procedures to prevent disproportionality or overidentification by race and ethnicity and provides for the collection and examination of data regarding disproportionality. This current legislation also outlines requirements when reviewing policies and procedures and extends opportunities for technical assistance, demonstration projects, dissemination of information, and implementation of scientifically based research.

The Problem-Solving Model in the Schools

Successful application of the aforementioned legislative guidelines within a school setting is predicated on three core assumptions (Shinn, 2002): (1) a problem is defined situationally as a discrepancy between what is expected and what occurs; (2) there are a subset of students within each school setting whose discrepancies are so significant that it may be unreasonable for them to achieve in general education unless their programs are modified; and (3) effective educators must "generate many possible plans of action prior to attempting problem solution" (Deno, 1989, p.11) and then evaluate the effects of the program actually implemented.

Canter (2005) describes the problem-solving model as a broad-sequenced model that seeks to determine what instructional supports are needed to solve student achievement problems. She notes that problem-solving models include early intervention components, general education classroom and school supports, and ongoing evaluation of student progress. Referral for special education evaluation is made only after these early supports fail to produce sufficient gains.

Merrell et al. (2006) add that the basis for the problem-solving model is that problems are not necessarily viewed as forms of pathology or disorder. The model is instead outcome focused, context specific, and driven by ongoing data collection. The emphasis is on a solution or outcome to the problem with the understanding that what constitutes a problem or a viable solution to it may differ across settings or contexts.

Problem-Solving Model Steps and Recommendations for Implementation with CLD Students

The stages utilized within the problem-solving model are intended to identify, validate, and analyze the problem and then develop, implement, and evaluate possible interventions. Each of the four steps as described by Merrell and colleagues (2006) is summarized here, and corresponding recommendations for implementing the problem-solving model with CLD students are provided.

Step 1: Problem Identification and Validation

During the problem-identification stage the problem is defined and validated as a quantifiable discrepancy between the student's current and desired performance. The problem is described in observable and measurable terms, and the frequency, duration, latency, and magnitude of the problem is recorded as appropriate. The problem is directly and repeatedly measured in the context in which it occurs. Key questions at this stage are, What is the problem? and How wide is the gap between actual and desired performance in this domain of functioning?

Particular care should be taken during this step to examine the cultural and linguistic demands required to meet the desired performance criteria. The language of instruction, the student's language proficiency, and the language demands of the task and method of measurement should be clearly understood and carefully evaluated. School psychologists working with CLD students should have an awareness of language acquisition and its impact on a student's response to instruction and intervention. This pervasive concern is perhaps best illustrated by the tremendous difference in language exposure often experienced by ELL students in comparison with their monolingual peers. Ortiz (1997) reports that English language learners with an average of as much as 2–3 hours per day of exposure to the English language will still be 15,000 total hours behind their monolingual English-speaking peers by kindergarten. By fifth grade, ELL students are nearly 24,000 total hours behind their monolingual English-speaking peers on average with respect to exposure and experience with the English language.

Cummins (1984) proposed basic interpersonal communication skills (BICS) and cognitive academic language proficiency (CALP) as two distinct types of language proficiency. BICS is the development of conversational language skills and is thought to take 2–3 years to acquire. CALP is the academic language skills that are necessary to fully understand instructions and produce verbal and written work unencumbered by issues of language acquisition and proficiency. CALP is a more advanced level of language acquisition and is estimated to take 5–7 years to develop.

In order to address issues of language proficiency in the context of the evaluation of academic performance, Ochoa (2005) recommends that evaluators compare when possible the educational trajectory of the student in question with his or her same-grade-level ELL peers. If the educational trajectories are similar and are within the time frame of BICS and CALP development, length of native language instructional programming and issues of language acquisition might be considered critical factors in the students' performance. However, there may be cause for concern if the educational trajectory of an ELL student across time is notably different from those of his or her ELL classmates who have been educated in a similar instructional setting for approximately the same number of years.

Familiarity with the process of second-language acquisition may be obtained through a review of several seminal studies in this area, including Cummins (1983, 1984), Ortiz and Polyzoi (1986), Collier (1987), and Thomas and Collier (1996, 1997, 2002). These and other studies provide critical information regarding the expected rate of second-language acquisition, the multiple factors that may influence language acquisition, the difference between basic communication and academic language skills, and the potential impact of second-language acquisition on academic achievement (Ochoa & Rhodes, 2005).

Step 2: Problem Analysis

During the problem-analysis stage the problem is directly measured with a focus on when, where, with whom, and during which activities the concern is more or less likely to occur or become exacerbated. The key question at this stage is, Why is the problem occurring? Information is gathered through multiple sources (student, teachers, parents, record review, etc.), and classroom and instructional factors are examined to determine what can be changed to enable learning and reduce the discrepancy between the student's current and desired performance.

Ochoa and Rhodes (2005) discuss information that should be gathered or reviewed when working with CLD students during this stage, including:

Educational History

Inquiry should be made through record review and parent interview about the country (or countries) in which the student has been educated, the language (or languages) of instruction, previous bilingual education services, reason for termination or exit from bilingual education services, grades repeated, number of schools attended, areas of academic success, and areas of academic difficulty or concern. If academic difficulties exist, it should be determined whether these difficulties are present across both languages or whether they are manifested only when the student is required to perform academic tasks in English. If they are present only when the student is required to perform tasks in English, then this may be an indication of second-language-acquisition issues rather than a specific content knowledge deficit or disability.

Language History

The language history of the child and family should be explored through record review (e.g., home language surveys; see Texas Education Agency, 2005, for examples of home language surveys across multiple languages) and parent interview. Potential questions for inclusion in a parent interview include: What language or languages are currently used at home? What language or languages have been used at home during the life of

the student? What language appears to be preferred by the student? In what language does the student prefer to read? In what language does the student watch TV or listen to music?

Bilingual and ESL Program Participation

Ochoa and Rhodes (2005) note that several different educational programs are used to educate ELL students in the United States, including English-only programs, pullout English as a second language (ESL), transitional bilingual programs, maintenance bilingual programs, and two-way or dual-language bilingual education programs. The amount of English and native language instruction that is used varies markedly across the programs, as does program effectiveness. The type of program(s) a student attended and the reason for exiting is key information for accurate problem analysis. For example, did the student attend a program that emphasized the development of English language skills only or did he or she attend a program that provided instruction in both the new and native languages? This programmatic difference will affect the rate of language acquisition and the knowledge of academic terms and concepts across both languages. Likewise, it is important to know whether the student met the exit criteria for a particular program or whether he or she exited simply because he or she moved from the school or district or because of a change in bilingual and ESL programming in the district.

Current Language Proficiency

The current language proficiency of the student should be examined through record review, teacher interview, and formal and informal assessment. The student's use of one particular language more frequently than another should not serve as an indicator of language proficiency. Recently administered language proficiency measures (no more than 6 months old) should be used to determine the student's level of proficiency across both languages. The student's current level of language proficiency should serve as a starting point for developing an assessment strategy that includes the appropriate combination of primary language (e.g.,

Spanish), secondary language (e.g., English), and nonverbal measures. Ochoa and Ortiz's multidimensional assessment model for bilingual individuals (Ortiz & Ochoa, 2005) provides a framework for considering these factors and an individual student's bilingual and ESL program participation when developing an assessment approach.

Level of Acculturation

The student's current level of acculturation in relation to the appropriateness of instruction and procedures should be assessed. Although less readily and intuitively understood by many school psychologists, the degree to which the student is acculturated to the mainstream of U.S. society has a significant impact on student progress and participation in the classroom and the decisions and procedures used in evaluation (Ortiz, 2005). For example, information on acculturation may be used to evaluate the student's fit within an instructional setting. A student may have a level of English proficiency sufficient to grasp the terms and concepts discussed within the instructional setting but may not have the societal and cultural knowledge necessary to use this information in the context required by an assignment or course objective. Bidimensional measurement of acculturation is recommended across cognitive styles, personality, identity, attitudes, and acculturative stress. See Kang (2006) for a review of instruments available for the assessment of acculturation.

Additional issues and concerns that should be carefully considered during the problem analysis stage are highlighted by Rhodes (2005):

- The extent to which the curricular content of the classroom or course is culturally representative of the student. Curricular additions and adjustments should be made as necessary.
- Known or suspected sensory or communicative impairments.
- The amount, type, and location of formal elementary and secondary schooling. Students who have immigrated to the United States, for example, may have experienced instruction in different countries and different languages, breaks in their educational time lines, and varied curricula.

- The student's mobility and attendance pattern and the potential impact on academic progress.
- Skills other than the targeted skill required to complete tasks or assignments. Does an assessment of motor skills require an understanding of verbal instructions? Are time factors such as speed of response a consideration in evaluating conceptual understanding?
- Experiences outside of the school setting that support or detract from academic success. Does the living situation of the student allow him or her to get an appropriate amount of sleep? Does the student have enough to eat? Is the student working a significant number of hours before or after school?

It is recommended that a structured format be used when reviewing "prereferral" concerns and conducting teacher, parent, and student interviews during this stage. The structured approach helps to ensure that key topics and issues are discussed and when translated is of assistance to bilingual practitioners and interpreters. Rhodes, Ochoa, and Ortiz (2005) provide an extensive list of prereferral questions and a structured interview format for teachers, parents, and students in English and Spanish. See Table 33.1 for an example of prereferral questions.

During the problem-analysis stage it is also important that the language spoken by the student or parent is not allowed to become a barrier to full participation. Bilingual practitioners should be employed to ensure that all necessary information is accurately gathered and conveyed. If a bilingual practitioner is unavailable, a trained interpreter should be employed. Guajardo Alvarado (2003) provides a recommended hierarchy for selecting and using bilingual personnel that is designed to help schools and practitioners move beyond the indiscriminate approach that has often been used when employing interpreters:

1. Trained bilingual evaluation specialists fluent in the student's native language using evaluation measures in the student's two languages
2. Bilingual evaluation specialists fluent in the student's native language using modified evaluation measures, translated

TABLE 33.1. Prereferral Team Considerations: Questions Pertaining to Second-Language Learners

General educational background history

1. Did child start his/her formal schooling in the United States?
2. How many years did the child attend school in native country?

Preschool experiences

3. Who was/were the child's primary caregiver(s)? What language(s) did each caregiver speak to the child? Obtain a percentage for each language spoken to the child by each caregiver.
4. Did child receive any preschool educational services (i.e., Head Start or private center)?

Schooling factors

Entrance to bilingual education and/or ESL program considerations
5. What does the child's Home Language Survey indicate?
6. Did bilingual education/ESL program personnel give language proficiency measures to child? If no, why not?

Bilingual education program factors
7. What type of bilingual education and/or ESL program does the school offer?
8. In what grades is bilingual education/ESL provided in this school?

Bilingual education exit considerations
9. What basis or criteria were used to exit child from bilingual education/ESL program?
10. Do these criteria meet state guidelines on exiting students from bilingual education/ESL program?

Considerations to review when no bilingual education/ESL program provided
11. What is the impact of this student not having received bilingual education/ESL services on his/her language development and academic performance?
12. What alternatives and strategies has the school used to address the language needs of the student?

Teacher factors
13. If child is currently in general education classroom setting with no bilingual education/ESL program being provided, what professional training and experiences does the child's general education teacher have with second-language learners?
14. What is the child's current teacher's track record on referring students to the prereferral team? In other words, does this teacher rarely refer students or is this a teacher who refers a significant number of his/her students each year?

Evaluating student's performance

15. How has/did the student perform(ed) across subjects and grade levels in bilingual education/ESL program instructional settings? Review grades provided on report card by subject area across grade levels. Please note whether these grades on based on grade-level material.
16. If student is no longer in or has never been in bilingual education/ESL program, how has the student performed across subjects and grade levels in general education? Review grades provided on report card by subject area across grade levels.

Language considerations

17. Are each of the suspected particular areas of difficulties noted in both the child's native language and in English?
18. Has the child obtained a Cognitive Academic Language Proficiency (CALP) level in his or her native/first language and in English?

Family and cultural factors

If family immigrated to the United States
19. What is the family's native country?
20. Why did the family immigrate to the U.S.? If they did not, specify the order and when each family member came to U.S. and who, if any, remain in the native country.

For migrant families
21. For how many years has the family migrated within a state or across state lines to find employment?
22. Does the family migrate between two specific locations? If so, from where to where and how long is the family at each location?

All families from culturally and linguistically diverse backgrounds
23. Who lives in the student's home?
24. What is each parent's educational level?
25. What literacy skills does the parent have in his or her native language and in English?

Note. Adapted from Rhodes, Ochoa, and Ortiz (2005, Form 5.1). Copyright 2005 by The Guilford Press. Adapted by permission.

tests, or tests with norming populations not representative of the student's background if it is clearly not feasible to use evaluation measures in the student's two languages
3. English-speaking evaluation specialists assisted by a trained bilingual ancillary examiner using standardized evaluation measures
4. English-speaking evaluation specialists assisted by a trained interpreter and using modified evaluation measures, translated tests, or tests with norming populations not representative of the student's background
5. Evaluation specialists using only nonverbal or performance intelligence evaluation measures for languages other than English or Spanish

See Rhodes (2000, 2005) for a discussion of selection, training, and use of interpreters.

Step 3: Intervention Development and Implementation

During the intervention development and implementation stage, the information gathered during the first two steps is used to select an appropriate intervention strategy with demonstrated empirical validity. The intervention strategy is selected based on functional relevance to the problem, contextual fit, and likelihood of success. The key question during this stage is, What should be done about it?

As determined by Steps 1 and 2, the intervention selected should consider the student's educational history, language history, participation in bilingual and ESL programs, level of language proficiency, level of acculturation, and other individual factors. A culturally and linguistically appropriate intervention designed to meet particular needs of the student should take into account whether data indicate that the student is likely to benefit from this type of intervention. The selection of an intervention with empirical validity or one that is evidence based is a particular challenge. Ingraham and Oka (2006) state that very few evidence-based interventions are currently available for use with CLD students and that the generalizability and portability of models validated

on other populations is unknown. They make the following observations regarding the use of interventions currently available:

1. The effectiveness of interventions that have not included diverse populations (among the intervention recipients, interventionists, and researchers) yet is as unknown.
2. More intervention research with other, more diverse groups must be conducted with designs that provide data regarding the transferability, generalization, and cultural validity of the intervention.
3. It is expected that adjustments may be needed for the intervention to be meaningful and successful for different cultural groups and/or in different contexts. Whether or not this will affect the outcome of the intervention is an empirical question that requires the collection and evaluation of data.

A serendipitous outgrowth from the intervention development and implementation stage is the possibility of systemic change if it becomes evident that many CLD students need the same types of intervention in order to reach their desired level of performance. The continuous monitoring of data within the problem-solving model also allows the practitioner to evaluate the individual effectiveness of interventions and make appropriate adjustments as needed. The clear pattern that may develop from this type of data collection could be instrumental in moving effective interventions into the general curriculum.

Step 4: Intervention Evaluation and Follow-Up

During this final stage, objective evidence is obtained through ongoing data collection in order to determine intervention effectiveness. The problem should be resolved in order for the process to be completed. The key question during this step is, Did it work? Single-subject design methods are often used to evaluate the effectiveness of treatment for an individual student (see Chapter 29).

Although seemingly perfunctory in nature, this stage is critical to the effectiveness of this model for CLD students. The intervention evaluation process should be based on objective measures of performance regarding the target behavior. The effectiveness of the intervention should not be determined by the number of documented trials and recalibrations of the intervention process but instead by the product that is produced. In other words, did it work? If not, why not? If so, to what extent did it work? The focus on problem resolution versus data compilation is paramount. Objective evidence of student failure is easy to obtain, categorize, and store. We have done that in various forms or fashions for years. What we need to know is whether it worked, and, if not, we need to persistently seek out true resolutions that incorporate the cultural, linguistic, and experiential background of the student.

Multicultural School Consultation within the Problem-Solving Model

Implementing the four steps of the problem-solving model with CLD students requires that school psychologists be proficient in providing consultative services in a multicultural and oftentimes multilingual environment. The concluding sections of this chapter provide a framework for providing multicultural school consultation and an overview of recommended competencies.

Multicultural School Consultation Framework

Ingraham (2000) proposed a multicultural school consultation (MSC) framework for selecting the appropriate approach when working with CLD families. The MSC framework is a guide to culturally appropriate school-based practice and may be utilized by both internal and external consultants using a variety of models (e.g., behavioral, ecological, instructional, mental health). The MSC framework is made up of five components that are designed to help guide the consultant through the decision-making process: (1) domains of consultant learning and development, (2) domains of consultee learning and development, (3) cultural variations in the consultation constellation, (4) contextual and power influences, and (5) hypothesized methods for supporting consultee and client success. By following this guided approach to MSC, school-based consultants addressing the issue of bilingual education may be better able to (1)

guide the conceptualization of issues in the consultation process, (2) develop approaches for consulting within a cultural context, and (3) identify a variety of areas for future empirical investigation (Ingraham, 2000).

Competencies Necessary for Effective Consultation

Rogers (2000) identified six competencies necessary for effective consultation regarding culturally and linguistically diverse students. These cross-cultural competencies include:

- *Understanding one's own and others' culture.* The consultant needs

> (a) [to] examine his or her own cultural/ethnic/racial heritage and identity to be able to develop greater self-awareness of beliefs, prejudices, and assumptions; and (b) to learn about the cultural and sociopolitical background of the consultee and client to better understand and respect their perspectives, values, and histories of oppression. (Rogers, 2000, p. 416)

- *Developing cross-cultural communication and interpersonal skills.* The consultant must develop the communication and interpersonal skills necessary to appropriately communicate the various bilingual education program options, the potential advantages and disadvantages of participating, and the rationale for recommendations in a way that is culturally and cross-culturally sensitive.
- *Examining the cultural embeddedness of consultation.* Each step in the consultative process should be viewed through the framework of the cultural perspective of the consultee or client.
- *Using qualitative methodologies.* The consultant should possess the skills necessary to utilize single-subject design methodologies, naturalistic data-gathering techniques, and ethnographic and case-study approaches to measure the effectiveness of bilingual education program participation and the related consultative process.
- *Acquiring culture-specific knowledge.* The consultant should have cultural-specific knowledge relevant for the particular consultee or client related to issues such as acculturation, immigration, parent's role in education, expected role of teachers, and bilingual education services.

• *Understanding of and skill in working with interpreters.* This extremely important competency for school-based consultants is often underdeveloped among practitioners. The limited number of culturally and linguistically diverse school psychologists often necessitates extensive use of interpretation services. School psychologists serving in the role of consultant should review the skills and competencies recommended for school-based interpreters. Lopez (2000, 2002) provides an expanded discussion of this topic.

Conclusion

Implemented correctly, with the thoughtful application of decades of theory, research, and legislative guidance, the problem-solving model holds great promise in helping differentiate cultural and linguistic difference from disability. Implemented without sufficient regard for cultural and linguistic factors and their relation to discrepancies between what is occurring and what is expected, it also has the potential to serve as the latest of many models that never quite put the pieces together in an attempt to service this complex and growing population. The pieces are aligned and the model is possible: the results are up to us.

References

Artiles, A. J., & Trent, S. C. (2000). Representation of culturally/linguistically diverse students. In C. R. Reynolds & E. Fletcher-Jantzen (Eds.), *Encyclopedia of special education* (Vol. 1, 2nd ed., pp. 513–517). New York: Wiley.

Artiles, A. J., Trent, S. C., & Palmer, J. (2004). Culturally diverse students in special education: Legacies and prospects. In J. A. Banks & C. M. Banks (Eds.), *Handbook of research on multicultural education* (2nd ed., pp. 716–735). San Francisco: Jossey-Bass.

Bergan, J. R. (1970). *Behavioral consultation.* Columbus, OH: Merrill.

Bergan, J. R., & Kratochwill, T. R. (1990). *Behavioral consultation and therapy.* New York: Plenum.

Canter, A. (2005). *Problem solving and RTI: New roles for school psychologists.* Bethesda, MD: National Association of School Psychologists.

Collier, V. (1987). Age and rate of acquisition of second language for academic purposes. *TESOL Quarterly, 21,* 617–641.

Cummins, J. (1983). Bilingualism and special education: Program and pedagogical issues. *Learning Disability Quarterly, 6,* 373–386.

Cummins, J. (1984). *Bilingualism and special education: Issues in assessment and pedagogy.* San Diego, CA: College Hill.

Deno, S. L. (1989). Curriculum-based measurement and alternative special education services: A fundamental and direct relationship. In M. R. Shinn (Ed.), *Curriculum-based measurement: Assessing special children* (pp. 1–17). New York: Guilford Press.

Fuchs, D., Mock, D., Morgan, P. L., & Young, C. L. (2003). Responsiveness to intervention: Definitions, evidence, and implications for the learning disabilities construct. *Learning Disabilities Research and Practice, 18*(3), 157–171.

Fuchs, L. S., & Fuchs, D. (1997). Use of curriculum-based measurement in identifying students with disabilities. *Focus on Exceptional Children, 30*(3), 1–16.

Guajardo Alvarado, C. (2003). *Best practices in the special education evaluation of culturally and linguistically diverse students.* Retrieved May 22, 2003, from *www.updc.org/oldsite/pdf/best.pdf.*

Ingraham, C. L. (2000). Consultation through a multicultural lens: Multicultural and cross-cultural consultation in schools. *School Psychology Review, 29,* 320–343.

Ingraham, C. L., & Oka, E. R. (2006). Multicultural issues in evidence-based interventions. *Journal of Applied School Psychology, 22*(2), 127–149.

Kang, S. M. (2006). Measurement of acculturation, scale formats, and language competence. *Journal of Cross-Cultural Psychology, 37*(6), 669–693.

Kindler, A. L. (2002). *Survey of the states' limited English proficient students and available educational programs and services 1999–2000 summary report.* Washington, DC: National Clearinghouse for English Acquisition and Language Instruction Educational Programs.

Lopez, E. C. (2000). Conducting instructional consultation through interpreters. *School Psychology Review, 29,* 378–388.

Lopez, E. C. (2002). Best practices in working with school interpreters to deliver psychological services to children and families. In A. Thomas & J. Grimes (Eds.), *Best practices in school psychology* (4th ed., pp. 1419–1432). Bethesda, MD: National Association of School Psychologists.

Losen, D. J., & Orfield, G. (Eds.). (2002). *Racial inequity in special education*. Cambridge, MA: Harvard Education Press.

Merrell, K. W., Ervin, R. A., & Gimpel Peacock, G. A. (2006). *School psychology for the 21st century*. New York: Guilford Press.

National Clearinghouse for English Language Acquisition and Language Instruction Educational Programs. (2002). *United States' most commonly spoken languages*. Retrieved September 10, 2007, from *www.ncbe.gwu.edu/askncela/05toplangs.html*.

National Clearinghouse for English Language Acquisition and Language Instruction Educational Programs. (2006). *United States' rate of LEP growth*. Retrieved September 10, 2007, from *www.ncbe.gwu.edu/states/stateposter.pdf*.

Noell, G. H., Gilbertson, D. N., VanDerHeyden, A. M., & Witt, J. C. (2005). Eco-behavioral assessment and intervention for culturally diverse at-risk students. In C. L. Frisby & C. R. Reynolds (Eds.), *Comprehensive handbook of multicultural school psychology* (pp. 904–927). New York: Jossey-Bass.

Ochoa, S. H. (2005). Bilingual education and second-language acquisition: Implications for assessment and school-based practice. In R. L. Rhodes, S. H. Ochoa, & S. O. Ortiz (Eds.), *Assessing culturally and linguistically diverse students: A practical guide* (pp. 57–75). New York: Guilford Press.

Ochoa, S. H., & Rhodes, R. L. (2005). Assisting parents of bilingual students to achieve equity in public schools. *Journal of Educational and Psychological Consultation, 16*(1&2), 75–94.

Ortiz, A. A., & Polyzoi, E. (1986). *Characteristics of limited English proficient Hispanic students in programs for the learning disabled: Implications for policy, practice and research: Part 1. Report summary*. Austin, TX: University of Texas. (ERIC Document Reproduction Service No. ED 267 578)

Ortiz, S. O. (1997). *Implications of English only instruction: When do English learners catch up?* Unpublished manuscript, St. John's University.

Ortiz, S. O. (2005). Language proficiency assessment: The foundation for psychoeducational assessment of second language learners. In R. L. Rhodes, S. H. Ochoa, & S. O. Ortiz (Eds.), *Assessing culturally and linguistically diverse students: A practical guide* (pp. 137–152). New York: Guilford Press.

Ortiz, S. O., & Ochoa, S. H. (2005). Cognitive assessment of culturally and linguistically diverse individuals: An integrated approach. In R. L. Rhodes, S. H. Ochoa, & S. O. Ortiz (Eds.), *Assessing culturally and linguistically diverse students: A practical guide* (pp. 18–201). New York: Guilford Press.

Perez, B., Skiba, R. J., & Chung, C. (2008). Latino students and disproportionality in special education. *Education Policy Brief, 6*(2), 1–8.

Rhodes, R. L. (2000). Legal and professional issues in the use of interpreters: A fact sheet for school psychologists. *National Association of School Psychologists Communiqué, 29*(1), 28.

Rhodes, R. L. (2005). Assessment of academic achievement: Practical guidelines. In R. L. Rhodes, S. H. Ochoa, & S. O. Ortiz (Eds.), *Assessing culturally and linguistically diverse students: A practical guide* (pp. 202–214). New York: Guilford Press.

Rhodes, R. L., Ochoa, S. H., & Ortiz, S. O. (2005). *Assessing culturally and linguistically diverse students: A practical guide*. New York: Guilford Press.

Rogers, M. R. (2000). Examining the cultural context of consultation. *School Psychology Review, 29*, 414–418.

Roseberry-McKibbin, C. (2002). *Multicultural students with special language needs* (2nd ed.). Oceanside, CA: Academic Communication Associates.

Rueda, R., & Windmueller, M. P. (2006). English language learners, LD, and overrepresentation: A multiple-level analysis. *Journal of Learning Disabilities, 39*, 99–107.

Sanchez, M., & Brisk, M. (2004). Teacher's assessment practices and understandings in a bilingual program. *NABE Journal of Research and Practice, 2*(1), 193–208.

Shinn, M. R. (2002). Best practices in using curriculum-based measurement in a problem-solving model. In A. Thomas & J. Grimes (Eds.), *Best practices in school psychology* (4th ed., Vol. 1, pp. 671–697). Bethesda, MD: National Association of School Psychologists.

Texas Education Agency. (2005). *Home language surveys: Multiple languages*. Retrieved December 28, 2008, from *http://ritter.tea.state.tx.us/curriculum/biling/homelangsurveys.html*.

Tharp, R. G., & Wetzel, R. J. (1969). *Behavior modifications in the natural environment*. New York: Academic Press.

Thomas, W., & Collier, V. (1996). *Language minority student achievement and program effectiveness*. Fairfax, VA: George Mason University, Center for Bilingual/Multicultural/ESL Education.

Thomas, W. P., & Collier, V. (1997). *School effectiveness for language minority students*. Washington, DC: National Clearinghouse for Bilingual Education.

Thomas, W. P., & Collier, V. P. (2002). *A national study of school effectiveness for language minority students' long-term academic achievement.* Retrieved September 4, 2002, from *www.crede.uscu.edu/research/llaa1.html.*

U.S. Census Bureau. (2001). *Percent of persons who are foreign born: 2000.* Washington, DC: Author.

U.S. Department of Education. (2007). *Disproportionality and overidentification.* Washington, DC: U.S. Government Printing Office.

U.S. Office of Education. (1977). Definition and criteria for defining students as learning disabled. *Federal Register, 42:250,* p. 65083.

Washington, DC: U.S. Government Printing Office.

Wan, G. (2008). *The education of diverse student populations: A global perspective* (Vol. 2). New York: Springer.

Watson, S. M., Rinaldi, C., Navarrete, L., Bianco, M., & Samson, J. (2007). *Addressing the educational needs of culturally and linguistically diverse learners with and without LD.* Retrieved August 20, 2007, from *www.cldinternational.org/Infosheets/DiverseLearning.asp.*

Witt, J. C. (2002). *STEEP RTI—response to intervention.* Retrieved June 30, 2008, from *www.isteep.com/steep_rti.html.*

Chapter 34

Making Problem-Solving School Psychology Work in Schools

W. David Tilly III
Bradley C. Niebling
Alecia Rahn-Blakeslee

Making problem-solving school psychology work in the real world of schools takes tenacity, commitment, and skill. At Heartland Area Education Agency 11, an intermediate service agency in central Iowa, we have been implementing a problem-solving model of school psychology for nearly 20 years (e.g., Ikeda et al., 2007). There are many benefits that accrue to students as a result of implementing this model. There are also significant implementation challenges that must be overcome to make it a reality. Previous chapters in this book have provided extensive information related to the different pieces of the problem-solving process, including assessment, analysis, intervention, and evaluation. In this chapter, we review the critical components necessary to initiate and implement a problem-solving model of school psychology with a focus on the model as a whole. Observations in this chapter are experience-based, research-referenced, and practical.

There are many ways to characterize the components necessary to implement a problem-solving model of school psychology. In this chapter, we discuss five major components that work together to support implementation of problem-solving school psychology. First, we describe a problem-solving method, which includes knowledge and skills regarding (1) defining problems empirically and environmentally, (2) analyzing problems functionally, (4) prescribing interventions that are directly and empirically linked to the defined problem and problem analysis, (4) supporting intervention implementation with fidelity, (5) monitoring student progress, and (6) formatively and summatively analyzing intervention effectiveness. Second, we describe the necessity of adopting a problem-solving framework that structures and supports professional problem-solving routines in schools. Third, we discuss assumptions and "ways of thinking" that are critical to successful implementation of problem solving in schools. Fourth, we discuss the training and critical skills necessary for problem-solving implementation. Fifth, we discuss the fundamental alignment that needs to be created within a problem-solving system to ensure sustained implementation across time.

System Foundations for Problem-Solving School Psychology

Two major foundational elements underlie problem-solving implementation in schools.

The first is a *problem-solving method*. The second is a *problem-solving framework*. The problem-solving method ensures that a validated process is used to address problems and that implementing psychologists have a theoretical framework to use when framing both problems and solutions. The problem-solving framework creates structures in schools that promote and support the application of the problem-solving method. The two are interdependent, and both are necessary to implement problem-solving school psychology practice.

Problem-Solving Method

At a basic level, the problem-solving method is a field-based application of the scientific method. It requires observation to drive problem identification and hypothesis generation, which in turn leads to a test of the hypothesis and an evaluation of the hypothesis test. Each of these steps has a direct analogue in problem-solving practice, resulting in a four-step problem-solving method.

For practical purposes, each of the four steps of the problem-solving method typically is guided by the process of answering a question. Four interrelated questions make up the problem-solving method: What is the problem? Why is it happening? What should be done about it? and Did the strategy work? The problem-solving method is graphically depicted in Figure 34.1. A summary of the

actions taken to answer each of the problem-solving questions is presented next.

• *Question 1: What is the problem?* In problem-solving practice, observation drives problem identification, just as it does in the scientific method. Problems are defined environmentally so that they can be scaled and measured. Most frequently, problems are framed as the difference between what is expected of student performance and what occurs. The resulting discrepancy represents the magnitude of the problem. To define problems as discrepancies, school psychologists must be skilled at (1) writing operational definitions of target behaviors, (2) scaling these behaviors for measurement and creating behavioral measurement systems, (3) defining operationally reasonable expectations for behavioral occurrence, and (4) directly measuring occurrence and nonoccurrence of the behavior in settings in which the behavior is problematic and settings in which it is not (Upah, 2008). That problems are represented by discrepancies, not as the behavior of concern, is a concept that is important. For example, hitting is not a problem if it occurs at the expected zero rate. However, in a second example, if Javier is expected to get to his math class before the bell rings at least 95% of the time and he only makes it 25% of the time, there is 70% discrepancy, a significant problem in most high schools. There are important benefits to defining problems

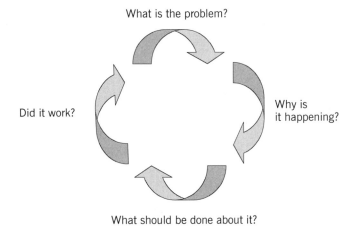

FIGURE 34.1. Problem-solving method.

as discrepancies. First, using discrepancies requires all involved parties to become objective about the nature of a problem. Problem-related variables are examined in ways that cause all parties involved to agree on "what the problem is," which significantly increases the probability that an effective solution might be found. Second, discrepancy-based definitions provide an objective context for understanding when the problem is improving. Third, discrepancy-based problem definitions allow direct scaling of problem magnitude. The greater the discrepancy between expectations and observed performance, the greater the problem. Fourth, discrepancy-based problem definitions most often are created based on naturally occurring units of behavior, which usually lend themselves directly to analysis and intervention (Tilly, 2008).

• *Question 2: Why is the problem occurring?* This second step is the analogue to hypothesis generation in the scientific method and is referred to as "problem analysis" in the problem-solving literature. The result from this second step of problem solving is a series of plausible hypotheses about factors contributing to the problem. This second step, perhaps the most complex, can be critical to solving student problems, as an accurate analysis will lead most directly to potentially effective interventions. To competently analyze problems in any domain, school psychologists must possess significant content-specific knowledge about that domain. They must work within a validated problem-analysis framework that is based on empirically validated practice. Problem analysis will require a series of assessments, and thinking is required on the part of the psychologist. That is, the test results themselves will not determine what to do. The analysis process itself is a structured thinking process, and tests are used only to assist in generating hypotheses about what might be effective at reducing the discrepancy (i.e., improving desired behaviors). A number of validated frameworks for problem analysis exist, including applied behavior analysis (ABA; Baer, Wolf & Risley, 1968; Sulzer-Azaroff & Mayer, 1991) and functional behavioral assessment (e.g., Tilly et al., 1998; Tilly, Knoster, & Ikeda, 2000; see also Jones & Wickstrom, Chapter 12, this volume) for

behavior and curriculum-based evaluation (Howell & Nolet, 2000; see also Marcotte & Hintze, Chapter 5, Burns & Klingbeil, Chapter 6, and Gansle & Noell, Chapter 7, this volume) for academics. No matter which framework is selected for problem analysis, they all share a series of characteristics, including: (1) Their assessments are direct and representative of student functioning in the real world, (2) their assessments are low inference in that they target skills rather than the traits or underlying characteristics that these skills or performances may represent, and (3) they yield plausible hypotheses regarding variables that maintain problem behavior that can be logically and empirically linked to validated interventions with a high likelihood for success. An extensive discussion of problem-analysis strategies is beyond the scope of this chapter, but excellent sources exist that provide greater detail and guidance (e.g., Shinn, Walker, & Stoner, 2002). In addition, a number of the earlier chapters in this volume provide extensive practical information on the assessment and analysis of individual and classwide academic problems, as well as emotional–behavioral problems (see Chapters 3–12).

• *Question 3: What should be done about the problem?* This step in problem solving is analogous to the process of hypothesis testing in the scientific method. In this case, the hypothesis that we are testing is whether the factors identified in our problem analysis are operational and whether manipulating them results in a reduction in the magnitude of the problem. More specifically, guided by the problem analysis, a series of planned modifications to the environment are made with the objective of changing performance in a prespecified way. If our problem analysis was accurate and if we selected interventions effectively, when these strategies are implemented, problem magnitude should be reduced. There are a series of components that should be attended to in intervention design. These are specified in Table 34.1 (Tilly, 2008). Every intervention will not have all of the components. However, all components should be considered when designing interventions for students. In Chapters 13–28 in this volume, various authors provide practical information on developing interventions for academic and emotional–

TABLE 34.1. Intervention Components

- *Antecedent interventions*: What changes can be made to the environment to prevent the problem from occurring?

- *Alternative skills instruction*: What skills can be taught to the individual that will reduce the occurrence of the problem?

- *Instructional consequent strategies*: What changes can be made to the instructional process to reinforce new skill acquisition and diminish problem occurrence?

- *Reduction-oriented consequent strategies*: What consequences, if any, need to be put in place to reduce the occurrence of the problem behavior?

- *Long-term prevention strategies*: What other individual or situational factors can we support to improve the individual's functioning?

- *Support for team members*: What support needs to be provided to team members to enable them to contribute to the intervention in an optimal way?

- *Antecedent interventions*: What changes can be made to the environment to prevent the problem from occurring?

Note. From Tilly, Knoster, et al. (1998). Reprinted with permission from the National Association of State Directors of Special Education.

behavioral problems that can be utilized within a problem-solving framework.

- *Question 4: Is what we are doing working?* This final step in the problem-solving process is analogous to the evaluation of hypothesis-testing data in the scientific method. Two types of data are examined. First, idiographic data on the individual's progress over time are compared to baseline performance to determine the progress that has been made. The second type of data are summative, expectation-referenced data that reflect the degree to which the problem has been lessened over time. Indeed, this step is similar to the process used during initial problem identification. The same units of behavior are used at this step, and the same or similar expectancy standards are used to index the magnitude of the problem after intervention. Daly, Barnett, Kupzyk, Hofstadter, and Barkley, Chapter 29, and Noell, Chapter 30 in this volume provide extensive details on issues related to the implementation and evaluation of interventions implemented in a problem-solving paradigm.

In nearly 20 years, we have learned a number of important lessons from implementing problem-solving practices. When we first implemented problem solving, we developed a 5-day, 357-step training program on how to implement the problem-solving method. We taught every single skill to criterion (e.g., behavioral definitions, scaling, behavioral measurement). It was an extremely rigorous process, and we expected our psychologists to implement these skills with fidelity for every case that they worked on. What we did not allow for was the various levels of intensity at which the problem-solving method needs to be applied to casework. What was lost by teaching the 357 microsteps was the general-case problem-solving method. Our staff learned specific skills and steps within a process. What we neglected to teach, in some cases, was the generalizeable thinking process that undergirds all problem-solving practice. In some cases, our staff understood the "what" of problem solving but did not understand the "why" of each step and the relative contribution to the overall model. Because of this situation, we modified our training significantly to teach both the practices and the thinking structures. We wrote a companion manual to our procedures manual, titled *Improving Children's Educational Results Through Data-Based Decision Making*, that illustrates and teaches the thinking process necessary when implementing the problem-solving method. This manual is available for download at *www. aea11.k12.ia.us/spedresources/modulefour. pdf*.

Problem-Solving Framework

A second major component necessary to implementing problem solving is a systems framework that supports, encourages, and reinforces problem-solving behaviors. In the early days of problem solving, systems structures were not available to support problem solving in schools. Instead, these skills were brought into the schools through implementation of consultation and problem-solving frameworks (e.g., Kratochwill & Bergan, 1990; Deno, 1985; Shinn, 1989). In short, these were individual implementations of the problem-solving method that were brought directly to the schoolhouse door. The expertise to run these frameworks was brought by highly skilled, specially trained practitioners who would lead implementation of problem solving one case at a time.

In the late 1980s and early 1990s, an initial problem-solving framework was created by Heartland to support individual problem solving for students. This model was based on working with single cases at a time and provided a context for implementing problem-solving practices in schools. This model is depicted in Figure 34.2. In the Heartland problem-solving approach, there were four interconnected iterations of the problem-solving method, with increasing levels of intensity represented in a Cartesian plane. The abscissa represents the varying intensities of problems that might occur in schools. The ordinate represents the appropriate amount of resources that might be applied to school-based problems in order to resolve them.

The Heartland problem-solving approach was unlike many other approaches. It was not considered a gated process, and explicit rules were not developed for students to move from one stage to the next. Instead, the problem-solving logic was applied to individual cases based on collaborative decision making. Decisions about moving levels included issues of discrepancy of student performance from local expectations on instructionally relevant curriculum-based assessments, student growth rates, and instructional need. In this way, locally specific resources could be applied to the intensity of student needs based on what was happening in the student's educational environment, as opposed to creating rigid, arbitrary decision-making criteria that had little instructional relevance to the student's day-to-day experiences in his or her school. A student's location within the method, as is further de-

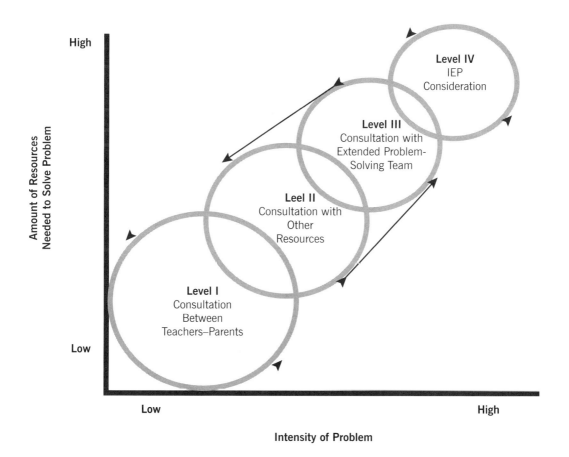

FIGURE 34.2. Heartland's initial problem-solving framework.

tailed subsequently, depends on a multitude of factors. Finally, there was no requirement that a student "start" in the first stage, then move to the second stage if the problem was not resolved, and so on. Instead, the intent of the approach was for those working with the student to examine the intensity of student needs and to match service delivery to the nature and intensity of those needs.

The first stage of implementation of the problem-solving method was consultation between parents and classroom teachers. Teachers and parents generally used the problem-solving logic, but their problem identification, problem analysis, intervention selection, and progress monitoring were informal and perception-based. If these initial attempts at problem resolution did not work, the second stage in problem solving was referral to the general-education building assistance team (BAT). These teams were composed of classroom teachers and based on the idea that the intensity of the problem behaviors would be best addressed by a collective body of experienced teachers supporting the student's classroom teacher. The BATs were trained to use the problem-solving method in their thinking, and, in most cases, the steps followed in implementing the problem-solving method were informal. If these more intensive efforts to remediate the student's problems were not successful, then a related services person, such as an educational consultant, a school social worker, or a school psychologist, would get involved in the case. These persons would review all of the work done to date and would set out to implement the problem-solving method with greater rigor. Formal consultation with teachers begins at this stage. The psychologist (or other related-service person) helps define the problem operationally, a formal problem analysis is conducted, a research-validated intervention is selected and implemented in the classroom, and formal progress monitoring occurs. It should be noted at this point that each of these three implementations of the problem-solving method is occurring in general education. There is no presumption that the problems being worked on represent a disability, and therefore no referral for special education is warranted.

The intervention implemented during the third stage of problem solving is evaluated after a reasonable implementation period. Data are used to compare the student's progress with baseline levels of performance, as well as environmental expectations. If the intervention appears to be working and the student is making adequate progress, the intervention can be continued. Alternatively, modifications to the intervention plan can be made and another phase of intervention can be implemented. Or it may be determined that additional resources beyond those available in general education are needed. In these situations, it is possible that problem solving may move to a fourth stage in which problem solving is still the focus but in which one of the questions that may be answered is whether the student in question has a disability and needs specially designed instruction to receive a free appropriate public education (i.e., whether the student qualifies for special education). The foregoing description provides an extremely limited treatment of a very detailed process. For greater depth of coverage, the reader can access the modules of Heartland AEA's Special Education Manual at *www.aea11.k12.ia.us/spedresources*.

Problem solving, when implemented through Heartland's original four-stage model, can be very effective for individual cases. However, implementation of problem solving within this framework has inherent limitations. First, case-by-case problem solving is not particularly efficient. Casework is done on an individual basis and interventions are prescribed for individual students, although quite often there are a number of students in a class with similar needs. We learned that, in most cases, even the best general education teachers could not implement more than one or two individual interventions well and continue to teach their entire classes of students. In these cases, group-level interventions might often be most appropriate from both efficiency and effectiveness standpoints. Second, case-by-case problem solving is reactive. It waits for academic or behavioral problems to occur in schools and then responds to them. As such, this approach is not positioned to be proactive and preventative in orientation. Finally, case-by-case problem solving, because of its reactive orientation, was often viewed by teachers as the new way to "get students into special education," which was never the purpose of the problem-solving framework.

Fortunately, new frameworks to support problem-solving practice in schools have become available in recent years.

Systems Framework

Given these emerging limitations of case-by-case problem solving, we began looking for ways to work more efficiently on problems with groups of students as opposed to the one-on-one for every case. For less intense problems, we began asking teachers to identify small groups as opposed to individual students experiencing difficulties. At the time this transformation was occurring, the Elementary and Secondary Education Act was reauthorized in 2002 as the No Child Left Behind Act, and many states and districts began working with the Reading First program that was a part of the federal law. The three Reading First technical assistance

centers (Oregon, Texas, and Florida) all had significant experience working with low-achieving readers and all began supporting a new framework, a three-tiered model, to use within schools.

The three-tiered model allows schools to arrange resources in a logical and rational way with regard to student need (Texas Education Agency, 2003). This model is depicted in Figure 34.3. The idea is that schools have limited resources and must deploy them in a way that provides the maximum benefit to the greatest numbers of students. Practice within a three-tiered model allows staff to dispense resources in direct relation to student need. The model makes the assumption that every child will become proficient in basic skills; however, what needs to vary is the amount of resources and intensity of instruction that will be required to get them there. The three tiers within the model re-

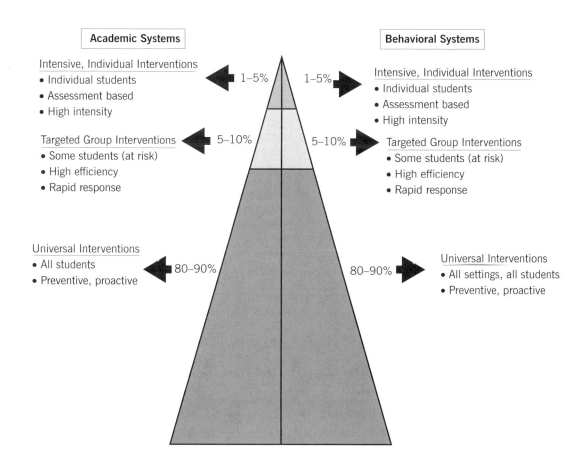

FIGURE 34.3. The three-tiered service-delivery model.

flect different levels of resource intensity for the full range of student needs, from students who require core instruction only to become proficient to students who need core plus supplemental instruction to a small number of students who will require intensive instruction to become proficient.

The three-tiered model follows similar logic to the four-tiered problem-solving model originally used at Heartland. Resources are deployed in direct relation to need, but it has a number of "engineering improvements" that make it attractive. First, it is a model that encompasses all children in a system, not only those experiencing problems. As such, problems can be identified much earlier and more objectively than in a teacher-referral-based system. Second, in this model the possibility exists that systems problems caused by poor or mismatched core curricula can be addressed, and many of the problems that would have historically found their way to individual problem solving can be resolved. Third, because the model is intended to be a general education model, it is less likely that classroom teachers will see it as the "new method" to get students into special education. Fourth, similar to Heartland's original problem-solving approach, although guidelines are given about student performance and intensity of needs across the different levels—or in this case tiers—of the model, no universally applied criteria are set for students' movement across tiers. Instead, the guidelines are used to help schools better understand how to allocate existing resources or in some cases make changes to existing practices to more accurately and efficiently match instruction and supports to student needs.

Assumptions/Beliefs of the Successful Problem Solver

As previously mentioned, the purpose of a problem-solving model is to find the educational strategy or intervention that will best meet the needs of the student. This service delivery model rests on several fundamental assumptions or beliefs related to assessment, intervention development and implementation, and evaluation at the individual student level and the systems level. Understanding and adopting these assumptions and beliefs

is critical in applying the thinking processes required to implement problem solving effectively in practice.

Our experience training many school psychologists to implement problem solving has taught us that it is necessary but not sufficient to teach specific problem-solving practices. School psychologists must also adopt a compatible set of assumptions about school psychology and educational practice (i.e., the purpose for engaging in problem-solving practices). Otherwise, the methods deployed will not be effective. Thus an initial step in teaching problem-solving practice is to teach the assumptions and beliefs underlying problem-solving implementation.

• *Assumption 1: The scientific method guides decision making.* As mentioned in a previous section, school psychologists committed to applying problem solving adopt the scientific method as a decision-making framework. Problem solving is an applied version of the scientific method; it is a set of practices or actions with a consistent logic set (Deno, 2002). Heartland's problem-solving process was adapted from several different models of problem solving, each with its own unique features, procedures, and vernacular (e.g., Barlow, Hayes, & Nelson, 1984; Bergan & Kratochwill, 1990; Bransford & Stein, 1984; Shinn, 1989). Despite the differences in the models, the four problem-solving questions identified earlier in this chapter guide thinking in each of these models. In general, the actions needed to answer each question include (1) observing and measuring the problem in the natural environment, (2) analyzing the problem etiology by creating and testing hypotheses, (3) using the problem-analysis results to design an intervention with a high probability of success, and (4) monitoring student progress to judge instructional/intervention effectiveness and provide feedback on whether the problem is resolved or must be reanalyzed or whether the intervention must be altered. The specific skills needed to successfully apply the thinking are detailed later.

• *Assumption 2: Direct, functional assessments provide the best information for decision making.* A second assumption is that assessments are conducted within a problem-solving system to provide the data necessary to make professional decisions about what interventions and resources will assist students. In other words, assessments are *functional* in that they are intended to answer questions about the reasons that a behavior of concern occurs and ultimately what might be done to improve it. Assessment materials are *direct* in that they are taken from the student's curriculum and require production-type responses (e.g., reading aloud, writing sentences), as opposed to selection-type responses (e.g., point to the … , circle the …). The focus of assessment should be on those environmental variables that can be measured and altered and that inform what to teach (curriculum) and how to teach (instruction). Low-level inferences predominate throughout the assessment process. That is, inferences are made about student skills rather than the abilities that these skills may be reflective of. Inferences are made about performances and behaviors rather than underlying traits. Assessment materials and processes are selected from materials and skills that the student is expected to perform in the classroom, as these are the most ecologically valid and educationally relevant to that student's schooling. The general rule is: Do not use a high-inference measure if a low-inference measure is available. At a basic level, the lower the level of inference, the higher the probability that assessment results will yield information that will be related to potentially effective interventions.

Functional assessment has several important characteristics. First, functional assessment is not a global screening or comprehensive battery; it is relevant to the identified problem. That is, assessments have high instructional utility and directly measure areas of concern, as opposed to broad constructs. Second, functional assessment is direct and repeatable; it uses material directly from the curriculum, which establishes a clear connection between the data gathered and the question being answered, as well as allowing frequent progress monitoring for making instructional changes or for judging overall evaluation of effectiveness. Third, functional assessment is multidimensional, allowing multiple sources of information (instruction, curriculum, environment, learner characteristics; ICEL) to be collected through multiple methodologies (records review, interview, observation, tests; RIOT). Fourth, function-

al assessment data are used to develop high-probability intervention activities (i.e., those likely to succeed) matched to individual student needs, not to characteristics or disabilities. Finally, because functional assessments are drawn from actual curricula and directly related to an identified problem, they match well with local expectations and thus are highly reliable and valid. See Chapter 2 of Module 4 in Heartland's decision-making manual for a discussion of functional assessment and Chapter 5 of Module 4 for a discussion of problem analysis (*www.aea11.k12.ia.us/spedresources/modulefour.pdf*).

• *Assumption 3: Learning is an interaction between curriculum, instruction, and the environment.* A third assumption is that learning is an interaction between curriculum, instruction, the environment, and the learner (Howell & Nolet, 2000). Each year, a significant number of students fail to profit from general education classroom instruction (Ysseldyke, Algozzine, & Thurlow, 2000). Although many presumed causes of failure exist (e.g., a student comes from a poor home situation, a student has ADHD, a student is lazy), a problem-solving system assumes that problems are situational, not within child (Deno, 1989). Problems are defined as a discrepancy or mismatch between what is expected and what occurs (Shinn, 1989). For example, a student who turns in only 50% of his homework on time when he is expected to turn in 90% of his homework would be viewed as having a problem by most teachers and parents. Because problems are defined situationally, the focus for ameliorating problems is on those variables that can be controlled and altered by the teacher (e.g., pacing of instruction, number of opportunities to respond, provision of corrective feedback, depth and breadth of content coverage). Problem analysis is a thinking process that integrates information from multiple sources to specify and test hypotheses regarding specific etiology of the observed problem and is an important action in identifying those variables that must be changed.

It is important to note at this juncture that framing problems situationally in no way implies that problem-solving school psychologists are blind to individual differences. To the contrary, individual differences are examined throughout the assessment and intervention process. However, these individual differences are not labeled with overly broad monikers, and the labels are not used to explain away the performance or skill problem. More important, there is no attempt to use these labels to prescribe general-level interventions that do not have observable relationships to results that are likely to be effective.

• *Assumption 4: All students can learn.* To work effectively with all students, school psychologists must assume that all students are capable of learning new skills and behaviors. As described previously, assessment data are collected not to diagnose disabilities but, rather, to diagnose the conditions under which the student's learning is *enabled* (Jeff Grimes, October 20, 1998, personal communication). We assume that the amount students can learn is limited only by how much students can learn. In other words, we cannot know how much an individual student may or may not be able to learn until we attempt to teach that student and monitor that student's response.

• *Assumption 5: Effective interventions are matched to unique student needs.* Once the behavior has been properly identified and appropriate functional assessment data have been collected, results can be used to match instruction to the student's specific needs. The importance of a correct match cannot be overstated, for "even the best intervention strategy is doomed if it is applied to an improperly defined target behavior" (Reynolds, Gutkin, Elliott, & Witt, 1984, p. 186).

A basic premise in all problem-solving implementations is that science-based practice will be implemented to the extent available. The increasing focus on evidence-based practice and using research-based programs and strategies has been strongly influenced by school psychologists (Ysseldyke et al., 2006). A variety of processes have been developed and used, such as those by The School Psychology Task Force on Evidence-Based Practice and What Works Clearinghouse, to determine the extent to which programs and strategies are evidence-based. Although the processes and criteria differ from group to group, all of these processes require researchers to employ the scientific method to examine the efficacy and/or effectiveness of a program or strategy. In Chapter 13 in this volume, Stoiber and DeSmet pro-

vide an overview of evidence-based practices in the selection of interventions.

Selecting an intervention that is based on the specific needs of the student is critical. In recent years, the emphasis on evidence-based strategies, materials, and programs has allowed school psychologists to become increasingly instrumental in the role of designing and implementing interventions. Recent meta-analyses have summarized intervention research and identified effective instructional practices (e.g., Swanson, 1999; Swanson & Hoskyn, 1998). Examples of evidence-based assessment and teaching practices that have demonstrated effectiveness include (1) curriculum-based measurement (CBM; Deno, 1985; Shinn, 1989), (2) Dynamic Indicators of Basic Early Literacy Skills (DIBELs; Good & Kaminski, 1996; Good, Gruba, & Kaminski, 2002), (3) curriculum-based evaluation (Howell & Nolet, 2000), (4) functional assessment and positive behavioral supports (Horner, Sugai, Todd, & Lewis-Palmer, 2005; Iwata, Dorsey, Slifer, Bauman, & Richman, 1982; O'Neill, Horner, Albin, Storey, & Sprague, 1997), (5) Direct Instruction (Engelmann & Carnine, 1982), (6) explicit instruction (Brophy & Good, 1986; Berliner, 1987), (7) peer-assisted learning strategies (Fuchs & Fuchs, 1998), and (8) strategy instruction (Schumaker, Deshler, & McKnight, 2002). Moreover, resources from which school psychologists can learn about evidence-based intervention strategies are more readily available (e.g., Shinn et al., 2002).

Although teaching and learning are functionally related (i.e., if students receive instruction that is matched to their needs, then learning will occur), the effectiveness of any intervention for any student cannot be determined prior to implementing that intervention. Indeed, no single approach is effective with all students (Reschly & Ysseldyke, 1995). Thus, whenever interventions are implemented, student performance must be monitored directly and objectively and adjustments made to interventions based on student performance gains.

Problem-Solving Skills

Although a core set of specific beliefs is necessary for successful problem solving, it is not alone sufficient. A wide range of knowledge and skills is necessary as well. These skills can be organized around the four problem-solving questions identified earlier and further subdivided into problem-solving steps. Thus a step-by-step process is created that can be explicitly taught to implementers. These skills can be acquired during preservice training, or they can be learned on the job, as is the case when new staff members begin employment at Heartland. However, effective problem solving cannot be accomplished without at least basic skills in each of the skill areas identified in Table 34.2. The steps identified in this table are the minimum steps necessary to implement problem solving in practice.

These skills, rooted in the foundations of the data-based program modification model (e.g., Deno & Mirkin, 1977) and the behavioral consultation model (e.g., Bergan, 1977), have applications in a variety of settings and situations, including supporting an individual student with reading difficulties and helping a school institute a schoolwide RTI decision-making system. Supporting staff in successfully learning and using problem-solving skills requires (1) training in both tool skills and the thinking process, (2) collecting and using data about staff skills, and (3) a system of ongoing support for implementation.

Train Tool Skills and the Thinking Process

Successful problem solving, as was previously mentioned, starts with accurately defining the problem. Without an accurate problem definition, all subsequent data collection and decisions will be targeted at the wrong problem. However, successfully engaging in problem solving requires accurate implementation of *all* the skills and thinking processes. For example, even if a student's reading difficulties are accurately defined as a skill deficit in the area of oral reading fluency, an inaccurate problem analysis that does not reveal whether that deficit is due to a lack of instruction may lead to the decision to place that student in an unnecessarily intense intervention when additional practice is all that is needed.

Ensuring that staff can successfully implement all steps of problem solving starts with training in the basic skills and thinking pro-

cess. An important component of training includes how to use problem-solving tools (e.g., problem-analysis forms, intervention plans). Increased tool skills have been demonstrated to lead to improved implementation of problem-solving steps (Flugum & Reschly, 1994). Although tool skills can improve the fidelity of implementing the problem-solving steps, it is less clear whether or not tool skills directly translate into a greater understanding and application of problem solving as a thinking process. Although problem solving can be described and applied in a relatively linear manner, different decisions can be made throughout the process. It is therefore important that, as implementation of problem solving is trained and monitored, the results of problem solving are discussed as well.

A key feature in Heartland's training of problem solving is that there is no specific problem-solving training per se. Instead, problem solving is integrated into the training of other skills required for a successful school psychologist. For example, problem solving is included in the training that all school psychologists new to Heartland receive in curriculum-based evaluation (CBE) and individualized education plans (IEPs). Other training opportunities available to staff that include problem-solving skills include learning to use DIBELS and to implement schoolwide positive behavior supports (PBS).

Collect and Use Data on Staff Skills

Similar to collecting data on student learning, it is critical to collect data on staff's acquisition and application of problem-solving skills. The goal is for staff members to be able to independently implement the entirety of the problem-solving process with a high level of fidelity and skill. The National Association of School Psychologists' (NASP) latest version of the Blueprint for Training and Practice (Ysseldyke et al., 2006) provides one helpful framework for understanding problem-solving skill levels. Heartland has developed a specific continuum of skill levels for each of the components outlined in Table 34.2. These skills, known as innovation configurations, operationalize specific problem-solving behaviors along a consistent 3-point continuum: (1) fully acceptable

TABLE 34.2. Problem-Solving Skills

Problem-solving question	Problem-solving step	Rationale for step	Skills
What is the problem?	Screening	• Screening allows the assessment process to be efficient. Not all concerns brought to the table turn out to be significant problems. The screening process allows us to collect a sample of problem-identification data in a quick, inexpensive way to determine whether additional assessment is warranted.	• Identify and select the appropriate domain(s) to assess. • Determine criteria for acceptable performance and select instrument or approach for data collection. • Implement screening activities. • Examine data for discrepancy. • Communicate results and define future actions.

	Problem identification	• Problem identification defines the problem environmentally as the difference between what is expected and what is occurring.	• Identify educationally relevant and alterable behavior(s) from the screening data.
			• Develop a clear, objective, and complete behavioral definition.
			• Collect baseline data that measures identified behavior.
			  • Establish the relevant behavioral dimension (e.g., frequency, accuracy, duration).
			  • Develop a feasible measurement strategy (e.g., who, how, what).
			• Validate the problem by selecting a standard of comparison and determining whether a discrepancy exists.
			• Determine whether the magnitude of the discrepancy (if one exists) is large enough to warrant intervention.

Why is the problem occurring?	Problem analysis	• Problem analysis helps the intervener in creating a plausible hypothesis linking observed behavior with the factor most likely related to the behavior's occurrence (or nonoccurrence). Based on this hypothesis, an intervention can be selected targeting those variables thought to be most related to the problem. The most critical dimension of the problem analysis step is to *match* the intervention with operational variables in the observed situation.	• Gather relevant information in the domains of instruction, curriculum, environment, and learner (ICEL) using multiple sources, such as reviews, interviews, observations, and tests (RIOT). • Develop assumed causes by generating hypotheses and predictions. • Validate hypotheses by collecting additional information, if necessary. • Use problem analysis results to identify a specific instructional target.

(cont.)

TABLE 34.2. *(cont.)*

Problem-solving question	Problem-solving step	Rationale for step	Skills
What should be done about the problem?	Intervention design	• A multicomponent intervention is created that takes into account multiple factors that may contribute to problem occurrence. Possible intervention components may include antecedent interventions, alternate skills instruction, instructional consequent strategies, reduction-oriented consequent strategies, long-term prevention strategies, and support for intervention implementers.	• Set an observable, measurable goal for desired performance level. • Develop a step-by-step intervention plan specifying the roles and procedures necessary to resolve the problem (i.e., who, what, when, where, how, how often). • Develop a plan for collecting treatment integrity data. • Develop a measurement strategy similar or identical to the strategy used to collect baseline data during problem identification. • Develop a decision-making plan for summarizing and evaluating progress toward the goal (e.g., frequency of data collection, rules for interpreting and making decisions about the data).
	Implementation	• The primary reason that most educational interventions fail is that they are not implemented, or are not implemented as planned. As such, it is important to monitor implementation of intervention strategies and ensure that they are in fact being provided as planned.	• Implement intervention according to intervention plan. • Collect progress monitoring data using measurement strategy. • Collect treatment integrity data according to plan.

Is what we are doing working?	Evaluation	• We cannot predict, with our current level of science and knowledge, whether an intervention will work for an individual prior to trying it. Hence, we must implement, measure, monitor and adjust our interventions based on progress monitoring data. These data tell us whether our interventions are working and whether we should keep or modify our interventions.	• Examine formative assessment data and use the decision-making rule to determine whether the intervention is working (i.e., formative evaluation).
			• Examine treatment integrity data to determine whether the intervention was implemented as planned.
			  • Use multiple sources of data to determine the outcome of the intervention (i.e., summative evaluation).
			  • The problem was resolved, and conditions that enable learning were identified.
			  • The problem was resolved, but the intervention cannot continue because resources cannot be sustained under current conditions.
			  • The problem was not resolved.

practice, (2) partially acceptable practice, and (3) unacceptable practice.

Data collected using innovation configurations such as these (e.g., see Figure 34.4) provides both staff and supervisors with information on staff skills. These data can be used to differentiate training and support for staff as they continue to improve their problem-solving skills. At Heartland, this is done primarily using a case review method. Specifically, staff present a case they worked on to peers and supervisors. Staff members rate their own work, as do supervisors. This provides an opportunity to have data-based, reflective dialogue not only on case results but also on the application of problem-solving skills and thinking. These data can then be used to provide staff with training and supports targeted at specific areas of need.

System of Support for Implementation

Training in problem-solving skills, as was previously mentioned, is not alone sufficient to ensure successful implementation. Heartland provides a variety of supports (e.g., mentoring, discipline meetings, a program assistant, psychologists in leadership positions) for staff in addition to training to ensure successful problem solving. At any given time, all psychologists at Heartland can quickly and easily access multiple forms of support.

For example, new psychologists are all paired with an experienced Heartland psychologist as part of the mentoring program. Mentors provide a wide variety of supports, including answering questions, modeling appropriate practices, reviewing work, and observing practice and providing coaching feedback. With this approach, psychologists new to Heartland can obtain differentiated support based on their needs. Support opportunities for all school psychologists at Heartland also occur at quarterly discipline meetings. These meetings provide an opportunity for psychologists to consult with each other on a wide range of job-related matters, including problem solving. Expert-level school psychologists also hold other positions at Heartland in areas such as leadership, assessment, research, curriculum, instruction, and training. Practicing school psychologists have access to these experts at intern meetings, at discipline meetings, and through committees and mentorship, and the experts can be contacted directly at any time for questions.

Opportunities such as these provide all school psychologists with job-embedded, naturally occurring support to improve their problem-solving skills. The combination of training and ongoing support has increased the problem-solving capacity of Heartland's school psychologists. It is also important to consider problem-solving supports within the larger structure of a system's functioning. For example, it is important to understand the connections between training needs and the staff evaluation system. To ensure that successful problem solving occurs, it is necessary to align all system components and structures so that problem solv-

Step or Element	Fully Acceptable Practice	Partially Acceptable Practice	Unacceptable Practice
Step 1. Implement measurement strategy	The measurement strategy develops as part of the intervention plan used. Assessment materials are organized, persons responsible designated, and time for data collection is arranged.	A different measurement strategy from than the one developed as part of the intervention plan is used. Materials, time, and personnel are all organized and available.	A measurement strategy is not implemented. Formative assessment data is haphazardly collected with no organization of material, time, or personnel.

FIGURE 34.4. Example innovation configuration.

ing is not only expected but also facilitated and reinforced.

Align the System to Ensure Consistent Application of Contingencies to Professional Behavior

The final critical component of implementing problem-solving school psychology is to align major elements of the system to reinforce the desired professional behaviors and to ensure long-term viability of the system. This component takes the longest to accomplish, usually a period of several years, but, when complete, it ensures that problem solving becomes business as usual rather than something new and different. Alignment in this case refers to the process of making the element explicit, usually in writing, and of ensuring that there is conceptual and operational consistency between each of the elements. The critical systems elements that must be aligned to support problem-solving practice are listed in the next section, with a brief description of each and a reference to completed documents from Iowa that illustrate the component.

Identify Principles of Effectiveness and Values

It is best to predicate practices on principles of effectiveness rather than on specific technologies or practices. In problem-solving systems, these principles both take into account the foundational values we hold about serving children and families and incorporate findings from the research literature. So, for example, a principle of effectiveness might be to "monitor progress frequently and make instructional changes as data warrant" instead of "to adopt curriculum-based measurement (CBM)." At the current time, CBM is one of the most effective progress monitoring technologies available, and Heartland schools use it extensively. However, our practices are based on the principle of progress monitoring, rather than the technology. This type of focus allows practices to improve over time as our knowledge base evolves. That is, although we use CBM extensively in our system, if better technologies become available to monitor student performance over time, we will adopt them, consistent with our basic

principles. The foundational principles that were used in Iowa during our major shift to problem-solving practices can be found at *www.aea11.k12.ia.us/spr/RSDSNeedsPrinciples.pdf.*

Align Professional Practices with Principles of Effectiveness

Once the principles of effectiveness are written, the next piece to align is specific practices. As systems transition from historical to problem-solving systems, the new assumptions and principles require new behaviors on the part of nearly everyone in schools, including school psychologists. Conversations must be held about which behaviors and professional practices are aligned with the system's principles of effectiveness. These are difficult discussions because, although past practices were based on the best available information and technologies, they cause us to look critically at those practices that we have implemented for many years. The difference is that we know more now, we have better research, and improved technologies are available to help us in professional practice. It would be a problem not to take advantage of what we have learned about instructional interventions since we started problem solving. An example of a clear definition of problem-solving practice was created by the Iowa AEA Directors of Special Education in 1994. This document, titled "Professional Practices in Problem Solving," can be accessed at *www.aea11.k12.ia.us/spr/ProfPracticesInProbSolving.pdf.*

Align Procedures Manuals with Expected Behaviors and Principles

Once professional practices have been defined, it is important that these practices find their way into policy and procedures at the agency level. This level of codification serves a number of purposes. It clarifies expectations and defines specifically what behaviors are expected of professionals within the agency. Procedures manuals also serve as one standard against which professional practice will be held, if ever challenged. Heartland has written an extensive procedures manual that supports comprehensive problem-solving practices. The modules can be accessed under "Special Education Manual" at *www.aea11.k12.ia.us/spedresources*.

Align Professional Development and Skills Coaching with Procedures Manual

When first implementing professional practices in problem solving, literally every professional in the system will need to develop new skills and competencies. The professional development to assist in this skill development must align closely with the procedures, practices, and principles that have been developed. It must be skill-focused, performance-based, and criterion-referenced. That is, it must incorporate a clear scope and sequence, it must allow for much practice in the new skills, there must be opportunities for coaching and feedback, and there must be a criterion of performance that all staff is trained to. One effective way to set this standard of performance is to create practice profiles (Hall & Hord, 2001) that identify different ways that specific skills might be implemented. Each of these different implementations represents a different level of proficiency along the road to competency. The "Professional Practices in Problem Solving" document identified earlier is written substantially as a set of practice profiles. The advantages of aligning your professional development with practice profiles are many. Primarily, however, practice profiles communicate to professionals that the skill development associated with problem solving exists on a continuum and that there is an expectation that skill development will occur over time. They communicate specific behaviors that are needed, and they give professionals a way to benchmark their progress across time as their skills grow.

Align Job Descriptions with Expected Behaviors

Once your system has committed to implementing a problem-solving model of service delivery, it is important to realign job descriptions and the hiring process with expected competencies for the new role. As more systems move toward implementation of problem-solving practices, it will become increasingly possible to hire school psychologists with proficiency in problem-solving practice. The questions on your job interviews should reflect the competencies from the job description, and the rating criteria for candidate's answers should reflect variation in knowledge and skills related to these competencies. Heartland's school psychologist job description can be reviewed at *www.aea11.k12.ia.us/employment/schoolpsychologist.html*.

Align Reinforcement Systems with Expected Behaviors

It is no secret that systems contingencies govern much professional behavior. As psychologists are learning new knowledge and skills, leaders must align contingencies in the system to reinforce the right behaviors. Many school psychologist behaviors are governed by contingencies associated with procedural compliance with federal and state laws (e.g., evaluation time lines, providing parents appropriate notices, holding meetings with the right participants). Some of these cannot be avoided. However, these are not the behaviors most related to improving student functioning. When transitioning to a problem-solving system, contingencies must be arranged to reinforce improved professional behaviors as well. For example, paying attention to the number of student graphs a staff member is involved with that demonstrate significant progress would be preferable to examining how many "assessments" a school psychologist completed in a given time period. Or asking staff to present to their colleagues some of the new practices they are implementing is preferable to having someone from one of the big testing companies come in and talk about the "new version" of a widely used, nationally normed test. The general rule is to align reinforcement opportunities with the behaviors that are expected in the new system and to ensure that the reinforcers are delivered contingent on the desired professional behavior.

Align Professional Staff Evaluation Process with Expected Behaviors

A final component to put in place that supports and fosters problem-solving practice in schools is an evaluation process that is predicated on and consistent with successful implementation of problem-solving processes in practice. Although this is an important component of overall systems alignment, it is probably the last component that should be put in place. Professionals need to have time to learn, implement, and experience problem-solving practice prior to being held accountable to those practices. As such, problem-solving training and coaching need to be in place for several years before aligning the evaluation system to allow professionals adequate time to grow and develop.

Summary

Implementing problem-solving school psychology in practice is a challenging and rewarding endeavor. It takes time, it takes tenacity, and it takes perseverance. The path to full implementation is not a straight one. Moreover, tremendous forces strive to maintain the "status quo." We all learned about the concept of "regression to the mean" in our introductory measurement classes, and the system has a tendency to want to regress to the mean whenever we work on changing it. Systems, however, can change in lasting ways. And moving our system toward problem-solving, science-based practice also holds tremendous benefits for the students and families that we serve. Isn't that why most of us became school psychologists in the first place?

References

Baer, D., Wolf, M., & Risley, R. (1968). Some current dimensions of applied behavior analysis. *Journal of Applied Behavior Analysis*, 1, 91–97.

Barlow, D. H., Hayes, S. C., & Nelson, R. O. (1984) *The scientist practitioner: Research and accountability in clinical and educational settings.* New York: Pergamon Press.

Bergan, J. R. (1977). *Behavioral consultation.* Columbus, OH: Merrill.

Bergan, J. R., & Kratochwill, T. R. (1990). *Behavioral consultation and therapy.* New York: Plenum Press.

Berliner, D. C. (1987). Simple views of effective teaching and a simple theory of classroom instruction. In D. C. Berliner & B. V. Rosenshine (Eds.), *Talks to teachers: A festschrift for N. L. Gage* (pp. 93–110). New York: Random House.

Bransford, J. D., & Stein, B. S. (1984). *The IDEAL problem solver.* New York: Freeman.

Brophy, J., & Good, T. (1986). Teacher behavior and student achievement. In M. Wittrock (Ed.), *Handbook of research on teaching* (pp. 340–370). New York: Macmillan.

Deno, S. (1985). Curriculum-based measurement: The emerging alternative. *Exceptional Children*, 52, 219–232.

Deno, S., & Mirkin, P. (1977). *Data-based program modification.* Minneapolis, MN: Leadership Training Institute for Special Education.

Deno, S. L. (1989). Curriculum-based measurement and special education services: A fundamental and direct relationship. In M. R. Shinn (Ed.), *Curriculum-based measurement: Assessing special children* (pp. 1–17). New York: Guilford Press.

Deno, S. L. (2002). Problem solving as "best practice." In A. Thomas & J. Grimes (Eds.), *Best practices in school psychology* (4th ed., Vol. 2, pp. 37–55). Bethesda, MD: National Association of School Psychologists.

Engelmann, S., & Carnine, D. (1982). *Theory of instruction: Principles and applications.* New York: Irvington.

Flugum, K. R., & Reschly, D. J. (1994). Prereferral interventions: Quality indices and outcomes. *Journal of School Psychology*, 32, 1–14.

Fuchs, D., & Fuchs, L. S. (1998). Researchers and teachers working together to adapt instruction for diverse learners. *Learning Disabilities Research and Practice*, 13, 126–137.

Good, R. H., Gruba, J., & Kaminski, R. A. (2002). Best practices in using Dynamic Indicators of Basic Early Literacy Skills (DIBELS) in an outcomes-driven model. In A. Thomas & J. Grimes (Eds.), *Best practices in school psychology* (4th ed., Vol. 1, pp. 679–700). Bethesda, MD: National Association of School Psychologist.

Good, R. H., & Kaminski, R. A. (1996). Assessment for instructional decisions: Toward a proactive/prevention model of decision-making for early literacy skills. *School Psychology Quarterly*, 11, 326–336.

Hall, G., & Hord, S. (2001). *Implementing change: Patterns, principles, and potholes.* Boston: Allyn & Bacon.

Horner, R. H., Sugai, G., Todd, A. W., & Lewis-Palmer, T. (2005). Schoolwide positive behavior support. In L. Bambara & L. Kern (Eds.), *Individualized support for students with problem behaviors: Designing positive behavior plans* (pp. 359–390). New York: Guilford Press.

Howell, K., & Nolet, V. (2000). *Curriculum-based evaluation: Teaching and decision making.* Belmont, CA: Wadsworth.

Ikeda, M. J., Rahn-Blakeslee, A., Niebling, B. C., Gustafson, J. K., Allison, R., & Stumme, J.

(2007). The Heartland Area Education Agency 11 problem-solving approach: An overview and lessons learned. In S. R. Jimerson, M. K. Burns, & A. M. VanDerHeyden (Eds.), *Handbook of response to intervention: The science and practice of assessment and intervention* (pp. 255–268). New York: Springer.

Iwata, B., Dorsey, M., Slifer, K., Bauman, K., & Richman, G. (1982). Toward a functional analysis of self-injury. *Analysis and Intervention in Developmental Disabilities, 2,* 3–20.

Kratochwill, T. R., & Bergan, J. R. (1990). *Behavioral consultation in applied settings: An individual guide.* New York: Plenum.

O'Neill, R. E., Horner, R. H., Albin, R. W., Storey, K., & Sprague, J. (1997). *Functional assessment and program development for problem behavior: A practical handbook.* Pacific Grove, CA: Brooks/Cole.

Reschly, D. J., & Ysseldyke, J. E. (1995). School psychology paradigm shift. In A. Thomas & J. Grimes (Eds.), *Best practices in school psychology* (3rd ed., pp. 17–31). Bethesda, MD: National Association of School Psychologists.

Reynolds, C. R., Gutkin, T. B., Elliott, S. N., & Witt, J. C. (1984). *School psychology: Essentials of theory and practice.* New York: Wiley.

Schumaker, J. B., Deshler, D. D., & McKnight, P. (2002). Ensuring success in the secondary general education curriculum through the use of teaching routines. In M. R. Shinn, H. M. Walker, & G. Stoner (Eds.), *Interventions for academic and behavior problems: II. Preventive and remedial approaches.* Bethesda, MD: National Association of School Psychologists.

Shinn, M. R. (Ed.). (1989). *Curriculum-based measurement: Assessing special children.* New York: Guilford Press.

Shinn, M. R., Walker, H. M., & Stoner, G. (Eds.). (2002). *Interventions for academic and behavioral problems: II. Preventive and remedial approaches.* Washington, DC: National Association of School Psychologists.

Sulzer-Azaroff, B., & Mayer, R. (1991). *Behavior analysis for lasting change.* Fort Worth, TX: Holt, Reinhart & Winston.

Swanson, H. L. (1999). Reading research for students with LD: A meta-analysis of intervention outcomes. *Journal of Learning Disabilities, 32,* 504–532.

Swanson, H. L., & Hoskyn, M. (1998). Experimental intervention research on students with learning disabilities: A meta-analysis of treatment outcomes. *Review of Educational Research, 68,* 277–321.

Tilly, W. D. (2008). The evolution of school psychology to science-based practice. In A. Thomas & J. Grimes (Eds.), *Best practices in school psychology* (5th ed., Vol. 1, pp. 17–36). Bethesda, MD: National Association of School Psychologists.

Tilly, W. D. III, Knoster, T., & Ikeda, M. J. (2000). Functional behavioral assessment: Strategies for positive behavioral support. In C. Telzrow & M. Tankersly (Eds.), *Issues in implementing IDEA '97.* Washington, DC: National Association of School Psychologists.

Tilly, W. D. III, Knoster, T. P., Kovaleski, J., Bambara, L., Dunlap, G., & Kincaid, D. (1998). *Functional behavioral assessment: Policy development in light of emerging research and practice.* Alexandria, VA: National Association of State Directors of Special Education.

University of Texas Center for Reading and Language Arts/Texas Education Agency. (2003). *3-tier reading model: Reducing reading difficulties for kindergarten through third grade students.* Austin, TX: Author.

Upah, K. F. (2008). Best practices in designing, implementing, and evaluating quality interventions. In A. Thomas & J. Grimes (Eds.), *Best practices in school psychology* (5th ed., Vol. 2, pp. 209–224). Bethesda, MD: National Association of School Psychologists.

Ysseldyke, J. E., Burns, M., Kelley, B., Morrison, D., Ortiz, S., Rosenfield, S., et al. (2006). *School psychology: A blueprint for training and practice: III.* Bethesda, MD: National Association of School Psychologists.

Ysseldyke, J. E., Algozzine, B., & Thurlow, M. L. (2000). *Critical issues in special education* (3rd ed.). Boston: Houghton Mifflin.

Author Index

Subject Index